Dry Eye Disease: The Clinician's Guide to Diagnosis and Treatment

Dry Eye Disease: The Clinician's Guide to Diagnosis and Treatment

Editor: Alfonso Dargie

AMERICAN
MEDICAL PUBLISHERS
www.americanmedicalpublishers.com

AMERICAN
MEDICAL PUBLISHERS
www.americanmedicalpublishers.com

Cataloging-in-Publication Data

Dry eye disease : the clinician's guide to diagnosis and treatment / edited by Alfonso Dargie.
p. cm.
Includes bibliographical references and index.
ISBN 979-8-88740-079-2
1. Dry eye syndromes. 2. Dry eye syndromes--Diagnosis. 3. Dry eye syndromes--Treatment.
4. Lacrimal apparatus--Diseases. I. Dargie, Alfonso.
RE216.D78 D79 2023
617.7--dc23

American Medical Publishers,
41 Flatbush Avenue,
1st Floor, New York,
NY 11217, USA

ISBN 979-8-88740-079-2 (Hardback)

Contents

Preface

A common condition that occurs when tears are unable to provide adequate lubrication to the eyes is known as dry eye disease. This inability of tears may lead to inflammation and damage to the eye's surface. The common symptoms include eye discomfort, stinging or burning or scratchy sensation in eyes, stringy mucus in or around eyes, sensitivity to light, eye redness, etc. Other symptoms include difficulty wearing contact lenses, difficulty in driving at night, watery eyes, and blurred vision or eye fatigue. There are several causes for tear film dysfunction including hormone changes, autoimmune disease, inflamed eyelid glands, or allergic eye disease. Some other reasons such as decreased tear production or increased tear evaporation may also result in this condition. Preventive measures involve taking eye breaks during long tasks, avoiding smoking, and humidifying the air. This book is a compilation of chapters that discuss the most vital concepts and emerging trends in dry eye disease. It will help the clinicians in keeping pace with the rapid changes in its diagnosis and treatment.

This book unites the global concepts and researches in an organized manner for a comprehensive understanding of the subject. It is a ripe text for all researchers, students, scientists or anyone else who is interested in acquiring a better knowledge of this dynamic field.

I extend my sincere thanks to the contributors for such eloquent research chapters. Finally, I thank my family for being a source of support and help.

Editor

1

Demodex folliculorum Infestation in Meibomian Gland Dysfunction Related Dry Eye Patients

Yiran Hao [1,2†], Xiaoyu Zhang [1,2†], Jiayu Bao [1,2], Lei Tian [1,2,3] and Ying Jie [1,2*]*

[1] Beijing Tongren Eye Center, Beijing Tongren Hospital, Beijing Institute of Ophthalmology, Capital Medical University, Beijing, China, [2] Beijing Ophthalmology and Visual Sciences Key Laboratory, Beijing Tongren Hospital, Capital Medical University, Beijing, China, [3] Beijing Advanced Innovation Center for Big Data-Based Precision Medicine, Beihang University & Capital Medical University, Beijing, China

***Correspondence:**
Ying Jie
jie_yingcn@aliyun.com
Lei Tian
tianlei0131@163.com

† These authors have contributed equally to this work and share first authorship

Objective: To report the influence of *Demodex folliculorum (D. folliculorum)* infestation in patients with meibomian gland dysfunction (MGD) related dry eye and the associations of the infestation with MGD related dry eye.

Methods: Eyelashes (three from the upper eyelid and three from the lower eyelid) from 119 eyes of 119 patients diagnosed with MGD related dry eye were examined under a light microscope. There were 68 eyes of 68 patients with MGD related dry eye and *D. folliculorum* infestation (*Demodex* positive group) and 51 eyes of 51 patients without infestation (*Demodex* negative group). All patients completed an Ocular Surface Disease Index (OSDI) questionnaire and underwent tests for dry eye and MGD. The tests included fluorescein tear breakup time (TBUT), corneal fluorescein staining, Schirmer I test (SIT), lid margin abnormalities, meibum expression assessment, and meibomian gland dropout.

Results: The scores for OSDI, corneal fluorescein staining, lid margin abnormalities, meibum expression, and meibomian gland dropout were significantly higher (all $P < 0.05$), while TBUT was significantly shorter in the *Demodex* positive group compared to the *Demodex* negative group ($P = 0.020$). The SIT values did not significantly differ between groups. Chalazion was significantly more prevalent in the *Demodex* positive group. The number of *D. folliculorum* was positively correlated with all three MGD parameters ($P \leq 0.035$), OSDI; corneal fluorescein scores, and it was inversely correlated with BUT. The correlation for SIT was $R^2 = 0.075$ ($P = 0.064$).

Conclusion: *Demodex folliculorum* infestation is possibly one of the key contributors in the pathogenesis of MGD related dry eye, and a higher prevalence of chalazion was found in *D. folliculorum* infected patients. The possible causal role of *D. folliculorum* infestation needs to be further studied.

Keywords: dry eye, *Demodex folliculorum* infestation, meibomian gland dysfunction, lid margin abnormality score, meibum expression, meibomian gland dropout, chalazion

INTRODUCTION

Demodex can have different effects on the ocular surface, including anterior blepharitis, posterior blepharitis accompanied by meibomian gland dysfunction (MGD), ocular rosacea, keratitis, and so on (1). There are two types of *Demodex* being identified in humans: *Demodex folliculorum* and *Demodex brevis*. *Demodex folliculorum (D. folliculorum)* is generally found around the root of the eyelashes as well as the lash follicles, while *Demodex brevis (D. brevis)* primarily infest the deeper sebaceous glands (2, 3). Previous studies have reported that *Demodex* infestation is related to ocular diseases including blepharitis, dry eye, conjunctivitis, corneal injury, and so on (4, 5). To be specific, *Demodex folliculorum* is more likely to cause anterior blepharitis with eyelash involvement while *Demodex brevis* may lead to posterior blepharitis more often, and the streptococci and staphylococci reside on the surface of the mites will lead to blepharitis both anteriorly and posteriorly (2, 3, 6). However, the role of *Demodex* infestation in the pathogenesis of chronic blepharitis is still controversial (1, 3, 6).

Dry eye disease (DED) is considered a type of multifactorial disease accompanied by various ocular symptoms. The pathogenesis of which mainly includes the imbalance of the microenvironment of the ocular surface and the instability of the tear film. According to the TFO DEWS II (2017), the condition could also be along with inflammation and damage of the ocular surface, as well as neurosensory disorders (7).

Meibomian glands, the largest sebaceous glands in the body, produce the main component of the tear film to maintain a stabilized ocular surface (8). They synthesize and secrete mixed lipids known as meibum, which are delivered through orifices located anterior to the mucocutaneous junction (9, 10). Diseases of the meibomian gland can be subdivided into focal lesions (hordeolum or chalazion) and diffuse lesions (MGD). MGD is a chronic disease of the meibomian glands, whose pathological basis includes the obstruction of the terminal duct of the glands with or without changes in the amount or quality of the meibum (11). When MGD happens, multiple factors including enhanced tear evaporation, hyperosmolarity, increased pro-inflammatory mediators in tears, and reduced lubrication between the eyelids and the eyeball will break the stability of tear film and disequilibrate the balance of the ocular surface, thus contributing to a series of ocular symptoms and signs, which overlap with DED (12). Therefore, MGD is considered to be a key factor of evaporative dry eye.

The reported prevalence of MGD was found to vary considerably. To be specific, the prevalence of which in the Shihpai Eye Study in Taiwan is 60.8%, in the Beijing Eye Study is 68.3%, and in the Singapore Malay Eye Study is 56.3% (13–15). MGD is more prevalent in the Asian populations and has been associated with pinguecula, anterior blepharitis, contact lens use, and infestation with *Demodex* mites (4, 13). Liang et al. reported a high prevalence of demodicosis, especially *Demodex brevis*, in patients with chalazion (4). However, the frequency of *Demodex* infestation in patients with dry eye accompanied by MGD and the association between *Demodex* infestation and Meibomian function have not been studied in detail.

As the detection rate of *D. brevis* is quite low in meibomian glands and could be affected by various factors, the objective of this study was to evaluate the function of meibomian glands and the ocular surface characteristics in MGD related dry eye patients with or without *Demodex folliculorum* infestation, to investigate the influence of anterior blepharitis on the ocular signs and symptoms of MGD related dry eye patients.

METHODS

All patients diagnosed with dry eye in the cornea clinic of the Tongren Eye Hospital, Beijing, between August 2020 and May 2021 were eligible for inclusion. Patients who are willing to participate in the study, with the same ethnicity (Chinese) and over 18 years old, were included after signing the informed consent. Subjects who previously underwent corneal or ocular surgery, had any ocular diseases other than DED, MGD, or *Demodex* infestation, had any other systemic, dermatologic, or rheumatologic diseases known to impact the tear film, had worn contact lens in the past 24 h, or underwent any treatment related to *Demodex* within 2 weeks, on medication recently were excluded from the study. A total of 119 eyes of 119 patients diagnosed with dry eye disease (DED) associated with meibomian gland dysfunction (MGD) who met the inclusion and exclusion criteria were included. The institutional review board of the Beijing Tongren Hospital, Beijing, China approved the study as TRECKY2021-065 in 2021, and all participants signed informed consent. The study was conducted in accordance with the Declaration of Helsinki.

The DED diagnosis was made according to the TFO DEWS II diagnostic methodology report (2017), which implies: (1) Ocular Surface Disease Index (OSDI) questionnaire $\geq$13 scores; (2) fluorescein tear film breakup time (TBUT) $\leq$5 s; (3) a non-anesthesia Schirmer I test value $\leq$5 mm/5 min; (4) being reported with corneal fluorescein staining (16).

The diagnosis of MGD was confirmed based on the international workshop on meibomian gland dysfunction: report of the diagnosis subcommittee (2011), which includes the following: (1) clinical signs: meibomian gland dropout, altered meibomian gland secretion, and changes in lid morphology; (2) symptoms of global discomfort including redness and swelling, itching, irritation, soreness, and so on (11).

All patients completed the OSDI survey and underwent the following ocular surface evaluation: (1) tear function assessment: fluorescein tear breakup time (TBUT), Schirmer I test (SIT); (2) assessment of meibomian gland function: lid margin examination, meibum quality, meibomian gland dropout, examination (or recorded diagnosis) of chalazion; (3) assessment of *Demodex* infestation as detailed below.

Ocular Surface Evaluation

Ocular Surface Disease Index

All patients were asked to complete the OSDI survey before clinical examinations, providing a score ranging from 0 (no symptoms) to 100 (severe symptoms).

Corneal Fluorescein Staining

Corneal fluorescein staining was determined after recording TBUT (described below) and was graded from 0 to 15 according to the National Eye Institute/Industry grading scale (NEI). Each section of the cornea was graded as 0 (no staining), 1 (mild, with <10 scattered staining dots), 2 (moderate, between 10 and 30 dots), and 3 (severe, with over 30 dots, confluent staining, or presence of corneal filaments), and the total of five sections was recorded (17).

Tear Function Assessment

Fluorescein Tear Breakup Time (TBUT)

Fluorescein dye was used to evaluate corneal staining and TBUT. A moistened aseptic fluorescein strip was dipped in the inferior fornix. The time interval between the last blink and the appearance of the first random dry spot on the corneal surface, being observed through a slit-lamp microscope with a cobalt-blue filter, was recorded by a stopwatch (16). The average of three consecutive TBUT tests was recorded. Corneal fluorescein staining was assessed after TBUT measurements and was graded according to the NEI scale.

Schirmer I Test (SIT)

A standard 5 × 40 mm Schirmer test strip was applied over the middle and outer third of the inferior lid. Patients were required to keep their eyes closed for 5 min, during which time the amount of wetting was recorded (18).

Assessment of Meibomian Gland Function

Meibomian gland assessment was carried out as previously described in the literature (19).

Lid Margin

The following lid margin abnormalities were recorded and scored from 0 to 4: irregularity, vascular engorgement, obstruction of meibomian gland orifices, anterior or posterior displacement of the mucocutaneous junction (20).

Meibum Expression

The quality of the meibum was semi-quantitatively graded in eight glands of the central third of the lower eyelids. To be specific, Grade 0: clear; Grade 1: cloudy; Grade 2: cloudy with particulate material and Grade 3: inspissated and toothpaste-like (11).

Meibomian Gland Dropout

All subjects underwent infrared imaging of the meibomian glands in both upper and lower eyelids with the Keratograph 5M (K5M; Oculus Optikgeräte GmbH, Wetzlar, Germany). After everting the upper and lower eyelids, the areas of partial or complete loss of the meibomian glands were scored according to criteria proposed by Arita et al. (20). The sum of the meiboscores for both upper and lower eyelids was recorded for each eye.

Demodex Examination

A modified sampling and counting method reported in the previous study (4) was used. Six eyelashes (3 each from the upper and lower eyelids) from the right eye of each patient were removed from and examined for *Demodex* species under a light microscope. The three lashes from each lid were selected from the nasal, middle, and temporal side; lashes were likely to have a higher tendency to harbor *Demodex*—those with cylindrical dandruff-like material at the base or those with a different color/brittle appearance were selected (21). Before epilation, the lash was rotated to bring any *Demodex* closer to the surface. The epilated lashes were placed on a glass slide, a drop of cedar oil was gently added to the lash, and the slide was examined under the microscope without a coverslip. A technician blinded to the clinical findings performed the microscopic examination and mite count. **Figure 1** shows images of *Demodex* seen on the root of a lash.

The patients were analyzed based on the presence or absence of *Demodex* on the eyelashes. The right eye from each patient was selected for analysis.

Statistical Analysis

All analyses were performed using SPSS version 17.0 (SPSS, Inc., Chicago, IL, USA). Data were tested for normality by the Kolmogorov-Smirnov test, and the mean and standard deviation (SD) were displayed. Welch's modified Student's two-sample *t*-test and the Wilcoxon rank-sum test were used to evaluating the differences between groups. A Chi-square test was carried out to assess the difference in gender distribution. Linear regression analysis was performed to estimate the association between various factors. A $P < 0.05$ was considered statistically significant.

RESULTS

Demographics

A total of 119 patients with MGD related dry eye who visited the Tongren Hospital were included in the study. After taking a series of ocular surface evaluations and *Demodex* examination described previously, subjects were subdivided into two groups according to the positivity of *Demodex* infestation. Sixty-eight eyes of 68 dry eye patients with MGD accompanied by *D. folliculorum* infestation were enrolled in the *Demodex* positive group, and 51 eyes of 51 dry eye patients with MGD related dry eye alone were enrolled in the *Demodex* negative group. The characteristics of the study population are shown in **Table 1**. The mean age of patients was 40.32 ± 12.88 years (range 19–65 years) with 22 men and 46 women in the *Demodex* positive group, while the mean age of patients was 39.65 ± 13.98 years (range 20–66 years) with 17 men and 34 women in the *Demodex* negative group. There was no difference between the mean age and gender composition between the two groups (age, $P = 0.785$; gender, $P = 0.910$).

All clinical indexes (OSDI, SIT, TBUT, and corneal staining) were significantly better in the *Demodex* negative group compared to the *Demodex* positive group. The prevalence of chalazion was significantly higher in patients with *Demodex* infection ($P = 0.033$).

Meibomian Gland Indices

The prevalence of MGD was significantly higher in patients with *Demodex* infection ($P = 0.002$). In addition, lid margin abnormality score and meiboscore were significantly higher, and the expressed meibum was significantly worse in the *Demodex* negative group compared to the *Demodex* positive group (all $P < 0.05$, **Table 2**).

Association Between Demodex Infestation, Ocular Surface, and Meibomian Gland Indexes

The number of *Demodex* was significantly associated with OSDI ($R^2 = 0.075$, $P = 0.024$) and corneal fluorescein score ($R^2 =$

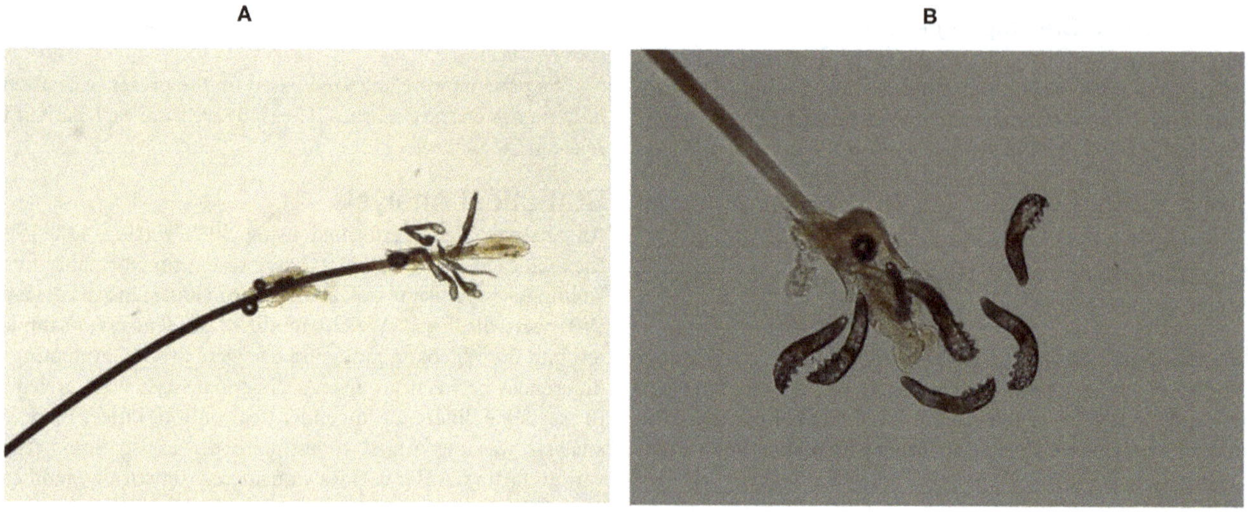

FIGURE 1 | *D. folliculorum* on the root of the eyelash. *Demodex* inside dandruff can be observed clearly both at low (×100) and high (×400) magnification.

TABLE 1 | Characteristics of the study population.

Parameters	*Demodex* positive group [range] (*n* = 68)	*Demodex* negative group [range] (*n*= 51)	*P*-value
Age (year)	40.32 ± 12.88 [19–65]	39.65 ± 13.98 [20–66]	0.785
Gender (male/female)	22/46	17/34	0.910
OSDI (score)	45.12 ± 18.53 [14–90]	35.78 ± 18.24 [12–65]	0.007
TBUT (s)	4.18 ± 1.79 [2–9]	5.01 ± 2.04 [1.96–9.85]	0.020
SIT (mm/5 min)	8.15 ± 4.06 [1–19]	7.16 ± 5.21 [1–17]	0.246
Fluorescein score	4.52 ± 2.4 [0–10]	2.19 ± 1.28 [0–4]	<0.001
Demodex number of eyelids	7.53 ± 4.43 [3–21]	–	–
Chalazion, n (%)	35.29%	17.65%	0.033

OSDI, the Ocular Surface Disease Index; TBUT, Fluorescein tear breakup time.

TABLE 2 | Meibomian Gland Function Indices in *Demodex* positive and *Demodex* negative group.

Parameters	*Demodex* positive group [range] (*n* = 68)	*Demodex* negative group [range] (*n* = 51)	*P*-value
Lid margin abnormality score	2.32 ± 0.72 [0–3]	1.53 ± 0.7 [0–3]	<0.001
Meibum score	2.06 ± 0.99 [0–3]	1.39 ± 1.02 [0–3]	<0.001
Meiboscore	3.54 ± 1.33 [2–6]	2.67 ± 1.74 [0–6]	0.0023

MGD, Meibomian gland dysfunction.

0.144, $P = 0.001$) and inversely correlated with TBUT ($R^2 = 0.072$, $P = 0.027$). The association with SIT was not statistically significant ($R^2 = 0.075$, $P = 0.064$). A significant positive correlation was observed between the number of *Demodex* and all three MGD parameters (Lid margin abnormality score, $R^2 = 0.065$, $P = 0.035$; meibum scores, $R^2 = 0.303$, $P < 0.001$; Meiboscore, $R^2 = 0.232$, $P < 0.001$).

DISCUSSION

It has been well-established that *Demodex* can infest eyelash follicles; however, its role in blepharitis remains controversial (22). Previous studies have shown that many infestations are asymptomatic, which could be related to the number of *Demodex* present (6, 23). *Demodex* may also worsen coexisting lid-margin diseases such as anterior blepharitis and posterior blepharitis, including MGD. A 60% prevalence of *Demodex* in lashes has been reported in patients with MGD vs. 18% in control subjects free of lid and margin disease (24). An over-reproduction of *Demodex* may cause lid-margin infestation, leading to irritation symptoms of ocular surface such as itching, a foreign-body sensation, or stinging (22). It has been recommended that *Demodex* infestation should be suspected in all patients with symptomatic advanced blepharitis, which is accompanied by abnormal fluorescein tear breakup time (22). As MGD is a key contributor to evaporative dry eye, a thorough examination of ocular symptoms, ocular signs, and meibomian gland function is necessary to evaluate the influence of *Demodex* infestation on MGD and dry eye to illuminate the role of *Demodex* in blepharitis.

Our study explored the relationship between the density of *Demodex* infestation with ocular symptoms and MGD function. We reported that the OSDI, corneal fluorescein score, the prevalence of chalazion and MGD, as well as the three MGD parameters measured, were significantly higher in the *Demodex* positive group, and the TBUT was significantly shorter in the *Demodex* positive group compared to the *Demodex* negative group. Our findings were consistent with the outcomes of previous studies (22, 25, 26), which indicated that ocular *Demodex* infection might be related to ocular discomfort and ocular surface damage. A previous study has clarified that *Demodex* can consume the lining of hair follicles and generate debris and waste accumulated at the root of the lashes, thus forming cylindrical dandruff (3). Another possible pathogenesis is that the mites mechanically obstruct the orifices of meibomian glands (1, 3). Both mechanisms lead to changes in the quality and quantity of glandular secretion, resulting in the alteration of the tear film, symptoms of eye irritation, clinically apparent inflammation, and ocular surface disease diagnosed as MGD or DED (27). Also, those abnormalities and dysfunction of the meibomian gland and ocular surface could be reflected by ocular parameters and meibomian gland indices that we have already studied. Apart from the causes of the mites themselves, the bacteria residing on the surface or inside themselves might be another possible pathogenesis. The staphylococci and streptococci on the surface of *Demodex* and the bacillus inside the *Demodex* as well as the toxins expressed by the organisms could activate the inflammatory cascade, contributing to the blepharitis both anteriorly and posteriorly and lead to the disorder of ocular surface and meibomian glands (1, 6, 28). Although previous studies reported that *D. folliculorum* and *D. brevis* were tend to parasite and cause blepharitis in different location, our results showed that the chronic blepharitis caused by *D. folliculorum* could also affect the function of ocular surface by the mechanisms discussed above and lead to a series of ocular signs and symptoms.

Our results also revealed that the number of *Demodex* was positively correlated with all MGD indices in the *Demodex* positive group. However, the minimum number required to produce symptoms is still unknown, and it is likely to be different in different patients.

In this study, we also tested the difference in the prevalence of chalazion with *Demodex* infestation. We found that the prevalence of chalazion was significantly higher in patients with *Demodex* infestation, which is consistent with the outcome from Liang et al. (4) who reported a high prevalence of demodicosis (69%) in those with chalazion compared to healthy controls (20.3%). They also reported an increased recurrence rate in those with infestation (33.3 vs. 10.3%) (4). Moreover, Yam et al. found a high prevalence of 72.9% of *Demodex* infestation in adult patients with recurrent chalazion (29). It has been shown that the chitinous exoskeleton of *Demodex* may act as a foreign body and produce granulomatous inflammation, which may implicate chalazion (4, 30). A recent study indicated that *Demodex* was also related to recurrence of chalazion after surgical excision (31). If *Demodex* is not radically eliminated, it cannot continue to clog the meibomian gland, resulting in abnormal meibum and leading to recurrent chalazion. Age is a key risk factor for MGD that has been proved to affect meibomian gland dropout, with the elderly showing a higher dropout rate (22, 32). To rule out the difference in age as a reason for the observed differences in the meibomian gland dropout between groups, we selected relatively young patients with a similar mean age between the two groups. While gender has also been associated with MGD dropout, there was a similar gender distribution between the two groups (33, 34).

The present study has several limitations. First, as it is an observational cross-sectional study, it cannot certainly assure whether *Demodex* infestation caused MGD and DED. Although the association between the number of mites and meibomian gland function indices and ocular surface parameters as well as biologic plausibility is suggestive of a causal role, it still merits further investigation. Also, we did not formally calculate the sample size. So, despite that our results are statistically significant, the sample could be considered relatively small. Apart from that, it is inevitable that false-negative results may appear during *Demodex* detection, for the six eyelashes removed from each patient is randomized and it is unavoidable to epilate uninfected lashes while infected lashes remained, which will cause false-negative result and affect the accuracy of the outcome.

In conclusion, our study indicated that all dry eye parameters and MGD indices were worse in the *Demodex* positive group than in the *Demodex* negative group. Specifically, the scores of OSDI, corneal fluorescein, lid margin abnormality, and meibum were significantly higher, and TBUT was significantly shorter in the *Demodex* positive group. *Demodex* infestation is possibly one of the key contributors to the pathogenesis of MGD related dry eye patients. In addition, it was associated with a higher prevalence of chalazion in those patients.

ETHICS STATEMENT

The studies involving human participants were reviewed and approved by Beijing Tongren Hospital, Capital Medical University, Beijing, China. The patients/participants provided their written informed consent to participate in this study.

AUTHOR CONTRIBUTIONS

YH: analysis and interpretation of data, drafting the article, final approval of the version to be published, and agreement to be accountable for all aspects of the work. XZ and JB: acquisition of data, drafting the article, final approval of the version to be published, and agreement to be accountable for all aspects of the work. LT: analysis and interpretation of data, revising it critically for important intellectual content, final approval of the version to be published, and agreement to be accountable for all aspects of the work. YJ: substantial contributions to conception and design, revising it critically for important intellectual content, final approval of the version to be published, and agreement to be accountable for all aspects of the work. All authors contributed to the article and approved the submitted version.

REFERENCES

1. Fromstein SR, Harthan JS, Patel J, Opitz DL. *Demodex* blepharitis: clinical perspectives. *Clin Optom.* (2018) 10:57–63. doi: 10.2147/OPTO.S142708
2. Elston CA, Elston DM. *Demodex* mites. *Clin Dermatol.* (2014) 32:739–43. doi: 10.1016/j.clindermatol.2014.02.012
3. Cheng AM, Sheha H, Tseng SC. Recent advances on ocular *Demodex* infestation. *Curr Opin Ophthalmol.* (2015) 26:295–300. doi: 10.1097/ICU.0000000000000168
4. Liang L, Ding X, Tseng S. High prevalence of *Demodex* brevis infestation in chalazia. *Am J Ophthalmol.* (2014) 157:342–8.e341. doi: 10.1016/j.ajo.2013.09.031

5. Gao YY, Di Pascuale MA, Elizondo A, Tseng SC. Clinical treatment of ocular demodecosis by lid scrub with tea tree oil. *Cornea.* (2007) 26:136–43. doi: 10.1097/01.ico.0000244870.62384.79
6. Liu J, Sheha H, Tseng SC. Pathogenic role of *Demodex* mites in blepharitis. *Curr Opin Allergy Clin Immunol.* (2010) 10:505–10. doi: 10.1097/ACI.0b013e32833df9f4
7. Bron AJ, de Paiva CS, Chauhan SK, Bonini S, Gabison EE, Jain S, et al. TFOS DEWS II pathophysiology report. *Ocul Surf.* (2017) 15:438–510. doi: 10.1016/j.jtos.2017.05.011
8. Knop E, Knop N, Millar T, Obata H, Sullivan DA. The international workshop on meibomian gland dysfunction: report of the subcommittee on anatomy physiology, and pathophysiology of the meibomian gland. *Invest Ophthalmol Vis Sci.* (2011) 52:1938–78. doi: 10.1167/iovs.10-6997c
9. Butovich IA. Meibomian glands, meibum, and meibogenesis. *Exp Eye Res.* (2017) 163:2–16. doi: 10.1016/j.exer.2017.06.020
10. Suzuki T, Teramukai S, Kinoshita S. Meibomian glands and ocular surface inflammation. *Ocul Surf.* (2015) 13:133–49. doi: 10.1016/j.jtos.2014.12.002
11. Tomlinson A, Bron AJ, Korb DR, Amano S, Paugh JR, Pearce EI, et al. The international workshop on meibomian gland dysfunction: report of the diagnosis subcommittee. *Invest Ophthalmol Vis Sci.* (2011) 52:2006–49. doi: 10.1167/iovs.10-6997f
12. Chhadva P, Goldhardt R, Galor A. Meibomian Gland Disease: The Role of Gland Dysfunction in Dry Eye Disease. *Ophthalmology.* (2017) 124(11S):S20–6. doi: 10.1016/j.ophtha.2017.05.031
13. Siak JJ, Tong L, Wong WL, Cajucom-Uy H, Rosman M, Saw SM, et al. Prevalence and risk factors of meibomian gland dysfunction: the Singapore Malay eye study. *Cornea.* (2012) 31:1223–8. doi: 10.1097/ICO.0b013e31823f0977
14. Jie Y, Xu L, Wu YY, Jonas JB. Prevalence of dry eye among adult Chinese in the Beijing Eye Study. *Eye.* (2009) 23:688–93. doi: 10.1038/sj.eye.6703101
15. Hassanzadeh S, Varmaghani M, Zarei-Ghanavati S, Heravian Shandiz J, Azimi Khorasani A. Global prevalence of meibomian gland dysfunction: a systematic review and meta-analysis. *Ocul Immunol Inflamm.* (2021) 29:66–75. doi: 10.1080/09273948.2020.1755441
16. Wolffsohn JS, Arita R, Chalmers R, Djalilian A, Dogru M, Dumbleton K, et al. TFOS DEWS II diagnostic methodology report. *Ocul Surf.* (2017) 15:539–74. doi: 10.1016/j.jtos.2017.05.001
17. Lemp MA. Report of the National Eye Institute/Industry workshop on clinical trials in dry eyes. *CLAO J.* (1995) 21:221–32.
18. Zeev MS, Miller DD, Latkany R. Diagnosis of dry eye disease and emerging technologies. *Clin Ophthalmol.* (2014) 8:581–90. doi: 10.2147/OPTH.S45444
19. Nichols KK, Foulks GN, Bron AJ, Glasgow BJ, Dogru M, Tsubota K, et al. The international workshop on meibomian gland dysfunction: executive summary. *Invest Ophthalmol Vis Sci.* (2011) 52:1922–9. doi: 10.1167/iovs.10-6997a
20. Arita R, Itoh K, Inoue K, Amano S. Noncontact infrared meibography to document age-related changes of the meibomian glands in a normal population. *Ophthalmology.* (2008) 115:911–5. doi: 10.1016/j.ophtha.2007.06.031
21. English FP. *Demodex* folliculorum and oedema of the eyelash. *Br J Ophthalmol.* (1971) 55:742–6. doi: 10.1136/bjo.55.11.742
22. Kabatas N, Dogan AS, Kabatas EU, Acar M, Bicer T, Gurdal C. The effect of *Demodex* infestation on blepharitis and the ocular symptoms. *Eye Contact Lens.* (2017) 43:64–7. doi: 10.1097/ICL.0000000000000234
23. Gao YY, Di Pascuale MA, Li W, Liu DT, Baradaran-Rafii A, Elizondo A, et al. High prevalence of *Demodex* in eyelashes with cylindrical dandruff. *Invest Ophthalmol Vis Sci.* (2005) 46:3089–94. doi: 10.1167/iovs.05-0275
24. Bhandari V, Reddy JK. Blepharitis: always remember *Demodex*. *Middle East Afr J Ophthalmol.* (2014) 21:317–20. doi: 10.4103/0974-9233.142268
25. Zhang XB, Ding YH, He W. The association between *Demodex* infestation and ocular surface manifestations in meibomian gland dysfunction. *Int J Ophthalmol.* (2018) 11:589–92. doi: 10.18240/ijo.2018.04.08
26. Pan S, Chen Y. A clinical study on the correlation between *Demodex* infestation and ocular surface changes in patients with meibomian gland dysfunction. *Indian J Ophthalmol.* (2021) 69:2389–94. doi: 10.4103/ijo.IJO_3641_20
27. Nelson JD, Shimazaki J, Benitez-del-Castillo JM, Craig JP, McCulley JP, Den S, et al. The international workshop on meibomian gland dysfunction: report of the definition and classification subcommittee. *Invest Ophthalmol Vis Sci.* (2011) 52:1930–7. doi: 10.1167/iovs.10-6997b
28. Nicholls SG, Oakley CL, Tan A, Vote BJ. *Demodex* species in human ocular disease: new clinicopathological aspects. *Int Ophthalmol.* (2017) 37:303–12. doi: 10.1007/s10792-016-0249-9
29. Yam JC, Tang BS, Chan TM, Cheng AC. Ocular demodicidosis as a risk factor of adult recurrent chalazion. *Eur J Ophthalmol.* (2014) 24:159–63. doi: 10.5301/ejo.5000341
30. Czepita D, Kuznagrygiel W, Czepita M, Grobelny A. *Demodex folliculorum* and *Demodex brevis* as a cause of chronic marginal blepharitis. *Ann Acad Med Stetinensis.* (2007) 53:63–7; discussion 67.
31. Luo X, Li J, Chen C, Tseng S, Liang L. Ocular demodicosis as a potential cause of ocular surface inflammation. *Cornea.* (2017) 36(Suppl 1):S9–14. doi: 10.1097/ICO.0000000000001361
32. Sato K, Nagayama H, Tadokoro K, Juji T, Takahashi TA. Association between meibomian gland changes and aging, sex, or tear function. *Cornea.* (2006) 25:651–5. doi: 10.1097/01.ico.0000227889.11500.6f
33. Schaumberg DA, Nichols JJ, Papas EB, Tong L, Uchino M, Nichols KK. The international workshop on meibomian gland dysfunction: report of the subcommittee on the epidemiology of, and associated risk factors for, MGD. *Invest Ophthalmol Vis Sci.* (2011) 52:1994–2005. doi: 10.1167/iovs.10-6997e
34. Darabad RR, Suzuki T, Richards SM, Jensen RV, Jakobiec FA, Zakka FR, et al. Influence of aromatase absence on the gene expression and histology of the mouse meibomian gland. *Invest Ophthalmol Vis Sci.* (2013) 54:987–98. doi: 10.1167/iovs.12-10992

2

Assessment of Eyelid Pressure Using a Novel Pressure Measurement Device in Patients With Moderate-to-Severe Dry Eye Disease

Jingyi Wang[1†], *Jiayu Bao*[1†], *Wenxiu Song*[2], *Siyuan Li*[1], *Yiran Hao*[1], *Lei Tian*[1,3*‡] *and Ying Jie*[1*‡]

[1] *Beijing Ophthalmology and Visual Sciences Key Laboratory, Beijing Tongren Eye Center, Beijing Institute of Ophthalmology, Beijing Tongren Hospital, Capital Medical University, Beijing, China,* [2] *Beijing Aier Intech Eye Hospital, Beijing, China,* [3] *Beijing Advanced Innovation Center for Big Data-Based Precision Medicine, Beihang University and Capital Medical University, Beijing, China*

Correspondence:
Lei Tian
tianlei0131@163.com
Ying Jie
jie_yingcn@aliyun.com

† *These authors have contributed equally to this work and share first authorship*

‡ *These authors have contributed equally to this work*

Objective: To assess a novel eyelid pressure measurement device and study the relationship between eyelid pressure and ocular surface parameters of moderate-to-severe dry eye disease (DED).

Methods: The present study included 70 eyes of 35 moderate-to-severe DED patients. All subjects were subjected to the following examinations for DED assessment: Ocular Surface Disease Index (OSDI) questionnaire, tear meniscus height (TMH), lipid layer thickness (LLT), number of partial blink (PB), total blink (TB) and partial blink rate (PBR), fluorescein tear breakup time (FBUT), corneal fluorescein staining (CFS), lid margin abnormality, meibum expression assessment (meibum score), meibomian gland dropout (MGd) and Schirmer I test. Pressure of the upper eyelid was measured thrice with the novel pressure measurement device. Repeatability of the device was evaluated by intraclass correlation coefficient (ICC). Safety of the device was evaluated by observing ocular adverse reactions of each subject prior to measurement, at day 1 and day 7 following measurement. Correlations between eyelid pressure and ocular surface parameters of moderate-to-severe DED were analyzed by using Pearson correlation coefficient and Kendall's tau-b correlation coefficient.

Results: ICC of the measurement results in our study was 0.86. There was no abnormality presenting in all subjects recorded prior to measurement, 1 and 7 days following measurement. The eyelid pressure was significantly correlated with PBR ($r = 0.286$, $P = 0.016$), FBUT ($r = -0.331$, $P = 0.005$), CFS ($r = 0.528$, $P = 0.000$), lid margin abnormality ($r = 0.408$, $P = 0.011$) and MGd ($r = 0.226$, $P = 0.016$) in moderate-to-severe DED patients, but not significantly correlated with OSDI score ($r = 0.016$, $P = 0.912$), TMH ($r = -0.002$, $P = 0.988$), meibum score ($r = 0.196$, $P = 0.317$), LLT ($r = 0.114$, $P = 0.346$), PB ($r = 0.116$, $P = 0.338$), TB ($r = 0.074$, $P = 0.544$), meibum score ($r = -0.196$, $P = 0.317$) and Schirmer I test ($r = 0.028$, $P = 0.821$).

Conclusion: The novel pressure measurement device exhibited good repeatability and safety in measuring eyelid pressure. Significant correlations were noted between the eyelid pressure and PBR, FBUT, CFS, lid margin abnormality and MGd in moderate-to-severe DED. The measurement of eyelid pressure combined with ocular surface parameters may be valuable for the assessment of DED.

Keywords: eyelid pressure, friction, tear film, ocular surface parameters, moderate-to-severe dry eye disease

INTRODUCTION

Dry eye disease (DED) has become a common health problem worldwide, which significantly influences the life quality of the patients (1). In 2017, the Tear Film and Ocular Surface Society (TFOS) Dry Eye Workshop (DEWS) updated the definition of DED as "a multifactorial disease of the ocular surface characterized by a loss of homeostasis of the tear film, and accompanied by ocular symptoms, in which tear film instability and hyperosmolarity, ocular surface inflammation and damage, and neurosensory abnormalities play etiological roles."(2). DED can cause a variety of ocular symptoms, such as dryness, burning and foreign body sensation, and even visual impairment in more severe cases (3). As a chronic ocular surface disease, DED not only affects the quality of life, but even causes harm to mental health (1). Therefore, it is very important to take early treatment and prevent the occurrence of DED. While there are many causes of DED, such as environmental changes, medication use, local inflammation, poor eye usage habits and so on. The friction between the eyelid and the eyeball during blinking and eye movement can also cause the occurrence of DED symptoms (4).

As an important eye appendage, the eyelid exerts a protective effect on the ocular surface. Normal anatomical structure and function of the eyelid can maintain its normal closure, reduce the evaporation of tears, and maintain the stability of the tear film. Blinking and eyelid dynamics play important roles in the distribution of tears and in the maintenance of the integrity of the ocular surface (5, 6). In 1986, Snella (7) reported that the pressure of the eyelid could alter the shape of the cornea, and the concept of eyelid pressure was initially proposed. During the blinking process, the movements of eyelids will generate friction on the ocular surface. Excessive eyelid pressure or increased blink rate can cause related damages to the cornea and conjunctiva (8). Mathers and Lem (9) used an optical interference microscope to demonstrate that the eyelid produced shear force on the cornea during blinking, resulting in corneal epithelial cell damages and changes. Cher (10) proposed the concept of "blink-related microtrauma" in 2003, which described the presence of ocular surface diseases caused by mechanical friction or lubrication disorders of the eye, such as superior limbic keratoconjunctivitis, filamentary keratitides and contact lens related damage. It seems that when the normal physiological state of eyelid changes, it will not only lose the protective effect on the ocular surface, but also cause damage to the ocular surface.

Tear film is the main refractive surface for light to enter the visual system, which can protect and moisten the ocular surface. Stability of tear film is an important indicator of ocular surface health (2). Therefore, when the stability of tear film is destroyed, it can lead to the occurrence of various ocular surface diseases, DED is one of them. Mechanical damage is one of the major causes affecting the stability of tear film, which can cause premature and rapid evaporation of tear. Barros et al. (11) found that under confocal microscopy, the number of stained corneal epithelial cells increased with the increase of mechanical friction, confirming the relationship between mechanical friction and corneal epithelial injury. In addition, long-term mechanical damage can also induce inflammation and destabilize the tear film (4). Tissues fibrosis caused by chronic inflammation can lead to changes in normal anatomical structure, such as lacrimal atresia, which affects the normal drainage of tear, resulting in epiphora. Meduri et al. (12, 13) found that patients with lacrimal atresia usually had ocular surface inflammatory diseases such as chronic blepharitis or chronic conjunctivitis, and showed significant symptoms and signs of epiphora. After punctoplasty surgery was performed to restore normal anatomical structure, the situation of epiphora was significantly improved. It suggests that mechanical damage and inflammatory reaction can be avoided by restoring normal anatomical structure, and then the stability of tear film can be maintained.

As a common ocular surface disease, DED is characterized by unstable tear film combined with a variety of ocular symptoms. Since increased eyelid pressure can lead to ocular surface damage and affect the tear film stability, eyelid pressure may be a cause of DED. To explore the relationship between eyelid pressure and DED, we developed a novel eyelid pressure measurement device. The aim of this study was to evaluate the repeatability and safety of the device and to investigate the correlations between eyelid pressure and ocular surface parameters of moderate-to-severe DED.

MATERIALS AND METHODS

Subjects

This prospective cross-sectional study was conducted from July 2021 to October 2021 at Beijing Tongren Hospital (<city>Beijing</city>, China). A total of 70 eyes were collected from 6 men (12 eyes) and 29 women (58 eyes). The subjects had an average age of 57 ± 9 (ranging from 32 to 66 years). The diagnosis of DED was based on the TFOS DEWS II definition and classification report. Any subject with any of the following conditions were excluded: (1) age lower than 18 years or higher than 70 years; (2) presence of eye diseases or systemic diseases involving the eyes; (3) a history of eye surgery or trauma to the eye; (4) with blepharoptosis, blepharospasm and other eyelid diseases that significantly affect eyelid pressure. All subjects provided informed consent for their participation in the study, and the entire process complied with the principles of the Declaration of Helsinki. This study was reviewed and approved by the Ethics Committee of Beijing Tongren hospital and registered in the Chinese Clinical Trial Registry (Clinical Trial Registration No. ChiCTR2100054636).

Eyelid Pressure Measurement

Eyelid Pressure Measurement Device

The eyelid pressure measurement device was composed of a control program, a data acquisition card, a drive amplifier circuit, and a membrane pressure sensor (**Figure 1**). Diameter of the sensor was 7.5 mm, the thickness was <0.1 mm, and the measurement range was 0–200 mN. Signal acquisition interval was set to 0.2 ms, and the sampling accuracy was 16 bit. By using a self-developed and designed control program (Labview 2012), the signal changes from the pressure sensor could be continuously recorded. Following setting up, a series of weights with different masses (5 g, 10 g, 20 g) were used to calibrate the system. The weights of different masses were placed on the sensor, and the data collected by the system were recorded, and linearly fit to the pressure in the sensor and the output electrical signal data to obtain the calibration parameters. It seemed that the sensor exhibited very high linearity and could be used for experimental testing.

Process of Measurement

Upper eyelids pressure was individually measured using the same sensor for each subject. The subject was allowed to sit and topical anesthesia eye drops (Proparacaine Hydrochloride, Alcon, Belgium) were instilled into the conjunctival sac for anesthesia. To protect the cornea, a sterile disposable soft contact lens (Soft Hydrophilic Contact Lens, Horien, China) was placed on the cornea of the subject. A pressure sensor was placed at the center of the upper eyelid. Subsequently, the subject was asked to close his eyes gently without squeezing and retain them closed for 10 sec. The record of the representative eyelid pressure is shown in **Figure 2**. Eyelid pressure was defined as the average of the values obtained during the 10 sec after the intersection point. After the measurement, one antibiotic eye drop (Chloramphenicol, Shenlong Pharmaceutical, China) was instilled into the patient's conjunctival sac to prevent infection.

Repeatability and Safety of the Device

To evaluate the repeatability of the device, an ophthalmologist was trained according to the protocol for the eyelid pressure measurement until proficiency with it. Our measurement was conducted in the same room (temperature 20–25°C and humidity 30–40%) between 10 a.m. and 2 p.m. in a single day. Measurement process was repeated thrice with an interval of no <10 min each time for both eyes of each subject in the same day. To evaluate the safety of the device, conjunctival congestion, secretion production, corneal epithelial injury and other ocular adverse reactions of each subject were observed prior to measurement, 1 and 7 days following measurement.

Ocular Surface Examinations

Process of All Examinations

According to DED clinical examination process, all subjects were examined in the following order: first, the completion of the Ocular Surface Disease Index (OSDI) questionnaire was performed prior to all examinations; after that, tear meniscus height (TMH) of the lower eyelid was measured with a Keratograph 5M (K5M) (OCULUS, Wetzlar, Germany); subsequently, the LipiView interferometer (TearScience, Morrisville, USA) was used to measure the lipid layer thickness of the tear film (LLT), the number of partial blink (PB) and total blink (TB) per 20 sec, and the partial blinking rate (PBR); then, 1–2% fluorescein sodium dye was placed into the conjunctival sac of the patient's lower eyelid, and the fluorescein tear breakup time (FBUT) and corneal fluorescein staining score (CFS) were measured; following that, the lid margin morphology and the meibum expression under the slit lamp were evaluated; after that, the images of the upper meibomian glands were obtained to record the situation of meibomian gland dropout (MGd) with the K5M. The subject was allowed to rest for 30 min, and Schirmer I test was performed for 5 min. To avoid the impact on the ocular surface following measurement, eyelid pressure was determined in the end (**Figure 3**). It had to be emphasized that the entire examination in the process of our study was performed by one examiner.

Evaluation of Ocular Surface Parameters

ODSI questionnaire consisted of 12 questions and the score ranged from 0 (no symptoms) to 100 (severe symptoms) (3). TMH was acquired by the measuring tool and recorded in millimeters (mm), based on the image photographed under white light in K5M. LLT, PB, TB and PBR were analyzed by LipiView interferometer based on a 20 sec video. FBUT of each eye was evaluated three times, and the average of three measurements was taken as the final result. CFS was scored according to American National Eye Institute/Industry (NEI) scale, with a total score of 0–15 (14). Eye lid margin abnormality was assessed with a 4-level scale based on the severity of the signs (grade 0–3) (15). Meibum score was assessed with a 4-level scale based on the secretory capacity and the quality in the 5 glands of central upper eyelids (grade 0–3) (16). MGd was assessed with a 4-level scale based on the images of the upper meibomian glands (grade 0–3) (17). The results of Schirmer I test were obtained from the wetted length of the test strip (18).

Statistical Analysis

All continuous variables were presented as mean ± standard deviations (SD). All categorical variables were presented as median. ICC was used to analyze the repeatability of the device. Pearson correlation coefficient was used to analyze the correlation between two continuous variables, and Kendall's tau-b correlation coefficient was used to analyze the correlation between continuous and categorical variables. A $P < 0.05$ was considered to indicate statistically significant difference. All analyses were performed with the Statistical Package for Social Sciences (SPSS) version 25.0.

RESULTS

Repeatability and Safety of the Device

ICC of the measurement results in our study was 0.86. No abnormalities in conjunctival congestion, secretion production,

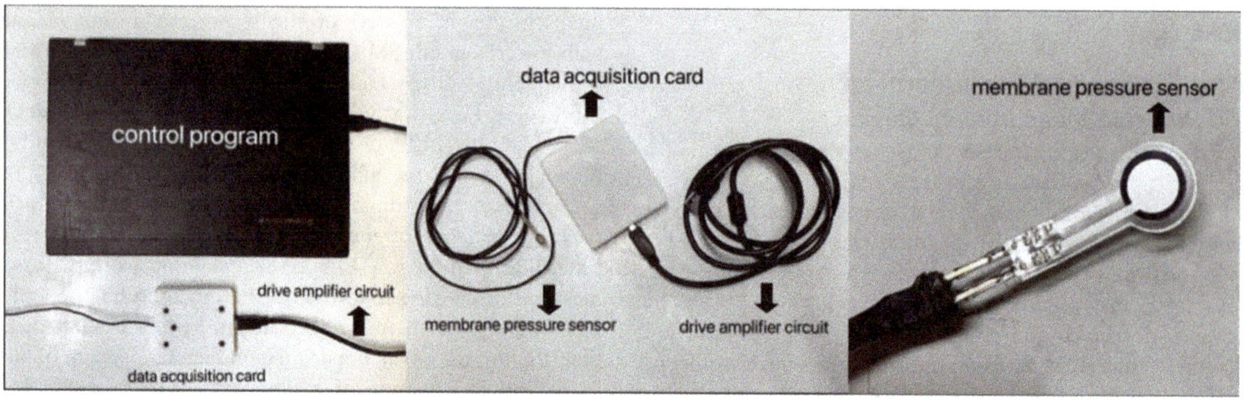

FIGURE 1 | The eyelid pressure measurement device.

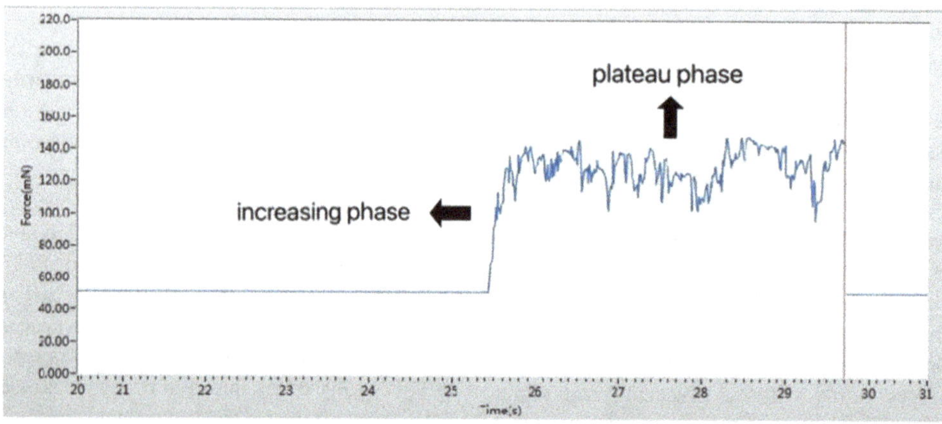

FIGURE 2 | Working interface of the pressure measurement device. The measured pressure was divided into two phases: an increasing phase and a plateau phase.

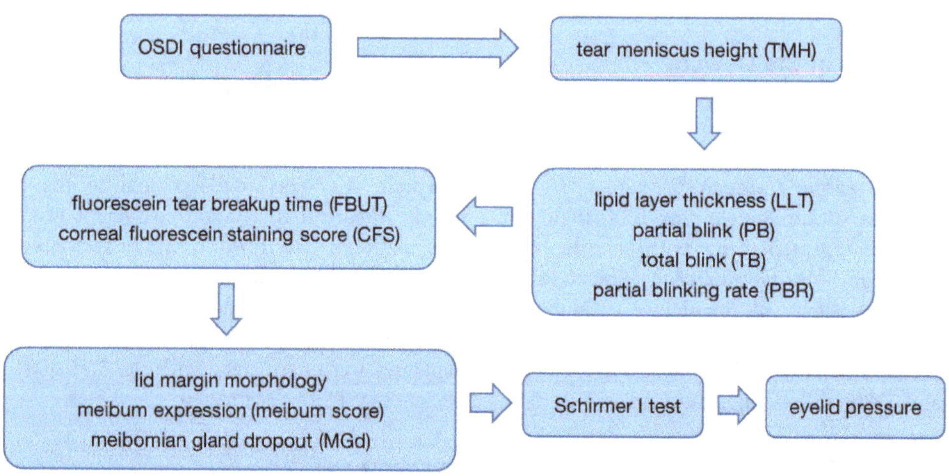

FIGURE 3 | The process of all examinations.

TABLE 1 | Descriptive statistics of 35 moderate-to-severe DED patients.

Parameters	Total eyes (n = 70)
Age (year)	57 ± 9
Eyelid pressure (mN)	92.20 ± 15.60
OSDI score	45.47 ± 17.23
TMH (mm)	0.23 ± 0.13
LLT (nm)	79.47 ± 20.40
PB	5.64 ± 4.32
TB	6.37 ± 4.45
PBR	0.89 ± 0.22
FBUT (s)	3.58 ± 0.67
CFS	4.80 ± 1.87
Lid margin abnormality	1.21 ± 0.41
Meibum score	1.25 ± 1.02
MGd	0.96 ± 0.95
Schirmer I test (mm)	5.26 ± 2.10

OSDI, Ocular Surface Disease Index; TMH, tear meniscus height; LLT, lipid layer thickness; PB, partial blink; TB, total blink; PBR, partial blink rate; FBUT, fluorescein tear breakup time; CFS, corneal fluorescein staining; MGd, meibomian gland dropout.

TABLE 2 | Relationship between eyelid pressure and ocular surface parameters.

Ocular parameters	Eyelid pressure (mN)	
	r	P-value
OSDI score	0.016	0.912
TMH (mm)	−0.002	0.988
LLT (nm)	0.114	0.346
PB	0.116	0.338
TB	0.074	0.544
PBR	0.286	0.016*
FBUT (s)	−0.331	0.005**
CFS	0.528	0.000**
Lid margin abnormality	0.408	0.011*
Meibum score	−0.196	0.317
MGd	0.226	0.016*
Schirmer I (mm)	0.028	0.821

$^{*}p < 0.05$; $^{**}p < 0.01$.
OSDI, Ocular Surface Disease Index; TMH, tear meniscus height; LLT, lipid layer thickness; PB, partial blink; TB, total blink; PBR, partial blink rate; FBUT, fluorescein tear breakup time; CFS, corneal fluorescein staining; MGd, meibomian gland dropout.

corneal epithelial injury and other ocular adverse reactions were presented in all subjects prior to measurement, 1 and 7 days following measurement.

Descriptive Statistics of the Subjects

Descriptive statistics of the 35 patients with moderate-to-severe DED are shown in **Table 1**, including age, eyelid pressure, OSDI score, TMH, LLT, PB, TB, PBR, FBUT, CFS, lid margin abnormality, meibum score, MGd and Schirmer I test.

Relationship Between Eyelid Pressure and Ocular Surface Parameters

Correlations between the eyelid pressure and ocular surface parameters of moderate-to-severe DED were assessed (**Table 2**). Upper eyelid pressure was significantly associated with PBR (**Figure 4**), FBUT (**Figure 5**), CFS (**Figure 6**), lid margin abnormality (**Figure 7**), and MGd (**Figure 8**). However, no significant correlation was noted between upper eyelid pressure and OSDI score, TMH, LLT, PB, TB, meibum score and Schirmer I test.

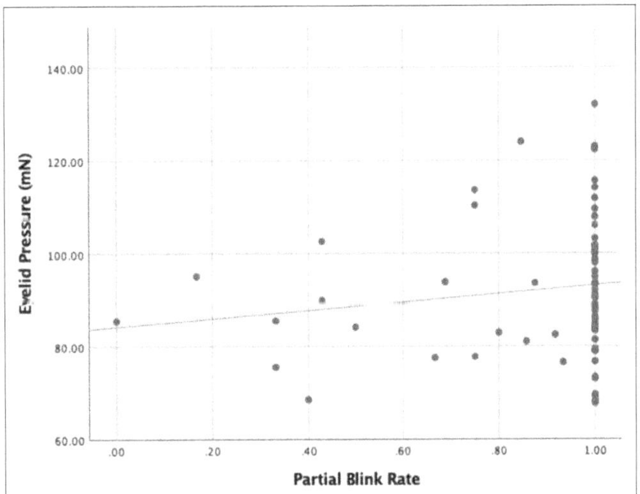

FIGURE 4 | The relationship between the eyelid pressure and the partial blink rate (PBR) (r = 0.286, P = 0.016).

DISCUSSION

Blink and eyelid dynamics play important roles in the distribution of tears and the maintenance of tear film integrity (19, 20). According to TFOS DEWS II, the friction caused by relative movement of the eyelid and eyeball is one of the important reasons for the destruction of the corneal epithelial barrier, which may lead to the development of DED symptoms (4). Several teams have done studies on DED and eyelid dynamics, and found that eyelid pressure in patients with DED was significantly higher than that in normal subjects, and was correlated with ocular surface staining scores and severity of lid-wiper epitheliopathy (LWE) (8, 21–23). The higher the CFS was, the higher the severity of DED became (19). To our knowledge, there were a few studies on the relationship between eyelid pressure and ocular surface parameters in patients with moderate-to-severe DED. Therefore, we selected moderate-to-severe DED patients with corneal epithelial injury to study the relationship between eyelid pressure and ocular surface parameters.

In this study, we developed a novel eyelid pressure measurement device, which was used to measure upper eyelid pressure in both eyes of 35 patients with moderate-to-severe DED three times, and the ICC was used to analyze the results. ICC of the measurement results in our study was 0.86, indicating that the device had good repeatability. No abnormality was noted in conjunctival congestion, secretion production, corneal

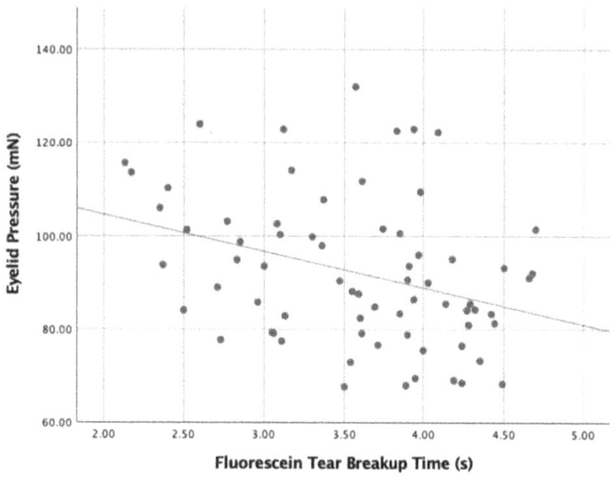

FIGURE 5 | The relationship between the eyelid pressure and the fluorescein tear breakup time (FBUT) (r = −0.331, P = 0.005).

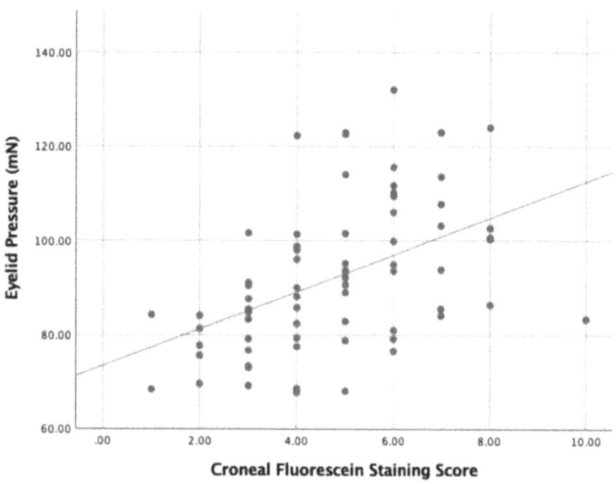

FIGURE 6 | The relationship between the eyelid pressure and the corneal fluorescein staining score (CFS) (r = 0.528, P = 0.000).

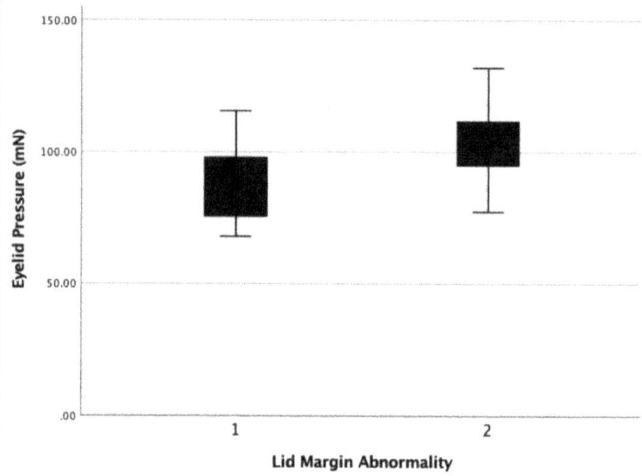

FIGURE 7 | The eyelid pressure of different levels of lid margin abnormality. Statistical significance was assessed between the 2 levels (r = 0.408, P = 0.011).

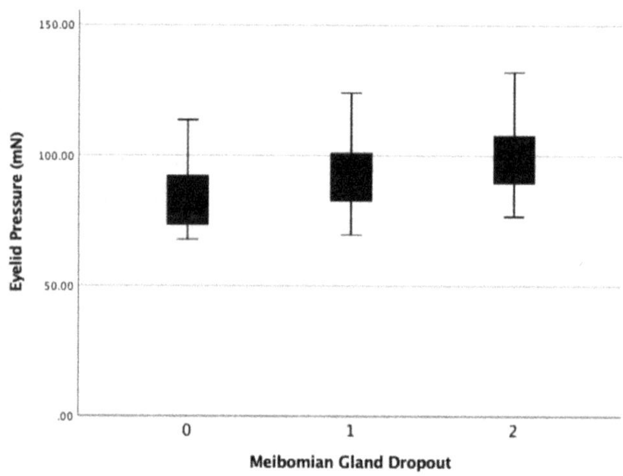

FIGURE 8 | The eyelid pressure of different levels of meibomain gland dropout (MGd). Statistical significance was assessed following comparison of the 3 levels (r = 0.226, P = 0.016).

epithelial injury and other ocular adverse reactions of all subjects prior to and following measurements, indicating that the device was safe for eyelid pressure measurement. We also found that eyelid pressure was significantly correlated with PBR, FBUT, CFS, lid margin abnormality and MGd, but not with OSDI score, TMH, LLT, PB, TB, meibum score and Schirmer I test.

The correlation between eyelid pressure and CFS was similar to the findings by Yoshioka et al. Their study discovered that patients with DED who had higher eyelid pressure showed more serious staining with corneal and conjunctival (24). In addition, they measured eyelid pressure in LWE patients and found that the severity of LWE increased significantly with elevated eyelid pressure (25). With the increase of eyelid pressure, the friction between eyelid and ocular surface during blinking and eye movement also increases, resulting in infiltration mechanical damage of the corresponding parts of the cornea and conjunctival, manifesting as increased CFS. At the same time, the increase of ocular surface friction leads to a series of inflammation, and increase of CFS (4). Although there have been many studies on CFS and FBUT in patients with DED, few studies on the relationship between eyelid pressure and FBUT at present are reported. We believed that the strong correlation between eyelid pressure and FBUT might be because the increase of eyelid pressure led to the enhancement of eyelid friction against the ocular surface, aggravating the instability of tear film and leading to the decline of FBUT.

Meibomian gland dysfunction (MGD) is the main cause of evaporative DED, and MGd, lid margin abnormality, and meibum are the main parameters to evaluate the Meibomian gland function (26). This study found that eyelid pressure was positively correlated with MGd and lid margin abnormality. Chronic high eyelid pressure can cause chronic mechanical irritation to the ocular surface, triggering a chain of inflammatory reactions (4). Atrophy or even loss of the meibomian gland may derive from chronic secretory difficulties and meibomian gland opening obstruction (27). The atrophy and loss of meibomian gland lead to the further reduction of meibum secretion. In order to increase the secretion of meibomian gland, orbicularis muscle will exert more extrusion pressure, which may lead to a corresponding increase in eyelid pressure (26). The increase of eyelid pressure leads to a further enhanced friction on the ocular surface, forming a vicious circle and aggravating the severity of DED.

In this study, eyelid pressure was significantly correlated with PBR. Wang et al. (28) found that an increase in incomplete blinks was positively associated with the risk of DED. Jie et al. (29) further confirmed that incomplete blink was associated with a higher OSDI score, more MGd, and decreased tear film stability. Compared with complete blink, the upper and lower eyelids do not fully contact during incomplete blink, resulting in uneven tear redistribution and aggravating the instability of tear film. Since the friction between the eyelid and ocular surface is related to the eyelid pressure and the contact area between the eyelid and the ocular surface, the higher the eyelid pressure is, the greater the friction is when the corneal area is assumed to be roughly the same (25). We hypothesized that due to the increase in friction, blinking patterns might be more prone to incomplete blink that required less eyelid power, manifesting as increased PBR. PB and TB were recorded in the blink frequency of subjects' normal gaze in the 20 sec video. Due to the influence of visual fatigue, task difficulty and other factors, there was a large individual difference in the blink mode (30). Therefore, we speculated that this was the reason why eyelid pressure had little correlation with PB and TB.

There were still some limitations to our study. First, due to the large size of the membrane pressure sensor, it could not be completely covered by the lower eyelid when put into the lower conjunctival sac, so it was difficult to accurately measure the eyelid pressure of the lower eyelid. Secondly, the pressure was not measured at multiple positions of the eyelid, so we could not get the correlation between the pressure and the staining condition in the corresponding area. Finally, we had limited number of subjects and the results needed to be further confirmed in studies with a large sample size.

CONCLUSION

We developed a novel pressure measurement device, which was used to measure the eyelid pressure in patients with moderate-to-severe DED, and analyzed the relationship between the eyelid pressure and ocular surface parameters. The device demonstrated good repeatability and safety. Furthermore, it was found that eyelid pressure in moderate-to-severe DED patients was significantly correlated with PBR, FBUT, CFS, lid margin abnormality and MGd, but not significantly correlated with OSDI score, TMH, LLT, PB, TB, meibum score and Schirmer I test. We believed that the measurement of eyelid pressure might be of important significance for the evaluation of DED, showing higher predictive value in combination with ocular surface parameters of DED.

ETHICS STATEMENT

The studies involving human participants were reviewed and approved by Ethics Committee of Beijing Tongren Hospital. The patients/participants provided their written informed consent to participate in this study.

DISCLOSURE

This manuscript has not been previously published, and all authors concur with the submission.

AUTHOR CONTRIBUTIONS

JW and JB performed the experiment, collected and recorded the data, and prepared the first draft. WS, SL, and YH contributed significantly to the data analysis and case collection. YJ and LT contributed to the concept of the study, helped supervise the project, and gave critical revision of the article. All authors contributed to the article and approved the submitted version.

REFERENCES

1. Zheng Y, Wu X, Lin X, Lin H. The prevalence of depression and depressive symptoms among eye disease patients: a systematic review and meta-analysis. *Sci Rep.* (2017) 7:46453. doi: 10.1038/srep46453
2. Craig JP, Nichols KK, Akpek EK, Caffery B, Dua HS, Joo CK, et al. TFOS DEWS II definition and classification report. *Ocul Surf.* (2017) 15:276–83. doi: 10.1016/j.jtos.2017.05.008
3. Wolffsohn JS, Arita R, Chalmers R, Djalilian A, Dogru M, Dumbleton K, et al. TFOS DEWS II diagnostic methodology report. *Ocul Surf.* (2017) 15:539–74. doi: 10.1016/j.jtos.2017.05.001
4. Bron AJ, de Paiva CS, Chauhan SK, Bonini S, Gabison EE, Jain S, et al. TFOS DEWS II pathophysiology report. *Ocul Surf.* (2017) 15:438–510. doi: 10.1016/j.jtos.2017.05.011
5. Bron AJ, Tiffany JM, Gouveia SM, Yokoi N, Voon LW. Functional aspects of the tear film lipid layer. *Exp Eye Res.* (2004) 78:347–60. doi: 10.1016/j.exer.2003.09.019
6. Goto E, Tseng SC. Kinetic analysis of tear interference images in aqueous tear deficiency dry eye before and after punctal occlusion. *Invest Ophthalmol Vis Sci.* (2003) 44:1897–905. doi: 10.1167/iovs.02-0818
7. Snellen. Die Richtung der Hauptmeridiane des astigmatischen Auges. *Archiv Für Ophthalmologie.* (1869) 15:199–207.
8. Sakai E, Shiraishi A, Yamaguchi M, Ohta K, Ohashi Y. Blepharo-tensiometer: new eyelid pressure measurement system using tactile pressure sensor. *Eye Contact Lens.* (2012) 38:326–30. doi: 10.1097/ICL.0b013e318268610a
9. Mathers WD, Lemp MA. Morphology and movement of corneal surface cells in humans. *Curr Eye Res.* (1992) 11:517–23. doi: 10.3109/02713689209001807
10. Cher I. Blink-related microtrauma: when the ocular surface harms itself.

Clin Exp Ophthalmol. (2003) 31:183–90. doi: 10.1046/j.1442-9071.2003.00633.x

11. Barros RC, Van Kooten TG, Veeregowda DH. Investigation of friction-induced damage to the pig cornea. *Ocul Surf.* (2015) 13:315–20. doi: 10.1016/j.jtos.2015.05.004
12. Meduri A, Inferrera L, Tumminello G, Delia G, Cicciù M, Aragona P. The application of a venous catheter for the surgical treatment of punctal occlusion. *J Craniofac Surg.* (2020) 31:1829–30. doi: 10.1097/scs.0000000000006536
13. Meduri A, Tumminello G, Oliverio GW, Inferrera L, Delia G, Aragona P, et al. Use of lacrimal symptoms questionnaire after punctoplasty surgery retrospective data of technical strategy. *J Craniofac Surg.* (2021) 32:2848–50. doi: 10.1097/scs.0000000000007813
14. Amparo F, Wang H, Yin J, Marmalidou A, Dana R. Evaluating corneal fluorescein staining using a novel automated method. *Invest Ophthalmol Vis Sci.* (2017) *58:* Bio168-bio173. doi: 10.1167/iovs.17-21831
15. Arita R, Minoura I, Morishige N, Shirakawa R, Fukuoka S, Asai K, et al. Development of definitive and reliable grading scales for meibomian gland dysfunction. *Am J Ophthalmol.* (2016) 169:125–37. doi: 10.1016/j.ajo.2016.06.025
16. Bron AJ, Benjamin L, Snibson GR. Meibomian gland disease. Classification and grading of lid changes. *Eye (Lond).* (1991) 5 (Pt 4):395–411. doi: 10.1038/eye.1991.65
17. Arita R, Itoh K, Inoue K, Amano S. Noncontact infrared meibography to document age-related changes of the meibomian glands in a normal population. *Ophthalmology.* (2008) 115:911–5. doi: 10.1016/j.ophtha.2007.06.031
18. Cho P, Yap M. Schirmer test. I. A review. *Optom Vis Sci.* (1993) 70:152–6. doi: 10.1097/00006324-199302000-00011
19. Branch., A.D.E.A.C., Ophthalmology department OC, Cross-strait Medical and Health Exchange Association., and Ophthalmology and Dry Ophthalmology Group OB. Chinese Medical Doctor Association. (2020). Expert consensus on dry eye in china: defination and classification (2020). *Chin J Ophthalmol.* 56:418–22. doi: 10.3760/cma.j.cn112142-20200316-00190
20. Rodriguez JD, Lane KJ, Ousler GW 3rd, Angjeli E, Smith LM, Abelson MB. Blink: characteristics, controls, and relation to dry eyes. *Curr Eye Res.* (2018) 43:52–66. doi: 10.1080/02713683.2017.1381270
21. Ehrmann K, Francis I, Stapleton F. A novel instrument to quantify the tension of upper and lower eyelids. *Cont Lens Anterior Eye.* (2001) 24:65–72. doi: 10.1016/s1367-0484(01)80015-1
22. Vihlen FS, Wilson G. The relation between eyelid tension, corneal toricity, and age. *Invest Ophthalmol Vis Sci.* (1983) 24:1367–73.
23. Yamamoto Y, Shiraishi A, Sakane Y, Ohta K, Yamaguchi M, Ohashi Y. Involvement of Eyelid Pressure in Lid-Wiper Epitheliopathy. *Curr Eye Res.* (2016) 41:171–8. doi: 10.3109/02713683.2015.1009636
24. Yoshioka E, Yamaguchi M, Shiraishi A, Kono T, Ohta K, Ohashi Y. Influence of eyelid pressure on fluorescein staining of ocular surface in dry eyes. *Am J Ophthalmol.* (2015) 160:685–92.e681. doi: 10.1016/j.ajo.2015.06.028
25. Yamaguchi M, Shiraishi A. Relationship between eyelid pressure and ocular surface disorders in patients with healthy and dry eyes. *Invest Ophthalmol Vis Sci.* (2018) 59:Des56–des63. doi: 10.1167/iovs.17-23586
26. Knop E, Knop N, Millar T, Obata H, Sullivan DA. The international workshop on meibomian gland dysfunction: report of the subcommittee on anatomy, physiology, and pathophysiology of the meibomian gland. *Invest Ophthalmol Vis Sci.* (2011) 52:1938–78. doi: 10.1167/iovs.10-6997c
27. Arita R, Itoh K, Maeda S, Maeda K, Furuta A, Fukuoka S, et al. Proposed diagnostic criteria for obstructive meibomian gland dysfunction. *Ophthalmology.* (2009) 116:2058–63.e2051. doi: 10.1016/j.ophtha.2009.04.037
28. Wang MTM, Tien L, Han A, Lee JM, Kim D, Markoulli M, et al. Impact of blinking on ocular surface and tear film parameters. *Ocul Surf.* (2018) 16:424–9. doi: 10.1016/j.jtos.2018.06.001
29. Jie Y, Sella R, Feng J, Gomez ML, Afshari NA. Evaluation of incomplete blinking as a measurement of dry eye disease. *Ocul Surf.* (2019) 17:440–6. doi: 10.1016/j.jtos.2019.05.007
30. Ousler GW 3rd, Abelson MB, Johnston PR, Rodriguez J, Lane K, Smith LM. Blink patterns and lid-contact times in dry-eye and normal subjects. *Clin Ophthalmol.* (2014) 8:869–74. doi: 10.2147/opth.S56783

3

Evaluation of the Ocular Surface and Meibomian Gland in Obstructive Sleep Apnea Hypopnea Syndrome

Shaohua Liu [1,2†], *Shisheng Li* [3†], *Mengmeng Li* [3], *Shiying Zeng* [3], *Baihua Chen* [1,2*] and *Liwei Zhang* [1,2*]

Department of Ophthalmology, The Second Xiangya Hospital of Central South University, Changsha, China, [2] *Hunan Clinical Research Centre of Ophthalmic Disease, Changsha, China,* [3] *Department of Otorhinolaryngology, The Second Xiangya Hospital of Central South University, Changsha, China*

Correspondence:
Liwei Zhang
liweizhang@csu.edu.cn
Baihua Chen
chenbaihua2017@csu.edu.cn;
chenbh2006@126.com

† *These authors share first authorship*

Purpose: To assess the ocular surface and meibomian gland (MG) of patients with obstructive sleep apnea hypopnea syndrome (OSAHS) and to explore the effects of surgery for OSAHS on the ocular surface and MG.

Methods: Based on the apnea hypopnea index (AHI), 21 patients with mild OSAHS (Group A, $5/h \leq AHI < 15/h$), 20 patients with moderate OSAHS (Group B, $15/h \leq AHI < 30/h$), 62 patients with severe OSAHS (Group C, $AHI \geq 30/h$) were examined. The ocular surface and MG were evaluated using Keratograph 5M. In addition, detailed Ophthalmic examination including visual acuity, refraction, slit-lamp examination of the anterior segment, corneal fluorescein staining (CFS), ocular surface disease index (OSDI) scoring, Schirmer I test (SIT) and serum lipid measurement was performed. For OSAHS patients with dry eye syndrome (DES) who underwent uvulopalatopharyngoplasty for improving AHI, the conditions of the ocular surface and MG were compared before surgery and 3 months after surgery. Only the data of the right eyes were analyzed.

Results: There were no significantly different in the OSDI score, tear meniscus height (TMH), or loss ratio of the lower eyelid (LRLE) among these groups. The first non-invasive tear film breakup time (fNIBUT), average non-invasive tear film breakup time (avNIBUT), bulbar redness index (BRI), lipid layer grading (LLG), CFS, plugged orifices and distortion in MG, the loss ratio of upper eyelid (LRUE), and the incidence of DES, floppy eyelid syndrome (FES) and meibomian gland dysfunction (MGD) showed significant differences between Groups A and C ($p = 0.015$, $p = 0.018$, $p < 0.001$, $p = 0.022$, $p = 0.036$, $p = 0.007$, $p = 0.019$, $p = 0.017$, $p = 0.045$, $p = 0.013$, and $p = 0.029$, respectively). The SIT in the Group A was significantly higher than in Group B ($p = 0.025$) and in Group C ($p < 0.001$). In the correlation analyses, the fNIBUT, avNIBUT, SIT and LLG had negative correlations with the AHI ($p = 0.013$, $p = 0.010$, $p = 0.003$, $p < 0.001$, and $p = 0.006$, respectively). The BRI, CFS and LRUE were positively correlated with the AHI ($p = 0.006$, $p = 0.007$, and $p = 0.046$, respectively). Three months after surgery, there were no significant differences in the ocular surface or MG.

Conclusion: Patients with severe OSAHS have poor stability of tear film and are prone to lipid-deficient dry eye as a result of the loss of meibomian gland. By improving the AHI, the ocular surface damage of OSAHS patients cannot be reversed in a short time.

Keywords: obstructive sleep apnea hypopnea syndrome, dry eye, ocular surface, meibomian gland, tear film

INTRODUCTION

Obstructive sleep apnea hypopnea syndrome (OSAHS) is a chronic intermittent hypoxic sleep-disordered breathing disease that is characterized by repeated apnea and hypopnea during sleep (1). The prevalence of OSAHS is 2–4% in symptomatic patients and 24% in asymptomatic patients, especially in middle-aged overweight men (2, 3). Long-term intermittent hypoxia, hypercapnia, heightened sympathetic nervous system activity and increased catecholamine levels constitute the pathophysiological mechanism of OSAHS (4). The systemic hypertension, atheromatosis and autonomic nerve dysfunction caused by OSAHS may give rise to a series of complications, such as coronary atherosclerotic heart disease, diabetes mellitus, heart failure and even death (5, 6). Ocular blood vessels are also affected by these mechanisms, including increased oxidative stress, systemic inflammation and sympathetic activity (4). OSAHS is associated with various eye diseases, including glaucoma, optic neuropathy, optic papilledema and ocular surface disease (7–15). This association can be explained that long-term intermittent hypoxia increases the levels of carbon dioxide in blood and causes hemodynamic changes, such as large nocturnal fluctuations in blood pressure, dilation and increased volume of cerebral vessels. It disturbs the normal ocular hemodynamics, resulting in a series of ocular disorders eventually (16, 17). The ocular surface manifestations of OSAHS present as floppy eyelid syndrome (FES), papillary conjunctivitis, punctate epithelial keratopathy, keratitis and keratoconus (7–11).

Previous studies have found that OSAHS is associated with reduced tear film breakup time (TBUT) and Schirmer values, and increased ocular surface disease (OSDI) scores and corneal fluorescein staining (CFS), these associations show that ocular surface parameters are impaired in OSAHS and suggest a tendency toward dry eye syndrome (DES) in these patients (18, 19). Meibomian gland dysfunction (MGD) is a common etiology of DES (20), and there are only two researches that have explored the relationship between meibomian gland (MG) and OSAHS. It has been demonstrated that MG are lost in OSAHS, especially severe OSAHS (21, 22). In recent years, non-invasive examination has begun to be frequently applied for the evaluation of dry eye and MG (23–25). Keratograph 5M is a non-invasive corneal topographer that measures non-invasive breakup time by the irregular change of ring pattern projected by the Placido disc onto the surface of the tear film (26). Compared with invasive examination, Keratograph 5M does not need to instill fluorescein, which can avoid physical interference following invasive procedures, such as reflex tearing, drop size and concentration of fluorescein (26–28). It has great reproductivity and reliability in dry eye tests as a non-invasive and objective examination (29–31), and can observe distinct morphological changes in MG with infrared imaging technology. We have also included more observation indices, including tear meniscus height, lipid layer and bulbar redness index.

The treatment of OSAHS includes conservative approaches, such as weight loss, avoiding smoking, excessive alcohol and sedatives, continuous positive airway pressure (CPAP) and surgical therapy (32–34). Although CPAP has always been the preferred therapy for moderate to severe OSAHS (33), the effects of CPAP for improving AHI on the ocular surface are unclear. Kadyan et al. and Acar et al. have found that ocular surface damage improves along with OSAHS severity after continuous positive airway pressure (CPAP) therapy (35, 36). However, Hayiric et al. found that ocular surface damage was exacerbated after CPAP therapy, although the severity of OSAHS improved (37). In the process of CPAP therapy, the opposite results may be affected by the air leakage or counterflow (38–40). Therefore, we will explore the effects of surgical therapy for improving AHI on the ocular surface and MG in this study.

METHODS

This study was conducted in the Department of Ophthalmology and Otorhinolaryngology at the Second Xiangya Hospital of Central South University between August 2019 and April 2021. This study was conducted according to the Declaration of Helsinki and approved by the Ethics Committee of the Second Xiangya Hospital of Central South University (Number: 2021205).

Participates

Patients who presented with snoring, nocturnal choking, and excessive daytime sleepiness underwent polysomnography (PSG) tests before their enrollment. According to the PSG results, a total of 103 patients (AHI $\geq$ 5) were included in our study. Based on the AHI, the severity of OSAHS was classified as follows: mild, 5/h $\leq$ AHI <15/h; moderate, 15/h $\leq$ AHI <30/h; severe, AHI $\geq$ 30/h (41). Twenty-one patients with mild OSAHS (Group A), 20 patients with moderate OSAHS (Group B) and 62 patients with severe OSAHS (Group C) were included in this study. Only the data of the right eyes were analyzed. Exclusion criteria included a history of ocular surgery and trauma, contact lens use, diabetes mellitus, glaucoma, thyroid-associated ophthalmopathy, chronic topical medication (anti-glaucoma eye drops), keratography, conjunctivitis, high myopia, rheumatic diseases and OSAHS patients receiving treatment. All subjects underwent detailed ophthalmological examinations. The examination was performed sequentially as follows: Keratograph 5M, visual acuity assessment, slit-lamp examination of the anterior segment, corneal fluorescein staining (CFS), ocular surface disease index (OSDI) questionnaire, Schirmer I test (SIT) and measurement of serum lipids. The results of PSG were blinded to the examiner during ophthalmic examination.

Keratograph 5M

Keratograph 5M was applied to non-invasively measure certain parameters of the ocular surface, including tear meniscus height (TMH), non-invasive break-up time of tear film (NIBUT), lipid layer grading (LLG), bulbar redness index (BRI) and infrared meibography (42–44). The TMH was measured with an integrated ruler on the vertical line through the pupil center. The NIBUT was comprised of the first NIBUT (fNIBUT) and the average NIBUT (avNIBUT). The level of NIBUT was classified as follows: normal 0 (fNIBUT $\geq$ 10 s and avNIBUT $\geq$ 14 s); borderline 1 (between 0 and 2) or Dry eye (fNIBUT $\leq$ 5 s or avNIBUT $\leq$ 6 s) (45). Based on structural clarity and color richness, the lipid layer grading was divided into three levels: thin (level 1 with fizzy structure and gray color), normal (level 2 with clear structure and rich color), and thick (level 3 with extremely clear structure and rich color) (42). The BRI, comprising nasal limbal, temporal limbal, temporal bulbar, nasal bulbar and global regions, appears together with the total area analyzed (mm^2), which is calculated by the equipment software as the area percentage ratio between the vessels and the rest of the analyzed area. The BRI ranges from 0.0 to 4.0, and the more blood vessels there are, the higher the score (46). Infrared images of the MG were taken after eyelid eversion, and the loss of the MG was calculated by Photoshop and Image J software as the area percentage ratio of dropout sections to the total area, including the upper and lower eyelids. Additionally, the distortion of ducts was defined as distortion of > 45° in at least one MG in the upper or lower eyelid (47).

Corneal Fluorescein Staining

The CFS was performed by placing a wet sodium fluorescein test strip in the lower conjunctival sac, and observed the dye under the blue light from a slit-lamp. The CFS was ranged from 0 to 12, which was the sum of the scores of the four corneal quadrants (superior nasal, inferior nasal, superior temporal and inferior temporal) scored individually as 0 (no staining), 1 (mild staining with 1–30 dots of stains), 2 (moderate staining between 1 and 3), or 3 (severe staining with confluent stains, filaments or ulcers) (48).

Ocular Surface Disease Index Questionnaire

The OSDI questionnaire is composed of three sections, involving eye symptoms, environmental factors and visual function. The score of each item on the questionnaire is 0 to 4. The OSDI score is the sum of the scores of 12 items, multiplied by 25, and then divided by the number of questions answered (49).

Schirmer I Test

After the subjects accomplished the corneal staining, they were given a 30 min rest. The Schirmer I test strip was placed into the lower eyelid one-third of the distance from the lateral canthus and the wetting distance was recorded after 5 min.

Diagnostic Criteria of LDDE, FES, and MGD

The diagnostical criteria of lipid-deficient dry eye (LDDE): LDDE is caused by the abnormal quality and quantity of the lipid layer, such as MGD, or various factors causing increased tear evaporation. The tear film stability decreased significantly (FBUT or NIBUT $\leq$ 5 s), and the tear secretion was slightly abnormal (10 mm/5 min $\leq$ SIT $\leq$ 12 mm/5 min), which tended to be considered as lipid-deficient dry eye (50). The floppy eyelid syndrome (FES) was defined as lid hyperlaxity, easily everted upper eyelids and reactive conjunctival changes (51). The diagnostic criteria of meibomian gland dysfunction (MGD) were abnormalities of the lid margin, meibomian gland orifices, meibum secretion and lipid layer thickness, dropout of the meibomian gland and ocular symptoms (52).

Statistical Analysis

Statistical analysis was executed with software package SPSS version 25.0 (SPSS Inc., Chicago, IL, USA). Descriptive variables are expressed as the mean $\pm$ standard deviation (SD). The normality distribution of the data was tested by the Kolmogorov-Smirnov test. The variables with a non-normal distribution were analyzed by means of a non-parametric test. The variables among the three groups were analyzed through the non-parametric Kruskal-Wallis H-test. The non-parametric Mann–Whitney U test was applied to compare two groups. The enumeration data was analyzed using Chi-square tests, including sex and the incidence of DES, FES and MGD. The paired Student's *T*-test was applied to compare the preoperative and postoperative

TABLE 1 | General information of the OSAHS patients.

	Group A ($n = 21$)	Group B ($n = 20$)	Group C ($n = 62$)
Age	35.6 ± 10.7	38.6 ± 7.3	40.1 ± 8.4
Sex (male/female)	17/4	18/2	61/1*
BMI (kg/m^2)	25.2 ± 2.5	26.6 ± 3.1	28.0 ± 3.0***
AHI	9.8 ± 3.1	24.8 ± 4.4	57.2 ± 15.8###
$mSaO_2$	82.1 ± 8.0	74.7 ± 7.8	63 ± 9.3###

*BMI, body mass index; AHI, apnea hypopnea index; $mSaO_2$, minimum oxygen saturation. Compared with Group A: *$P < 0.05$, ***$P < 0.001$, Mann-Whitney U test. ###$P < 0.001$, Kruskal-Wallis H-test.*

TABLE 2 | The serum lipid levels of the OSAHS patients.

Serum lipids	Group A ($n = 19$)	Group B ($n = 15$)	Group C ($n = 48$)
TC (2.90–5.20)	4.74 ± 0.58	4.81 ± 0.88	5.28 ± 0.84*
TG (<1.71)	2.56 ± 2.15	2.34 ± 1.19	2.80 ± 1.61
HDL (>1.04)	1.10 ± 0.27	1.12 ± 0.21	1.06 ± 0.22
LDL (<3.12)	3.08 ± 0.62	3.17 ± 0.78	3.55 ± 0.76*

*TC, total cholesterol; TG, triglycerides; HDL, high density lipoprotein; LDL, low density lipoprotein. Compared with Group A: *$P < 0.05$, Mann–Whitney U test.*

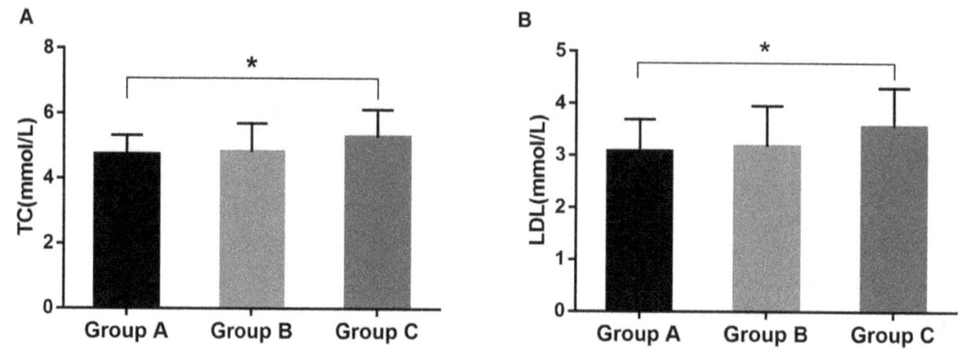

FIGURE 1 | The significant difference in serum lipids among these groups. The difference was significant for TC **(A)** and LDL **(B)** between Groups A and C. $^*P < 0.05$.

differences. Spearman's correlation was applied to analyze the relationship between the variables. P-value < 0.05 was considered as statistically significant.

RESULTS

The general information of the subjects is shown in **Table 1**. The ratio of males to females was 96–7 and body mass index (BMI) was 28.0 ± 3.0 kg/m^2 in severe OSAHS patients, which was significantly higher in Group C than in Group A ($p < 0.001$). Some patients were taking hypolipidemic drugs or had a lack of results, resulting in the partial loss of serum lipid data (**Table 2**). The total cholesterol (TC) values were 4.74 ± 0.58 mmol/L, 4.81 ± 0.88 mmol/L, and 5.28 ± 0.84 mmol/L for Groups A, B, and C, respectively. The low-density lipoprotein (LDL) values were 3.08 ± 0.62 mmol/L, 3.17 ± 0.78 mmol/L, and 3.55 ± 0.76 mmol/L for Groups A, B, and C, respectively. These values were significantly different between Groups A and C ($p = 0.014$ and $p = 0.020$) (**Table 2; Figure 1**). The high-density lipoprotein (HDL) or triglyceride (TG) levels was not significantly different among these groups.

The ocular surface parameters are presented in **Table 3** and **Figure 2**. The OSDI score and TMH were not significant difference among the groups ($p = 0.291$ and $p = 0.287$, respectively). The fNIBUT and avNIBUT were significantly different between the group A and Group C. In Group C, fNIBUT and avNIBUT were shorter than in Group A ($p = 0.015$ and $p = 0.018$, respectively). Similarly, the BRI, LLG and CFS has significant difference among these groups. In Group A, both BRI and CFS were lower and LLG was higher than in Group C ($p < 0.001$, $p = 0.022$ and $p = 0.036$, respectively). The Schirmer values were 14.7 ± 1.5 mm, 13.7 ± 1.4 mm, and 12.4 ± 1.5 mm, respectively. The Schirmer in the Group A was significantly higher than in Group B ($p = 0.025$) and in Group C ($p < 0.001$).

The morphology of MG was significantly altered in severe OSAHS patients (**Figure 3**). Plugged orifices and distortion of ducts were observed in 70.97 and 58.06% of patients with severe OSAHS, respectively ($p = 0.007$, $p = 0.019$). In the Group C, the loss ratio of the upper eyelid was more severe than that in the Group A ($p = 0.017$). However, that of the lower eyelid was much higher but not significantly different. The incidence of DES and MGD was higher in Group C than in the Group A ($p = 0.045$ and $p = 0.013$, respectively), and all of dry eye was lipid-deficient dry eye (LDDE). The FES was observed more frequently in severe OSAHS patients ($p = 0.029$) (**Table 4**).

The correlation analyses are described in detail in **Tables 5, 6**. The fNIBUT, avNIBUT, Schirmer values and LLG were significantly negatively correlated with the AHI ($R = -0.263$, $p = 0.006$; $R = -0.200$, $p = 0.038$; $R = -0.200$, $p < 0.001$; $R = -0.211$, $p = 0.029$, respectively). Moreover, the BRI, CFS and LRUE were found to be significantly positively correlated with the AHI ($R = 0.284$, $p = 0.003$; $R = 0.256$, $p = 0.008$; $R = 0.176$, $p = 0.040$). The TC and LDL levels were significantly correlated with MGD ($R = 0.221$, $p = 0.041$; $R = 0.246$, $p = 0.023$, respectively) (**Figure 4**).

TABLE 3 | The ocular surface parameters of the OSAHS patients.

	Group A (n = 21)	Group B (n = 20)	Group C (n = 62)
OSDI score	3.4 ± 4.6	3.6 ± 4.3	5.2 ± 6.0
TMH (mm)	0.25 ± 0.06	0.24 ± 0.05	0.23 ± 0.05
fNIBUT (mm)	12.01 ± 5.98	12.55 ± 5.24	$8.27 \pm 4.18^*$
avNIBUT (mm)	14.94 ± 5.83	12.55 ± 5.24	$11.52 \pm 4.81^*$
BRI	1.0 ± 0.4	1.2 ± 0.4	$1.4 \pm 0.4^{***}$
LLG	2.1 ± 0.9	1.8 ± 0.7	$1.6 \pm 0.7^*$
Plugged orifices (n, %)	8 (38.10%)	11 (55%)	44 (70.97%)**
Distortion (n, %)	6 (28.57%)	9 (45%)	36 (58.06%)*
LRUE (%)	25.71 ± 12.50	30.40 ± 13.07	$36.38 \pm 18.08^*$
LRLE (%)	26.45 ± 16.54	26.87 ± 25.57	27.03 ± 23.22
CFS	0.2 ± 0.4	0.4 ± 0.5	$0.6 \pm 0.6^*$
Schirmer (mm)	$14.7 \pm 1.5^{\#}$	$13.7 \pm 1.4^*$	$12.4 \pm 1.5^{***\#\#}$

OSDI, ocular surface disease index; TMH, tear meniscus height; fNIBUT, first non-invasive breakup time; avNIBUT, average non-invasive breakup time; BRI, bulbar redness index; LLG, lipid layer grading; LRUE, loss ratio of the upper eyelid; LRLE, loss ratio of the lower eyelid; CFS, corneal fluorescein staining; Compared with Group A: $^*P < 0.05$, $^{**}P < 0.01$, $^{***}P < 0.001$, *Mann–Whitney U test. Compared with Group B:* $^{\#}P < 0.05$, $^{\#\#}P < 0.01$, *Mann–Whitney U test.*

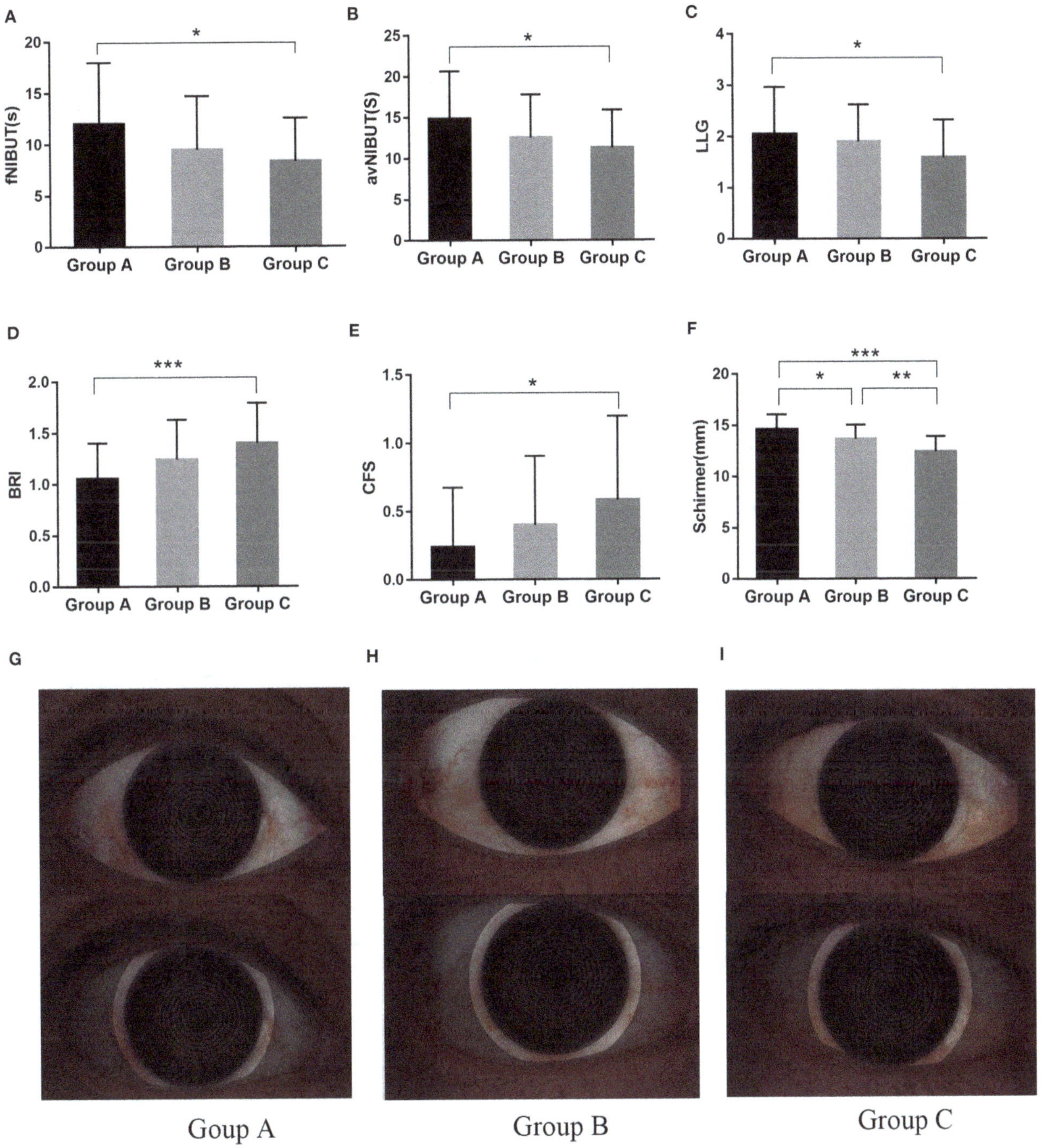

FIGURE 2 | The significant difference in Ocular Surface Parameters and bulbar redness index among these groups. The fNIBUT **(A)**, avNIBUT **(B)**, and LLG **(C)** were lower in severe OSAHS patients. The difference was significant between Groups A and C for BRI **(D)**, as well as for CFS **(E)**. The Schirmer in the Group A was significantly higher than in Group B ($P = 0.025$) and in Group C **(F)**. The bulbar redness index in mild **(G)**, moderate **(H)**, and severe **(I)** OSAHS patients. $^{*}P < 0.05$; $^{**}P < 0.01$; $^{***}P < 0.001$.

A total of 103 OSAHS patients were enrolled in our study, of these patients, 66 cases were diagnosed with DES. 5 cases who underwent uvulopalatopharyngoplasty for OSAHS were followed up in 3 months, of which 3 cases were moderate OSAHS patients and 2 cases were severe OSAHS patients. The characteristics of the postoperative ocular surface are shown in **Table 7**. The AHI values were significantly different from the preoperative values, but no significant differences were found among other ocular surface characteristics.

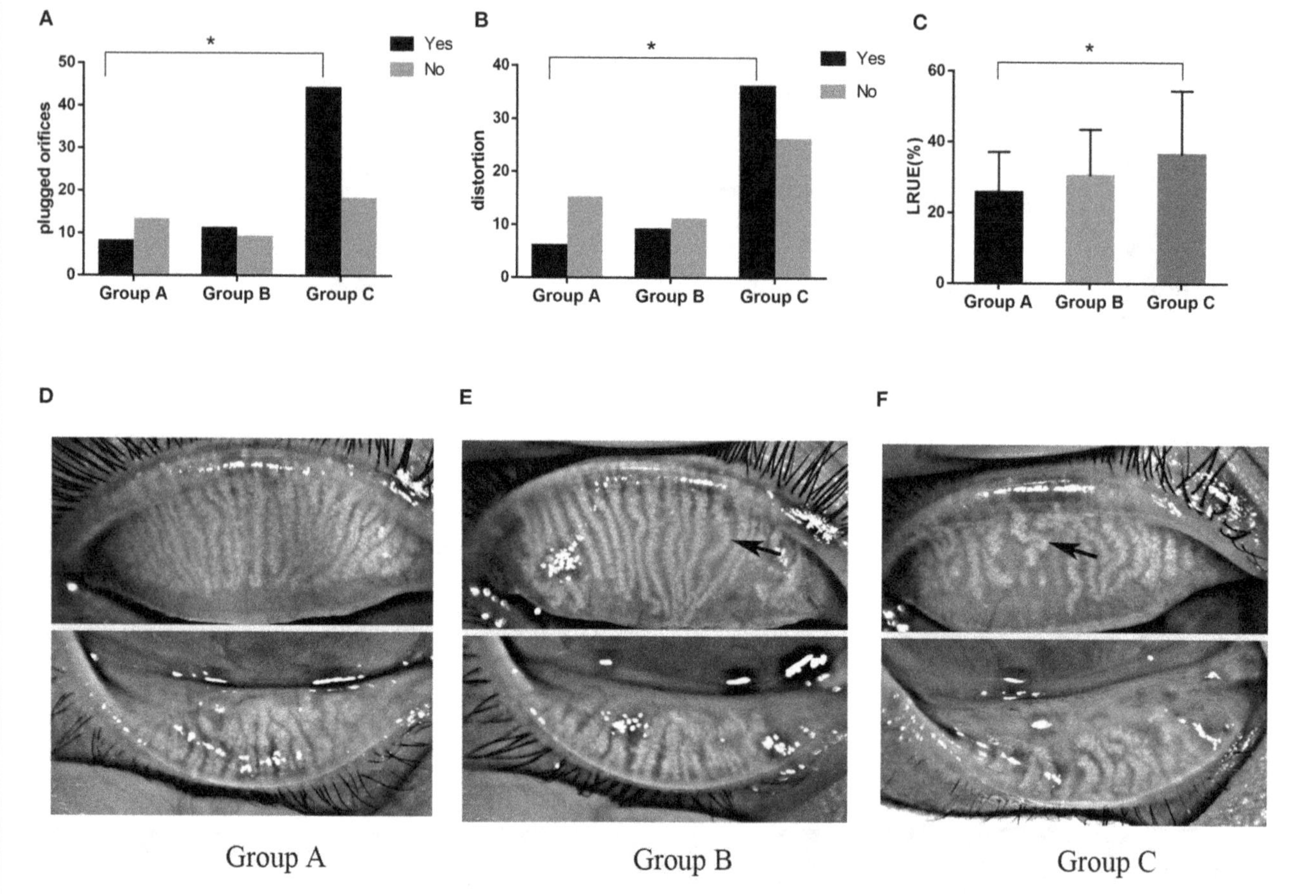

FIGURE 3 | The morphological changes of MG. The number of plugged orifices **(A)** and distortion **(B)** of the MG was higher in severe OSAHS patients. The loss ratio of the upper eyelid **(C)** was significantly different between Groups A and C. The loss of meibomian gland in mild **(D)**, moderate **(E)**, and severe **(F)** OSAHS patients. Black arrows demonstrate the distortion in the duct. *$P < 0.05$.

TABLE 4 | The incidence of DES, FES and MGD in patients.

	Group A (n = 21)	Group B (n = 20)	Group C (n = 62)
DES (n, %)	4 (19.1%)	6(30%)	27 (43.6%)*
LDDE/ATD	4/0	6/0	27/0
FES (n, %)	0	0	12 (19.4%)*
MGD (n, %)	7 (33.3%)	9 (45%)	40 (64.5%)*

*DES, dry eye syndrome; LDDE, lipid-deficient dry eye; ATD, aqueous tear deficiency; FES, floppy eyelid syndrome; MGD, meibomian gland dysfunction. Compared with Group A: *$P < 0.05$, Chi-square test.*

DISCUSSION

To our knowledge, this is the first study to evaluate certain parameters of the ocular surface for OSAHS patients by a non-invasive instrument, and to analyze the correlation between the ocular surface and the severity of OSAHS in terms of AHI. In our study, we found that the patients with severe OSAHS had higher BRI and CFS scores, which were positively correlated with the AHI. The BRI may be a potential objective index to estimate the severity of OSAHS in the clinic. In OSAHS patients, long-term chronic intermittent hypoxia has been found to increase oxidative stress, resulting in an upregulation of stress signaling cascades, such as HIF-1, NF-KB and Nrf2 (53). These pathways further incite a systematic chronic inflammatory response and immunological alterations (54), and increase the expression of proinflammatory cytokines and adhesion molecules, including IL-6, IL-8, TNFα, and Fas recptor-positive lymphocytes (55). Dilated conjunctival vessels and damaged epithelial cells release cytokines, resulting in a persistent inflammatory state that ultimately causes the apoptosis of goblet cells and keratoconjunctival epithelial cells (56). Therefore, inflammation may contribute to ocular surface damage in OSAHS patients. Local anti-inflammatory treatments may improve the ocular surface damage caused by OSAHS, but this needs further research.

Additionally, the loss ratio of the upper eyelid MG was higher in severe OSAHS patients, and the incidence of gland distortion, FES and MGD were positively correlated with the AHI. The proportion of OSAHS patients with FES varies from 2 to 40%, and the occurrence of FES in OSAHS patients indicates that

TABLE 5 | The correlation between ocular surface parameters and the apnea hypopnea index.

	R	*P*
OSDI score	0.103	0.156
TMH	0.102	0.305
fNIBUT	−0.245	0.013**
avNIBUT	−0.253	0.010*
BRI	0.268	0.006**
LLG	−0.267	0.006**
LRUE (%)	0.197	0.046*
LRLE (%)	0.062	0.534
CFS	0.263	0.007**
Schirmer I	−0.366	<0.001***

*OSDI, ocular surface disease index; TMH, tear meniscus height; fNIBUT, first non-invasive breakup time; avNIBUT, average non-invasive breakup time; LLG, lipid layer grading; BRI, bulbar redness index; LRUE, loss ratio of the upper eyelid; LRLE, loss ratio of the lower eyelid; CFS, corneal fluorescein staining; R, Spearman's correlation coefficient, $-1 \leq R \leq 1$; P: Spearman's correlation analysis significance value. *P-value < 0.05; **P-value < 0.01; ***P-value < 0.001.*

TABLE 6 | The correlation between MGD and serum lipids.

	R	*P*
TC	0.182	0.041*
TG	0.092	0.399
HDL	−0.165	0.128
LDL	0.224	0.038*

*TC, total cholesterol; TG, triglycerides; LDL, low density lipoprotein; HDL, high density lipoprotein. R, Spearman's correlation analysis coefficient, $-1 \leq R \leq 1$, P: Spearman's correlation analysis significance value. *P value < 0.05.*

the disease severity is more serious (57). This may be related to the increase in elastase activity in eyelid connective tissue caused by longstanding hypoxia, resulting in the degradation and fracture of eyelid elastic fibers (18, 57). We hypothesize that the reason for the above change in OSAHS patients may be due to the long-term intermittent hypoxia that leads to an increase in matrix metalloproteinase activity in eyelid connective tissue, the degradation of elastic fibers, a decrease in eyelid tension, and the weakening of the squeeze-driving effect of the orbicularis oculi muscle on the MG, resulting in stasis of the meibum. With the accumulation of meibum, the pressure in the conduct gradually increases, which contributes to the atrophy and dropout of the MG eventually. An additional reason could be that intermittent hypoxia increases the degradation of the MG matrix, causing the gland duct to be distorted and irregular. This could result in the increased resistance to meibum secretion, causing the stasis of meibum. This may be followed by its accumulation and degeneration, which would change the quantity and quality of meibum secretion.

Furthermore, the plugged orifices increase the intraluminal pressure, forming a vicious circle that leads to atrophy and dropout of the MG. Finally, another reason could be due to the lower androgen level in OSAHS patients than that in normal people (58). The MG contains the androgen receptor, which can improve the quality of meibum secretion (59). Therefore, the decreased androgen level may be one of the reasons for the abnormal morphology and function of the MG.

In 2019, Karaca et al. observed dropout and morphological changes in the MG in OSAHS patients with a slit-lamp biomicroscope (19). They first reported that compared with mild OSAHS patients, severe OSAHS patients had a higher degree of upper meiboscore and morphological alterations, such as thinning, dilatation and distortion. However, the lower meiboscore was not significantly different. Similarly, our findings were in accordance with their results. Muhafiz et al. found that the loss of the MG in both the upper and lower eyelid was more severe in the OSAHS group than that in the control group (22). Research has found that the loss of MG was significantly different in the upper eyelid and lower eyelid between Sjögren's syndrome and non-Sjögren's syndrome (45). Heiko and Youngsub et al. observed that the loss of MG in the lower eyelid was more severe than that in the upper eyelid in MGD patients (60, 61). This phenomenon can be explained by the evident action of orbicularis oculi muscles in the upper eyelid during blinking. In addition, the direction of meibum delivery of the upper eyelid is consistent with the direction of gravity, while that of the lower eyelid is the opposite. Therefore, the meibum from the lower eyelid is more easily stagnate in the orifices, leading to duct dilation, acinar atrophy and eventual loss of MG. In OSAHS patients, the pathogenesis of FES is mainly related to the elastin located in the tarsal plate of the upper eyelid (7), and long-term hypoxia decreases the amount of elastin, causing prominent upper eyelid laxity (62, 63). This may result in a relative deterioration in easy and persistent secretion of meibum from the upper eyelid. Thus, as shown in this study, the loss of the MG in the upper eyelid appears to be more prominent.

The tear film has a complex structure, and it is followed by a lipid layer, aqueous layer, and mucin layer from the outside to inside. The normal function of various tear functional units is vital to a stable tear film and heathy ocular surface (64). The MG is a type of sebaceous gland with tubule acinar structure and holocrine function. MG secrete meibum to the ocular surface, where it coats the aqueous layer and prevents tear evaporation and provides tear stability (65). Studies have shown that TBUT and Schirmer values were lower in OSAHS patients, and much more in moderate and severe OSAHS (18, 19, 21). Similarly, we also found these results in moderate and severe OSAHS, and they were associated with increasing OSAHS severity. Previous researches have found that the values of NIBUT were higher than FBUT (31, 66, 67). The reason could be that the fluorescein affects the stability of tear film, and has low Reproducibility (64), while Keratograph 5M is considered as a non-invasive and objective method that measure BUT by the analysis of disruption of the reflection of Placido rings onto the tear film, with good repeatability and reliability (29). Additionally, the lipid layer was thinner and the incidence of DES was higher in severe OSAHS patients, and the DES was lipid-deficient dry eye caused by MGD. As mentioned above, in patients with OSAHS, long-standing intermittent hypoxia causes systematic inflammation, resulting in distortion and dropout of the MG and subsequent

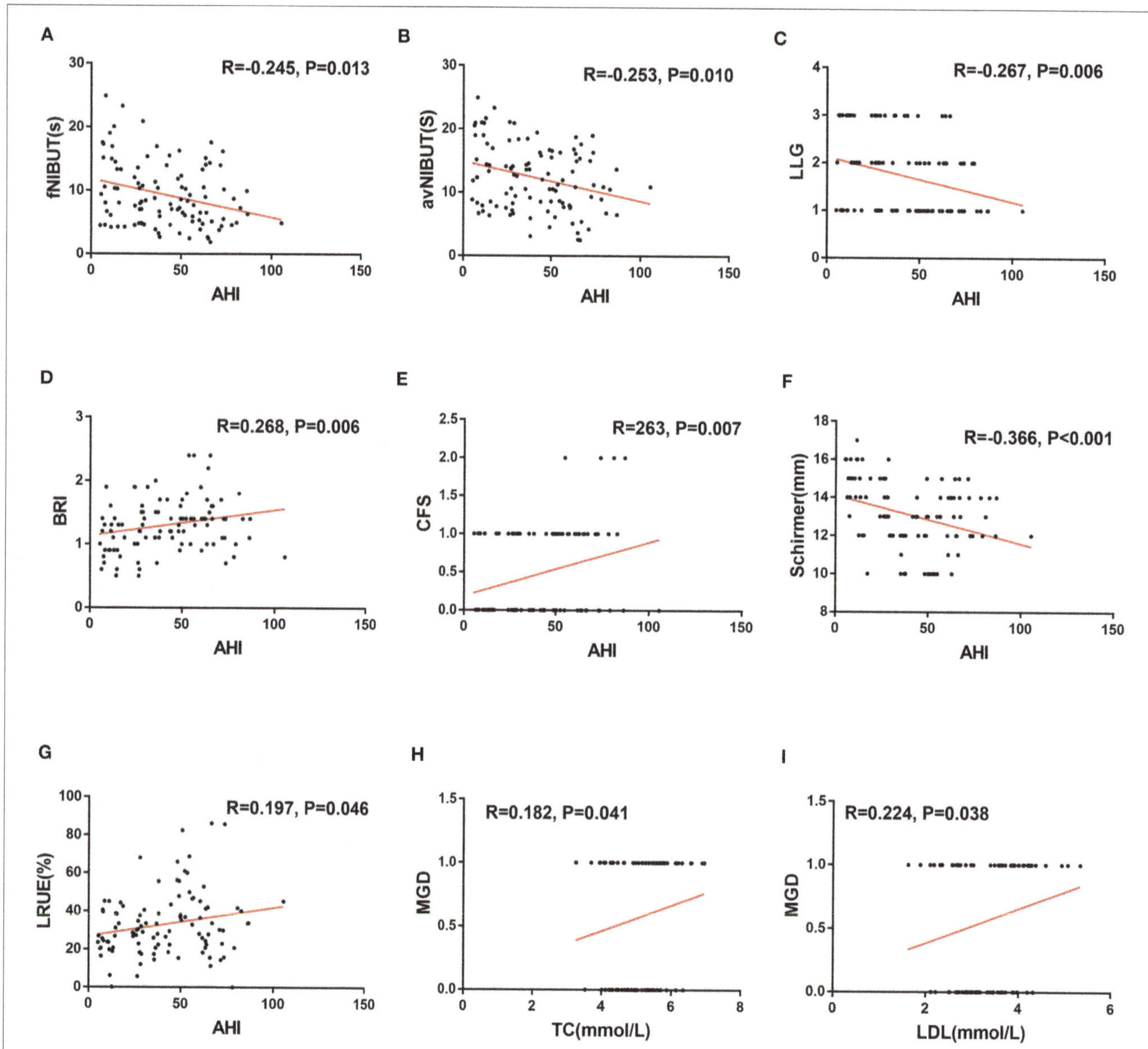

FIGURE 4 | Correlations between the AHI and ocular surface parameters, MGD and serum lipids. The fNIBUT **(A)**, avNIBUT **(B)**, LLG **(C)**, and Schirmer **(F)** were significantly negatively correlated with the AHI. The BRI **(D)**, CFS **(E)**, and LRUE **(G)** were positively correlated with the AHI. The TC **(H)** and LDL**(I)** were positively correlated with MGD. R, Spearman's correlation coefficient, $-1 \leq R \leq 1$. A *P*-value < 0.05 was considered to be statistically significant.

MGD. MGD affects the quality of meibum, causing accelerated tear evaporation and decreased stability of tear film and tear hyperosmotic pressure. These conditions lead to ocular surface damage through a series of inflammatory cascade responses and are the main causes of lipid-deficient dry eye.

Studies have shown that elevations in TC, TG and LDL, and decreases in HDL in patients with OSAHS, and those alterations may be exacerbated with the increasing of OSAHS severity (68, 69). A possible reason is that long-standing intermittent hypoxia stimulates the production of stearoyl-coenzyme A desaturase-1 and reactive oxygen species. Increase production of these cause lipid peroxidation and sympathetic system dysfunction, resulting in disorders of lipid metabolism and dyslipidemia (69). In this study, TC and LDL levels were higher in severe OSAHS patients than in mild OSAHS patients. Meibum is mainly composed of wax and neutral sterol esters, with low amounts of polar lipids, triglycerides, and cholesterol, which have been reported to range from 1 to 2% (70). Alterations in the quality of meibum and plugged ducts are considered the core of MGD. Research has found that high levels of TG, TC and LDL are associated with MGD (71, 72). The melting point of normal meibum ranges from 30 to 34°C, but the melting point of cholesterol is 148°C because of structural differences (73). Therefore, meibum would have a

TABLE 7 | The ocular surface parameters of Pre- and Post-operation in patients.

	Pre-operation ($n = 5$)	Post-operation ($n = 5$)	*P*-value
AHI	40.48 ± 25.38	16.42 ± 9.19	0.030*
OSDI score	2.27 ± 2.88	1.52 ± 1.86	0.363
TMH (mm)	0.25 ± 0.07	0.25 ± 0.04	0.932
fNIBUT (s)	7.49 ± 3.42	7.95 ± 6.28	0.905
avNIBUT (s)	11.17 ± 6.22	11.28 ± 6.78	0.977
LLG	1.8 ± 0.8	1.8 ± 0.8	-
BRI	1.58 ± 0.26	1.35 ± 0.32	0.319
LRUE (%)	34.22 ± 25.80	32.72 ± 24.65	0.316
LRLE (%)	24.43 ± 33.33	23.45 ± 32.98	0.294
CFS	0.83 ± 0.98	0.67 ± 0.82	0.363
Schirmer I (mm)	12.83 ± 2.82	13.33 ± 1.86	0.580

*AHI, apnea hypopnea index; TMH, tear meniscus height; fNIBUT, first non-invasive breakup time; avNIBUT, average non-invasive breakup time; LLG, lipid layer grading; BRI, bulbar redness index; LRUE, loss ratio of the upper eyelid; LRLE, loss ratio of the lower eyelid; CFS, corneal fluorescein staining. *P-value < 0.05, paired Student's T-test.*

higher melting point and be more viscous due to a higher concentration of cholesterol, thus plugging the ducts and resulting in MGD.

Currently, CPAP and surgery are the two major treatment modalities for OSAHS. CPAP is considered as the first-ling treatment for OSAHS, but patient compliance has been notably poor result from mask discomfort, nasal dryness and congestion, and difficulty adopting to the pressure, which decrease the usage and efficacy (74, 75). In the literature, there are 3 prospective studies on ocular surface problems in patients with OSAHS after CPAP therapy. Kadyan et al. and Acar et al. have reported that TBUT and ocular irritative symptoms were improved in OSAHS patients after CPAP therapy (35, 36). This may be explained by reduced displacement of mask due to OSAHS patients were in a supine position during CPAP. The blood oxygen levels were increased after long-term treatment, and the mechanical injury to the eyelid was reduced accordingly, thereby improving the ocular surface health. Hayiric et al. has demonstrated that the TBUT was decreased only in the right eyes between pre-CPAP and post-CPAP (37). They speculated that the inconsistency between the left and right eyes may be caused by the sleep posture. When in the left-lying position, air leakage promotes tear evaporation due to the shift of the CPAP mask, resulting in decreased TBUT and increased ocular irritative symptoms. The evaluation of the effects of CPAP therapy for improving AHI on the ocular surface has been influenced by a variety of factors, the following conclusions were controversial. Therefore, we sought to explore the changes of the ocular surface parameters in OSAHS patients after surgical treatment. In the present study, the OSAHS severity was significantly improved 3 months after surgery, but the ocular surface characteristics were not significantly different. The ocular surface damage in OSAHS patients cannot be reversed in a short time by improving the severity of OSAHS. However, there are some limitations in demonstrating the effects of surgery on ocular surface parameters due to small samples and short period of follow-up. It may be necessary to follow up with more cases and longer treatment cycles to observe the changes in ocular surface parameters to explain whether improving the severity of OSAHS by surgery can help to improve the ocular surface condition. This could thereby achieve the purpose of clinically intervening in the progression of dry eye in OSAHS patients or treating dry eye in OSAHS patients.

ETHICS STATEMENT

The studies involving human participants were reviewed and approved by the Ethics Committee of the Second Xiangya Hospital of Central South University. The patients/participants provided their written informed consent to participate in this study.

AUTHOR CONTRIBUTIONS

SLiu and SLi: analysis and interpretation of data and drafting and revising the article. ML and SZ: participate in survey and data collection. LZ and BC: substantial contributions to conception and design and revising it critically for important intellectual content. All authors approved the final manuscript.

REFERENCES

1. Guilleminault C, Abad V. Obstructive sleep apnea syndromes. *Med Clin North Am.* (2004) 88:611–30. doi: 10.1016/j.mcna.2004.01.002
2. Lee W, Nagubadi S, Kryger M, Mokhlesi B. Epidemiology of obstructive sleep apnea: a population-based perspective. *Expert Rev Respir Med.* (2008) 2:349–64. doi: 10.1586/17476348.2.3.349
3. Finkel K, Searleman A, Tymkew H, Tanaka C, Saager L, Safer-Zadeh E, et al. Prevalence of undiagnosed obstructive sleep apnea among adult surgical patients in an academic medical center. *Sleep Med.* (2009) 10:753–8. doi: 10.1016/j.sleep.2008.08.007
4. Kohler M, Stradling J. Mechanisms of vascular damage in obstructive sleep apnea. *Nat Rev Cardiol.* (2010) 7:677–85. doi: 10.1038/nrcardio.2010.145
5. Kohler M. Deleterious systemic effects of OSA: how much evidence do we need? *Thorax.* (2015) 70:817–8. doi: 10.1136/thoraxjnl-2015-207247
6. Stansbury R, Strollo P. Clinical manifestations of sleep apnea. *J Thorac Dis.* (2015) 7:E298–310. doi: 10.3978/j.issn.2072-1439.2015.09.13
7. Culbertson W, Ostler H. The floppy eyelid syndrome. *Am J Ophthalmol.* (1981) 92:568–75. doi: 10.1016/0002-9394(81)90652-8
8. Mojon D, Goldblum D, Fleischhauer J, Chiou A, Frueh B, Hess C, et al. Eyelid, conjunctival, and corneal findings in sleep apnea syndrome. *Ophthalmology.* (1999) 106:1182–5. doi: 10.1016/S0161-6420(99)90256-7
9. Mastrota K. Impact of floppy eyelid syndrome in ocular surface and dry e disease. *Optom Vis Sci.* (2008) 85:814–6. doi: 10.1097/OPX.0b013e3181852777
10. Culbertson W, Tseng S. Corneal disorders in floppy eyelid syndrome. *Cornea.* (1994) 13:33–42. doi: 10.1097/00003226-199401000-00007
11. Donnenfeld E, Perry H, Gibralter R, Ingraham H, Udell I. Keratoconus associated with floppy eyelid syndrome. *Ophthalmology.* (1991) 98:1674–8. doi: 10.1016/S0161-6420(91)32070-0

12. Sergi M, Salerno D, Rizzi M, Blini M, Andreoli A, Messenio D, et al. Prevalence of normal tension glaucoma in obstructive sleep apnea syndrome patients. *J Glaucoma.* (2007) 16:42–6. doi: 10.1097/01.ijg.0000243472.51461.24
13. Tsang C, Chong S, Ho C, Li M. Moderate to severe obstructive sleep apnoea patients is associated with a higher incidence of visual field defect. *Eye.* (2006) 20:38–42. doi: 10.1038/sj.eye.6701785
14. Seif G, Trope G. Impact of 10 years of glaucoma research funding: the glaucoma research society of Canada. *Can J Ophthalmol.* (2010) 45:132–4. doi: 10.3129/i09-240
15. Peter L, Jacob M, Krolak-Salmon P, Petitjean T, Bastuji H, Grange J, et al. Prevalence of papilloedema in patients with sleep apnoea syndrome: a prospective study. *J Sleep Res.* (2007) 16:313–8. doi: 10.1111/j.1365-2869.2007.00598.x
16. Dhillon S, Shapiro C, Flanagan J. Sleep-disordered breathing and effects on ocular health. *Can J Ophthalmol.* (2007) 42:238–43. doi: 10.3129/can.j.ophthalmol.i07-029
17. Grover D. Obstructive sleep apnea and ocular disorders. *Curr Opin Ophthalmol.* (2010) 21:454–8. doi: 10.1097/ICU.0b013e32833f00dc
18. Acar M, Firat H, Acar U, Ardic S. Ocular surface assessment in patients with obstructive sleep apnea-hypopnea syndrome. *Sleep Breath.* (2013) 17:583–8. doi: 10.1007/s11325-012-0724-0
19. Karaca E, Akçam H, Uzun F, Özdek S, Ulukavak Çiftçi T. Evaluation of ocular surface health in patients with obstructive sleep apnea syndrome. *Turk J Ophthalmol.* (2016) 46:104–8. doi: 10.4274/tjo.57778
20. Baudouin C, Messmer E, Aragona P, Geerling G, Akova Y. Benítez-del-Castillo J, et al. Revisiting the vicious circle of dry eye disease: a focus on the pathophysiology of meibomian gland dysfunction. *Br J Ophthalmol.* (2016) 100:300–6. doi: 10.1136/bjophthalmol-2015-307415
21. Karaca I, Yagci A, Palamar M, Tasbakan M, Basoglu O. Ocular surface assessment and morphological alterations in meibomian glands with meibography in obstructive sleep apnea syndrome. *Ocul Surf.* (2019) 17:771–6. doi: 10.1016/j.jtos.2019.06.003
22. Muhafiz E, Ölçen M, Erten R, Bozkurt E. Evaluation of meibomian glands in obstructive sleep apnea-hypopnea syndrome. *Cornea.* (2020) 39:685–90. doi: 10.1097/ICO.0000000000002252
23. Wang X, Lu X, Yang J, Wei R, Yang L, Zhao S, et al. Evaluation of dry eye and meibomian gland dysfunction in teenagers with myopia through noninvasive keratograph. *J Ophthalmol.* (2016) 2016:6761206. doi: 10.1155/2016/6761206
24. Arita R, Fukuoka S, Morishige N. New insights into the lipid layer of the tear film and meibomian glands. *Eye Contact Lens.* (2017) 43:335–9. doi: 10.1097/ICL.0000000000000369
25. Vigo L, Pellegrini M, Bernabei F, Carones F, Scorcia V, Giannaccare G. Diagnostic performance of a novel noninvasive workup in the setting of dry eye disease. *J Ophthalmol.* (2020) 2020:5804123. doi: 10.1155/2020/5804123
26. Wolffsohn J, Arita R, Chalmers R, Djalilian A, Dogru M, Dumbleton K, et al. TFOS DEWS II diagnostic methodology report. *Ocul Surf.* (2017) 15:539–74. doi: 10.1016/j.jtos.2017.05.001
27. Johnson M, Murphy P. The effect of instilled fluorescein solution volume on the values and repeatability of TBUT measurements. *Cornea.* (2005) 24:811–7. doi: 10.1097/01.ico.0000154378.67495.40
28. Mooi J, Wang M, Lim J, Müller A, Craig J. Minimising instilled volume reduces the impact of fluorescein on clinical measurements of tear film stability. *Cont Lens Anterior Eye.* (2017) 40:170–4. doi: 10.1016/j.clae.2017.01.004
29. Tian L, Qu J, Zhang X, Sun X. Repeatability and reproducibility of noninvasive keratograph 5M measurements in patients with dry eye disease. *J Ophthalmol.* (2016) 2016:8013621. doi: 10.1155/2016/8013621
30. Hong J, Sun X, Wei A, Cui X, Li Y, Qian T, et al. Assessment of tear film stability in dry eye with a newly developed keratograph. *Cornea.* (2013) 32:716–21. doi: 10.1097/ICO.0b013e3182714425
31. Wang M, Craig J. Comparative evaluation of clinical methods of tear film stability assessment: a randomized crossover trial. *JAMA Ophthalmol.* (2018) 136:291–4. doi: 10.1001/jamaophthalmol.2017.6489
32. Goldberg R. Treatment of obstructive sleep apnea, other than with continuous positive airway pressure. *Curr Opin Pulm Med.* (2000) 6:496–500. doi: 10.1097/00063198-200011000-00006
33. Sullivan C, Issa F, Berthon-Jones M, Eves L. Reversal of obstructive sleep apnoea by continuous positive airway pressure applied through the nares. *Lancet.* (1981) 1:862–5. doi: 10.1016/S0140-6736(81)92140-1
34. Lin H, Friedman M, Chang H, Gurpinar B. The efficacy of multilevel surgery of the upper airway in adults with obstructive sleep apnea/hypopnea syndrome. *Laryngoscope.* (2008) 118:902–8. doi: 10.1097/MLG.0b013e31816422ea
35. Kadyan A, Asghar J, Dowson L, Sandramouli S. Ocular findings in sleep apnoea patients using continuous positive airway pressure. *Eye.* (2010) 24:843–50. doi: 10.1038/eye.2009.212
36. Acar M, Firat H, Yuceege M, Ardic S. Long-term effects of PAP on ocular surface in obstructive sleep apnea syndrome. *Can J Ophthalmol.* (2014) 49:217–21. doi: 10.1016/j.jcjo.2013.11.010
37. Hayirci E, Yagci A, Palamar M, Basoglu O, Veral A. The effect of continuous positive airway pressure treatment for obstructive sleep apnea syndrome on the ocular surface. *Cornea.* (2012) 31:604–8. doi: 10.1097/ICO.0b013e31824a2040
38. Harrison W, Pence N, Kovacich S. Anterior segment complications secondary to continuous positive airway pressure machine treatment in patients with obstructive sleep apnea. *Optometry.* (2007) 78:352–5. doi: 10.1016/j.optm.2006.12.015
39. Stauffer J, Fayter N, MacLurg B. Conjunctivitis from nasal CPAP apparatus. *Chest.* (1984) 86:802. doi: 10.1378/chest.86.5.802a
40. Fayers T, Simcock D, Wilkins M. Reactivation of recurrent corneal erosion syndrome by continuous positive pressure ventilation. *Cornea.* (2007) 26:1292. doi: 10.1097/ICO.0b013e31814923aa
41. Grigg-Damberger M. The AASM scoring manual four years later. *J Clin Sleep Med.* (2012) 8:323–32. doi: 10.5664/jcsm.1928
42. Li N, Wang T, Wang R, Duan X. Tear film instability and meibomian gland dysfunction correlate with the pterygium size and thickness pre- and postexcision in patients with pterygium. *J Ophthalmol.* (2019) 2019:5935239. doi: 10.1155/2019/5935239
43. Ren Y, Chen J, Zheng Q, Chen W. Short-term effect of a developed warming moist chamber goggle for video display terminal-associated dry eye. *BMC Ophthalmol.* (2018) 18:33. doi: 10.1186/s12886-018-0700-y
44. Li J, Ma J, Hu M, Yu J, Zhao Y. Assessment of tear film lipid layer thickness in patients with meibomian gland dysfunction at different ages. *BMC Ophthalmol.* (2020) 20:394. doi: 10.1186/s12886-020-01667-8
45. Zang S, Cui Y, Cui Y, Fei W. Meibomian gland dropout in Sjögren's syndrome and non-Sjögren's dry eye patients. *Eye.* (2018) 32:1681–7. doi: 10.1038/s41433-018-0149-5
46. Pérez-Bartolomé F, Sanz-Pozo C. Martínez-de la Casa J, Arriola-Villalobos P, Fernández-Pérez C, García-Feijoó J. Assessment of ocular redness measurements obtained with keratograph 5M and correlation with subjective grading scales. *J Fr Ophtalmol.* (2018) 41:836–46. doi: 10.1016/j.jfo.2018.03.007
47. Arita R, Itoh K, Maeda S, Maeda K, Tomidokoro A, Amano S. Association of contact lens-related allergic conjunctivitis with changes in the morphology of meibomian glands. *Jpn J Ophthalmol.* (2012) 56:14–9. doi: 10.1007/s10384-011-0103-6
48. Lemp M. Report of the national eye institute/industry workshop on clinical trials in dry eyes. *CLAO J.* (1995) 21:221–32.
49. Zheng B, Liu X, Sun Y, Su J, Zhao Y, Xie Z, et al. Development and validation of the Chinese version of dry eye related quality of life scale. *Health Qual Life Outcomes.* (2017) 15:145. doi: 10.1186/s12955-017-0718-5
50. Yeh T, Lin M. Meibomian gland contrast sensitivity and specificity in the diagnosis of lipid-deficient dry eye: a pilot study. *Optom Vis Sci.* (2021) 98:121–6. doi: 10.1097/OPX.0000000000001636
51. Salinas R, Puig M, Fry C, Johnson D, Kheirkhah A. Floppy eyelid syndrome: a comprehensive review. *Ocul Surf.* (2020) 18:31–9. doi: 10.1016/j.jtos.2019.10.002
52. Arita R, Itoh K, Maeda S, Maeda K, Furuta A, Fukuoka S, et al. Proposed diagnostic criteria for obstructive meibomian gland dysfunction. *Ophthalmology.* (2009) 116:2058–63.e1. doi: 10.1016/j.ophtha.2009.04.037
53. Toffoli S, Roegiers A, Feron O, Van Steenbrugge M, Ninane N, Raes M, et al. Intermittent hypoxia is an angiogenic inducer for endothelial cells: role of HIF-1. *Angiogenesis.* (2009) 12:47–67. doi: 10.1007/s10456-009-9131-y
54. Vakil M, Park S, Broder A. The complex associations between obstructive sleep apnea and auto-immune disorders: a review. *Med Hypotheses.* (2018) 110:138–43. doi: 10.1016/j.mehy.2017.12.004
55. de Lima F, Mazzotti D, Tufik S, Bittencourt L. The role inflammatory response genes in obstructive sleep apnea syndrome: a review. *Sleep Breath.* (2016) 20:331–8. doi: 10.1007/s11325-015-1226-7

56. Stern M, Gao J, Schwalb T, Ngo M, Tieu D, Chan C, et al. Conjunctival T-cell subpopulations in Sjögren's and non-Sjögren's patients with dry eye. *Invest Ophthalmol Vis Sci.* (2002) 43:2609–14.
57. Muniesa M, Huerva V. Sánchez-de-la-Torre M, Martínez M, Jurjo C, Barbé F. The relationship between floppy eyelid syndrome and obstructive sleep apnoea. *Br J Ophthalmol.* (2013) 97:1387–90. doi: 10.1136/bjophthalmol-2012-303051
58. Molina F, Suman M, Carvalho T, Piatto V, Taboga S, Maniglia J, et al. Evaluation of testosterone serum levels in patients with obstructive sleep apnea syndrome. *Braz J Otorhinolaryngol.* (2011) 77:88–95. doi: 10.1590/S1808-86942011000100015
59. Krenzer K, Dana M, Ullman M, Cermak J, Tolls D, Evans J, et al. Effect of androgen deficiency on the human meibomian gland and ocular surface. *J Clin Endocrinol Metab.* (2000) 85:4874–82. doi: 10.1210/jc.85.12.4874
60. Pult H, Riede-Pult B, Nichols J. Relation between upper and lower lids' meibomian gland morphology, tear film, and dry eye. *Optom Vis Sci.* (2012) 89:E310–5. doi: 10.1097/OPX.0b013e318244e487
61. Eom Y, Choi K, Kang S, Lee H, Kim H, Song J. Comparison of meibomian gland loss and expressed meibum grade between the upper and lower eyelids in patients with obstructive meibomian gland dysfunction. *Cornea.* (2014) 33:448–52. doi: 10.1097/ICO.0000000000000092
62. Netland P, Sugrue S, Albert D, Shore J. Histopathologic features of the floppy eyelid syndrome. *Involv Tarsal Elastin Ophthalmol.* (1994) 101:174–81. doi: 10.1016/S0161-6420(94)31368-6
63. Ezra D, Beaconsfield M, Sira M, Bunce C, Wormald R, Collin R. The associations of floppy eyelid syndrome: a case control study. *Ophthalmology.* (2010) 117:831–8. doi: 10.1016/j.ophtha.2009.09.029
64. Rolando M, Zierhut M. The ocular surface and tear film and their dysfunction in dry eye disease. *Surv Ophthalmol.* (2001) 45(Suppl. 2):S203–10. doi: 10.1016/S0039-6257(00)00203-4
65. Bron A, de Paiva C, Chauhan S, Bonini S, Gabison E, Jain S, et al. TFOS DEWS II pathophysiology report. *Ocul Surf.* (2017) 15:438–510. doi: 10.1016/j.jtos.2017.05.011
66. Lan W, Lin L, Yang X, Yu M. Automatic noninvasive tear breakup time (TBUT) and conventional fluorescent TBUT. *Optom Vis Sci.* (2014) 91:1412–8. doi: 10.1097/OPX.0000000000000418
67. Sutphin J, Ying G, Bunya V, Yu Y, Lin M, McWilliams K, et al. Correlation of measures from the OCULUS keratograph and clinical assessments of dry eye disease in the dry eye assessment and management study. *Cornea.* (2021). doi: 10.1097/ICO.0000000000002804 [Epub ahead of print].
68. Liu A, Cardell J, Ariel D, Lamendola C, Abbasi F, Kim S, et al. Abnormalities of lipoprotein concentrations in obstructive sleep apnea are related to insulin resistance. *Sleep.* (2015) 38:793–9. doi: 10.5665/sleep.4678
69. Adedayo A, Olafiranye O, Smith D, Hill A, Zizi F, Brown C, et al. Obstructive sleep apnea and dyslipidemia: evidence and underlying mechanism. *Sleep Breath.* (2014) 18:13–8. doi: 10.1007/s11325-012-0760-9
70. Butovich I. The Meibomian puzzle: combining pieces together. *Prog Retin Eye Res.* (2009) 28:483–98. doi: 10.1016/j.preteyeres.2009.07.002
71. Kuriakose R, Braich P. Dyslipidemia and its association with meibomian gland dysfunction: a systematic review. *Int Ophthalmol.* (2018) 38:1809–16. doi: 10.1007/s10792-017-0633-0
72. Guliani B, Bhalla A, Naik M. Association of the severity of meibomian gland dysfunction with dyslipidemia in Indian population. *Indian J Ophthalmol.* (2018) 66:1411–6. doi: 10.4103/ijo.IJO_1256_17
73. Butovich I, Millar T, Ham B. Understanding and analyzing meibomian lipids–a review. *Curr Eye Res.* (2008) 33:405–20. doi: 10.1080/02713680802018419
74. Pépin J, Woehrle H, Liu D, Shao S, Armitstead J, Cistulli P, et al. Adherence to positive airway therapy after switching from CPAP to ASV: a big data analysis. *J Clin Sleep Med.* (2018) 14:57–63. doi: 10.5664/jcsm.6880
75. Inoue A, Chiba S, Matsuura K, Osafune H, Capasso R, Wada K. Nasal function and CPAP compliance. *Auris Nasus Larynx.* (2019) 46:548–58. doi: 10.1016/j.anl.2018.11.006

4

The Association Between Sleep Disorders and Incidence of Dry Eye Disease in Ningbo: Data from an Integrated Health Care Network

Qinxiang Zheng [1,2†], Saiqing Li [2†], Feng Wen [1†], Zhong Lin [2], Kemi Feng [2], Yexiang Sun [3], Jie Bao [2], Hongfei Weng [1], Peng Shen [3], Hongbo Lin [3*] and Wei Chen [1,2*]*

[1] The Affiliated Ningbo Eye Hospital of Wenzhou Medical University, Ningbo, China, [2] Eye Hospital and School of Ophthalmology and Optometry, Wenzhou Medical University, Wenzhou, China, [3] Department of Chronic Diseases and Health Promotion, Yinzhou District Center for Disease Control and Prevention, Ningbo, China

***Correspondence:**
Peng Shen
shen-peng@foxmail.com
Hongbo Lin
lin673160@163.com
Wei Chen
chenweimd@wmu.edu.cn

†These authors have contributed equally to the study

Purpose: To investigate the association between sleep disorders and dry eye disease (DED) in Ningbo, China.

Methods: Our data came from the Yinzhou Health Information System (HIS), including 257932 patients and was based on a 1:1 matching method (sleep disorder patients vs. patients without sleep disorders) during 2013–2020. Sleep disorders and DED were identified using ICD-10 codes. Cox proportional hazards regression was used to identify the association between sleep disorders and DED.

Results: The eight-year incidence of DED was significantly higher in participants with diagnosis of sleep disorders (sleep disorders: 50.66%, no sleep disorders: 16.48%, $P< 0.01$). Sleep disorders were positively associated with the diagnosis of DED (HR: 3.06, 95% CI: 2.99–3.13, $P < 0.01$), when sex, age, hypertension, diabetes and other systemic diseases were adjusted. In the sleep disorders patients, advancing age, female sex, and presence of coexisting disease (hypertension, diabetes, hyperlipidemia, thyroid disease, depression, heart disease, and arthritis) were significantly associated with the development of DED by the multivariate cox regression analysis (all $P < 0.05$).In addition, there was a significantly positive association between estazolam and the incidence of DED in both sleep disorder and non-sleep disorder groups (all $P < 0.05$).

Conclusions : Sleep disrder was associated with a three-time increased risk of DED. This association can be helpful in effective management of both sleep disorders and DED.

Keywords: sleep disorders, dry eye disease, risk factor, sleep medicine, coexisting disease

INTRODUCTION

Sleep disorder, defined as an abnormality in sleep quality or quantity, has become a major social health concern throughout the world (1–3). Sleep quality and duration of sleep are important for physical and mental health, and sleep dysfunction damages autonomic nerve and endocrine function, leading to extensive changes in many aspects of the body system (3). Numerous evidence show that sleep disorders increase the risk of obesity, hypertension, diabetes, dementia, and cardiovascular disease (4–9).

Dry eye disease (DED) is a multifactorial disease of the ocular surface characterized by a loss of tear film homeostasis, causing tear film instability and hyperosmolarity, as well as ocular surface inflammation and damage, and neurosensory abnormalities play etiological roles (10). The incidence of DED was estimated to range from 5 to 50% worldwide (11). DED causes a variety of ocular surface discomfort (such as pain, foreign body sensation, irritation, and photophobia) and visual dysfunction, which not only impedes daily activities, but also exerts psychological impacts (12–14).

Previous studies have found that aging, female sex, systemic diseases (hypertension, diabetes, thyroid disease, anxiety, depression, and so on) are associated with DED development (11, 12, 15, 16). The association between DED and sleep disorders has recently attracted attention (11, 17, 18). It was found that DED patients sleep poorly, and patients with sleep disorders are more likely to have DED (17, 19–28). Some studies were conducted in community populations or cohort populations by collecting questionnaires on sleep and dry eye symptoms (19, 20, 26, 27), however these studies may have drawbacks of selection bias and recall bias. There are also studies suggesting that sedative antidepressants would promote dry eye symptoms and signs (17, 29–31). In the current study, we would like to compare the incidence of DED that developed in participants with or without sleep disorders, using the integrated health care network system data, and evaluate whether sleep disorders was a risk factor for DED.

MATERIALS AND METHODS

Study Population

Yinzhou District, located in the Yangtze River Delta, is one of the core areas of Ningbo. According to the statistical yearbook of Yinzhou District, by the end of 2018, there were 1.34 million permanent residents in Yinzhou District. Data on hospital visits were obtained from the Yinzhou Health Information System (YHIS), which seamlessly links the health information archives, chronic disease registration system, resident death registration system and hospital outpatient system of permanent residents in Yinzhou District, and can provide real-time treatment information of patients in 2 general hospitals, 3 specialized hospitals, 24 community health service centers and 248 community service stations in the whole district. The health information of each resident living in Yinzhou is integrated into YHIS. Detailed information about this system has been described in the previous research (32).

Medical information was classified according to the ICD-10 (International Classification of Diseases, 10th Revision). In this study, we first excluded all patients who were deceased, we selected hospital visits for sleep disorders (ICD-10: G47) and DED (ICD-10: H04.103, H11.104, H16.202 and H18.803) during 2013–2020. We excluded patients diagnosed with DED before sleep disorders. Finally, we identified 128,966 patients with sleep disorders between 2013 and 2020. To design the matched cohort study using the sleep disorder patients as the case group, we established the control group by propensity score matching by adjusting for same sex, same age range and same date of diagnosis for sleep disorders. We used a 1:1 matching method to select the control group (128,966 patients) who were not diagnosed with sleep disorders. Finally, the data used in this study included 257,932 patients from 2013 to 2020.

Variables

The outcome variable of this study is whether DED will occur after patients were diagnosed with sleep disorders. If

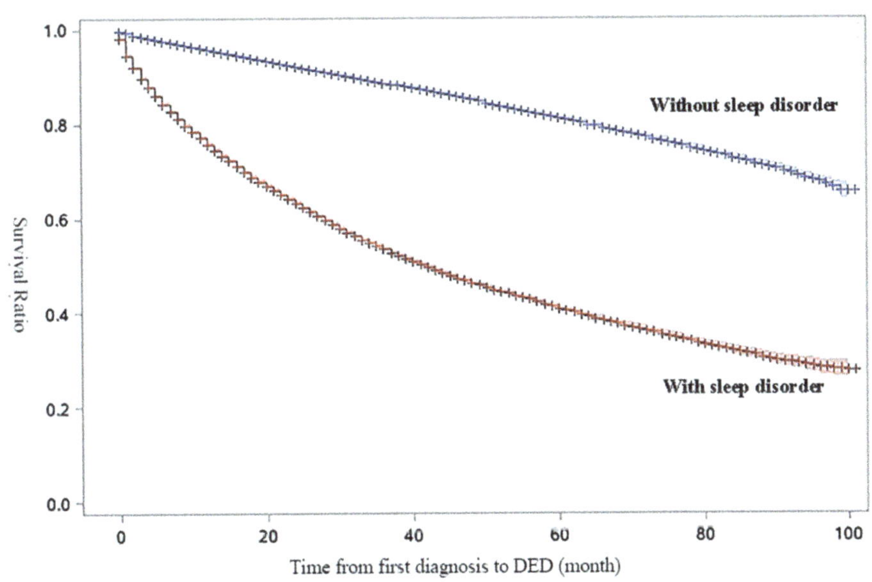

FIGURE 1 | Survival curve for survival-ratio of dry eye disease (DED). The results of log-rank test for time to DED by diagnosis of sleep disorders were statistically significant (HR: 3.81, 95%CI:3.75–3.87, $P < 0.01$).

diagnosis of DED (ICD-10: H04.103, H11.104, H16.202, and H18.803), it was defined as DED diagnosis, and classified the patient as the DED diagnosis group. In this study, sleep disorders were defined as organic sleep disorders (ICD-10: G47), including insomnia, hypersomnia, narcolepsy/cataplexy, sleep apnea, disorders of the sleep-wake schedule and other sleep disorders. In the study, we included the following independent variables: gender, age, medical history (hypertension, diabetes, thyroid disease, anxiety, depression, heart disease, and arthritis), and medication history of sleep disorders. The ages were classified at 10-year intervals: under 29 years, 30–39 years, 40–49 years, 50–59 years, 60–69 years, over 70 years. At present, the clinical drugs for insomnia mainly include benzodiazepine receptor agonists (BZRAs), melatonin receptor agonists, orexin receptor antagonists, antidepressants and etc. (33, 34). We studied the using condition of sleep medicine in patients with sleep disorders, excluding the drugs mentioned in the guide but not found in the YHIS. Finally, we mainly included BZRAs (estazolam, diazepam, alprazolam, lorazepam), antidepressants (trazodone, mirtazapine, doxepin), and other sedatives (gabapentin, olanzapine).

Statistical Analysis

In order to study the relationship between DED and sleep disorders, we first determined the frequency and percentage of people with DED diagnosis. Next, we performed a log rank test and generated a survival curve to compare the diagnostic rate of DED between patients with and without sleep disorders. Finally, we performed survival analysis using the univariate cox regression analysis, and then variables with $P < 0.20$ in univariate regression analysis were included in multivariate cox regression analysis to determine the association between sleep disorders and DED, and studied the association of other independent variables with DED. All statistical analyses were performed using SAS statistical software version 9.2 (SAS company, Cary, North Carolina, USA). A $P < 0.05$ was considered to be statistically significant.

RESULTS

Using the 1:1 propensity score matching method (patients with sleep disorder vs. patients without sleep disorders), we analyzed 257,932 patients with or without sleep disorders between 2013 and 2020. **Supplemental Table 1** shows the distribution of the study population for each variable and the 8-year incidence of DED among different variable subgroups. The 8-year incidence of DED was 50.66 and 16.48% in participants with and without sleep disorders, respectively. About 33.57% of patients in our study were diagnosed with DED over 8 years, and incidence

TABLE 1 | Results of survival analysis using Cox regression analysis for association between sleep disorders and dry eye disease (DED) in the study population (n = 257,932).

Variables	Model 1		Model 2		Model 3	
	HR (95%CI)	*P*	HR (95%CI)	*P*	HR (95%CI)	*P*
Sleep disorder	3.81 (3.75, 3.87)	<0.01	3.28 (3.23, 3.34)	<0.01	3.06 (2.99, 3.13)	<0.01
Sex						
Male	1.00 (-)	-	-	-	1.00 (-)	-
Female	1.20 (1.17, 1.23)	<0.01	-	-	1.25 (1.22, 1.29)	<0.01
Age (years)						
<30	1.0 (-)	-	-	-	1.0 (-)	-
30–39	1.86 (1.71, 2.04)	<0.01	-	-	1.94 (1.77, 2.12)	<0.01
40–49	2.00 (1.88, 2.13)	<0.01	-	-	2.04 (1.92, 2.18)	<0.01
50–59	1.71 (1.62, 1.82)	<0.01	-	-	1.73 (1.63, 1.84)	<0.01
60–69	1.44 (1.36, 1.53)	<0.01	-	-	1.46 (1.38, 1.55)	<0.01
≥70	1.18 (1.11, 1.26)	<0.01	-	-	1.18 (1.11, 1.26)	<0.01
Medical history						
Hypertension	1.12 (1.17, 1.23)	<0.01	1.04 (0.98, 1.10)	0.21	1.02 (0.96, 1.08)	0.51
Diabetes	1.07 (0.98, 1.16)	0.12	0.96 (0.88, 1.04)	0.33	0.95 (0.87, 1.03)	0.19
Hyperlipidemia	1.22 (1.12, 1.34)	<0.01	1.10 (1.01, 1.20)	0.04	1.09 (0.99, 1.19)	0.07
Thyroid disease	0.91 (0.70, 1.17)	0.44	0.85 (0.66, 1.10)	0.21	-	-
Anxiety	1.13 (0.76, 1.69)	0.54	0.98 (0.65, 1.46)	0.90	-	-
Depression	1.19 (0.91, 1.56)	0.19	1.15 (0.88, 1.50)	0.31	1.14 (0.87, 1.50)	0.33
Heart disease	1.38 (1.22, 1.56)	<0.01	1.20 (1.07, 1.36)	<0.01	1.18 (1.05, 1.34)	<0.01
Arthritis	1.39 (1.01,1.93)	0.04	1.23 (0.89, 1.70)	0.21	1.23 (0.89, 1.70)	0.21

HR, Hazard ratio; CI, Confidence interval.
Model 1: Univariate cox regression analysis, and no variables were adjusted.
Model 2: Sex and age were adjusted.
Model 3: Variables with P < 0.20 in univariate cox regression analysis were included for multivariate cox regression analysis.

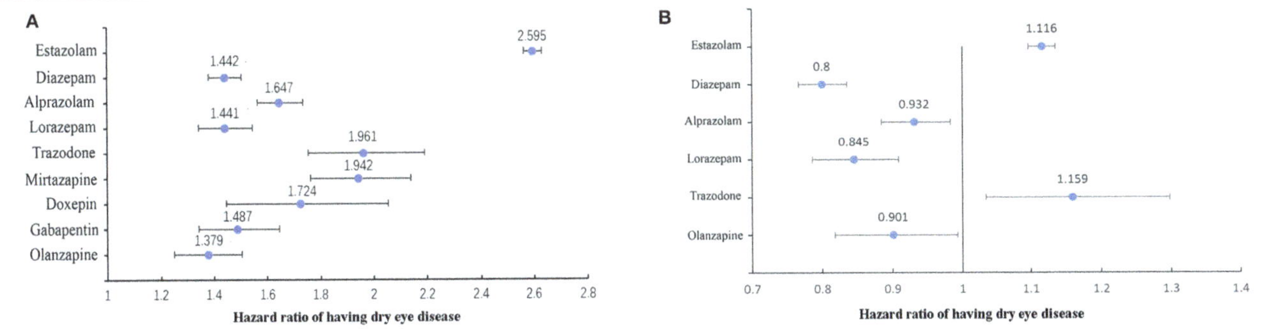

FIGURE 2 | The association between sleep medicine and DED in general population ($n = 257{,}932$). **(A)** Results of univariate cox regression analysis, all drugs in the figure were statistically significant ($P < 0.01$). **(B)** Results of multivariate cox regression analysis, all drugs in the figure were statistically significant ($P < 0.05$).

TABLE 2 | The distribution of the sleep disorders population ($n = 128{,}966$) for each sleep medicine.

Medicine	Total		DED		P-value
	N	%	*N*	%	
Estazolam					<0.01
Yes	81,539	63.23	44,116	54.10	
No	47,427	36.77	21,222	44.75	
Diazepam					<0.01
Yes	3,626	2.81	2,188	60.34	
No	125,340	97.19	63,150	50.38	
Alprazolam					<0.01
Yes	2,346	1.82	1,429	60.91	
No	126,620	98.18	63,909	50.47	
Lorazepam					<0.01
Yes	1,288	1.00	775	60.17	
No	127,678	99.00	64,563	50.57	
Trazodone					<0.01
Yes	505	0.39	311	61.58	
No	128,461	99.61	65,027	50.62	
Mirtazapine					<0.01
Yes	616	0.48	402	65.26	
No	128,350	99.52	64,936	50.59	
Doxepin					<0.01
Yes	174	0.13	124	71.26	
No	128,792	99.87	65,214	50.64	
Gabapentin					<0.01
Yes	502	0.39	293	58.37	
No	128,464	99.61	65,045	50.63	
Olanzapine					<0.01
Yes	754	0.58	429	56.90	
No	128,212	99.42	64,909	50.63	

The proportion of DED for different sleep medicine in sleep disorders population ($n = 128{,}966$).
DED, Dry eye disease.
**Chi square test was used to compare the incidence of DED with the use of individual drug.*

was higher in patients with sleep disorders (with sleep disorders: 50.66%, without sleep disorders: 16.48%).

Figure 1 shows the survival curve to compare the survival rate of DED in patients with sleep disorders and without sleep disorders during the study period. In the survival curve, patients with sleep disorders were more likely to be diagnosed with DED than patients without sleep disorders ($P < 0.05$ for log rank test).

Table 1 shows the results of survival analysis using the Cox proportional hazard model to determine the association between DED and sleep disorders after adjusting other independent variables. Univariate regression analysis showed that sleep disorders, age, gender and coexisting systemic diseases (hypertension, hyperlipidemia, heart disease, and arthritis) were significantly associated with the development of DED (all $P < 0.05$). Then we included variables with $P < 0.20$ from the model 1 for multivariate cox regression analysis. By the multivariate regression analysis, sleep disorders were positively associated with the diagnosis of DED (HR: 3.06, 95% CI: 2.99–3.13, $P < 0.01$), with a three-time increased risk. Among the independent variables, the risk of diagnosing DED was higher in women than in men (HR: 1.25, 95% CI: 1. 22–1.29, $P < 0.01$). Compared with young people who were <30 years, increased age was associated with DED diagnosis ($P < 0.01$), and the risk was the highest in the population aged 40–49 years (HR: 2.04, 95% CI: 1.92–2.18, $P < 0.01$). In addition, only heart disease was positively associated with the diagnosis of DED ($P < 0.01$). At the same time, other coexisting systematic diseases did not have significant association with the diagnosis of DED ($P > 0.05$).

Next, we analyzed the effect of sleep drugs on DED in the general population. **Figure 2A** shows the results of univariate cox regression analysis, all sleep medicine increase the risk of DED (all $P < 0.01$). The sleep medicine with statistical significance ($P < 0.05$) in multivariate cox regression analysis are shown in **Figure 2B**. It can be seen that estazolam and trazodone were positively associated with the DED.

Additionally, we analyzed the using condition of sleep medicine and its association with DED in sleep disorders

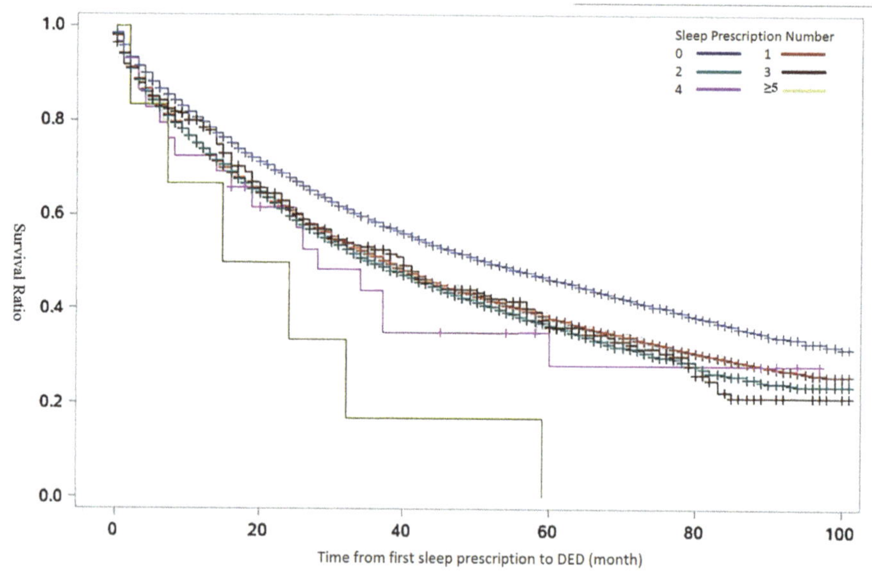

FIGURE 3 | Kaplan-Meier curves for survival-ratio of dry eye disease (DED) over time by the number of sleep prescriptions. The results of log-rank test for time to DED by sleep prescriptions number were statistically significant ($P < 0.01$). The number of sleep prescription refers to the cumulative number of sleep drugs used by the patient.

patients. **Table 2** shows the distribution of the sleep disorders population for each sleep medicine with the Chi square test. The number of cases in **Table 2** refers to the person who uses this sleep drug, regardless of whether they use other type sleep drugs or not. Among the sleep disorders, the frequency of estazolam was 63.23%, which was most common in the patients. Compared with patients not using sleep medicine, the incidence of DED significantly increased in the sleep medicine using group (all $P < 0.01$). **Figure 3** shows that the incidence of DED over time raised with the increasing of the sleep prescription number used in the sleep disorders.

Similarly, we performed Cox proportional hazard model in the sleep disorder group to determine the relationship between the independent variable and DED. The results of regression analysis are presented in the **Table 3**. In the model 3 (variables with $P < 0.20$ in univariate cox analysis were included for multivariate cox analysis), the variables of female and 30–39 years significantly increased the DED diagnosis ($P < 0.01$) in the sleep disorders patients. However, the results comparing anxiety with DED were not statistically significant ($P = 0.08$). As is shown in **Table 3**, the estazolam and trazodone were positively associated with the DED ($P < 0.05$). Contrarily, diazepam and lorazepam showed negative correlation with DED ($P < 0.05$).

In the same way, we analyzed the relationship between the independent variable and DED in the patients without sleep disorder by performing Cox proportional hazard model. The results of regression analysis are presented in the **Table 4**. We can see the variables of female and 40–49 years significantly increased the DED diagnosis ($P < 0.01$) when using multivariate cox analysis. Among the coexisting systemic diseases, only heart disease was significantly correlated with the incidence of DED ($P = 0.01$). **Table 4** showed the estazolam, diazepam and gabapentin were all positively associated with the DED ($P < 0.05$).

DISCUSSION

In the current study, we found that sleep disorder is a risk factor of DED, with a three-time increased risk to the subjects without sleep disorders. Besides, the use of estazolam increased the risk of DED regardless of the presence of sleep disorder.

In our study, the 8-year incidence of DED in the study population was 33.57%. Many previous population-based studies have indicated a correlation between sleep disorders and DED (19, 20, 24–27, 35). Han et.al reported that sleep disorders were related to dry eye incidence rate (HR:1.32), and sleep had a greater impact on DED in male and young patients (36). In a nationally population-based survey in Korea, people with sleep duration shorter than 5 h were found to be 20% more likely to suffer from DED, compared to those with more than 6 h of sleep (35).Hanyuda et al. also showed that sleep deprivation and poor sleep quality were significantly related to DED in a Japanese population (26). Additionally, two large studies conducted in Hangzhou and Singapore also revealed that poor sleep quality and short sleep time were significantly correlated with DED (19, 20). Our results are similar with the above studies, compared with patients without sleep disorders, patients with sleep disorders have a higher risk of DED (HR:3.06).

The association between sleep disorders and DED are based on physiological findings. Sleep disorders are often related to autonomic nerve dysfunction, which could affect

TABLE 3 | Results of survival analysis using Cox proportional hazard model for association between independent variables and dry eye disease (DED) in the sleep disorder patients (n = 128,966).

Variables	Model 1		Model 2		Model 3	
	HR (95%CI)	*P*	HR (95%CI)	*P*	HR (95%CI)	*P*
Sex						
Male	1.00 (-)	-	-	-	1.00 (-)	-
Female	1.14 (1.12, 1.16)	<0.01	-	-	1.15 (1.13, 1.17)	<0.01
Age (years)						
<30	1.00 (-)	-	-	-	1.00 (-)	-
30–39	1.84 (1.74, 1.95)	<0.01	-	-	1.70 (1.60, 1.81)	<0.01
40–49	1.80 (1.70, 1.90)	<0.01	-	-	1.67 (1.57, 1.77)	<0.01
50–59	1.51 (1.42, 1.60)	<0.01	-	-	1.42 (1.33, 1.50)	<0.01
60–69	1.32 (1.25, 1.40)	<0.01	-	-	1.28 (1.21, 1.36)	<0.01
≥70	1.23 (1.15, 1.31)	<0.01	-	-	1.20 (1.13, 1.28)	<0.01
Medical history						
Hypertension	1.10 (1.08, 1.12)	<0.01	0.94 (0.93, 0.96)	<0.01	0.87 (0.86, 0.89)	<0.01
Diabetes	1.07 (1.05, 1.09)	<0.01	0.99 (0.97, 1.01)	0.32	0.97 (0.95, 0.99)	<0.01
Hyperlipidemia	1.22 (1.20, 1.24)	<0.01	1.13 (1.11, 1.15)	<0.01	1.11 (1.09, 1.13)	<0.01
Thyroid disease	1.10 (1.04, 1.17)	<0.01	1.12 (1.05, 1.19)	<0.01	1.10 (1.04, 1.17)	<0.01
Anxiety	1.09 (1.08, 1.11)	<0.01	1.04 (1.02, 1.06)	<0.01	0.98 (0.96, 1.00)	0.08
Depression	1.18 (1.15, 1.20)	<0.01	1.15 (1.13, 1.18)	<0.01	1.13 (1.10, 1.16)	<0.01
Heart disease	1.27 (1.25, 1.29)	<0.01	1.16 (1.15, 1.18)	<0.01	1.15 (1.13, 1.17)	<0.01
Arthritis	1.18 (1.14, 1.23)	<0.01	1.15 (1.10, 1.20)	<0.01	1.12 (1.08, 1.17)	<0.01
Sleep medicines						
Estazolam	1.21 (1.19, 1.23)	<0.01	1.12 (1.10, 1.20)	<0.01	1.12 (1.10, 1.14)	<0.01
Diazepam	0.87 (0.83, 0.90)	<0.01	0.84 (0.81,0.88)	<0.01	0.80 (0.77, 0.83)	<0.01
Alprazolam	1.01 (0.96, 1.06)	0.80	0.98 (0.93, 1.03)	0.36	-	-
Lorazepam	0.94 (0.87, 1.00)	0.06	0.92 (0.85, 0.98)	<0.01	0.83 (0.78, 0.90)	<0.01
Trazodone	1.26 (1.12, 1.40)	<0.01	1.25 (1.11, 1.40)	<0.01	1.15 (1.03, 1.29)	0.02
Mirtazapine	1.20 (1.09, 1.33)	<0.01	1.18 (1.06, 1.30)	<0.01	1.09 (0.99, 1.21)	0.09
Doxepin	1.04 (0.87, 1.24)	0.65	0.96 (0.80, 1.15)	0.66	-	-
Gabapentin	1.12 (1.05, 1.30)	0.27	1.09 (0.97, 1.22)	0.12	-	-
Olanzapine	0.98 (0.89, 1.08)	0.72	0.96 (0.88, 1.06)	0.44	-	-

HR, Hazard ratio; CI, Confidence interval.
Model 1: Univariate cox regression analysis, and no variables were adjusted.
Model 2: Sex and age adjusted.
Model 3: Variables with P < 0.20 in univariate cox analysis were included for multivariate cox analysis.

the parasympathetic fibers in the lacrimal gland, resulting in reduced tear secretion (37, 38). Sleep deprivation may also inhibit peroxisome proliferator-activated receptor alpha (PPARα) signaling which increase oxidative stress leading to DED (39). In addition, the activation of the hypothalamic–pituitary–adrenal axis during sleep may lead to a relatively dehydrated state, thereby reducing tear secretion (40, 41).

Our results also found that use of sleep medications in the sleep disorders was significantly associated with DED. Kawashima et al. have demonstrated that sedative antidepressants could significantly decreased tear break-up time of DED patients (29). Antidepressants could promote dry eye symptoms through anticholinergic side effects (inhibition of cholinergic nerve fibers in meibomian and lacrimal glands) or other potential pharmacological mechanisms to reduce tear secretion (17, 30). Using the multivariate cox regression analysis, we found that there was a significantly positive association between estazolam and the incidence of DED in both sleep disorder and non-sleep disorder participants. Estazolam, a kind of benzodiazepine drugs (BZDs), can non selectively activate different γ subunits on γ-aminobutyric acid receptor A and has pharmacological effects of sedation, hypnosis, antianxiety, muscle relaxation and anti-convulsion (42). Estazolam has side effects of anticholinergic activity (43), which reduces the secretion of tears, resulting in DED. In the present study, the ratio of estazolam use amounts to 63.23% in the subjects with sleep disorders, while the ratio of other sleep medicine were below 3%, which may limit the power of detection small effect. Therefore, the association between other sleep medicines and dry eye needs to be evaluated in a larger study with sufficient sleep medication users.

TABLE 4 | Results of survival analysis using Cox proportional hazard model for association between independent variables and dry eye disease (DED) in the patients without sleep disorder (n = 128,966).

Variables	Model 1		Model 2		Model 3	
	HR (95%CI)	*P*	HR (95%CI)	*P*	HR (95%CI)	*P*
Sex						
Male	1.00 (-)	-	-	-	1.00 (-)	-
Female	1.20 (1.17, 1.23)	<0.01	-	-	1.25 (1.22, 1.29)	<0.01
Age (years)						
<30	1.00 (-)	-	-	-	1.00 (-)	-
30–39	1.86 (1.71, 2.04)	<0.01	-	-	1.92 (1.75, 2.10)	<0.01
40–49	2.00 (1.88, 2,13)	<0.01	-	-	2.03 (1.90, 2.16)	<0.01
50–59	1.71 (1.62, 1.82)	<0.01	-	-	1.72 (1.62, 1.83)	<0.01
60–69	1.44 (1.36, 1.53)	<0.01	-	-	1.46 (1.38, 1.54)	<0.01
≥70	1.18 (1.11, 1.26)	<0.01	-	-	1.18 (1.11, 1.26)	<0.01
Medical history						
Hypertension	1.13 (1.07, 1.20)	<0.01	1.04 (0.98, 1.10)	0.21	1.02 (0.96, 1.08)	0.58
Diabetes	1.07 (0.98, 1.16)	0.12	0.96 (0.88, 1.04)	0.33	0.95 (0.87, 1.03)	0.18
Hyperlipidemia	1.22 (1.12, 1.34)	<0.01	1.10 (1.01, 1.20)	0.04	1.09 (1.00, 1.20)	0.06
Thyroid disease	0.91 (0.70, 1.17)	0.44	0.85 (0.66, 1.10)	0.21	-	-
Anxiety	1.13 (0.76, 1.69)	0.54	0.98 (0.65, 1.46)	0.90	-	-
Depression	1.19 (0.91, 1.56)	0.19	1.15 (0.88, 1.50)	0.31	1.11 (0.85, 1.45)	0.45
Heart disease	1.38 (1.22, 1.56)	<0.01	1.20 (1.07, 1.36)	<0.01	1.17 (1.04, 1.33)	0.01
Arthritis	1.39 (1.01, 1.93)	0.04	1.23 (0.89, 1.70)	0.21	1.21 (0.88, 1.67)	0.25
Sleep medicines						
Estazolam	1.59 (1.43, 1.77)	<0.01	1.44 (1.29, 1.60)	<0.01	1.42 (1.27, 1.59)	<0.01
Diazepam	2.01 (1.49, 2.72)	<0.01	1.76 (1.30, 2.38)	<0.01	1.69 (1.24, 2.28)	<0.01
Alprazolam	0.82 (0.44, 1.53)	0.54	0.74 (0.40, 1.38)	0.34	-	-
Lorazepam	1.14 (0.82, 1.58)	0.44	1.01 (0.73, 1.41)	0.95	-	-
Trazodone	0.83 (0.35, 1.99)	0.68	0.82 (0.34, 1.97)	0.66	-	-
Mirtazapine	1.11 (0.46, 2.66)	0.82	1.25 (0.52, 2.99)	0.62	-	-
Doxepin	2.31 (0.33, 16.33)	0.40	1.85 (0.26, 13.08)	0.54	-	-
Gabapentin	1.75 (1.41, 2.17)	<0.01	1.51 (1.22, 1.88)	<0.01	1.51 (1.22,1.88)	<0.01
Olanzapine	0.78 (0.53, 1.14)	0.20	0.75 (0.51, 1.10)	0.14	-	-

HR, Hazard ratio; CI, Confidence interval.
Model 1: Univariate cox regression analysis, and no variables were adjusted.
Model 2: Sex and age adjusted.
Model 3: Variables with P < 0.20 in univariate cox analysis were included for multivariate cox analysis.

The advantage of current study lies in the large sample size based on data from an integrated health care network covering a whole district in southeast China. Most of the previous studies used questionnaires (19, 20, 26, 27), which would cause recall bias. Our data from the medical information system can avoid such bias. The Cox proportional hazards model used in the current study is a reliable method to analyze the incidence of dry eye in sleep disorders patients, since it took the impact of time into consideration, which is different from the previous cross-sectional population studies (19, 20, 26, 27). Besides, the paired cohort design using propensity score matching (1:1) increased the reliability of our study. However, limitations are unavoidable, and the main one is the diagnosis of DED and sleep disorder may not be in consistency among the hospitals and community health centers during the 8-year period. However, the paired cohort design made up for this drawback to a certain degree.

In conclusion, our findings suggest that sleep disorders is a potential risk factor for DED and the use of sleep medicines might be associated with dry eye development. Patients with sleep disorders or those using sleep medicines should be monitored for development of dry eye.

ETHICS STATEMENT

The studies involving human participants were reviewed and approved by Institutional Review Board of the affiliated Ningbo Eye Hospital of Wenzhou Medical University. Written informed consent for participation was not required for this study in accordance with the national legislation and the institutional requirements.

AUTHOR CONTRIBUTIONS

QZ designed the study. SL, FW, ZL, and KF analyzed the data. YS and JB checked the data. QZ and SL wrote the manuscript. HW revised the manuscript. PS, HL, and WC instructed the whole study and revised the manuscript. All authors contributed to the article and approved the submitted version.

REFERENCES

1. Kerkhof GA. Epidemiology of sleep and sleep disorders in The Netherlands. *Sleep Med.* (2017) 30:229–39. doi: 10.1016/j.sleep.2016.09.015
2. Govindarajan A, Urbach DR, Kumar M, Li Q, Murray BJ, Juurlink D, et al. Outcomes of daytime procedures performed by attending surgeons after night work. *N Engl J Med.* (2015) 373:845–53. doi: 10.1056/NEJMsa1415994
3. Altevogt BM CH. Sleep disorders and sleep deprivation: An unmet public health problem. *J Am Acad Child Adolescent Psychiatry.* (2008) 47:473–4. doi: 10.1097/01.CHI.0000270812.55636.3b
4. Sabia S, Fayosse A, Dumurgier J, van Hees VT, Paquet C, Sommerlad A, et al. Association of sleep duration in middle and old age with incidence of dementia. *Nat Commun.* (2021) 12:2289. doi: 10.1038/s41467-021-22354-2
5. Shahrbabaki SS, Linz D, Hartmann S, Redline S, Baumert M. Sleep arousal burden is associated with long-term all-cause and cardiovascular mortality in 8001 community-dwelling older men and women. *Eur Heart J.* (2021) 42:2088–99. doi: 10.1093/eurheartj/ehab151
6. Vorona RD, Winn MP, Babineau TW, Eng BP, Feldman HR, Ware JC. Overweight and obese patients in a primary care population report less sleep than patients with a normal body mass index. *Arch Intern Med.* (2005) 165:25–30. doi: 10.1001/archinte.165.1.25
7. Meng L, Zheng Y, Hui R. The relationship of sleep duration and insomnia to risk of hypertension incidence: a meta-analysis of prospective cohort studies. *Hypertens Res.* (2013) 36:985–95. doi: 10.1038/hr.2013.70
8. Cappuccio FP, D'Elia L, Strazzullo P, Miller MA. Quantity and quality of sleep and incidence of type 2 diabetes: a systematic review and meta-analysis. *Diabetes Care.* (2010) 33:414–20. doi: 10.2337/dc09-1124
9. Aurora RN, Kim JS, Crainiceanu C, O'Hearn D, Punjabi NM. Habitual sleep duration and all-cause mortality in a general community sample. *Sleep.* (2016) 39:1903–9. doi: 10.5665/sleep.6212
10. Craig JP, Nichols KK, Akpek EK, Caffery B, Dua HS, Joo CK, et al. TFOS DEWS II definition and classification report. *Ocul Surf.* (2017) 15:276–83. doi: 10.1016/j.jtos.2017.05.008
11. Stapleton F, Alves M, Bunya VY, Jalbert I, Lekhanont K, Malet F, et al. TFOS DEWS II epidemiology report. *Ocul Surf.* (2017) 15:334–65. doi: 10.1016/j.jtos.2017.05.003
12. Kawashima M. Systemic health and dry eye. *Invest Ophthalmol Vis Sci.* (2018) 59:Des138–42. doi: 10.1167/iovs.17-23765
13. Vehof J, Sillevis Smitt-Kamminga N, Kozareva D, Nibourg SA, Hammond CJ. Clinical characteristics of dry eye patients with chronic pain syndromes. *Am J Ophthalmol.* (2016) 162:59–65.e2. doi: 10.1016/j.ajo.2015.11.017
14. Yu J, Asche CV, Fairchild CJ. The economic burden of dry eye disease in the United States: a decision tree analysis. *Cornea.* (2011) 30:379–87. doi: 10.1097/ICO.0b013e3181f7f363
15. Wang MTM, Vidal-Rohr M, Muntz A, Diprose WK, Ormonde SE, Wolffsohn JS, et al. Systemic risk factors of dry eye disease subtypes: a New Zealand cross-sectional study. *Ocul Surf.* (2020) 18:374–80. doi: 10.1016/j.jtos.2020.04.003
16. Vehof J, Snieder H, Jansonius N, Hammond CJ. Prevalence and risk factors of dry eye in 79,866 participants of the population-based Lifelines cohort study in the Netherlands. *Ocul Surf.* (2021) 19:83–93. doi: 10.1016/j.jtos.2020.04.005
17. Ayaki M, Tsubota K, Kawashima M, Kishimoto T, Mimura M, Negishi K. Sleep disorders are a prevalent and serious comorbidity in dry eye. *Invest Ophthalmol Vis Sci.* (2018) 59:Des143–50. doi: 10.1167/iovs.17-23467
18. Monjan AA. Perspective on sleep and aging. *Front Neurol.* (2010) 1:124. doi: 10.3389/fneur.2010.00124
19. Yu X, Guo H, Liu X, Wang G, Min Y, Chen SS, et al. Dry eye and sleep quality: a large community-based study in Hangzhou. *Sleep.* (2019) 42:zsz160. doi: 10.1093/sleep/zsz160
20. Lim EWL, Chee ML, Sabanayagam C, Majithia S, Tao Y, Wong TY, et al. Relationship between sleep and symptoms of tear dysfunction in singapore malays and Indians. *Invest Ophthalmol Vis Sci.* (2019) 60:1889–97. doi: 10.1167/iovs.19-26810
21. Wu M, Liu X, Han J, Shao T, Wang Y. Association between sleep quality, mood status, and ocular surface characteristics in patients with dry eye disease. *Cornea.* (2019) 38:311–7. doi: 10.1097/ICO.0000000000001854
22. Ayaki M, Kawashima M, Negishi K, Kishimoto T, Mimura M, Tsubota K. Sleep and mood disorders in women with dry eye disease. *Sci Rep.* (2016) 6:35276. doi: 10.1038/srep35276
23. Kawashima M, Uchino M, Yokoi N, Uchino Y, Dogru M, Komuro A, et al. The association of sleep quality with dry eye disease: the Osaka study. *Clin Ophthalmol.* (2016) 10:1015–21. doi: 10.2147/OPTH.S99620
24. Ayaki M, Kawashima M, Negishi K, Kishimoto T, Mimura M, Tsubota K. Sleep and mood disorders in dry eye disease and allied irritating ocular diseases. *Sci Rep.* (2016) 6:22480. doi: 10.1038/srep22480
25. Ayaki M, Kawashima M, Negishi K, Tsubota K. High prevalence of sleep and mood disorders in dry eye patients: survey of 1,000 eye clinic visitors. *Neuropsychiatr Dis Treat.* (2015) 11:889–94. doi: 10.2147/NDT.S81515
26. Hanyuda A, Sawada N, Uchino M, Kawashima M, Yuki K, Tsubota K, et al. Relationship between unhealthy sleep status and dry eye symptoms in a Japanese population: the JPHC-NEXT study. *Ocul Surf.* (2021) 21:306–12. doi: 10.1016/j.jtos.2021.04.001
27. Magno MS, Utheim TP, Snieder H, Hammond CJ, Vehof J. The relationship between dry eye and sleep quality. *Ocul Surf.* (2021) 20:13–9. doi: 10.1016/j.jtos.2020.12.009
28. Kim KI, Park YS, Kim RH, Kim JH. Factors associated with dry eye symptoms in elderly Koreans: the fifth Korea National Health and nutrition examination survey 2010–2012. *Korean J Fam Med.* (2019) 40:22–30. doi: 10.4082/kjfm.17.0058
29. Kawashima M, Yamada M, Shigeyasu C, Suwaki K, Uchino M, Hiratsuka Y, et al. Association of systemic comorbidities with dry eye disease. *J Clin Med.* (2020) 9:2040. doi: 10.3390/jcm9072040
30. Koçer E, Koçer A, Özsütçü M, Dursun AE, Krpnar I. Dry eye related to commonly used new antidepressants. *J Clin Psychopharmacol.* (2015) 35:411–3. doi: 10.1097/JCP.0000000000000356
31. Zhang S, Hong J. Risk factors for dry eye in Mainland China: a multi-center cross-sectional hospital-based study. *Ophthalmic Epidemiol.* (2019) 26:393–9. doi: 10.1080/09286586.2019.1632905
32. Wang JB, Huang QC, Hu SC, Zheng PW, Shen P, Li D, et al. Baseline and longitudinal change in blood pressure and mortality in a Chinese cohort. *J Epidemiol Community Health.* (2018) 72:1083–90. doi: 10.1136/jech-2018-211050
33. Aurora RN, Zak RS, Auerbach SH, Casey KR, Chowdhuri S, Karippot A, et al. Best practice guide for the treatment of nightmare disorder in adults. *J Clin Sleep Med.* (2010) 6:389–401. doi: 10.5664/jcsm.27883
34. Okun ML, Ebert R, Saini B. A review of sleep-promoting medications used in pregnancy. *Am J Obstet Gynecol.* (2015) 212:428–41. doi: 10.1016/j.ajog.2014.10.1106
35. Lee W, Lim SS, Won JU, Roh J, Lee JH, Seok H, et al. The association between sleep duration and dry eye syndrome among Korean adults. *Sleep Med.* (2015) 16:1327–31. doi: 10.1016/j.sleep.2015.06.021
36. Han KT, Nam JH, Park EC. Do sleep disorders positively correlate with dry eye syndrome? Results of national claim data. *Int J Environ Res Public Health.* (2019) 16:878. doi: 10.3390/ijerph16050878
37. Li S, Ning K, Zhou J, Guo Y, Zhang H, Zhu Y, et al. Sleep deprivation disrupts the lacrimal system and induces dry eye disease. *Exp Mol Med.* (2018) 50:e451. doi: 10.1038/emm.2017.285
38. Palma JA. Autonomic dysfunction in sleep disorders: introduction to the series. *Clin Auton Res.* (2018) 28:507–8. doi: 10.1007/s10286-018-0571-6
39. Tang L, Wang X, Wu J, Li SM, Zhang Z, Wu S, et al. Sleep deprivation induces

dry eye through inhibition of PPARα expression in corneal epithelium. *Invest Ophthalmol Vis Sci.* (2018) 59:5494–508. doi: 10.1167/iovs.18-24504
40. Dartt DA. Regulation of tear secretion. *Adv Exp Med Biol.* (1994) 350:1–9. doi: 10.1007/978-1-4615-2417-5_1
41. Dartt DA. Neural regulation of lacrimal gland secretory processes: relevance in dry eye diseases. *Prog Retin Eye Res.* (2009) 28:155–77. doi: 10.1016/j.preteyeres.2009.04.003
42. Sleep disorders group soN, Chinese Medical Association. Guidelines for the diagnosis and treatment of insomnia in Chinese adults. *Chin J Neurol.* (2018) 51:324–35. doi: 10.21037/jtd.2019.06.09
43. Richa S, Yazbek JC. Ocular adverse effects of common psychotropic agents: a review. *CNS Drugs.* (2010) 24:501–26. doi: 10.2165/11533180-000000000-00000

5

Dry Eye Disease in Patients With Schizophrenia

*Qiankun Chen [1], Zhengjiang Wei [2], Leying Wang [1], Xizhan Xu [1], Zhenyu Wei [1], Panpan Zheng [3], Kai Cao [1], Zijun Zhang [1], Kexin Chen [1] and Qingfeng Liang [1]**

[1] Beijing Institute of Ophthalmology, Beijing Tongren Eye Center, Beijing Tongren Hospital, Capital Medical University, Beijing Key Laboratory of Ophthalmology and Visual Sciences, Beijing, China, [2] Beijing Miyun Mental Health Prevention and Treatment Hospital, Beijing, China, [3] National Center for Children's Health, Beijing Children's Hospital, Capital Medical University, Beijing, China

***Correspondence:**
Qingfeng Liang
lqflucky@163.com

Objective: To evaluate the clinical features and inflammatory cytokines of dry eye disease (DED) in patients with schizophrenia.

Methods: This is a case-control study. The modified self-rating depression scale (M-SDS) and the ocular surface disease index (OSDI) were used to evaluate the symptoms of depression and DED, respectively. Lipid layer thickness (LLT), partial blink rate (PBR), meibomian gland loss (MGL), tear break-up time (TBUT), corneal fluorescein staining, Schirmer I-test, and eyelid margin abnormalities were also measured. A multiplex ELISA Quantibody array was used to detect the inflammatory cytokines in the tears of all participants.

Results: Forty schizophrenic patients and 20 control subjects were included. The mean age was 45.0 ± 9.5 years (range, 22–63 years) in schizophrenic patients and 45.4 ± 16.2 years (range, 23–76 years) in controls ($P = 0.914$). The ratio of male to female was 1.1 in schizophrenic patients and 1.0 in controls ($P = 0.914$). Ten women (52.6%) with schizophrenia and 2 (20%) in the control group ($P = 0.096$) were menopausal or post-menopausal. The OSDI [0.0 (0.0–4.2) vs. 7.3 (2.1–14.6)] and TBUT [4.5 (3.0–6.0) vs. 10.0 (3.5–11.0)] were significantly lower in patients with schizophrenia than in controls ($P = 0.003$ and $P = 0.009$, respectively). The rate of MGL [36.5 (17.5–47.5) vs. 8.5 (0.0–17.5)] increased in schizophrenic patients ($P < 0.001$). Among pro-inflammatory cytokines, the levels of interleukin (IL)-1α, IL-6, IL-11, IL-12A, IL-15, IL-17A, and granulocyte colony-stimulating factor (G-CSF) in tears were elevated in the schizophrenia group (all $P < 0.01$). Most of the chemokines examined were at increased levels in the tears of schizophrenics (all $P < 0.05$). The levels of matrix metalloproteinases-9 (MMP-9) and intercellular adhesion molecule-1 (ICAM-1) were also higher in the schizophrenic patients (all $P < 0.001$). The concentrations of IL-1Ra, tissue-inhibitor of metalloproteinase-1 (TIMP-1), and TIMP-2 in the schizophrenia group were decreased (all $P < 0.001$). In schizophrenic patients, the level of CCL2 in tears was positively correlated with OSDI ($R = 0.34$, $P = 0.03$). The increasing TIMP-1 and decreasing IL-5 were correlated with increasing LLT ($R = 0.33$, $P = 0.035$; $R = -0.35$, $P = 0.027$, respectively). The level of ICAM-1 was then positively correlated with partial blink rate (PBR) ($R = 0.33$, $P = 0.035$). There was a negative correlation between IL-8 and the Schirmer *I*-test ($R = -0.41$, $P = 0.009$).

Conclusions: Patients with schizophrenia were more likely to experience asymptomatic DED, with mild symptoms and obvious signs. The inflammatory cytokines in the tears of schizophrenic patients differed greatly from that of non-schizophrenic patients.

Keywords: dry eye disease, schizophrenia, cytokine, inflammation, tear

INTRODUCTION

Dry eye disease (DED) is one of the most common ocular surface diseases and has been recognized as a major public health problem (1). Based on the report of Dry Eye Workshop II (DEWS II) from the Tear Film & Ocular Surface Society, DED was defined as a multifactorial disease of the tear film and ocular surface, including three core parts: tear film instability, ocular surface inflammation, and neurosensory abnormalities (2). We have always emphasized that the symptoms were the main features of DED, but the symptoms of DED were often inconsistent with the signs (3). Some researchers, however, tried to explain it with the theory that mental health conditions could be one of the considerable contributing factors for DED symptoms and undiagnosed mental diseases could have similar symptoms in some special types of DED (4). In addition, psychiatric medications could influence the stability of the tear film and were considered as a risk factor for DED (5). In recent years, numerous studies have focused on the relationship between DED and psychiatric disorders, such as depression, anxiety, post-traumatic stress disorders, and sleep disorders (6–11).

Although some DED patients present psychiatric or mood disorders, it remains unclear whether psychiatric patients also experience the symptoms or clinical signs of DED. As a severe psychotic disorder, schizophrenia is characterized by varying degrees of cognitive impairments, emotional aberrations, and behavioral anomalies (12). So, It may be a good model to evaluate the relationship between DED and psychiatric disorders because schizophrenia always disrupts the processes of perception, reasoning, judgment. The medications for schizophrenia may also induce the signs of DED (13). Although a study conducted in Taiwan, China, found that patients with DED may be more likely to develop schizophrenia (10), the symptoms of DED were not associated with schizophrenia according to a population-based study in the Netherlands (14). Until now, there have been few studies to analyze the DED status of schizophrenic patients and detect the relationship between DED and schizophrenia. So, with the existing epidemiological investigations, the relationship between DED and schizophrenia was investigated at both the clinical and molecular levels.

MATERIALS AND METHODS

Study Design

A case-control study was performed at Beijing Tongren Hospital, Capital Medical University, and Beijing Miyun Mental Health Prevention and Treatment Hospital between December 2020 and April 2021. This study was registered in the Chinese Clinical Trial Registry (Registration number: ChiCTR-RDD-17013855), and ethical approval was obtained from the Medical Ethics Committee of Beijing Tongren Hospital (TRECKY2019-130). All participants obtained written informed consent in accordance with the Declaration of Helsinki.

Participants

All enrolled schizophrenic patients were hospitalized in the Beijing Miyun Mental Health Prevention and Treatment Hospital, whose diagnoses were conducted by professional psychiatrists (ZJ W) using international criteria for schizophrenia listed in the *Diagnostic and Statistical Manual of Mental Disorders* (Fourth Edition). The inclusion criteria were that the patients should be over 18 years old, their conditions should be under control, and they should be able to complete the questionnaires and ocular examinations. The exclusion criteria included current pregnancy or lactation, and any ocular surface disease that may affect the integrity of the cornea (for example, past corneal chemical injury, recurrent corneal epithelial erosion, corneal epithelial defect, and map-dot-fingerprint dystrophy). Cases with ocular topical treatment within the past 6 months, history of ocular trauma, previous ocular laser or surgical treatment, and other common ocular diseases were also excluded.

The inclusion criteria for the control group were that the patients should be older than 18 years with no ocular discomfort. Exclusion criteria of the control group included: (1) abnormality of lid margin and cornea under slit lamp microscopy; (2) conjunctival inflammation; (3) systemic diseases or medications that may cause DED; (4) contact lens wear in the month prior to enrollment; (5) other ocular diseases; (6) pregnant or lactating women.

Demographic Information Collection

Demographic information was obtained from questionnaires based on the previous study (15). These questionnaires included basic information (age and gender), systemic medical history (such as hypertension, hyperlipidemia, diabetes mellitus, and coronary heart disease), and smoking and alcohol intake history.

Depression Symptoms Evaluation

The symptoms of depression were assessed using the modified self-rating depression scale (M-SDS) adapted from the 1965 self-rating depression scale by Zung, which had been applied in the Beijing Eye Study (15, 16). The M-SDS consisted of 20 questions, each carrying a score of 1 to 4. Definite depression was defined as having an M-SDS score of 40 or higher.

Ocular Surface Evaluation

The ocular surface symptoms of each participant were quantified by the ocular surface disease index (OSDI) questionnaire (range,

0–100) (17). OSDI contained 12 questions, which included DED symptoms (sensitivity to light, foreign body sensation eye pain or sore eyes, blurred vision and poor vision), restrictions on daily activities (reading, driving at night, working on the computer or automatic teller machine, and watching TV), and environmental factors (wind, low humidity, and air conditioning). Each question consisted of 5 levels, which were as follows: 0, none; 1, sometimes; 2, half the time; 3, most of the time; and 4, all the time. The higher the score, the more severe the symptoms. An OSDI score of 13 or higher was considered as a symptom of DED (18).

All ocular surface examinations were performed on the left eye of the participants.

The LipiView interferometer (TearScience Inc, Morrisville, North Carolina, USA) was used to measure lipid layer thickness (LLT), capture infrared photography of the meibomian gland, and analyze blink pattern as previously described (19). Interferometry color units (ICU) represent the amount of lipid distribution, and 1 ICU is about 1 nm of LLT. Conformance factor (CF) represents the quality of the measured data. If the CF is lower than 0.7, it must be re-tested to ensure the correctness of the data. Partial blink rate (PBR) was calculated by the ratio of partial blinks to total blinks (20). ImageJ software was used to semi-automatically analyze the loss rate of the lower lid meibomian glands.

Tear break-up time (TBUT) was calculated according to the previous description (21). In brief, the fluorescein strip (Tianjin Jingming New Technological Development Co., Ltd., China) was wetted with saline, and then a drop was put into the lower fornix. Participants were asked to blink several times before being observed under a cobalt blue filter at the slit lamp. The time gap between participants starting to open their eyes and the appearance of the first dark spot on the tear film was recorded. The average of three consecutive measurements was regarded as TBUT. TBUT <10 s was considered abnormal (18).

Corneal staining was conducted according to the Oxford scheme to assess the integrity of corneal epithelium after TBUT evaluation (22). In brief, the Oxford score was graduated with points ranging from 0 to 5, based on the staining dots of cornea as follows: 0 for ≤1 dot; 1 for ≤10 dots; 2 for ≤32 dots; 3 for ≤100 dots; 4 for ≤316 dots; and 5 for >316 dots.

Schirmer *I*-test was carried out as described previously (23). A 5 × 35 mm sterile filter paper strip (Tianjin Jingming New Technological Development Co., Ltd., China) with one end folded at a right angle at 5 mm was placed at the middle and outer 1/3 of the inferior fornix. The subject was then asked to close the eyes, and the soaked length of the filter paper was measured after 5 min.

Eyelid margin abnormalities (including irregularity, telangiectasia, plugging of orifices, and Marx line location) were evaluated under slit-lamp microscopy with 1 point for each item, and the total score of eyelid margin was added up (24).

Tear Collection and Cytokine Detection

A total quantity of 60 μl of tears were extracted from the temporal area of the meniscus under the left eye of each participant using 20 μl microcaps (Drummond Scientific Company, Broomall, PA, USA) and stored at −80°C.

Multiplex ELISA Quantibody array kits (QAH-DED-1, RayBiotech) were used to detect the cytokines in tears, including interleukins (ILs), chemokines, matrix metalloproteinases (MMPs) and inhibitors, and other cytokines related to DED. The Quantibody array was carried out according to the manual provided by the company. To be brief, the 16-well glass chip was dried completely and incubated at room temperature for 1 h with 100 μl sample dilution in each well. The diluent was removed and cleaned two times by Wellwash Versa (Thermo Fisher Scientific, Waltham, MA, USA) with wash buffer I and II, respectively. Samples of 60 μl volume were added and incubated overnight at 4°C. Detection antibody cocktails of 80 μl were then added and incubated at room temperature for 2 h on a shaker. After cleaning again as before, 80 μl of Cy3 equivalent dye-conjugated streptavidin was put into each well and incubated on a shaker at room temperature, away from light, for 1 h. After the third cleaning, a laser scanner (InnoScan 300 Microarray Scanner, Innopsys, Carbonne, France) was used for detection. Finally, QAH-DED-1 data analysis software was used for data analysis. Standard substances with eight concentration gradients were used as controls.

Statistical Analysis

Statistical analysis was performed with SPSS 26.0. A Kolmogorov-Smirnov test was used to assess for normality of continuous variables. The *t*-test was used for measurement data that followed a normal distribution, described by mean ± standard deviation. For non-normal distribution parameters, the Mann–Whitney *U*-test was used, and the values of parameters were described in terms of median and inter-quartile range. Chi-square test was used for enumeration date. Moreover, Spearman's correlation coefficient was calculated. The value of $P < 0.05$ was considered statistically significant.

RESULTS

Demographic Characteristics

A total of 60 participants were included—40 patients with schizophrenia and 20 control subjects. The demographic information and medical history of the schizophrenic patients and controls were summarized in **Table 1**. The mean age was 45.0 ± 9.5 years (range, 22–63 years) in the schizophrenic group and 45.4 ± 16.2 years (range, 23–76 years) in the control group ($P = 0.914$). The number of men in the schizophrenic group and control group were 21 (52.5%) and 10 (50%), respectively ($P = 0.802$). Ten women (52.6%) with schizophrenia and two (20%) in the control group ($P = 0.096$) were menopausal or post-menopausal. The length of hospital stay in patients with schizophrenia was 33.4 ± 65.2 months (range, 1–315 months). Twenty-six (65%) patients took one kind of antipsychotic drug and 14 (35%) patients took a combination of antipsychotic drugs. These antipsychotic drugs included rispehdone, olanzapine, zopiclone, clonazepam, sodium valproate, trihexyphenidyl, lorazepam, haloperidol, quetiapine fumarate, magnesium valproate, sertraline, escitalopram oxalate, and estazolam.

TABLE 1 | Characteristics and basic medical history of schizophrenic patients and normal controls.

Parameters	Schizophrenia group (n = 40)	Normal controls (n = 20)	P-value
Age (years)	45.0 ± 9.5	45.4 ± 16.2	0.914
Gender [n (%)]			0.802
Male	19 (47.5%)	10 (50%)	
Female	21 (52.5%)	10 (50%)	
Systemic diseases [n (%)]			
Hypertension	6 (15%)	1 (5%)	0.407
Hyperlipidemia	8 (20%)	1 (5%)	0.249
Diabetes mellitus	5 (12.5%)	2 (10%)	1.000
Coronary heart disease	3 (7.5%)	1 (5%)	1.000
Others	10 (25%)	6 (30%)	0.542
Smoking [n (%)]	19 (47.5%)	3 (15%)	0.022*
Alcohol intake [n (%)]	4 (10%)	2 (10%)	0.089
M-SDS	26.0 (22.0–32.5)	26.5 (23.0–30.5)	0.597

*P < 0.05 was considered statistically significant.

TABLE 2 | Ocular surface clinical outcomes in controls and schizophrenia group.

Parameters	Schizophrenia group (n = 40)	Normal controls (n = 20)	P-value
OSDI	0.0 (0.0–4.2)	7.3 (2.1–14.6)	0.003*
LLT (nm)	75 (58.5–84)	89.5 (63.0–100.0)	0.229
PBR (%)	50.0 (25.0–77.5)	77.4 (33.3–100.0)	0.229
MGL (%)	36.5 (17.5–47.5)	8.5 (0.0–17.5)	<0.001*
TBUT (s)	4.5 (3.0–6.0)	10.0 (3.5–11.0)	0.009*
Oxford score	0.0 (0.0–0.0)	0.0 (0.0–0.0)	0.294
Schirmer I-test (mm)	10.0 (6.0–16.0)	7.0 (2.5–17.5)	0.509
Eyelid margin [n (%)]			
Irregularity	14 (35.0)	1 (5.0)	0.009*
Telangiectasia	24 (60.0)	9 (45.0)	0.204
Orifice plugging	30 (75.0)	11 (55.0)	0.102
Marx line location	22 (55.0)	10 (50.0)	0.463
Score of eyelid	2.0 (1.0–3.0)	1.5 (1.0–2.0)	0.032*

*OSDI, ocular surface disease index; LLT, lipid layer thickness; PBR, partial blink rate; TBUT, tear brake-up time; MGL, meibomian gland loss. *P < 0.05 was considered statistically significant.*

There was no significant difference in the prevalence of systemic diseases (such as hypertension, hyperlipidemia, diabetes mellitus, and coronary heart disease) (all $P < 0.05$). Nineteen (47.5%) patients with schizophrenia smoked more than 5 cigarettes a day, far more than the 3 (15%) patients in the controls ($P = 0.022$). Four (10%) schizophrenic patients and 2 (10%) of the control subjects consumed alcohol everyday ($P = 0.089$). The median score of M-SDS in the schizophrenia group was 26.0 (22.0–32.5), which was similar to 26.5 (23.0–30.5) of the controls ($P = 0.597$).

Clinical Manifestations

Compared with normal controls, schizophrenic patients had lower OSDI score [median 0.0 (0.0–4.2) vs. 7.3 (2.1–7.6); $P = 0.003$, **Table 2**]. Three (7.5%) patients with schizophrenia showed DED symptoms, which was <5 (25%) patients in the controls ($P = 0.073$). However, the rate of meibomian gland loss (MGL) was 36.5 (17.5–47.5) percent in schizophrenic patients compared with 8.5 (0.0–17.5) percent in controls ($P < 0.001$). In the assessment of tear film stability, TBUT was significantly reduced in schizophrenia group ($P = 0.009$). Notably, 39 (97.5%) of schizophrenics and 9 (45%) of controls presented abnormalities in TBUT ($P < 0.001$). There was no significant difference between the two groups in LLT, PBR, Oxford score, and the Schirmer *I*-test (all $P > 0.05$). Therefore, among schizophrenic patients, 36 (90%) cases presented DED signs without symptoms, which were more than 5 (25%) from the control group ($P < 0.001$). In evaluation of eyelid margin, 14 (35.0%) schizophrenic patients and 1 (5.0%) in the control group ($P = 0.009$) presented irregularity. There was no significant difference in telangiectasia, plugging of orifices, and Marx line location between the two groups ($P = 0.204$; $P = 0.102$; $P = 0.463$, respectively). The total score of eyelid margin was higher in schizophrenic patients than controls (median, 2.0 vs. 1.5; $P = 0.032$).

Cytokine Expression in Tears

The expression levels of cytokines in tears were measured between the two groups and clustered into several categories according to previous studies (25, 26). Principal component analysis (PCA) and the heatmap showed obvious separation of cytokines from the two cohorts (**Figure 1**), suggesting that the ocular surface status of the two populations may be different.

Among pro-inflammatory cytokines, the levels of interleukin (IL)-1α, IL-6, IL-11, IL-12A, IL-15, IL-17A, and granulocyte colony-stimulating factor (G-CSF) in tears were significantly higher in patients with schizophrenia than that in normal controls (all $P < 0.01$; **Figure 2**). No significant differences in IL-2 and IL-7 levels were observed between the two groups ($P = 0.107$; $P = 0.163$, respectively). Among anti-inflammatory cytokines, IL-1Ra was decreased and IL-10 was increased in tears of schizophrenic patients compared with that of controls (all $P < 0.001$).

The cytokines of tears released by T helper (Th) cells were also measured. The cytokines secreted by Th1 were significantly higher in the tears of schizophrenic patients than that of normal controls, including IL-1β, tumor necrosis factor (TNF)-α, and interferon (IFN)-γ (all $P < 0.001$; **Figure 2**). The cytokines produced by Th2 (IL-4, IL-5, and IL-13) were also increased in patients with schizophrenia ($P < 0.001$; $P < 0.001$; $P = 0.012$, respectively).

In chemokines, the expression levels of chemokine (C-C motif) ligand 2 (CCL2), CCL4, CCL5, CCL11, CCL15, IL-8, chemokine (C-X-C motif) ligand 9 (CXCL9), and CXCL10 in tears of schizophrenic patients were significantly higher

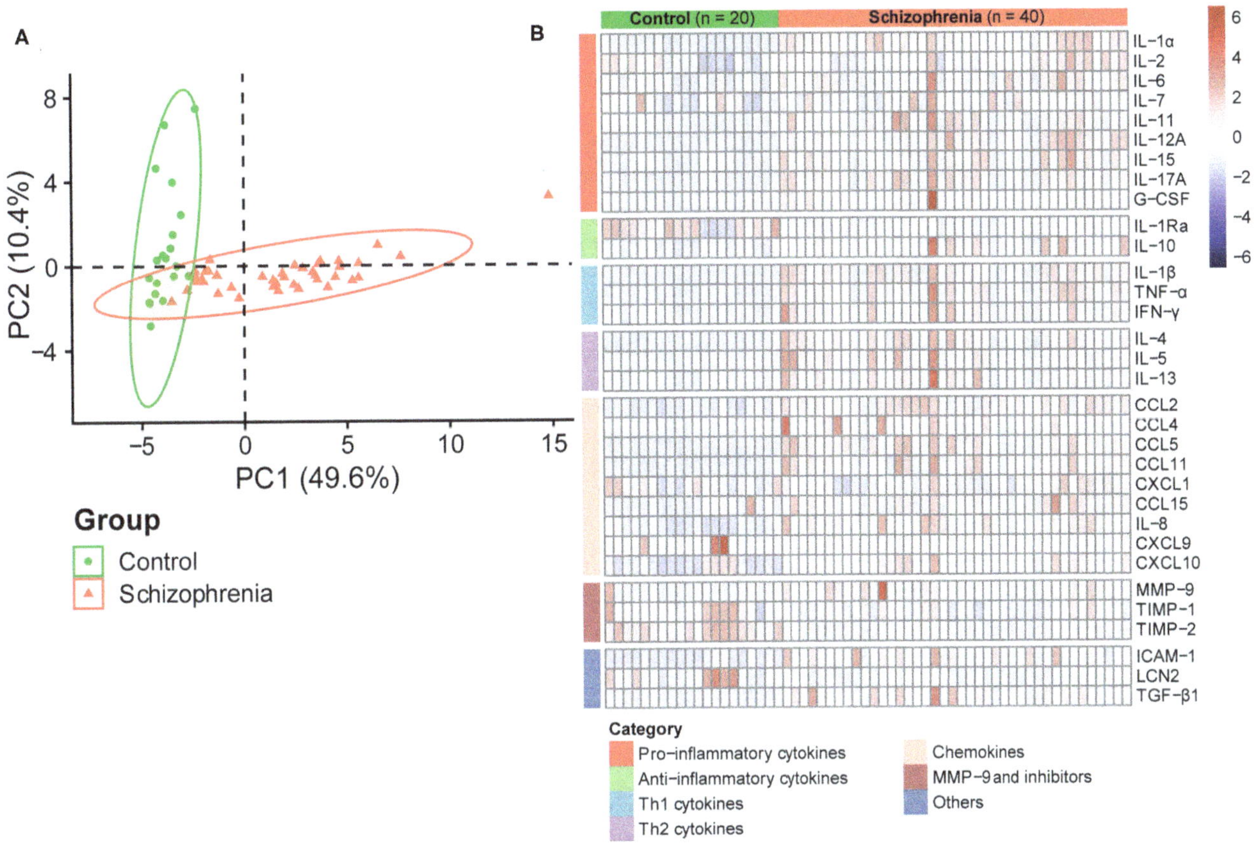

FIGURE 1 | Cytokines profile in tears of subjects with and without schizophrenia. **(A)** Principal component analysis was performed by the concentration of 32 cytokines in tears. Scatter plot of principal component 1 (PC1) and PC2 were represented, and each dot represented a sample projected in them. The orange and green dots represented schizophrenia and control groups, respectively. **(B)** Heatmap of high and low concentrations of tear cytokines. The groups evaluated were controls ($n = 20$) and patients with schizophrenia ($n = 40$). High levels of cytokines were shown in red on the heatmap, while low levels were shown in blue.

than that of normal controls (all $P < 0.05$; **Figure 2**). There was no significant difference in CXCL1 level of tears between schizophrenic patients and controls ($P = 0.589$).

Additionally, we also found that the expression of matrix metalloproteinases-9 (MMP-9) and their inhibitors in tears were different between the two groups. The level of MMP-9 was increased in schizophrenic patients ($P < 0.001$; **Figure 2**). However, the concentration of tissue-inhibitor of metalloproteinase-1(TIMP-1) and TIMP-2 in patients was much lower than that of controls (all $P < 0.001$). Finally, other cytokines outside the above classification, including intercellular adhesion molecule-1 (ICAM-1) and transforming growth factor-beta 1 (TGF-β1), were also elevated in the tears of schizophrenic patients (all $P < 0.001$).

Correlation Between Clinical Parameters and Cytokines

Among schizophrenic patients, the concentration of CCL2 in tears was positively correlated with OSDI ($R = 0.34$, $P = 0.03$; **Figure 3**). The levels of IL-13, IFN-γ, and IL-5 were positively correlated with TBUT ($R = 0.43$, $P = 0.005$; $R = 0.36$, $P = 0.023$; $R = 0.32$, $P = 0.045$, respectively). The increasing TIMP-1 and decreasing IL-5 were correlated with increasing LLT in schizophrenic patients ($R = 0.33$, $P = 0.035$; $R = -0.35$, $P = 0.027$, respectively). The increasing level of ICAM-1 was positively correlated with increasing PBR in patients with schizophrenia ($R = 0.33$, $P = 0.035$). There was a negative correlation between IL-8 and Schirmer *I*-test ($R = -0.41$, $P = 0.009$). In addition, we also found the correlation of cytokines in the tears of patients with schizophrenia (**Supplementary Figure S1**).

DISCUSSION

In the current study, we found an increase in DED (mainly asymptomatic DED) in patients with schizophrenia. Compared to controls, most inflammatory cytokines of tears were significantly increased in schizophrenic patients. Correlation between the concentration of cytokines and clinical parameters was also observed.

The results of this study showed that OSDI and TBUT were decreased, and the rate of MGL was elevated in patients with schizophrenia. These indicated that the symptoms and signs of DED in schizophrenic patients were inconsistent, with mild

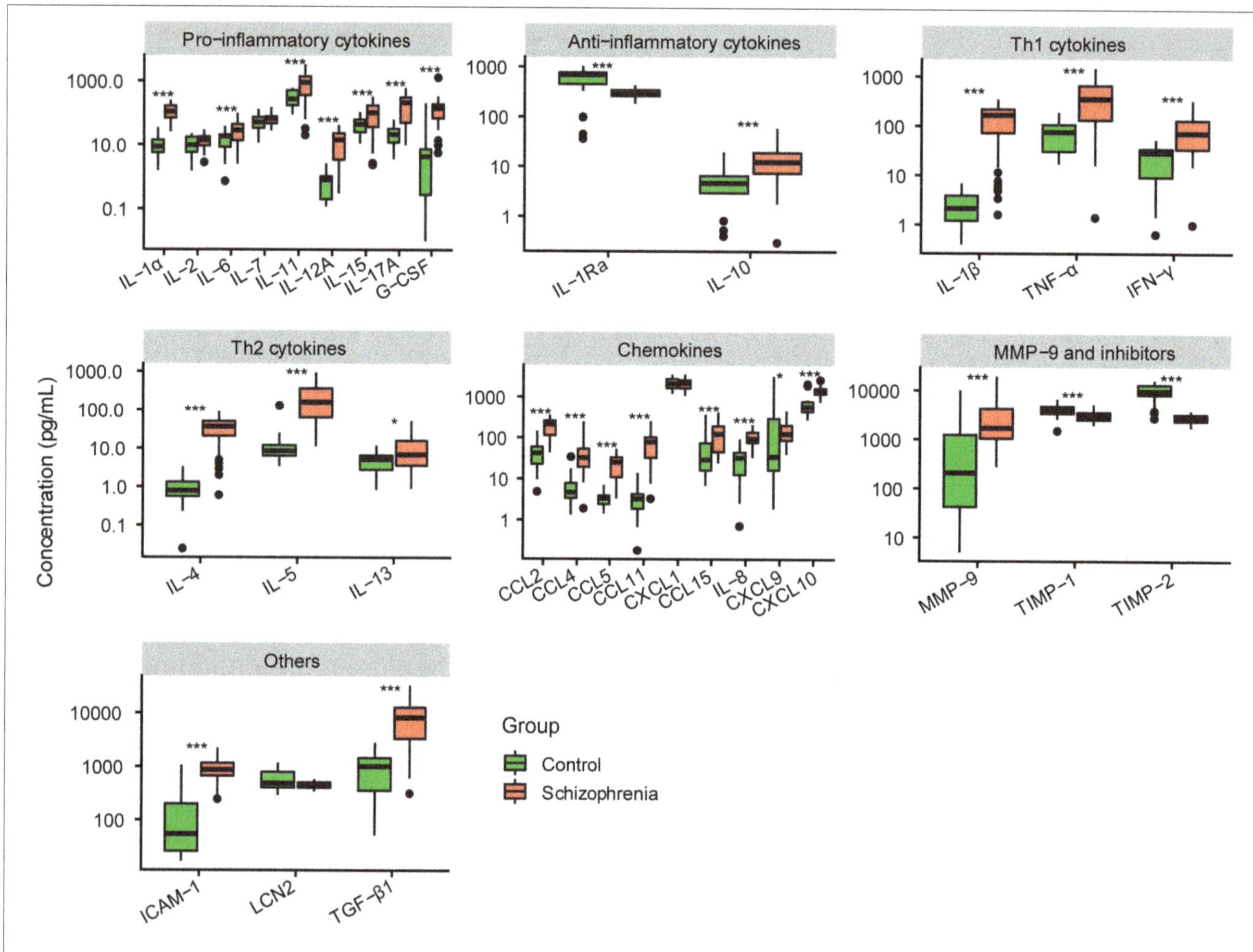

FIGURE 2 | Comparative analysis of expression level of 32 cytokines in tears between normal controls and schizophrenia group. *$P < 0.05$; ***$P < 0.001$.

symptoms and severe signs. Moreover, low TBUT, high MGL, and normal Schirmer *I*-test suggested that DED in schizophrenic patients was more likely to be evaporative rather than aqueous-deficient. A study conducted by Tiskaoglu et al. (27) showed that patients with newly diagnosed depressive disorder had lower Schirmer score and TBUT, while DED symptoms were not different from the control group. Kim et al. (28) suggested that depression was related to DED symptoms rather than signs. A review by McMonnies (29) also showed that dry eye features in patients with mental disorders were mostly severe symptoms and relatively mild signs. In addition, other studies have found that patients with depression, anxiety, and obsessive-compulsive disorder had more severe signs and symptoms of DED than the controls (11, 30). Unlike previous studies, our study involved patients with schizophrenia. Moreover, the patients in the previous studies were outpatients, whereas we focused on inpatients. In the current study, all schizophrenic patients took antipsychotic drugs, which could induce side-effects on the ocular surface, including pigmentary deposits of conjunctiva and cornea, reduction of tear secretion and tear film stability, damage of corneal epithelium, reduction of corneal thickness, and ocular toxicity (13, 31, 32). The absence of DED symptoms in patients with schizophrenia may be due to cognitive abnormalities and hypoesthesia (33). Moreover, the obvious signs of DED in schizophrenic patients could be due to the lack of activities and use of antipsychotic drugs (13).

Cytokines are key signal molecules of the immune system, which play important roles in the inflammatory response of the ocular surface and whole body. Among the tear cytokines examined, increased levels of pro-inflammatory cytokines (IL-1α, IL-6, IL-11, IL-12A, IL-15, IL-17A, and G-CSF), anti-inflammatory cytokines (IL-10), Th1 cytokines (IL-1β, TNF-α, and IFN-γ), Th2 cytokines (IL-4, IL-5, and IL-13), chemokines (CCL2, CCL4, CCL5, CCL11, CCL15, IL-8, CXCL9, and CXCL10), MMP-9, and others (ICAM-1 and TGF-β1) were observed in patients with schizophrenia. While the concentration of IL-1Ra of anti-inflammatory cytokines, TIMP-1 and TIMP-2 were decreased in tears of schizophrenic patients. A meta-analysis showed increased levels of IL-6, IL-8, IL-10, IL-12, IL-1β, IFN-γ, TNF-α, and TGF-β in the blood of patients with schizophrenia, which was similar to our findings (34). The levels of IL-2, IL-4, IL-10, TGF-β, and IL-17 in blood were

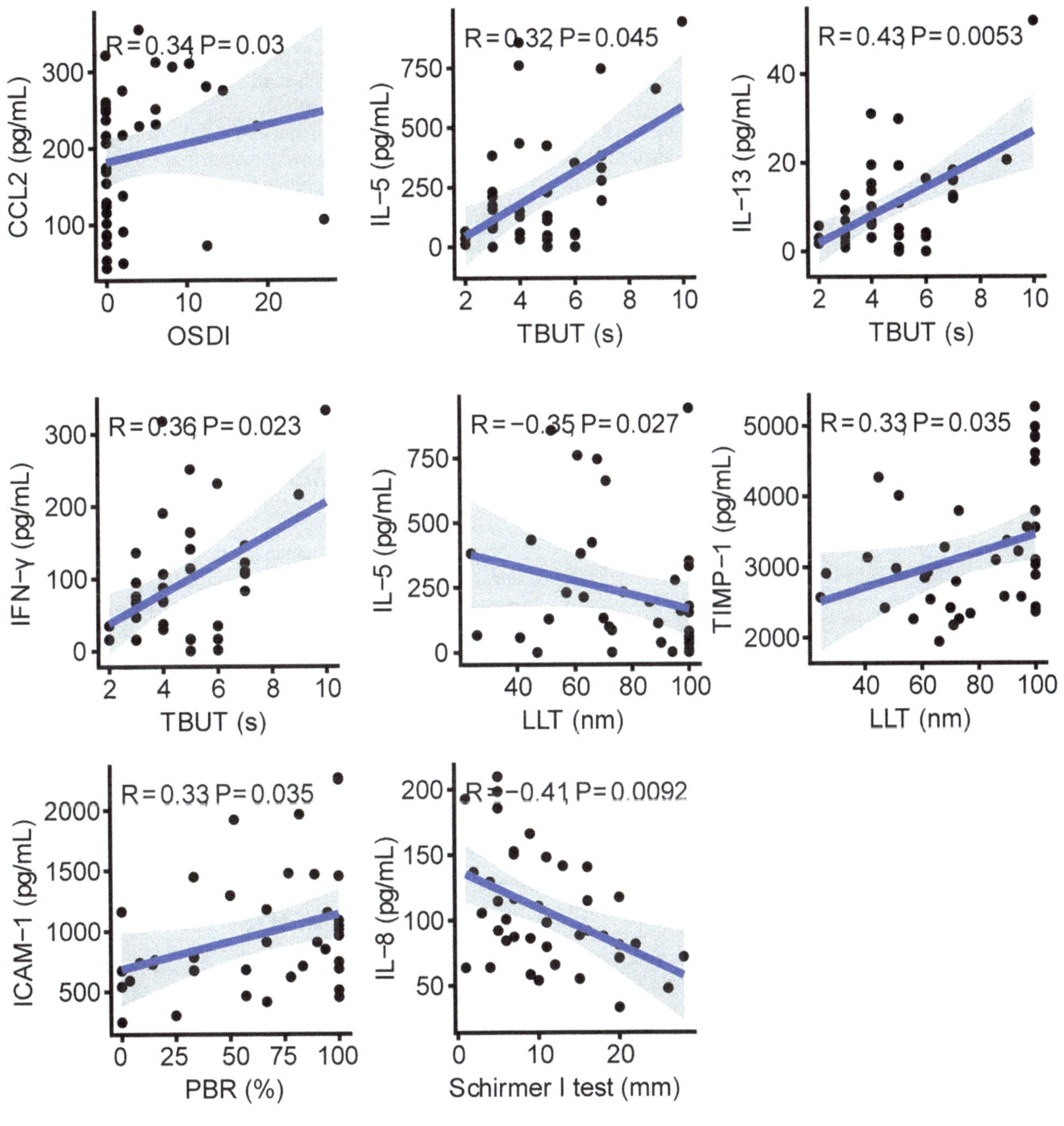

FIGURE 3 | Correlation between cytokines and clinical parameters in schizophrenic patients.

also detected to be elevated in schizophrenic patients (35). Some studies found an increased level of IL-1Ra in the serum of patients with schizophrenia, while another study showed decreased expression of IL-1Ra in the prefrontal cortex (34–36). In chemokines, the levels of CCL2, CCL3, CCL4, CCL5, CCL11, and IL-8 in serum were increased in patients compared to controls, but CXCL9 and CXCL10 were similar between the two groups (37, 38). MMP-9, as a novel role involved in pathological synaptic plasticity in schizophrenia, was highly expressed in serum and brain tissues of patients with schizophrenia and could be regulated by TIMP-1 and TIMP-2 (39). The ratio of MMP-9/TIMP-1 in serum was higher in schizophrenic patients compared to healthy controls, which was similar to our study (40). As inflammation of the ocular surface is one of the core mechanisms of DED, increased inflammatory cytokines in the tears of schizophrenic patients could potentially cause ocular surface damage and promote the occurrence of DED. In a meta-analysis of 13 studies, there were strong pieces of evidence that the concentrations of IL-1β, IL-6, IL-10, IFN-γ, and TNF-α were significantly elevated in the tears of DED patients (41). The levels of IL-1α, IL-4, IL-11, IL-12A, IL-13, IL-15, IL-17A, and G-CSF were also increased in the tears of DED patients according to previous studies (42–45). Additionally, IL-1Ra was reduced in patients with DED, and topical treatment with IL-1Ra was effective in improving the clinical signs and reducing underlying inflammation of DED (46). During the inflammation response of DED, chemokines such as CCL2, CCL3, CCL5, CCL15, IL-8, CXCL9, and CXCL10 could recruit and bind macrophages, dendritic cells, neutrophils, and activated T cells (47–49). MMP-9 was a recognized cytokine that activated other inflammatory cytokines, leading to a vicious cycle of inflammation, impaired tear secretion, ocular surface damage, and worsening DED symptoms (50). Matrix metalloproteinase inhibitors, TIMP-1 and TIMP-2, could mediate corneal regeneration by inducing corneal epithelium proliferation and inhibiting apoptosis (51). Another study showed that the ratio of MMP-9/TIMPs was higher in evaporative dry eye, which was consistent with the current study (52). ICAM-1 and TGF-β1 were also highly expressed in the ocular surface of patients with DED (53, 54).

Further study found the correlation between tear cytokine levels and DED clinical parameters. As a well-known monocyte chemotactic protein-1 (MCP-1), the increase in CCL2 concentration was positively correlated with the increase of OSDI score in this study, suggesting that CCL2 could be an aggravating factor for the symptoms of DED. Similar to our findings, Perez et al. (55) found a significant increase of CCL2 in DED patients with mild signs but exaggerated symptoms. IL-8, a chemokine that recruited immune cells, was increased in the tears of patients with DED and has been found to be negatively associated with the Schirmer *I*-test, the same as in our study (56). As a natural endogenous inhibitor of MMP-9, TIMP-1 improved the symptoms and signs of DED, which was consistent with the positive correlation between the increase in TIMP-1 and the increase in LLT in the current study (57). IL-13 and IFN-γ were associated with the damage of corneal epithelial integrity and decrease of tear secretion in evaporative dry eye (58, 59). However, the levels of IL-13 and IFN-γ in tears were positively correlated with TBUT, as observed by us. Increased concentration of IL-5 in tears was inversely associated with TBUT, OSDI, and Oxford score in patients with DED, whereas we observed a positive association between IL-5 and TBUT, and a negative correlation between IL-5 and LLT in patients with schizophrenia (59, 60). In addition, we also observed that ICAM-1 concentration was positively correlated with PBR in patients. ICAM-1, an adhesion molecule that recruited and assisted in the migration of inflammatory cells during inflammation response of DED, has been a target for dry eye therapy (55). Also, partial blink was reported to be associated with DED (61). The correlation between cytokines and clinical parameters was somewhat different from previous studies, possibly because the ocular surface conditions of patients with schizophrenia may be different from those of patients with ordinary DED.

There were some limitations in this study. First, the relationship of inflammatory cytokines between blood and tears was not comparatively analyzed because of ethical issues. Second, all patients with schizophrenia were treated with antipsychotic medicines, which may have a potential effect on the results. Third, more patients with schizophrenia smoked than controls, which was consistent with the results of a meta-analysis that smoking may be associated with the risk of dry eye (62). Finally, a small number of cases were included in this study. There is a requirement for a prospective study with a large sample size to verify our findings.

In conclusion, patients with schizophrenia were more likely to be accompanied by asymptomatic DED, which presented mild symptoms and obvious signs. DED in patients with schizophrenia was a mixed type, but mainly evaporative. The cytokine profiles in tears of schizophrenic patients differed from that of non-schizophrenic patients. Correlations between tear cytokines and ocular surface clinical parameters were also observed. Further studies of DED in untreated schizophrenic patients are needed.

ETHICS STATEMENT

The studies involving human participants were reviewed and approved by Medical Ethics Committee of Beijing Tongren Hospital (TRECKY2019-130). The patients/participants provided their written informed consent to participate in this study.

AUTHOR CONTRIBUTIONS

QL performed the study design. QC analyzed the data and wrote the manuscript. QC, ZJW, LW, XX, ZW, PZ, KC, ZZ, and KXC collected and analyzed data. All authors approved the final manuscript.

ACKNOWLEDGMENTS

We are extremely grateful to all the participants and their authorized relatives who participated in this study, as well as the entire psychiatric medical teams.

REFERENCES

1. Stapleton F, Alves M, Bunya VY, Jalbert I, Lekhanont K, Malet F, et al. TFOS DEWS II epidemiology report. *Ocul Surf.* (2017) 15:334–65. doi: 10.1016/j.jtos.2017.05.003
2. Craig JP, Nichols KK, Akpek EK, Caffery B, Dua HS, Joo CK, et al. TFOS DEWS II definition and classification report. *Ocul Surf.* (2017) 15:276–83. doi: 10.1016/j.jtos.2017.05.008
3. Baudouin C, Aragona P, Van Setten G, Rolando M, Irkeç M, Benítez del Castillo J, et al. Diagnosing the severity of dry eye: a clear and practical algorithm. *Br J Ophthalmol.* (2014) 98:1168–76. doi: 10.1136/bjophthalmol-2013-304619
4. Kaštelan S, Bakija I, Bogadi M, Gverović Antunica A, Gotovac M, Šimunović Filipčić I. Mental disorders as influencing factors for discordances in the signs and symptoms of dry eye disease. *Psychiatr Danub.* (2021) 33(Suppl 4):588-595.

5. Acan D, Kurtgoz P. Influence of selective serotonin reuptake inhibitors on ocular surface. *Clin Exp Optom.* (2017) 100:83–6. doi: 10.1111/cxo.12415
6. Galor A, Feuer W, Lee DJ, Florez H, Faler AL, Zann KL, et al. Depression, post-traumatic stress disorder, and dry eye syndrome: a study utilizing the national United States Veterans Affairs administrative database. *Am J Ophthalmol.* (2012) 154:340–6.e2. doi: 10.1016/j.ajo.2012.02.009
7. Wen W, Wu Y, Chen Y, Gong L, Li M, Chen X, et al. Dry eye disease in patients with depressive and anxiety disorders in Shanghai. *Cornea.* (2012) 31:686–92. doi: 10.1097/ICO.0b013e3182261590
8. Hallak JA, Tibrewal S, Jain S. Depressive symptoms in patients with dry eye disease: a case-control study using the beck depression inventory. *Cornea.* (2015) 34:1545–50. doi: 10.1097/ICO.0000000000000641
9. Han SB, Yang HK, Hyon JY, Wee WR. Association of dry eye disease with psychiatric or neurological disorders in elderly patients. *Clin Interv Aging.* (2017) 12:785–92. doi: 10.2147/CIA.S137580
10. Liang CY, Cheang WM, Wang CY, Lin KH, Wei LC, Chen YY, et al. The association of dry eye syndrome and psychiatric disorders: a nationwide population-based cohort study. *BMC Ophthalmol.* (2020) 20:123. doi: 10.1186/s12886-020-01395-z
11. Eroglu FC, Gediz BS, Ozturk M, Kazanci B. Association between dry eye disease and newly diagnosed obsessive-compulsive disorder. *Cornea.* (2021) 40:817–21. doi: 10.1097/ICO.0000000000002724
12. Owen MJ, Sawa A, Mortensen PB. Schizophrenia. *Lancet.* (2016) 388:86–97. doi: 10.1016/S0140-6736(15)01121-6
13. Ceylan E, Ozer MD, Yilmaz YC, Kartal B, Yildiz Ekinci D, Çinici E, et al. The ocular surface side effects of an anti-psychotic drug, clozapine. *Cutan Ocul Toxicol.* (2016) 35:62–6. doi: 10.3109/15569527.2015.1018387
14. Vehof J, Snieder H, Jansonius N, Hammond CJ. Prevalence and risk factors of dry eye in 79,866 participants of the population-based Lifelines cohort study in the Netherlands. *Ocul Surf.* (2021) 19:83–93. doi: 10.1016/j.jtos.2020.04.005
15. Labbé A, Wang YX, Jie Y, Baudouin C, Jonas JB, Xu L. Dry eye disease, dry eye symptoms and depression: the Beijing Eye Study. *Br J Ophthalmol.* (2013) 97:1399–403. doi: 10.1136/bjophthalmol-2013-303838
16. Zung WW. A self-rating depression. Scale. *Arch Gen Psychiatry.* (1965) 12:63–70. doi: 10.1001/archpsyc.1965.01720310065008
17. Schiffman RM, Christianson MD, Jacobsen G, Hirsch JD, Reis BL. Reliability and validity of the ocular surface disease index. *Arch Ophthalmol.* (2000) 118:615–21. doi: 10.1001/archopht.118.5.615
18. Wolffsohn JS, Arita R, Chalmers R, Djalilian A, Dogru M, Dumbleton K, et al. TFOS DEWS II diagnostic methodology report. *Ocul Surf.* (2017) 15:539–74. doi: 10.1016/j.jtos.2017.05.001
19. Eom Y, Lee JS, Kang SY, Kim HM, Song JS. Correlation between quantitative measurements of tear film lipid layer thickness and meibomian gland loss in patients with obstructive meibomian gland dysfunction and normal controls. *Am J Ophthalmol.* (2013) 155:1104–10.e2. doi: 10.1016/j.ajo.2013.01.008
20. Su Y, Liang Q, Su G, Wang N, Baudouin C, Labbé A. Spontaneous eye blink patterns in dry eye: clinical correlations. *Invest Ophthalmol Vis Sci.* (2018) 59:5149–56. doi: 10.1167/iovs.18-24690
21. Lemp MA. Report of the national eye institute/industry workshop on clinical trials in dry eyes. *CLAO J.* (1995) 21:221–32.
22. Bron AJ, Evans VE, Smith JA. Grading of corneal and conjunctival staining in the context of other dry eye tests. *Cornea.* (2003) 22:640–50. doi: 10.1097/00003226-200310000-00008
23. Aragona P, Aguennouz M, Rania L, Postorino E, Sommario MS, Roszkowska AM, et al. Matrix metalloproteinase 9 and transglutaminase 2 expression at the ocular surface in patients with different forms of dry eye disease. *Ophthalmology.* (2015) 122:62–71. doi: 10.1016/j.ophtha.2014.07.048
24. Tomlinson A, Bron AJ, Korb DR, Amano S, Paugh JR, Pearce EI, et al. The international workshop on meibomian gland dysfunction: report of the diagnosis subcommittee. *Invest Ophthalmol Vis Sci.* (2011) 52:2006–49. doi: 10.1167/iovs.10-6997f
25. Jabeen S, Espinoza JA, Torland LA, Zucknick M, Kumar S, Haakensen VD, et al. Noninvasive profiling of serum cytokines in breast cancer patients and clinicopathological characteristics. *Oncoimmunology.* (2019) 8:e1537691. doi: 10.1080/2162402X.2018.1537691
26. Boshtam M, Asgary S, Kouhpayeh S, Shariati L, Khanahmad H. Aptamers against pro- and anti-inflammatory cytokines: a review. *Inflammation.* (2017) 40:340–9. doi: 10.1007/s10753-016-0477-1
27. Tiskaoglu NS, Yazici A, Karlidere T, Sari E, Oguz EY, Musaoglu M, et al. Dry eye disease in patients with newly diagnosed depressive disorder. *Curr Eye Res.* (2017) 42:672–6. doi: 10.1080/02713683.2016.1236966
28. Kim KW, Han SB, Han ER, Woo SJ, Lee JJ, Yoon JC, et al. Association between depression and dry eye disease in an elderly population. *Invest Ophthalmol Vis Sci.* (2011) 52:7954–8. doi: 10.1167/iovs.11-8050
29. McMonnies CW. Why the symptoms and objective signs of dry eye disease may not correlate. *J Optom.* (2021) 14:3–10. doi: 10.1016/j.optom.2020.10.002
30. Ulusoy MO, Işik-Ulusoy S, Kivanç SA. Evaluation of dry eye disease in newly diagnosed anxiety and depression patients using anterior segment optical coherence tomography. *Eye Vis.* (2019) 6:25. doi: 10.1186/s40662-019-0149-y
31. Sadykov E, Studnička J, Hosák L, Siligardou MR, Elfurjani H, Hoikam JL, et al. The interface between psychiatry and ophthalmology. *Acta Medica.* (2019) 62:45–51. doi: 10.14712/18059694.2019.104
32. Choy BNK, Ng ALK, Shum JWH, Fan MCY, Lai JSM. A case report: anti-psychotic agents related ocular toxicity. *Medicine.* (2016) 95:e3360. doi: 10.1097/MD.0000000000003360
33. Jakubaschk J, Böker W. Disorders of pain perception in schizophrenia. *Schweiz Arch Neurol Psychiatr.* (1985). 142:55–76.
34. Goldsmith DR, Rapaport MH, Miller BJ. A meta-analysis of blood cytokine network alterations in psychiatric patients: comparisons between schizophrenia, bipolar disorder and depression. *Mol Psychiatry.* (2016) 21:1696–709. doi: 10.1038/mp.2016.3
35. Reale M, Costantini E, Greig NH. Cytokine Imbalance in Schizophrenia. From research to clinic: potential implications for treatment. *Front Psychiatry.* (2021) 12:536257. doi: 10.3389/fpsyt.2021.536257
36. Toyooka K, Watanabe Y, Iritani S, Shimizu E, Iyo M, Nakamura R, et al. A decrease in interleukin-1 receptor antagonist expression in the prefrontal cortex of schizophrenic patients. *Neurosci Res.* (2003) 46:299–307. doi: 10.1016/S0168-0102(03)00093-2
37. Stuart MJ, Baune BT. Chemokines and chemokine receptors in mood disorders, schizophrenia, and cognitive impairment: a systematic review of biomarker studies. *Neurosci Biobehav Rev.* (2014) 42:93–115. doi: 10.1016/j.neubiorev.2014.02.001
38. Teixeira AL, Reis HJ, Nicolato R, Brito-Melo G, Correa H, Teixeira MM, et al. Increased serum levels of CCL11/eotaxin in schizophrenia. *Prog Neuropsychopharmacol Biol Psychiatry.* (2008) 32:710–4. doi: 10.1016/j.pnpbp.2007.11.019
39. Lepeta K, Kaczmarek L. Matrix metalloproteinase-9 as a novel player in synaptic plasticity and schizophrenia. *Schizophr Bull.* (2015) 41:1003–9. doi: 10.1093/schbul/sbv036
40. Rahimi S, Sayad A, Moslemi E, Ghafouri-Fard S, Taheri M. Blood assessment of the expression levels of matrix metalloproteinase 9 (MMP9) and its natural inhibitor, TIMP1 genes in Iranian schizophrenic patients. *Metab Brain Dis.* (2017) 32:1537–42. doi: 10.1007/s11011-017-0043-z
41. Roda M, Corazza I, Bacchi Reggiani ML, Pellegrini M, Taroni L, Giannaccare G, et al. Dry eye disease and tear cytokine levels-a meta-analysis. *Int J Mol Sci.* (2020) 21:3111. doi: 10.3390/ijms21093111
42. Massingale ML Li X, Vallabhajosyula M, Chen D, Wei Y, Asbell PA. Analysis of inflammatory cytokines in the tears of dry eye patients. *Cornea.* (2009) 28:1023–7. doi: 10.1097/ICO.0b013e3181a16578
43. Zhao H, Li Q, Ye M, Yu J. Tear luminex analysis in dry eye patients. *Med Sci Monit.* (2018) 24:7595–602. doi: 10.12659/MSM.912010
44. Mrugacz M, Ostrowska L, Bryl A, Szulc A, Zelazowska-Rutkowska B, Mrugacz G. Pro-inflammatory cytokines associated with clinical severity of dry eye disease of patients with depression. *Adv Med Sci.* (2017) 62:338–44. doi: 10.1016/j.advms.2017.03.003
45. Ramamoorthy P, Khanal SJJN. Inflammatory proteins associated wit contact lens-related dry eye. *Cont Lens Anterior Eye.* (2021) 3:101442. doi: 10.1016/j.clae.2021.101442
46. Okanobo A, Chauhan SK, Dastjerdi MH, Kodati S, Dana R. Efficacy of topical blockade of interleukin-1 in experimental dry eye disease. *Am J Ophthalmol.* (2012) 154:63–71. doi: 10.1016/j.ajo.2012.01.034
47. Na KS, Mok JW, Kim JY, Rho CR, Joo CK. Correlations between tea cytokines, chemokines, and soluble receptors and clinical severit of dry eye disease. *Invest Ophthalmol Vis Sci.* (2012) 53:5443–50. doi: 10.1167/iovs.11-9417

48. Lam H, Bleiden L, de Paiva CS, Farley W, Stern ME, Pflugfelder SC. Tear cytokine profiles in dysfunctional tear syndrome. *Am J Ophthalmol.* (2009) 147:198–205.e1. doi: 10.1016/j.ajo.2008.08.032
49. Bron AJ, de Paiva CS, Chauhan SK, Bonini S, Gabison EE, Jain S, et al. TFOS DEWS II pathophysiology report. *Ocul Surf.* (2017) 15:438–510. doi: 10.1016/j.jtos.2017.05.011
50. Lanza NL, Valenzuela F, Perez VL, Galor A. The matrix metalloproteinase 9 point-of-care test in dry eye. *Ocul Surf.* (2016) 14:189–95. doi: 10.1016/j.jtos.2015.10.004
51. Sendon-Lago J, Seoane S, Martinez-Ordoñez A, Eiro N, Saa J, Vizoso FJ, et al. Corneal regeneration by conditioned medium of human uterine cervical stem cells is mediated by TIMP-1 and TIMP-2. *Exp Eye Res.* (2019) 180:110–21. doi: 10.1016/j.exer.2018.12.004
52. Khamar P, Nair AP, Shetty R, Vaidya T, Subramani M, Ponnalagu M, et al. Dysregulated tear fluid nociception-associated factors, corneal dendritic cell density, and vitamin D levels in evaporative dry eye. *Invest Ophthalmol Vis Sci.* (2019) 60:2532–42. doi: 10.1167/iovs.19-26914
53. Chotikavanich S, de Paiva CS Li de Q, Chen JJ, Bian F, Farley WJ, et al. Production and activity of matrix metalloproteinase-9 on the ocular surface increase in dysfunctional tear syndrome. *Invest Ophthalmol Vis Sci.* (2009) 50:3203–9. doi: 10.1167/iovs.08-2476
54. Shetty R, Sethu S, Chevour P, Deshpande K, Pahuja N, Nagaraja H, et al. Lower vitamin D level and distinct tear cytokine profile were observed in patients with mild dry eye signs but exaggerated symptoms. *Transl Vis Sci Technol.* (2016) 5:16. doi: 10.1167/tvst.5.6.16
55. Perez VL, Pflugfelder SC, Zhang S, Shojaei A, Haque R. Lifitegrast, a novel integrin antagonist for treatment of dry eye disease. *Ocul Surf.* (2016) 14:207–15. doi: 10.1016/j.jtos.2016.01.001
56. Nair S, Vanathi M, Mahapatra M, Seth T, Kaur J, Velpandian T, et al. Tear inflammatory mediators and protein in eyes of post allogenic hematopoeitic stem cell transplant patients. *Ocul Surf.* (2018) 16:352–67. doi: 10.1016/j.jtos.2018.04.007
57. Li Q, Liu J, Liu C, Piao J, Yang W, An N, et al. Effects of intense pulsed light treatment on tear cytokines and clinical outcomes in meibomian gland dysfunction. *PLoS ONE.* (2021) 16:e0256533. doi: 10.1371/journal.pone.0256533
58. Jackson DC, Zeng W, Wong CY, Mifsud EJ, Williamson NA, Ang CS, et al. Tear interferon-gamma as a biomarker for evaporative dry eye disease. *Invest Ophthalmol Vis Sci.* (2016) 57:4824–30. doi: 10.1167/iovs.16-19757
59. Wang S, Zhang H. Upregulation of the IL-33/ST2 pathway in dry eye. *Mol Vis.* (2019) 25:583–92.
60. Luo G, Xin Y, Qin D, Yan A, Zhou Z, Liu Z. Correlation of interleukin-33 with Th cytokines and clinical severity of dry eye disease. *Indian J Ophthalmol.* (2018) 66:39–43. doi: 10.4103/ijo.IJO_405_17
61. Jie Y, Sella R, Feng J, Gomez ML, Afshari NA. Evaluation of incomplete blinking as a measurement of dry eye disease. *Ocul Surf.* (2019) 17:440–6. doi: 10.1016/j.jtos.2019.05.007
62. Xu L, Zhang W, Zhu XY, Suo T, Fan XQ, Fu Y. Smoking and the risk of dry eye: a meta-analysis. *Int J Ophthalmol.* (2016) 9:1480–6. doi: 10.18240/ijo.2016.10.19

6

Semiautomated and Automated Quantitative Analysis of Corneal Sub-Basal Nerves in Patients With DED With Ocular Pain Using IVCM

*Yu Zhang, Yaying Wu, Wenbo Li and Xiaodan Huang**

Eye Center, School of Medicine, The Second Affiliated Hospital of Zhejiang University, Hangzhou, China

Correspondence:
Xiaodan Huang
huangxiaodan@zju.edu.cn

Purpose: Investigate the correlation and agreement between the results of semiautomated and fully automated quantitative analysis of the corneal sub-basal nerve plexus (SNP) in patients with dry eye disease (DED) with ocular pain using *in vivo* confocal microscopy (IVCM).

Method: A total of 50 voluntary participants were enrolled in this study, i.e., 25 DED patients with ocular pain and 25 healthy controls. Each patient underwent an evaluation of ocular symptoms that utilized: the Ocular Surface Disease Index (OSDI), the Ocular Pain Assessment Survey (OPAS), the tear film breakup time (TBUT) test, the Schirmer test, corneal staining, and IVCM. Five SNP images of the cornea of each eye were selected and analyzed using a semiautomated analysis software (NeuronJ) and a fully automated method (ACCMetrics) to quantify corneal nerve fiber density (CNFD), corneal nerve branch density (CNBD), and corneal nerve fiber length (CNFL).

Results: The intraclass correlation coefficient (ICC) of the CNFD (0.460 [0.382–0.532], $p < 0.001$), CNBD (0.608 [0.545–0.665], $p < 0.001$), and CNFL (0.851 [0.822–0.875], $p < 0.001$) represents the repeatability and consistency of measurements by the NeuronJ and ACCMetrics software. The CNFL values ($r = 0.881$, $p < 0.001$) obtained using the two methods have extremely high correlation, and similarly, the CNFD values ($r = 0.669$, $p < 0.001$) and CNBD values ($r = 0.703$, $p < 0.001$) are highly correlated. The CNFL had the biggest area under the curve (AUC; 0.747 [0.700–0.793], $p < 0.001$) when using ACCMetrics. In DED patients with ocular pain, the mean CNFD values for semiautomated and fully automated quantization were 23.5 ± 8.1 and 23.8 ± 8.6 n/mm^2; the mean CNBD values were 46.0 ± 21.3, 35.7 ± 23.3 n/mm^2; and the mean CNFL values were 19.3 ± 4.3 and 15.2 ± 3.8 mm/mm^2, which were significantly lower than healthy subjects ($p < 0.001$).

Conclusion: There is a significant correlation between the measurements obtained via ACCMetrics and NeuronJ, especially for CNFL, which can be considered as the primary indicator in the diagnosis of DED with ocular pain. The SNP of the disease was significantly lower than that of healthy subjects.

Keywords: dry eye disease, ocular pain, *in vivo* confocal microscopy, corneal subbasal nerve plexus, NeuronJ, ACCMetrics

INTRODUCTION

Dry eye disease (DED) is one of the most often reported ocular diseases, with a global incidence of 5–50% by symptoms (1–3). Ocular surface inflammation and injury, tear film instability, hyperosmolarity, and neurosensory abnormalities are all factors that contribute to DED, as defined by the International Dry Eye Workshop in 2017 (4). Along with abnormalities of the tear film and ocular surface, the revised DED criteria include neurosensory dysfunction as a contributing component. Ocular pain, such as burning, aching, and itching, is a frequent symptom of moderate-to-severe DED. It is commonly accepted that DED combined with ocular pain alters the structure and function of the ocular surface's sensory nerves, resulting in the appearance of unpleasant sensations ranging from mild discomfort and dryness to scorching pain (5).

With an abundant supply of nerve fibers, the cornea is one of the most highly innervated tissues in the body. The human cornea is filled with sensory nerve fibers originating from the trigeminal nerve's ophthalmic branch and sympathetic and parasympathetic nerve fibers. Nerve fibers in the human cornea flow radially from the periphery of the anterior part of the stroma to its center. These nerve fibers penetrate the Bowman's layer and then branch vertically and horizontally between the epithelium of the Bowman's layer and the basal epithelium to create a network of nerve fibers known as the sub-basal nerve plexus (SNP) (6). Numerous scientific investigations have been conducted on the corneal nerve's structural and functional anomalies in the setting of a range of ocular and systemic illnesses (7).

Corneal *in vivo* confocal microscopy (IVCM) is a noninvasive technique for obtaining high-resolution images of the SNP at the cellular level with image quality equivalent to that obtained using histochemical techniques. Oliveira-Soto and Efron were the first to utilize IVCM to describe corneal nerves (8). Previous research has revealed variations in the morphology of the corneal nerves in patients having DED, such as considerably decreased nerve density and relatively high reflectivity, beading, and tortuosity. Shetty et al. observed a substantial reduction in SNP characteristics (corneal nerve fiber length [CNFL], fiber density, fiber width, total branch density, nerve branch density, and fiber area) in DED with ocular pain patients (9). Yavuz-Saricay et al. discovered a significant decrease in main and branch nerve densities, an increase in dendritic cell density, and the existence of microneuromas in DED patients with ocular pain (10).

Notwithstanding the growing use of IVCM in DED clinical practice, there have only been a few pertinent advances in available software tools that facilitate automated corneal nerve analysis. To date, the majority of IVCM image analyses of corneal nerves have been performed manually or semiautomatically, which has a lot of drawbacks, such as being time-consuming, subjective, prone to observer bias, and having low repeatability and consistency (6). According to the latest the dry eye workShop II (DEWS II) of the tear film and ocular surface society (TFOS) Pain and Sensation Subcommittee Report, automating quantitative IVCM assessments would significantly improve research technique and interpretation of the results (5).

At the present, quantitative applications for evaluating corneal nerves range from fully manual (CCMetrics, University of Manchester, Manchester, UK) to semiautomated (NeuronJ, with ImageJ plugin, National Institutes of Health, Bethesda, MA, USA) to fully automated (ACCMetrics, University of Manchester, Manchester, UK), all of which generate varying degrees of quantitative nerve evaluation (11). Due to the laborious and time-consuming nature of applying fully automated CCMetrics software, the fully automated CCMetrics approach has been replaced with the semiautomated NeuronJ technique (12). The NeuronJ software traces the structure of the nerve semiautomatically with a smooth line, providing total length measurements. However, the operator's ability to discern the nerve's beginning and end impacts the accuracy of the measurements (13). ACCMetrics is a fully automated image analysis program that reduces the time required to evaluate an image to 15 s per image. ACCMetrics evaluates neural morphometric characteristics, such as corneal nerve fiber density (CNFD), CNFL, and corneal nerve branch density (CNBD), and nerve fiber total branch density, nerve fiber area, and nerve fiber width. As a result, it is particularly advantageous for major studies analyzing a massive amount of IVCM images (14).

The objective of this study is to evaluate the diagnostic performance of ACCMetrics, a fully automated software, with that of NeuronJ, a semiautomated program, in distinguishing patients with DED with ocular pain from healthy controls via IVCM morphometric analysis of the corneal SNP. The correlations between DED with ocular pain and several characteristics of the corneal SNP, such as the CNFD, CNBD, and CNFL, were also investigated to identify which was the more significant diagnostic parameter.

MATERIALS AND METHODS

Subjects

We conducted this prospective observational study in 2019 and 2020 at the outpatient clinics of the Second Affiliated Hospital, Zhejiang University School of Medicine, in adherence to the precepts of the Declaration of Helsinki. The study was authorized by the Ethics Committee of the Second Affiliated Hospital at Zhejiang University School of Medicine (2019-283). All participants freely signed an informed consent form. A total of 50 participants comprised DED patients (n = 25) and healthy controls ($n = 25$).

An OSDI score of $\geq$13 points, a Schirmer I test score of $<$10 mm/5 min, and a tear film breakup time (TBUT) of $<$10 s, associated with Ocular Pain Assessment Survey (OPAS) scores of 10–27, were used as diagnostic criteria for DED with ocular pain.

An OSDI score of $<$7 points, a Schirmer I test score of $\geq$10 mm/5 min, or a TBUT score of $\geq$10 s, associated with OPAS scores of 0–9, is considered healthy.

Individuals who met the following criteria were all excluded from the study: (1) inability or unwillingness to sign an informed consent form, (2) a history of eye surgery, (3) a history of wearing contact lenses during the previous 30 days, (4) a history of eye diseases other than DED, (5) a history of using any eye medication other than eye lubricant during the previous 3 months, and (6) severe systemic disease.

In vivo Confocal Microscopy

In this study, all participants underwent an IVCM examination. The remote center of motion (RCM) module of the *in vivo* confocal microscope (HRT-3, Heidelberg Engineering GmbH, Heidelberg, Germany) was used to observe the center of the corneal epithelium. The IVCM has a helium-neon diode laser with a wavelength of 670 nm, a ×60 objective lens (Olympus, Tokyo, Japan), a numerical aperture of 0.9, and a working distance of 0.0–3.0 mm relative to the flat cap (Tomo-Cap, Heidelberg Engineering GmbH, Germany). The images were two-dimensional, with a field size of 400 × 400 μm and a resolution of 384 × 384 pixels. An expert technician performed all operations. Before beginning the examination, the technician placed a drop of carbomer gel (Bausch & Lomb, Germany) on the microscope lens and then covered it with a disposable corneal contact cap. Next, a drop of topical anesthetic was applied to the eye (Proparacaine Hydrochloride Eye Drops, Alcon, United States), and the participant was instructed to place their chin and forehead in a bracket. Participants were instructed to look at a blip of light directly from the machine in front of them. The lens was zeroed out before being pushed toward the cornea of the participant's eye. The SNP of the cornea was then targeted at a depth of 50–80 μm. The participants were then instructed to move their center of attention across their visual field to capture images of the corneal nerves from the central, upper, lower, nasal, and temporal orientations. A minimum of five clean, wrinkle-free, nonoverlapping, and representative photos were taken in each direction. The five most representative photos for each eye were selected and examined using NeuronJ and ACCMetrics. NeuronJ is a Java-based image analysis software package that includes a nerve-tracing plugin module. ACCMetrics is a software application for autonomous image analysis and processing developed by the University of Manchester in Manchester, United Kingdom. All images were manually assessed using NeuronJ by two experienced *blind observers* (YZ and WL). CNFD, CNBD, and CNFL were chosen as measurement indicators.

Ocular Surface Disease Index (OSDI)

The OSDI consists of six questions on visual disturbance and visual function. Each response is graded on a 5-point scale, with the total OSDI score ranging from 0 (no symptoms) to 100 (maximum symptoms). Patients with a score >13 are diagnosed with symptomatic DED.

Ocular Pain Assessment Survey

We assessed average eye pain severity and frequency, aggravating causes, related factors, and symptomatic alleviation over the preceding 2 weeks using a 32-question ocular pain questionnaire designed by Yureeda Qazi using numerical rating scales (15).

Tear Film Breakup Time

The TBUT test assesses the amount of time between a full blink and the appearance of the first tear film break.

Corneal Fluorescein Staining

Corneal fluorescein staining was conducted after the TBUT test. The Oxford Scale was used to assess corneal stains under a yellow filter. Positive scores were defined as those that exceeded zero points.

Statistics

All statistical analyses, excluding Bland-Altman plots, were conducted using version 26 of the IBM Statistical Package for the Social Sciences (SPSS) software package for Windows (IBM, Chicago, IL, USA). Bland-Altman plots were created via an online website: https://spssau.com. IVCM and SPSS were used to construct the figures used in this study. The descriptive statistics are summarized as mean ± SD. A Kolmogorov-Smirnov test was used to assess the normality of continuous variables, and the Bland-Altman plots were employed to determine the interobserver agreement between the measurements. The repeatability and reproducibility values were calculated in terms of mean bias and 95% limits of agreement (LoA). The intraclass correlation coefficient (ICC) was determined as an index of repeatability and reproducibility between measurements. Paired *t*-tests were used to assess the differences between the two sets of measurements being compared. The receiver operating characteristic (ROC) curve, area under the ROC curve (AUC), cutoff point, sensitivity, and specificity were also calculated. Correlation between the results obtained using NeuronJ and ACCMetrics was explored using logarithmic Pearson's correlation coefficient (r). The analysis was double-sided, and a $p < 0.05$ was considered statistically significant.

RESULTS

Demographics and Medical Status

A total of 50 voluntary participants were enrolled in this study, comprising 25 patients with DED with ocular pain (7 men and 18 women, mean age: 43.8 ± 14.7 years) and 25 healthy controls (6 men and 19 women, mean age: 44.2 ± 11.0 years). The clinical test results of patients with DED with ocular pain were as follows: average pain time of 1.89 ± 1.1 years, average OSDI score of 62.73 ± 20.73, average OPAS score of 12.84 ± 5.77, average TBUT of 2.24 ± 1.27 s, average Schirmer test score of 8.18 ± 7.36

TABLE 1 | The intraclass correlation coefficient (ICC) for measurements of NeuronJ and ACCMetrics.

ICC	Neuron J		ACCMetrics	
	Interobserver	*p* value	Comparison with NeuronJ*	*p* value
CNFD	0.933 (0.914–0.948)	<0.001	0.460 (0.382–0.532)	<0.001
CNBD	0.921 (0.898–0.938)	<0.001	0.608 (0.545–0.665)	<0.001
CNFL	0.918 (0.895–0.937)	<0.001	0.851 (0.822–0.875)	<0.001

Comparisons between ACCMetrics and mean measurements from two observers. Results are expressed as mean ± SD, statistically significant difference using ANOVA. In brackets are the 95% CIs.

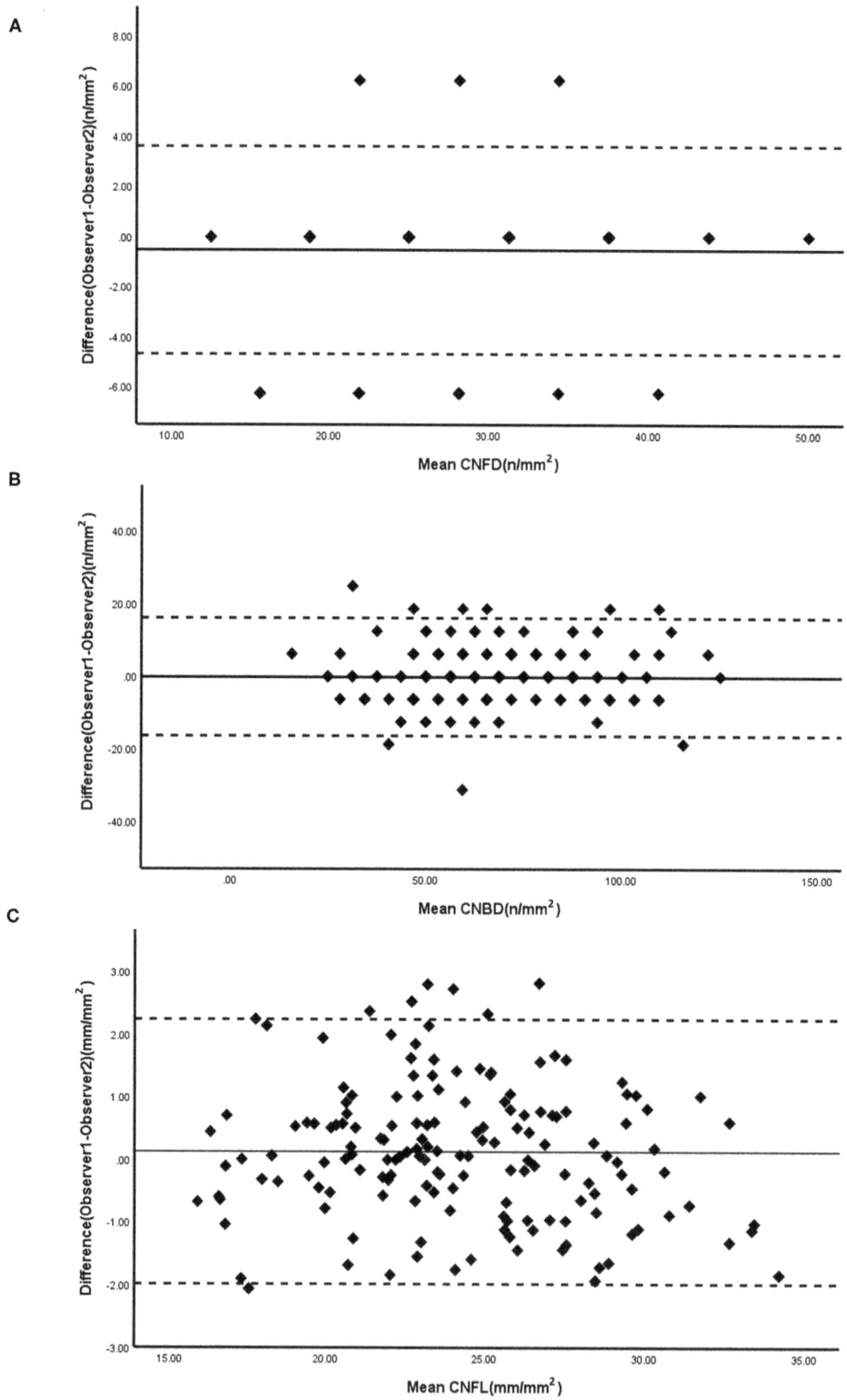

FIGURE 1 | Bland-Altman plots for CNFD **(A)**, CNBD **(B)**, and CNFL **(C)** were measured by two masked observers. Solid line, mean difference; Dashed lines, 95% CI. CNFD, corneal nerve fiber density; CNBD, corneal nerve branch density; CNFL, corneal nerve fiber length.

mm/5', and average corneal staining score of 1.89 ± 1.59. These indicators were within normal limits in the healthy controls.

Interobserver Agreement for NeuronJ and ACCMetrics Measurements

All the images were measured by two blind observers (YZ and WL), semiautomatically using NeuronJ and automatically using ACCMetrics.

Table 1 presents a summary of the ICC for interobserver measures obtained using NeuronJ and ACCMetrics to show the amount of agreement between the two observers. As can be seen in **Table 1**, all three parameters had an excellent interobserver agreement. With an ICC value of 0.933 (95% CI: 0.914–0.948, $p < 0.001$), CNFD had the most agreement, followed by CNBD, with an ICC value of 0.921 (95% CI: 0.898–0.938, $p < 0.001$), and CNFL, with an ICC value of 0.918 (95% CI: 0.895–0.937, $p < 0.001$).

Figure 1 presents Bland-Altman plots of differences vs. the averages of the CNFD, CNBD, and CNFL in images of the healthy controls obtained by the blind observers, YZ and WL. The solid lines indicate the average difference, while the dashed lines represent the 95% LoA. The mean difference (±SD) between the two observers was as follows: CNFD, −0.533 ± 2.113; CNBD, 0.147 ± 5.202; and CNFL, 0.130 ± 1.078. The coefficients of repeatability (CoR) for CNFD, CNBD, and CNFL were 4.262, 10.176, and 2.121, respectively.

Differences in CNFD, CNBD, and CNFL Between the Semiautomated and Automated Methods

A total of 500 images obtained from the entire cohort were analyzed using NeuronJ and ACCMetrics. The data on CNFD, CNBD, and CNFL are presented in **Table 2**. The mean CNFDs quantified via NeuronJ and ACCMetrics were 25.0 ± 7.6 and 27.4 ± 9.4 n/mm^2, respectively (paired-samples *t*-test, $t = -5.619$, $p < 0.001$). The mean CNBDs quantified via NeuronJ and ACCMetrics were 57.1 ± 23.3 and 41.1 ± 24.2 n/mm^2, respectively (paired-samples *t*-test, $t = 15.740$, $p < 0.001$), and the mean CNFL quantified via NeuronJ and ACCMetrics were 21.6 ± 4.7 and 17.0 ± 4.0 mm/mm^2, respectively (paired-samples *t*-test, $t = 40.385$, $p < 0.001$). As can be seen in **Table 2**, there is a substantial difference between the results obtained *via* the two strategies. The CNFD calculated by ACCMetrics was significantly higher than that assessed via NeuronJ, while the CNBD and CNFL estimated by ACCMetrics were clearly lower than those calculated via NeuronJ.

TABLE 2 | Mean ± SD of parameters of the entire cohort measured by NeuronJ and ACCMetrics.

TOTAL	NeuronJ	ACCMetrics	t Value	*p* Value
CNFD (n/mm^2)	25.0 ± 7.6	27.4 ± 9.4	−5.619	<0.001
CNBD (n/mm^2)	57.1 ± 23.3	41.1 ± 24.2	15.740	<0.001
CNFL (mm/mm^2)	21.6 ± 4.7	17.0 ± 4.0	40.385	<0.001

Results are expressed as mean ± SD.

As illustrated in **Figure 2**, the nerve fibers traced in NeuronJ are colored purple, and NeuronJ is capable of calculating the sum of the fiber lengths (CNFL). However, the CNFD and CNBD values need to be manually recorded by the observers. In the images analyzed using ACCMetrics, CNFD values were traced in red, CNBD values were denoted as green dots, and CNFL is the sum of all nerve tracings, i.e., red-colored tracings and blue-colored tracings. To a certain extent, some of the CNBD and CNFL values were not detected and are indicated by arrows and circles in the images.

Agreement in CNFD, CNBD, and CNFL Between NeuronJ and ACCMetrics

Table 1 presents a summary of the ICC for the two methods: NeuronJ and ACCMetrics. An ICC value of 0.460 (95% CI: 0.382–0.532, $p < 0.001$) was the lowest value for the CNFD. The CNBD has an ICC value of 0.608 (95% CI: 0.545–0.665, $p < 0.001$), while the CNFL has an ICC value of 0.851 (95% CI: 0.822–0.875, $p < 0.001$). We can speculate that the CNFL has strong agreement and repeatability.

The scatterplots (**Figure 3**) of the CNFD, CNBD, and CNFL showed correlations between NeuronJ and ACCMetrics. The CNFD values ($r = 0.471$, $p < 0.001$) are moderately related, the CNBD values ($r = 0.609$, $p < 0.001$) are strongly related, and the CNFL values ($r = 0.864$, $p < 0.001$) are highly related, based on manual and automated analysis.

The Bland-Altman plots (**Figure 4**) for the CNFD, CNBD, and CNFL present the agreements between the results obtained via NeuronJ and ACCMetrics. The results show differences in CNFD (−2.4 ± 8.9), CNBD (16.0 ± 21.0), and CNFL (4.7 ± 2.4); the 95% LoA of CNFD (−19.903 - 15.058), CNBD (−25.207 - 57.193), and CNFL (−0.013 - 9.348); and the repeatability coefficient (RC) of CNFD (18.094), CNBD (51.730), and CNFL (10.273). The majority of the scatter plots fall within the 95% CI, indicating that the two detection methods are consistent.

The ROC curves and relevant analysis convincingly demonstrate the ability of each parameter to diagnose DED with ocular pain. **Table 3** presents a summary of the AUC, cutoff, sensitivity, and specificity values, while **Figure 5** presents the ROC curves. Using ACCMetrics, the CNFL most effectively distinguishes patients with DED with ocular pain from healthy controls (AUC = 0.747 [0.700–0.793], cutoff = 0.384, sensitivity = 0.884, specificity = 0.500, $p < 0.001$). Using NeuronJ, the CNBD had the highest AUC of 0.773 (0.728–0.818), followed by the CNFL (0.769 [0.725–0.813]) and CNFD (0.608 [0.555–0.662]).

Significantly Lower CNFD, CNBD, and CNFL in Patients With DED With Ocular Pain Than in Healthy Controls *via* Both NeuronJ and ACCMetrics

To investigate the correlation between SNP and patients with DED with ocular pain, we compared the mean differences

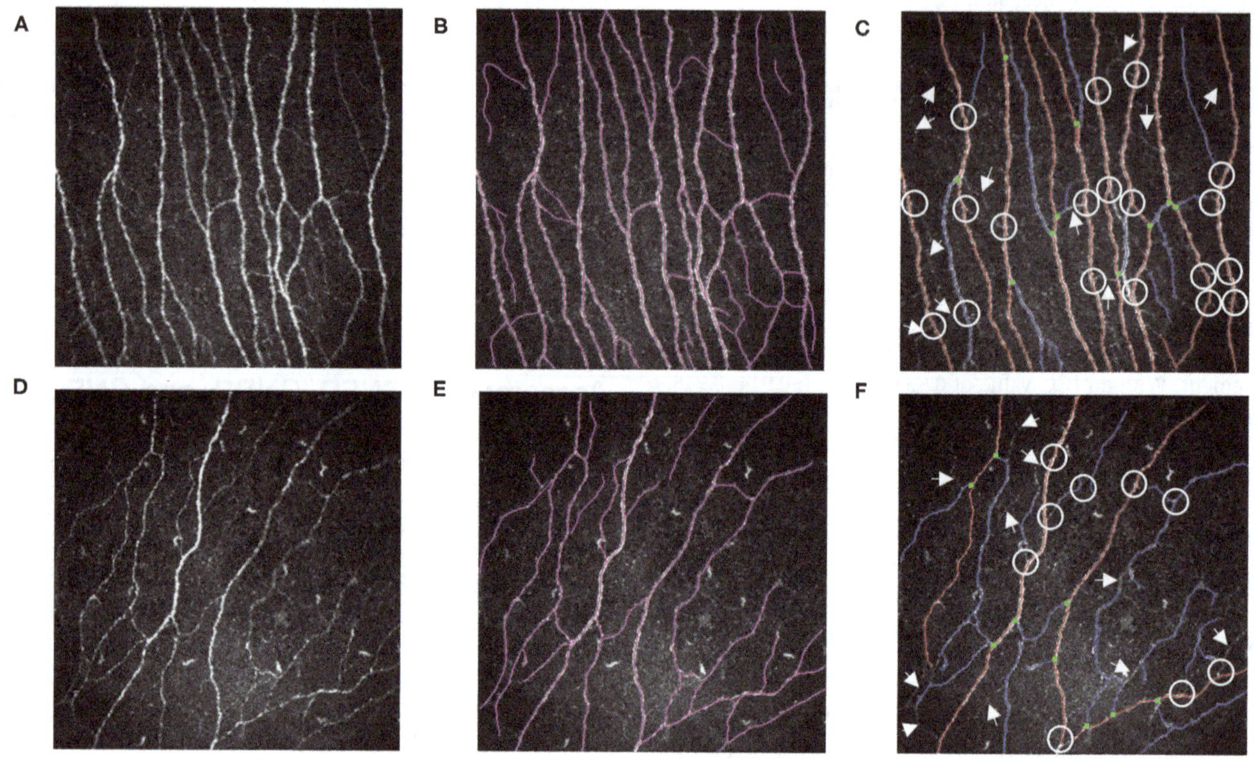

FIGURE 2 | Illustrations are examples of SNP measurements. **(A)** A representative raw IVCM image from a healthy control and **(D)** a patient of DED with ocular pain. **(B,E)** were measured by NeuronJ; **(C,F)** were automatically analyzed by ACCMetrics. Nerve fibers which failed to be identified were marked as arrows. Nerve branches that were unable to be detected were marked as circles. DED, dry eye disease; SNP, sub-basal nerve plexus; IVCM, *in vivo* confocal microscopy.

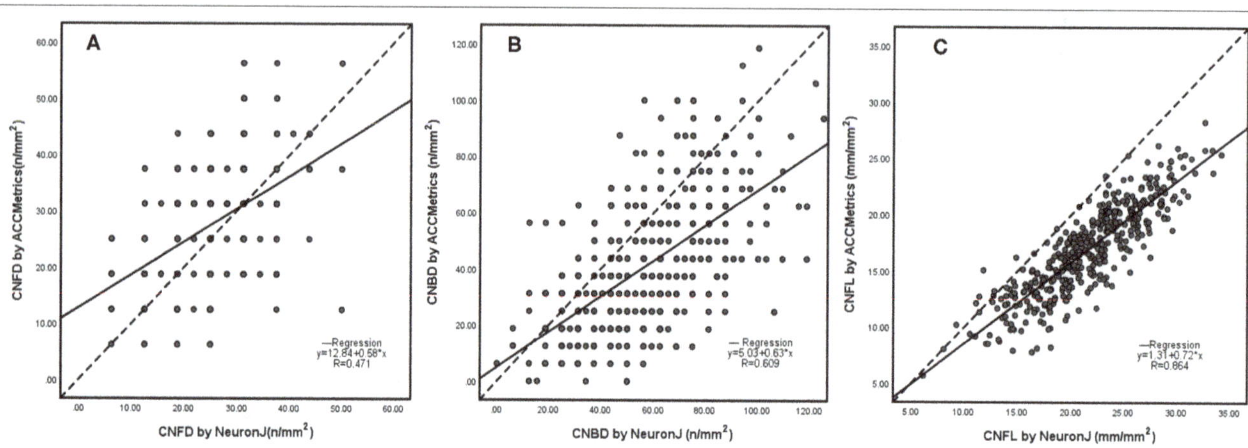

FIGURE 3 | Scatterplots of CNFD **(A)**, CNBD **(B)**, and CNFL **(C)** using NeuronJ vs. ACCmetrics on the whole images ($n = 500$). CNFD, corneal nerve fiber density; CNBD, corneal nerve branch density; CNFL, corneal nerve fiber length.

between the results obtained using NeuronJ and ACCMetrics for healthy controls and DED with ocular pain patients. As illustrated in **Table 4**, the patients with DED with ocular pain had significantly fewer SNP than healthy controls. When using NeuronJ, the values for the CNFD, CNBD, and CNFL were 26.5 ± 6.9 vs. 23.5 ± 8.1 n/mm^2, $p < 0.001$; 67.0 ± 20.4 vs. 46.0 ± 21.3 n/mm^2, $p < 0.001$; and 23.7 ± 4.1 vs. 19.3 ± 4.3 mm/mm^2, $p < 0.001$, respectively. When ACCMetrics is utilized, the values for CNFD, CNBD, and CNFL were 30.7 ± 8.9 vs. 23.8 ± 8.6 n/mm^2, $p < 0.001$; 46.0 ± 24.0 vs. 35.7 ± 23.3 n/mm^2, $p < 0.001$; and 18.6 ± 3.4 vs. 15.2 ± 3.8 mm/mm^2, $p < 0.001$, respectively.

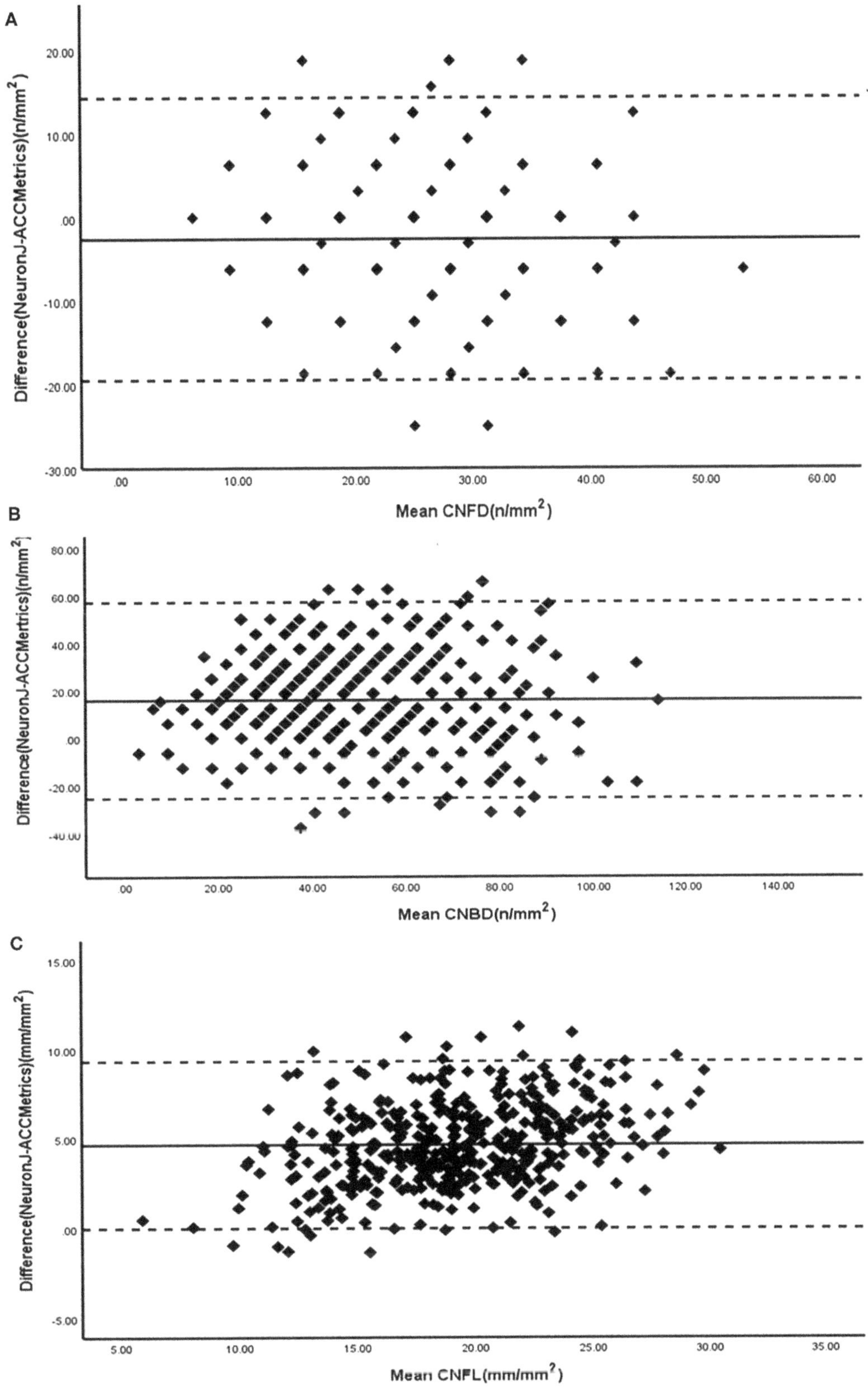

FIGURE 4 | Bland-Altman plots for CNFD **(A)**, CNBD **(B)**, and CNFL **(C)** measured by NeuronJ and ACCMetrics. Solid lines, mean difference; Dashed lines, 95% CI. CNFD, corneal nerve fiber density; CNBD, corneal nerve branch density; CNFL, corneal nerve fiber length.

TABLE 3 | AUC indicators for the discrimination of DED with ocular pain.

Parameter	AUC & 95%CI	Cutoff	Sensitivity	Specificity	*p* Value
ACCMetrics -CNFD	0.705 (0.656–0.754)	0.328	0.609	0.719	<0.001
ACCMetrics -CNBD	0.629 (0.577–0.682)	0.183	0.631	0.552	<0.001
ACCMetrics -CNFL	0.747 (0.700–0.793)	0.384	0.884	0.500	<0.001
NeuronJ–CNFD	0.608 (0.555–0.662)	0.177	0.409	0.768	<0.001
NeuronJ–CNBD	0.773 (0.728–0.818)	0.490	0.889	0.601	<0.001
NeuronJ–CNFL	0.769 (0.725–0.813)	0.420	0.791	0.629	<0.001

AUC, area under the ROC curve; DED, dry eye disease.

DISCUSSION

In this study, we compared two distinct assessment techniques for IVCM images and the difference in SNP between DED with ocular pain patients and healthy subjects. We used ACCMetrics, a fully automated measurement software, and NeuronJ, a semiautomated method, to identify SNP and detect ocular pain symptoms associated with DED with ocular pain.

Previous research studies have shown that patients with DED with ocular pain have fewer SNP than healthy controls and that ACCMetrics can partially replace the manual method. The semiautomated measurements were particularly well correlated with the measurements obtained via the manual methods for the same image (16). According to a study by Giannaccare et al., the ACCMetrics software can detect alternations in SNP and distinguish DED patients (6). In patients with DED with ocular pain, Kheirkhah et al. discovered a significantly low number and density of sub-basal nerves (17). However, research studies on the relationship between SNP and ocular pain symptoms in DED with ocular pain patients, and the corresponding measurement indicators, were hard to obtain. Simultaneously, it is necessary to demonstrate the specific efficacy of fully automated software over the traditional method.

The ACCMetrics software can partially replace semiautomated methods (18). The traditional semiautomated method has a high ICC and CoR between observers for the CNFD, CNBD, and CNFL (**Table 1** and **Figure 1**). In **Table 1**, it can also be seen that the CNFL (ICC $= 0.851$, $p < 0.001$) has the highest ICC between ACCMetrics and Neuron J, whereas the CNBD (ICC $= 0.608$, $p < 0.001$) has a medium ICC. Between the two methods, the CNFL has the highest correlation ($r = 0.864$, $p < 0.001$), followed by the CNBD ($r = 0.609$, $p < 0.001$). The difference in the CNFL (4.7 ± 2.4) is apparent on the Bland-Altman plot, and the majority of the scatter plots are distributed within the 95% CI. Based on the foregoing, we propose the CNFL as one of the measurement indicators to replace semiautomated methods.

Furthermore, when the ACCMetrics software is compared to the traditional method, there are negligible differences in the results. In **Table 1**, it can be seen that the ACCMetrics software recorded higher CNFD values, lower CNBD values, and lower CNFL values. Conversely, the CNFD has a weak correlation (ICC $= 0.460$, $p < 0.001$, $r = 0.471$, $p < 0.001$) between the two approaches. **Figure 2** presents the reasons behind some differences, e.g., some nerve trunks were misidentified and a certain number of nerve bands and fibers were missed, as indicated by the arrows and circles in the images. Consequently, we must acknowledge that the two methods differ, and we do not recommend CNFD as the primary parameter to be measured.

However, we recommend combining the CNFD, CNBD, and CNFL to support the diagnosis of DED with ocular pain, with the CNFL serving as the most critical parameter. Patients with ocular pain have fewer SNP, such as lower CNFD, CNBD, and CNFL values, regardless of whether the data are obtained via NeuronJ or ACCMetrics (17). From **Table 4**, it is apparent that when NeuronJ was used, CNFD was decreased by 11.32%, CNBD was decreased by 31.19%, and CNFL was decreased by 18.99%. Following the implementation of ACCMetrics, CNFD was decreased by 22.48%, CNBD was decreased by 22.39%, and CNFL was decreased by 18.28%. The ROC parameters (**Figure 5**) also demonstrate that the three indexes are all highly efficient diagnostic tools. In addition, we recommend the CNFL obtained via NeuronJ and ACCMetrics as the recommended parameter. DED patients with ocular pain exhibit distinctive pathological changes in the SNP, which can be detected using IVCM, and nerve quantification can be used to confirm the diagnosis.

It is widely accepted that manual and semiautomated methods have some advantages, such as the highest degree of consistency and efficacy. The observers can obtain additional pathological details on factors, such as inflammatory cells, nerve ganglion, neuroma, and nerve endpoint, which helps them make a more accurate diagnosis of the situation (19). However, these methods are not only time and energy consuming, but also challenging to apply in a medical environment, particularly, when analyzing large amounts of data (18).

A fully automated method is well suited to clinical applications because it is operated automatically, allowing clinicians to conserve time and energy. A significantly large number of clinical samples can be assessed and the values of parameters can be calculated, facilitating a deeply comprehensive understanding of the symptoms, and consequently, highly effective treatment for the patients (20). Nevertheless, there are some disadvantages, such as the extremely high image quality requirements, such as image representativeness, clarity, and contrast. As indicated in **Figure 2**, the ACCMetrics software recognizes fewer nerve fibers and is not very capable of distinguishing nerve branches, inflammatory cells, nerve ganglions, neuromas, nerve endpoints, and other such entities in the cornea (16).

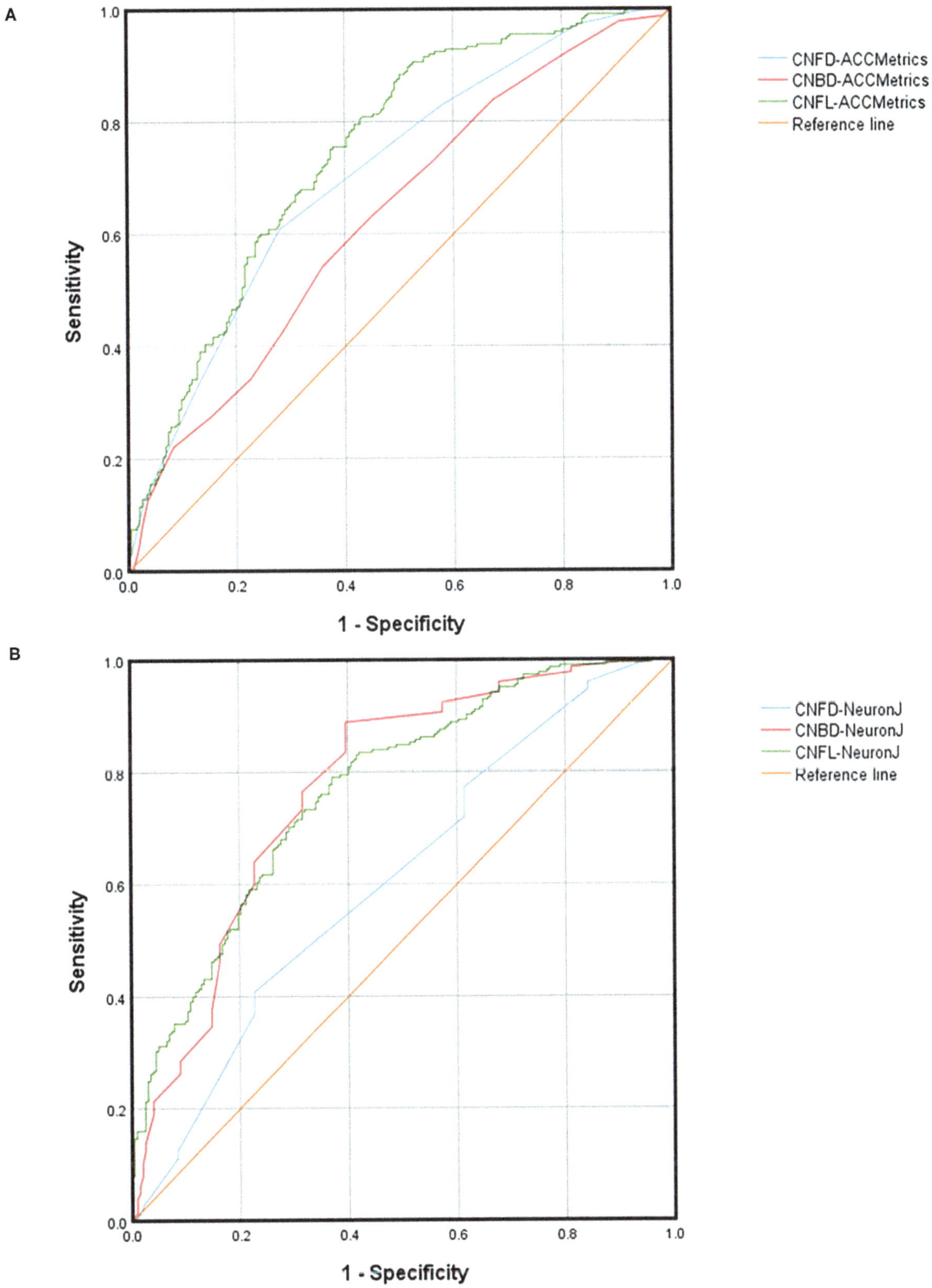

FIGURE 5 | ROC parameters of CNFD, CNBD, and CNFL dividing by DED with ocular pain using ACCMetrics **(A)** and NeuronJ **(B)**. DED, dry eye disease; CNFD, corneal nerve fiber density; CNBD, corneal nerve branch density; CNFL, corneal nerve fiber length.

TABLE 4 | Mean ± SD of parameters measured by NeuronJ and ACCMetrics.

		Control	DED with ocular pain	Mean difference & 95%CI	*t* Test	
					t Value	*P* Value
CNFD (n/mm^2)	NeuronJ	26.5 ± 6.9	23.5 ± 8.1	3.0 (1.6–4.4)	4.1	<0.001
	ACCMetrics	30.7 ± 8.9	23.8 ± 8.6	6.9 (5.2–8.6)	8.1	<0.001
CNBD (n/mm^2)	NeuronJ	67.0 ± 20.4	46.0 ± 21.3	20.9 (16.9–24.9)	10.4	<0.001
	ACCMetrics	46.0 ± 24.0	35.7 ± 23.3	10.3 (5.8–14.8)	4.5	<0.001
CNFL (mm/mm^2)	NeuronJ	23.7 ± 4.1	19.3 ± 4.3	4.5 (3.7–5.3)	11.0	<0.001
	ACCMetrics	18.6 ± 3.4	15.2 ± 3.8	3.4 (2.7–4.1)	9.7	<0.001

Results are expressed as mean ± SD. DED, dry eye disease.

Simultaneously, our research does have some limitations. Standard IVCM generates narrow-field images of the cornea (400 × 400 μm) that each display an extremely small area (<1%). According to the study of Winter et al., averaging parameters from multiple IVCM images may not result in very well accurate predictions for the whole image region (21). Additionally, it requires manual selection of non-overlapping IVCM images from a larger pool of images acquired during the image acquisition phase. Meanwhile, Allgeier et al. developed a novel automated approach that incorporates directed eye movements to rapidly expand the captured SNP region and axial focus plane oscillations to ensure complete imaging of the SNP (22). Moreover, we learned from their work on CNFL that expanding the mosaic image area stabilizes the CNFL values and decreases the movement variation (23). Currently, there have been a number of reports using wide-field imaging tools to study SNP-related diseases, such as the study of severe diabetic foot deformity by Herlyn et al. (24), Andreasson et al.'s research on Parkinson's disease with restless legs syndrome (25), Sterenczak et al.'s research on atypical cellular elements of unknown origin of a diabetic cornea (26), Koschmieder et al.'s research on multiple myeloma (27), and so on. A significant advantage of the wide-field technique is its capacity to offer imaging data with a wider field of view, possibly allowing the physician to analyze identical tissue sections repeatedly (22). Moreover, it prevents subjective field selection, resulting in an objective perspective of the whole SNP architecture, enabling accurate analysis of SNP patterns and precise quantification of SNP parameters (28). However, the wide-field technique for mosaic images is generally more time-consuming and difficult to implement in terms of software and hardware (e.g., three connected PCs) configuration. In our study, due to a lack of appropriate software and hardware, we relied on the widely used standard IVCM image extraction approach (29). Our study applied the well-accepted method of averaging the values of the five sites to represent the overall SNP of the eye (11). In the process of photographing and image selection, we tried to select images containing non-repeating SNP. The study of Ahmad Kheirkhah supported that there are no significant variations in the mean sub-basal nerve and dendritic cell densities between the average values of three representative standard IVCM images and wide-field mosaic composite images (29). However, given that the images we analyzed were of cases of decreased nerve density, the wide-field composite images may more accurately represent the entire cornea. We anticipate further studies on the application of wide-field techniques on DED with ocular pain.

Our expectations and recommendations for the future of the ACCMetrics software are as follows: we anticipate that the structure will improve software detection while simultaneously increasing recognition in images with low contrast and poor clarity; improved detection of nerve bands, weak nerve fibers, inflammatory cells, nerve ganglions, neuromas, nerve endpoints, and other abnormalities in the nervous system, and detection of other irregularities in the corneal stroma.

In summary, the fully automated software ACCMetrics can be used to partly replace semiautomated method NeuronJ. For instance, a relatively precise measurement of the CNFL can denote a significant degree of corneal nerve loss in patients, which can be used as a reference for the diagnosis of DED with ocular pain. Present status demonstrates the clinical importance in various fields of medicine and not only in DED with ocular pain. It may be turned out as an early biomarker for many neurodegenerative diseases, such as diabetic peripheral neuritis, Parkinson's disease, and so on. Nevertheless, current software often incorrectly recognizes and underestimates nerve fibers and is unable to identify biological details in images (e.g., inflammatory cells). Therefore, we anticipate that the ACCMetrics software will be upgraded and further developed to meet the demands of clinical practice.

ETHICS STATEMENT

The studies involving human participants were reviewed and approved by the Ethics Committee of The Second Affiliated Hospital at Zhejiang University School of Medicine. The patients/participants provided their written informed consent to participate in this study.

AUTHOR CONTRIBUTIONS

YZ wrote the manuscript. XH designed the research. YW and XH collected the data. YZ, YW, and WL analyzed the data. All authors contributed to the article and approved the submitted version.

ACKNOWLEDGMENTS

The authors would like to express our gratitude to Prof. Rayaz Malik and colleagues at the University of Manchester (UK) for granting us permission to utilize the ACCMetrics program for automated analysis of the *in vivo* confocal microscopy images in this study.

REFERENCES

1. Farrand K, Fridman M, Stillman I, Schaumberg D. Prevalence of diagnosed dry eye disease in the United States among adults aged 18 years and older. *Am J Ophthalmol.* (2017) 182:90–8. doi: 10.1016/j.ajo.2017.06.033
2. Rouen P, White M. Dry eye disease: prevalence, assessment, and management. *Home Healthc Now.* (2018) 36:74–83. doi: 10.1097/NHH.00000000000000652
3. Song P, Xia W, Wang M, Chang X, Wang J, Jin S, et al. Variations of dry eye disease prevalence by age, sex and geographic characteristics in China: a systematic review and meta-analysis. *J Global Health.* (2018) 8:020503. doi: 10.7189/jogh.08.020503
4. Craig J, Nichols K, Akpek E, Caffery B, Dua H, Joo C, et al. TFOS DEWS II definition and classification report. *Ocul Surf.* (2017) 15:276–83. doi: 10.1016/j.jtos.2017.05.008
5. Belmonte C, Nichols J, Cox S, Brock J, Begley C, Bereiter D, et al. TFOS DEWS II pain and sensation report. *Ocul Surf.* (2017) 15:404–37. doi: 10.1016/j.jtos.2017.05.002
6. Giannaccare G, Pellegrini M, Sebastiani S, Moscardelli F, Versura P, Campos EC. In vivo confocal microscopy morphometric analysis of corneal subbasal nerve plexus in dry eye disease using newly developed fully automated system. Graefe's archive for clinical and experimental. *Ophthalmology.* (2019) 257:583–9. doi: 10.1007/s00417-018-04225-7
7. Patel S, Hwang J, Mehra D, Galor A. Corneal Nerve Abnormalities in Ocular and Systemic Diseases. *Exp Eye Res.* (2021) 202:108284. doi: 10.1016/j.exer.2020.108284
8. Oliveira-Soto L, Efron N. Morphology of corneal nerves using confocal microscopy. *Cornea.* (2001) 20:374–84. doi: 10.1097/00003226-200105000-00008
9. Shetty R, Sethu S, Deshmukh R, Deshpande K, Ghosh A, Agrawal A, et al. Corneal dendritic cell density is associated with subbasal nerve plexus features, ocular surface disease index, and serum vitamin d in evaporative dry eye disease. *Biomed Res Int.* (2016) 2016:4369750. doi: 10.1155/2016/4369750
10. Yavuz-Saricay L, Bayraktutar B, Kenyon B, Hamrah P. Concurrent ocular pain in patients with neurotrophic keratopathy. *Ocul Surf.* (2021). doi: 10.1016/j.jtos.2021.08.003
11. Chin J, Yang L, Ji A, Nubile M, Mastropasqua L, Allen J, et al. Validation of the use of automated and manual quantitative analysis of corneal nerve plexus following refractive surgery. *Diagnostics (Basel, Switzerland).* (2020) 10. doi: 10.3390/diagnostics10070493
12. Tavakoli M, Ferdousi M, Petropoulos IN, Morris J, Pritchard N, Zhivov A, et al. Normative values for corneal nerve morphology assessed using corneal confocal microscopy: a multinational normative data set. *Diabetes Care.* (2015) 38:838–43. doi: 10.2337/dc14-2311
13. Henley R, Chandrasekaran V, Giulivi C. Computing neurite outgrowth and arborization in superior cervical ganglion neurons. *Brain Res Bullet.* (2019) 144:194–9. doi: 10.1016/j.brainresbull.2018.12.001
14. Liu Y, Lin M, Mehta J. Analysis of corneal nerve plexus in corneal confocal microscopy images. *Neural Regen Res.* (2021) 16:690–1. doi: 10.4103/1673-5374.289435
15. Qazi Y, Hurwitz S, Khan S, Jurkunas U, Dana R, Hamrah P. Validity and reliability of a novel ocular pain assessment survey (OPAS) in quantifying and monitoring corneal and ocular surface pain. *Ophthalmology.* (2016) 123:1458–68. doi: 10.1016/j.ophtha.2016.03.006
16. Dehghani C, Pritchard N, Edwards K, Russell AW, Malik RA, Efron N. Fully automated, semiautomated, and manual morphometric analysis of corneal subbasal nerve plexus in individuals with and without diabetes. *Cornea.* (2014) 33:696–702. doi: 10.1097/ICO.00000000000000152
17. Kheirkhah A, Dohlman TH, Amparo F, Arnoldner MA, Jamali A, Hamrah P, et al. Effects of corneal nerve density on the response to treatment in dry eye disease. *Ophthalmology.* (2015) 122:662–8. doi: 10.1016/j.ophtha.2014.11.006
18. Wu PY, Wu JH, Hsieh YT, Chen LC, Cheng T, Wu PY, et al. Comparing the results of manual and automated quantitative corneal neuroanalysing modules for beginners. *Sci Rep.* (2021) 11:18208. doi: 10.1038/s41598-021-97567-y
19. Wu LQ, Mou P, Chen ZY, Cheng JW, Le QH, Cai JP, et al. Altered corneal nerves in Chinese thyroid-associated ophthalmopathy patients observed by in vivo confocal microscopy. *Med Sci Monit.* (2019) 25:1024–31. doi: 10.12659/MSM.912310
20. Recchioni A, Sisó-Fuertes I, Hartwig A, Hamid A, Shortt AJ, Morris R, et al. Short-term impact of FS-LASIK and SMILE on dry eye metrics and corneal nerve morphology. *Cornea.* (2020) 39:851–7. doi: 10.1097/ICO.0000000000002312
21. Winter K, Scheibe P, Köhler B, Allgeier S, Guthoff RF, Stachs O. Local variability of parameters for characterization of the corneal subbasal nerve plexus. *Curr Eye Res.* (2016) 41:186–98. doi: 10.3109/02713683.2015.1010686
22. Allgeier S, Bartschat A, Bohn S, Peschel S, Reichert KM, Sperlich K, et al. 3D confocal laser-scanning microscopy for large-area imaging of the corneal subbasal nerve plexus. *Sci Rep.* (2018) 8:7468. doi: 10.1038/s41598-018-25915-6
23. Allgeier S, Winter K, Bretthauer G, Guthoff RF, Peschel S, Reichert KM, et al. A novel approach to analyze the progression of measured corneal sub-basal nerve fiber length in continuously expanding mosaic images. *Curr Eye Res.* (2017) 42:549–56. doi: 10.1080/02713683.2016.1221977
24. Herlyn A, Prakasam RK, Peschel S, Allgeier S, Kohler B, Winter K, et al. Corneal subbasal nerve plexus changes in severe diabetic charcot foot deformity: a pilot study in search for a DNOAP biomarker. *J Diabetes Res.* (2018) 2018:5910639. doi: 10.1155/2018/5910639
25. Andréasson M, Lagali N, Badian RA, Utheim TP, Scarpa F, Colonna A, et al. Parkinson's disease with restless legs syndrome-an in vivo corneal confocal microscopy study. *NPJ Parkinson's Disease.* (2021) 7:4. doi: 10.1038/s41531-020-00148-5
26. Sterenczak KA, Stachs O, Marfurt C, Matuszewska-Iwanicka A, Stratmann B, Sperlich K, et al. Atypical cellular elements of unknown origin in the subbasal nerve plexus of a diabetic cornea diagnosed by large-area confocal laser scanning microscopy. *Diagnostics (Basel).* (2021) 11:154. doi: 10.3390/diagnostics11020154
27. Koschmieder A, Stachs O, Kragl B, Stahnke T, Sterenczak KA, Henze L, et al. Non-invasive detection of corneal sub-basal nerve plexus changes in multiple myeloma patients by confocal laser scanning microscopy. *Biosci Rep.* (2020) 40:BSR20193563. doi: 10.1042/BSR20193563
28. Badian RA, Allgeier S, Scarpa F, Andréasson M, Bartschat A, Mikut R, et al. Wide-field mosaics of the corneal subbasal nerve plexus in Parkinson's disease using in vivo confocal microscopy. *Sci Data.* (2021) 8:306. doi: 10.1038/s41597-021-01087-3
29. Kheirkhah A, Muller R, Mikolajczak J, Ren A, Kadas EM, Zimmermann H, et al. Comparison of standard versus wide-field composite images of the corneal subbasal layer by in vivo confocal microscopy. *Investig Ophthalmol Visual Sci.* (2015) 56:5801–7. doi: 10.1167/iovs.15-17434

7

Ocular Surface Ion-Channels are Closely Related to Dry Eye: Key Research Focus on Innovative Drugs for Dry Eye

*Shuo Yang†, Yaying Wu†, ChunYang Wang and Xiuming Jin**

Eye Center, Second Affiliated Hospital, School of Medicine, Zhejiang University, Hangzhou, China

***Correspondence:**
Xiuming Jin
lzyjxm@zju.edu.cn

These authors share first authorship

†

Abundant ion-channels, including various perceptual receptors, chloride channels, purinergic receptor channels, and water channels that exist on the ocular surface, play an important role in the pathogenesis of dry eye. Channel-targeting activators or inhibitor compounds, which have shown positive effects in *in vivo* and *in vitro* experiments, have become the focus of the dry eye drug research and development, and individual compounds have been applied in clinical experimental treatment. This review summarized various types of ion-channels on the ocular surface related to dry eye, their basic functions, and spatial distribution, and discussed basic and clinical research results of various channel receptor regulatory compounds. Therefore, further elucidating the relationship between ion-channels and dry eye will warrant research of dry eye targeted drug therapy.

Keywords: ocular surface, dry eye, ion channels, compounds, targeted therapy

INTRODUCTION

Ion channels are crucial for sensing temperature and mechanical and chemical stimuli and are important structures for transmitting information between cells (1–3). Dry eye (DE) is a multifactorial ocular surface syndrome that mainly manifests as a series of sensory abnormalities on the ocular surface, including pain, burning sensation, and increased sensitivity to foreign bodies (4, 5). Abnormal physiological functions of the corneal epithelium and nerve endings also contribute to DE pathogenesis (5–10). These abnormalities, along with the dysfunctional expression and function of ion channels on the surface of the eye, further aggravate subjective symptoms of discomfort from DE (11, 12).

Many ion channels exist in the cornea, conjunctival epithelial cells, and corneal nerve fibers (4, 11). Their main physiological function is to maintain the internal and external ecological balance of the cells, sense chemical, temperature, and pressure stimuli, and transmit information (11). At present, many studies have revealed the key role of ion channels present in ocular surface cells in the pathogenesis of DE, and some ion channel activators or inhibitors have shown promise in the targeted treatment of DE (11–17). This review focused on the research status and progress of studying ion channels related to the ocular surface and DE and summarized the importance of ion channels in the DE to provide insights on DE-targeted drugs.

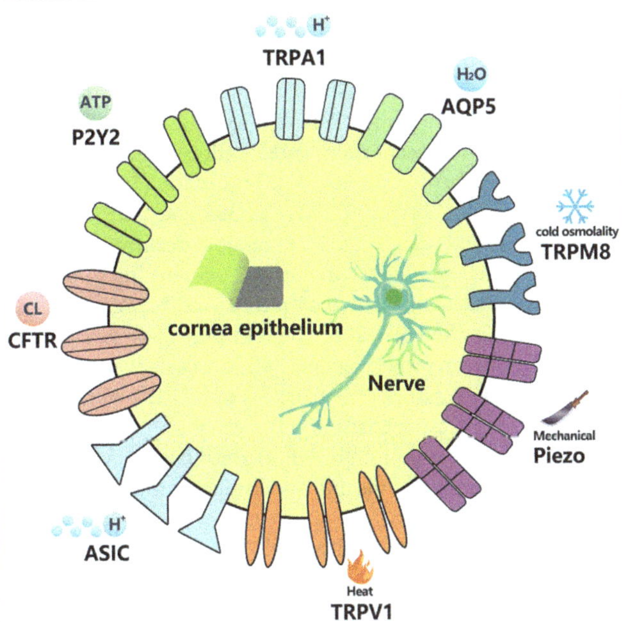

FIGURE 1 | Ion-channels that exist in the cornea, conjunctival epithelial cells, and corneal nerve fibers. The specific stimuli activating each receptor channel class is shown (11, 18–20).

DISTRIBUTION OF DE-RELATED ION-CHANNELS ON THE OCULAR SURFACE

The stability of the ocular surface environment is an important factor in the pathological mechanisms of DE (5–9). The physiological state of the cornea, conjunctiva, and corneal nerve plays a considerable role in the occurrence and development of the DE, and the information transmission of related physiological functions depends on various ion channels at the cellular level (**Figure 1**) (11).

The trigeminal ganglion (TG) is distributed widely on the ocular surface through the eye meridian, especially in the cornea. There are multimodal nociceptors (~70%), mechanical nociceptors (15–20%), and temperature receptors (10–15%) at nerve endings, which can sense mechanical, thermal, and chemical stimuli within or near a harmful threshold (4, 11). At present, many studies have reported that the expression of ion channels is influenced by DE in corneal nerve endings, mainly including transient receptor potential (TRP) channels (TRPV1, TRPA1, and TRPM8), acid-sensing ion channels (ASICs), and mechanically gated ion channels (piezo2) (11–17).

Many ion channel receptor proteins also appear in corneal epithelial cells. At present, the ion channels related to DE include TRPV1, TRPM8, TRPA1, cystic fibrosis transmembrane conductance regulator (CFTR), chloride channels, among others (11, 13–16). In addition, receptor proteins closely related to the physiological functions of ion channels, such as purine and purinergic receptors [G protein coupled adenosine receptors (ARS), P2Y receptors (p2yrs), and ATP gated P2X receiver ion channels (p2xrs)], show potential in DE-targeted therapy (17). Aquaporins (AQPs), proteins involved in the balance and stability of the water inside and outside the cells, also exist in the corneal epithelium. Recently, it has been found that they are closely related to the pathogenesis of DE (21).

Goblet cells in the conjunctival epithelium secrete mucin (MUC5AC) and some non-mucin proteins, including peroxidase, trefoil factor, and defensin. As an important component of tear film formation, mucin maintains the conjunctival and corneal epithelial microenvironment (22–25). Studies have shown that purinergic gated ion channel proteins are expressed in the conjunctival epithelium and goblet cells and participate in the inflammatory response of NLRP3 (26). Mergler et al. detected human conjunctival cells and found that conjunctiva expressed TRPV1, TRPV2, and TRPV4 channels, implying novel drug targets for DE therapeutics (27).

POLYMODAL NOCICEPTORS AND DE

Polymodal nociceptors are widely present in cornea and nerve fibers. They can be activated by external stimuli, such as harmful mechanical factors, heat, and chemical stimuli. Simultaneously, they are also sensitive to endogenous chemical mediators and inflammatory cells (11). In DEs, polymodal nociceptors can sense changes of temperature, inflammatory stimulation, and osmotic pressure caused by DEs, and regulate the wetting of the ocular surface. According to these characteristics, the screening of TRP family receptor block or activation-related compounds is of great significance for the development of DE-related ocular surface-targeted drugs. It has been reported that these receptors are closely related to DE, as described in the following paragraphs.

Transient Receptor Potential A1 (TRPA1)

TRPA1, also known as ANKTM1, is an ion channel receptor of TRP that participates in nociceptive temperature and mechanical perception (28–30). TRPA1 activation causes calcium influx and plays a role in persistent and allergic inflammation (30, 31). Katagiri et al. found that TRPA1 mechanisms are involved in the sensitivity of ocular responsive trigeminal brain neurons in the model for tear defect DE (32).

TRP Cation Channel Subfamily V Member 1 (TRPV1)

TRPV1 participates in polymodal nociceptors' sensory conduction (33). Previous studies have confirmed that TRPV1 is an ion channel related to sensations including pain and pruritus, and diseases like asthma (34–38). As a multi-sensory receptor, TRPV1 is activated by capsaicin, acidity, heat damage, and a hypertonic external environment (33). Eye irritation is a common clinical symptom of DE, and the TRPA1 inhibitor has shown great potential in easing peripheral nerve pain (39). Masuoka et al. have reported that chronic lacrimal deficiency sensitizes the response mediated by TRPV1 in corneal epithelial cells, which may be related to hyperalgesia caused by noxious stimulation in water-deficient DEs (40). In the DE model, overexpression of TRPV1 in TRPM8+ sensory neurons leads to cold hyperalgesia in corneal and non-corneal tissues without affecting their thermal sensitivity and promotes the release of neuropeptide P to signal cold response nociception (41). The increase in tear permeability and ocular surface inflammatory reactions are important mechanisms for the pathogenesis of DE (4–9). In addition, hyperosmotic stress (HOS) induces EGFR, MAPK, and NF signaling pathways through the TRPV1 channel and further mediates the increase of the pro-inflammatory cytokine interleukin (IL)-6 and chemokine IL-8 (42). Hua et al. found that the TRPV1 inhibitor capsaicin significantly reduced inflammatory tumor necrosis factor (TNF)-α, IL-1β, and IL-6 stimulated by human corneal endothelial cells (HCECs) (43). They further reported osmo-protectors to suppress inflammatory responses via the TRPV1 pathway in HCECs exposed to HOS (43). The targeted drug regulation of TRPV1 activity or its signal medium may be utilized as a novel method to inhibit the inflammatory response of DE syndrome. The mRNA expression levels of TRPA1, TRPV1, ASIC1, and ASIC3 were upregulated in the TG ocular branches of rigorously treated DE mice. After the intervention of the DE disease (DED) mouse model with the TRPV1 blocker (capsazepine), a reduction in the multimodal response of the cornea to heat, cold, and acid stimulation, and a further reduction in eye pain-associated anxious states were observed (44). Another study found that 1.125% syl1001, a novel short interfering RNA targeting TRPV1, can greatly improve ocular surface disease index scores and is tolerated well (45). Bereiter et al. clarified that TRPV1 plays an important role in mediating the enhanced nociceptive behavior in DE, which is beneficial for treating ocular surface stimulation pain in patients with moderate to severe DEs (46). These data support the effectiveness of blocking TRPV1 in treating tear deficiency and relieving chronic eye pain in DED, and is a potential choice for DED-targeted therapy.

ASIC3

ASICs are hydrogen ion–gated cation channels that are easily activated and opened by extracellular H^+ ions, instigate Na^+ ion influx, lead to cell depolarization and excitation, and participate in the sensitization process of moderate acid stimulation (47–51). Previous ASIC-related studies have mostly focused on the protection of the optic nerve and retinal injury. Inhibition of ASICs can reduce retinal ischemia-reperfusion and optic nerve injury (52, 53). In DE research, the possible role of the ASIC channel was recognized during a recent study. ASIC3 was shown to activate several corneal multimode sensory nerve fibers, significantly increase the blink and tear rate, and mediate acid stimulation and inflammatory pain on the ocular surface (54). ASICs are present in corneal sensory neurons. An acidic pH depolarizes these neurons to stimulate the action potential. ASIC blockers eliminate nociceptive behaviors caused by moderate acid stimulation (54). Even in the allergic keratoconjunctivitis model, ASIC3 blocking can also significantly reduce nociceptive behavior and reduce nociceptor sensitization during inflammation (54).

MECHANO-NOCICEPTORS AND DE

In the corneal nerve fiber axons, 20–30% of the receptors are mechanical nociceptors sensitive to mechanical pressure and activated by pressure perception (11, 55). Piezo channel protein, a member of the mechanically gated cation channel family, is the main baroreceptor on the ocular surface (56). It can be divided into two subtypes: piezo1/fam38a and piezo2/fam38b. Bron et al. found that piezo2 expression occurred in ~26% of TG neurons and 30% of corneal afferent neurons (55). Morozumi et al. confirmed that piezo1 and especially piezo2 are common in the corneal epithelium and optic nerves (57). Piezo inhibitors can protect against optic nerve damage caused by high intraocular pressure (57). Corneas of patients with DEs are sensitive to temperature changes and mechanical stimulation. As a common clinical symptom of DE, corneal pain may be related to the influence of chronic inflammation on the corneal pain conduction pathway. The piezo2 channel existing in the corneal nerve is directly involved in alleviating acute corneal mechanical injury, and local regulation of piezo2 helps ease the related pain caused by ocular surface mechanical stimulation (58).

COLD RECEPTORS AND DE

Cold receptors account for 10.15% of corneal neurons. They are sensitive to ocular surface temperature, continuously produce action potentials, and are regulated by dynamic changes in temperature (11). TRPM8 is a member of the cation channel family of TRP. As a cold sensory receptor, TRPM8 mainly senses temperature changes on the ocular surface and participates in temperature sensing, thermoregulation, and sensing pain caused by cold (11, 14, 16, 59). TRPM8 is also involved in the pathophysiology of DE and has anti-hypersensitivity and antipruritic effects (15, 60). On the ocular surface, evaporation of tears and changes in temperature lead to the activation of TRPM8, which further regulates basic tear secretion (61).

A study has found that in corneal refractive surgery and moderate DE, cold-heat receptors seem to mainly be affected, which can cause the major unpleasant feeling of DE (39). The corneal cold-sensitive neurons were closely related to the function of the TRPM8 channel in the injury response. The enhanced functional expression of the TRPM8 channel in primary sensory neurons of the trigeminal nerve could lead to an increase in tear rate and DE sensation (62). The dry conditions changed the sensitivity of neurons to menthol (its activator), resulting in desensitization to a cold-induced response, which could lead to reduced tear production that is harmful to patients with DEs (63). Moreover, certain interactions exist between TRP pathways. Khajavi et al. showed that the activation of TRPM8 can reduce TRPV1 activity, which may play a therapeutic role in the treatment of TRPV1-mediated inflammatory hyperalgesia, colitis, and DE syndrome (64). Arcas et al. reported the direct agonistic effect of tacrolimus on TRPM8 activity, which explains the anti-inflammatory effect of TRPM8 channels on the ocular surface of DEs (65). In related clinical studies, it was communicated that TRPM8 activation had a positive effect on DEs. A TRPM8 receptor agonist called cryosim-3 (C3, 1-diisopropylphosphorylnonane) can significantly increase tear secretion and improve DE symptoms (66). Yoon et al. also confirmed that C3 can significantly improve the symptoms of DE associated with menstrual pain, which is ineffective in routine treatments (67). In addition, a warm compress containing menthol can continuously increase the amount of tears and tear film stability in patients with DEs (68).

However, it seems paradoxical that patients with DED are more sensitive to cold compared to patients with non-DED. The duration of DED, rather than age, is an important factor in sensitivity to cold. Corneal cold receptor sensitivity decreased with an increase in DED duration (69). Fakih et al. found that severe DED mice had cold hyperalgesia, which was consistent with the high expression of TRPM8 mRNA in the TG. Chronic m8-b (TRPM8 antagonist) instillations significantly reversed the corneal mechanical hyperalgesia and spontaneous eye pain. M8-b also reduced the sustained spontaneous and cold-induced ciliary nerve activity observed in DED mice, as well as inflammation in the cornea and TG (60). In this regard, Kaido et al. further studied the cold perception of the TRPM8 pathway in DEs and found that activating TRPM8 only at the peripheral level was not enough to explain the manifestations of DE-related symptoms of discomfort (70). Higher brain levels may be involved in the occurrence and progression of DE symptoms.

CHLORIDE CHANNEL-CFTR AND DE

CFTR is an important chloride ion and water secretion channel (18, 71). In corneal epithelial cells, CFTR channel activation is important for maintaining the balance of chloride transport and promoting tear secretion (72). It has potential value in the treatment of DEs. The protective effect of CFTR channel-related activators on DEs has been observed in DE animal experiments. Nandoskar et al. found that CFTR was also present in lacrimal gland cells, in which CFTR was significantly expressed in ductal cells, while the expression of CFTR was significantly reduced in an autoimmune dacryoadenitis rabbit model (73). There is an obvious imbalance between the osmotic pressure and chloride ions in the ocular surface of DED. However, the combined administration of CFTR activator (genistein) and vitamin D (calcitriol) can reduce HOS-induced TonEBP (Tonicity—responsive enhancer binding protein), inflammatory gene expression, p-p38, and vitamin D receptor (VDR) degradation in HCECs (74). Furthermore, CFTR activators can significantly improve the ocular surface of mice with DE and even accelerate the repair of damaged corneal epithelium (75). Lee et al. screened a new CFTR activator, isorhamnetin, and reported that it could significantly increase the tear secretion in a mouse DE model, improve the ocular surface injury in mice, and inhibit the expression of IL-1β, IL-8, and TNF-α (76). Flores et al. also screened aminophenyl-1,3,5-triazine, CFTRact-K089, and fully activated CFTR, which can double tear secretion in a DE mouse model (77). In the tear deficiency mouse DE model induced by lacrimal ablation, it is interesting to note that 0.1 nmol CFT act-k089 can restore the tear secretion level by administering drops three times a day (77). Felix et al. conducted pharmacological experiments on New Zealand white rabbits with CFTR activator cftract-k267 and found that CFTR channel activation significantly increased tear production. At the same time, no obvious long-term toxicity affected the ocular surface after continuous treatment for 28 days (78). These data further suggest the relative safety and potential advantages of CFTR-related activators in DE treatment.

AQPS AND DE

AQPs were previously thought to be selective only to water, but recent studies have found that they have more complex regulatory mechanisms and a range of permeability. They also have characteristics of double water channels and gated ion channels and play an important role in maintaining the homeostasis of internal and external balance (21, 79). AQPs are closely related to the transport of Na^+ and K^+ on the cell membrane. They can maintain the osmotic gradient of corneal cells, further maintain the water balance of corneal cells, and play an important role in corneal transparency (21, 79). In the corneal epithelium, aquaporins 3 and 5 (AQP3 and 5) have been identified (19, 72, 80–82). Tear film hypertonicity and ocular surface inflammation are the main pathogenic factors of DE, and the AQP5 protein channel plays a role in the pathological process. AQPs and anti-AQPs autoantibodies have been confirmed to be involved in the pathogenesis of Sjögren's syndrome (83). Liu et al. reported that AQP5-/- mice can spontaneously develop DE symptoms, in which AQP5 deficiency changes the structure of lacrimal gland epithelial cells (84). Mucin secreted by conjunctival goblet cells (mainly MUC5AC) is a key condition for tear film stability. The co-immunoprecipitation of conjunctival AQP5 and MUC5AC suggested a possible physical interaction between the two molecules in response to acute DE stress (85). Nakamachi et al. found that pituitary adenylate cyclase-activating polypeptide (PACAP)–deficient mice can have DE-like symptoms, such as corneal keratosis and reduced tears. PACAP eye drops can increase the level of AQP5 in the tear film and p-AQP5 in the infraorbital lacrimal gland. Inhibition of AQP5 can reduce PACAP-induced tear secretion (86). In the study of new DE alternative drugs, it was revealed that the internal mechanism might be related to the upregulation of AQP5. Yu et al. found that ambroxol significantly increased tear secretion and upregulated the expression of AQP5 (87). AQP5 can also be used as a predictor of DE. Mani et al. detected that the expression of AQP4 increased and the expression of AQP5 decreased in conjunctival cells of patients after vitreoretinal surgery, indicating that the changes in these factors may suggest the prognosis of surgically sourced DE (88). Interestingly, Ren et al. found that hyperosmolarity-induced AQP5 upregulation promoted inflammation and caused corneal cell apoptosis (89), which seems to be a contradictory result and may be related to the overall internal imbalance of AQP5.

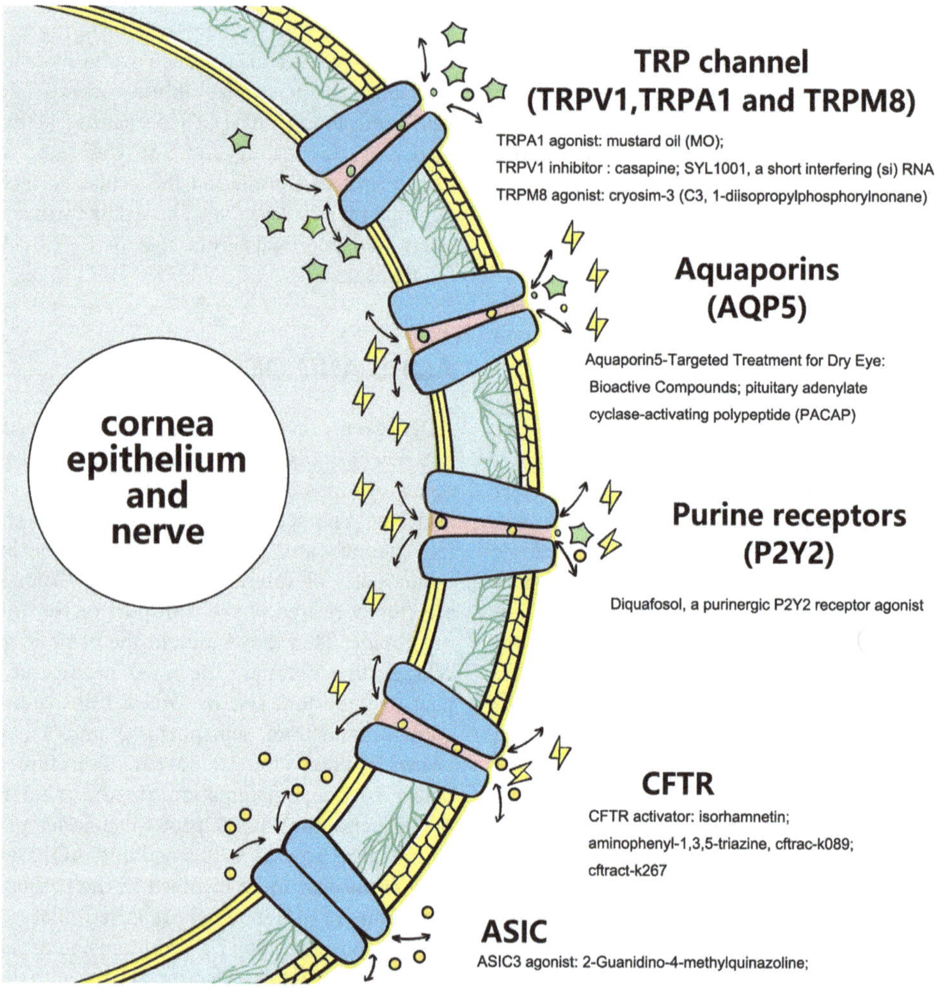

FIGURE 2 | Ion-channels target activating or inhibiting compounds as substrates for these specific receptors affect subsequent ions and intra- and extracellular information transmission.

PURINE AND PURINERGIC RECEPTORS AND DE

Purine receptors are widely distributed in neuronal and non-neuronal cells and mediate important signals such as cell proliferation, differentiation, and death, and participate in physiological and pathological activities such as immune response, exocrine and endocrine, inflammation, pain, platelet aggregation, and endothelial-mediated vasodilation (20, 90, 91). Purine receptors mainly include G protein-coupled adenosine receptors (ARS), P2Y receptors (p2yrs), and ATP-gated P2X receptor ion channels (p2xrs).

There are few studies on G protein coupled adenosine receptors (ARS) and P2X receptors in the field of DE (13). A key adaptive response to tear film hyperosmolarity induced by excessive evaporation is the reflective release of mucin by conjunctival goblet cells. The P2X7 receptor/channel is also activated during continuous extracellular hyperosmolarity. The activation of P2X7 not only damages the viability of goblet cells but also enhances exocytosis activity (26).

The P2Y receptor is a purinergic receptor, a G protein coupled receptor of extracellular nucleotides, and participates in physiology and pathophysiology, including inflammatory response and neuropathic pain (92, 93). At present, the P2Y2 subtype in the P2Y receptor (p2yrs) family is closely related to DEs (13). Research has found that the number of purinergic receptors P2Y1, P2Y11, and P2Y13 in lacrimal gland MEC (myoepithelial cells) of TSP1-/- mice (a mouse model of Sjögren's syndrome) decreased significantly, and the regulatory ability of cholinergic agonists, VIP, and purinergic receptors decreased, accompanied by increased expression of inflammatory factors (94). Dogru et al. reported that the tear stability, quantity, and ocular surface health of aged mice decreased with age, but the mRNA expression level of the P2Y2 receptor in the conjunctiva increased significantly, which may be used as compensation for the decline of age-related tear function (95).

Diquafosol is a purinergic P2Y2 receptor agonist that stimulates the conjunctiva to secrete water and mucin. It has achieved positive results in basic and clinical research in the field of DE. The diquafosol tetrasodium (DQS) was found to stimulate meibocytes to release lipids through the P2Y2 receptor and possibly facilitate holocrine secretion in isolated rabbit Meibomian gland cells (96). Diquafosol significantly reduced the levels of reactive oxygen species, apoptosis, and inflammation in corneal cells caused by DE in *in vivo* and *in vitro* DE models (97). In a one-year clinical study, the researchers used diquafosol to treat 580 patients with DEs for 12 months and found that it significantly improved the kerato-conjunctival staining score, tear film break-up time, and Dry Eye-related Quality of Life Score (DEQS) (98). This demonstrated that diquafosol 3.0% ophthalmic solution was tolerated well and was effective in the long-term treatment of DED. Utsunomiya et al. further confirmed that diquafosol was more effective in patients with DEs with foreign body sensation and problems when reading and using visual display terminals (99, 100). In a large randomized, double-blind clinical study, diquafosol improved the ocular surface Rose Bengal staining score more than sodium hyaluronate ophthalmic solution (101).

CONCLUSIONS

As an important intercellular information-mediated pathway, ion channels play an important role in various physiological and pathological processes. As the main component of the ocular surface, many ion channels with various functions exist in the corneal nerve, corneal epithelium, and conjunctival epithelium. DE is a common ocular surface disease, and the ion channels play an important role in its pathogenesis. This review summarized the current research status and progress of TRP channels, AQPs, CFTR chloride channels, and purine and purified receptors closely related to DE. Notably, the development of antagonists and activators for these key channels may help with their further popularization and clinical applications. However, from other studies, we have recognized that there may also be possible biological functional variability behind relevant antagonists or activators, which may be related to the overall stability of the internal environment and the interaction between different channel signals. The eye surface receptor protein family has a wide range of members, and its corresponding physiological functions are also diverse. Selection of the best receptor channel, finding the best specific receptor channel targeted drugs, and reducing the impact on other physiological functions will be the focus areas of ion channel research. Therefore, pharmacologists need to screen channel-targeted compounds that are more stable, simple, and have fewer side effects to provide more choices for the over-the-counter treatment of DE. In conclusion, a new and broad treatment protocol for treating DEs by developing ocular surface ion receptor channel-targeted therapy is in our future (**Figure 2**).

AUTHOR CONTRIBUTIONS

SY and XJ conceived the idea and wrote the manuscript. SY, YW, CW, and XJ prepared and reviewed the manuscript. All authors have read and approved the final version of the manuscript.

ACKNOWLEDGMENTS

We would like to thank Editage (www.editage.com) for English language editing.

REFERENCES

1. Kefauver JM, Ward AB, Patapoutian A. Discoveries in structure and physiology of mechanically activated ion channels. *Nature.* (2020) 587:567–76. doi: 10.1038/s41586-020-2933-1
2. Kondratskyi A, Kondratska K, Skryma R, Klionsky DJ, Prevarskaya N. Ion channels in the regulation of autophagy. *Autophagy.* (2018) 14:3–21. doi: 10.1080/15548627.2017.1384887
3. Imbrici P, Nicolotti O, Leonetti F, Conte D, Liantonio A. Ion channels in drug discovery and safety pharmacology. *Methods Mol Biol.* (2018) 1800:313–26. doi: 10.1007/978-1-4939-7899-1_15
4. Belmonte C, Nichols JJ, Cox SM, Brock JA, Begley CG, Bereiter DA, et al. TFOS DEWS II pain and sensation report. *Ocul Surf.* (2017) 15:404–37. doi: 10.1016/j.jtos.2017.05.002
5. Clayton JA. Dry eye. *N Engl J Med.* (2018) 378:2212–23. doi: 10.1056/NEJMra1407936
6. Bron AJ, de Paiva CS, Chauhan SK, Bonini S, Gabison EE, Jain S, et al. TFOS DEWS II pathophysiology report [published correction appears in Ocul Surf. 2019 Oct;17(4):842]. *Ocul Surf.* (2017) 15:438–510. doi: 10.1016/j.jtos.2017.05.011
7. Baiula M, Spampinato S. Experimental pharmacotherapy for dry eye disease: a review. *J Exp Pharmacol.* (2021) 13:345–58. doi: 10.2147/JEP.S237487
8. O'Neil EC, Henderson M, Massaro-Giordano M, Bunya VY. Advances in dry eye disease treatment. *Curr Opin Ophthalmol.* (2019) 30:166–78. doi: 10.1097/ICU.0000000000000569
9. Messmer EM. The pathophysiology, diagnosis, and treatment of dry eye disease. *Dtsch Arztebl Int.* (2015) 112:71–82. doi: 10.3238/arztebl.2015.0071
10. Guerrero-Moreno A, Baudouin C, Melik Parsadaniantz S, Réaux-Le Goazigo A. Morphological and functional changes of corneal nerves and their contribution to peripheral and central sensory abnormalities. *Front Cell Neurosci.* (2020) 14:610342. doi: 10.3389/fncel.2020.610342
11. Giblin JP, Comes N, Strauss O, Gasull X. Ion channels in the eye: involvement in ocular pathologies. *Adv Protein Chem Struct Biol.* (2016) 104:157–231. doi: 10.1016/bs.apcsb.2015.11.006
12. Kabra M, Pattnaik BR. Sensing through non-sensing ocular ion channels. *Int J Mol Sci.* (2020) 21:6925. doi: 10.3390/ijms21186925
13. Jacobson KA, Civan MM. Ocular purine receptors as drug targets in the eye. *J Ocul Pharmacol Ther.* (2016) 32:534–547. doi: 10.1089/jop.2016.0090
14. Liu Y, Mikrani R, He Y, Faran Ashraf Baig MM, Abbas M, Naveed M, et al. TRPM8 channels: A review of distribution and clinical role. *Eur J Pharmacol.* (2020) 882:173312. doi: 10.1016/j.ejphar.2020.173312
15. Yang JM, Wei ET, Kim SJ, Yoon KC. TRPM8 channels and dry eye. *Pharmaceuticals (Basel).* (2018) 11:125. doi: 10.3390/ph11040125
16. González-Muñiz R, Bonache MA, Martín-Escura C, Gómez-Monterrey I. Recent progress in trpm8 modulation: an update. *Int J Mol Sci.* (2019) 20:2618. doi: 10.3390/ijms20112618
17. Burnstock G. Introduction to purinergic signaling. *Methods Mol Biol.* (2020) 2041:1–15. doi: 10.1007/978-1-4939-9717-6_1
18. Hwang TC, Kirk KL. The CFTR ion channel: gating, regulation, and anion permeation. *Cold Spring Harb Perspect Med.* (2013) 3:a009498. doi: 10.1101/cshperspect.a009498

19. Schey KL, Wang Z, L Wenke J, Qi Y. Aquaporins in the eye: expression, function, and roles in ocular disease. *Biochim Biophys Acta.* (2014) 1840:1513–23. doi: 10.1016/j.bbagen.2013.10.037
20. Müller CE, Baqi Y, Namasivayam V. Agonists and Antagonists for Purinergic Receptors. *Methods Mol Biol.* (2020) 2041:45–64. doi: 10.1007/978-1-4939-9717-6_3
21. Ahmed T, Ghafoor S. Aquaporins; systemic, functional and therapeutic correlations in health and disease. *J Pak Med Assoc.* (2021) 71:1228–33. doi: 10.47391/JPMA.01-063
22. Watanabe H. Significance of mucin on the ocular surface. *Cornea.* (2002) 21:S17–S22. doi: 10.1097/00003226-200203001-00005
23. Baudouin C, Rolando M, Benitez Del Castillo JM, Messmer EM, Figueiredo FC, Irkec M, et al. Reconsidering the central role of mucins in dry eye and ocular surface diseases. *Prog Retin Eye Res.* (2019) 71:68–87. doi: 10.1016/j.preteyeres.2018.11.007
24. Puro DG. Role of ion channels in the functional response of conjunctival goblet cells to dry eye. *Am J Physiol Cell Physiol.* (2018) 315:C236–46. doi: 10.1152/ajpcell.00077.2018
25. Hori Y. Secreted mucins on the ocular surface. *Invest Ophthalmol Vis Sci.* (2018) 59:DES151-DES156. doi: 10.1167/iovs.17-23623
26. Puro DG. Impact of P2X7 purinoceptors on goblet cell function: implications for dry eye. *Int J Mol Sci.* (2021) 22:6935. doi: 10.3390/ijms22136935
27. Mergler S, Garreis F, Sahlmüller M, Lyras EM, Reinach PS, Dwarakanath A, et al. Calcium regulation by thermo- and osmosensing transient receptor potential vanilloid channels (TRPVs) in human conjunctival epithelial cells. *Histochem Cell Biol.* (2012) 137:743–61. doi: 10.1007/s00418-012-0924-5
28. Meents JE, Ciotu CI, Fischer MJM. TRPA1: a molecular view. *J Neurophysiol.* (2019) 121:427–43. doi: 10.1152/jn.00524.2018
29. Souza Monteiro de Araujo D, Nassini R, Geppetti P, De Logu F. TRPA1 as a therapeutic target for nociceptive pain. *Expert Opin Ther Targets.* (2020) 24:997–1008. doi: 10.1080/14728222.2020.1815191
30. Talavera K, Startek JB, Alvarez-Collazo J, Boonen B, Alpizar YA, Sanchez A, et al. Mammalian transient receptor potential trpa1 channels: from structure to disease. *Physiol Rev.* (2020) 100:725–803. doi: 10.1152/physrev.00005.2019
31. McMahon SB, Wood JN. Increasingly irritable and close to tears: TRPA1 in inflammatory pain. *Cell.* (2006) 124:1123–5. doi: 10.1016/j.cell.2006.03.006
32. Katagiri A, Thompson R, Rahman M, Okamoto K, Bereiter DA. Evidence for TRPA1 involvement in central neural mechanisms in a rat model of dry eye. *Neuroscience.* (2015) 290:204–13. doi: 10.1016/j.neuroscience.2015.01.046
33. Bevan S, Quallo T, Andersson DA. TRPV1. *Handb Exp Pharmacol.* (2014) 222:207–45. doi: 10.1007/978-3-642-54215-2_9
34. Bujak JK, Kosmala D, Szopa IM, Majchrzak K, Bednarczyk P. Inflammation, cancer and immunity-implication of TRPV1 channel. *Front Oncol.* (2019) 9:1087. doi: 10.3389/fonc.2019.01087
35. Aghazadeh Tabrizi M, Baraldi PG, Baraldi S, Gessi S, Merighi S, Borea PA. Medicinal chemistry, pharmacology, and clinical implications of trpv1 receptor antagonists. *Med Res Rev.* (2017) 37:936–83. doi: 10.1002/med.21427
36. Dai Y. TRPs and pain. *Semin Immunopathol.* (2016) 38:277–91. doi: 10.1007/s00281-015-0526-0
37. Huang YK, Lu YG, Zhao X, Zhang JB, Zhang FM, Chen Y, et al. Cytokine activin C ameliorates chronic neuropathic pain in peripheral nerve injury rodents by modulating the TRPV1 channel. *Br J Pharmacol.* (2020) 177:5642–57. doi: 10.1111/bph.15284
38. Wang Y, Gao Y, Tian Q, Deng Q, Wang Y, Zhou T, et al. TRPV1 SUMOylation regulates nociceptive signaling in models of inflammatory pain [published correction appears in Nat Commun. 2018 Jun 28;9(1):2593]. *Nat Commun.* (2018) 9:1529. doi: 10.1038/s41467-018-05022-w
39. Belmonte C, Acosta MC, Merayo-Lloves J, Gallar J. What causes eye pain?. *Curr Ophthalmol Rep.* (2015) 3:111–21. doi: 10.1007/s40135-015-0073-9
40. Masuoka T, Yamashita Y, Nakano K, Takechi K, Niimura T, Tawa M, et al. Chronic tear deficiency sensitizes transient receptor potential vanilloid 1-mediated responses in corneal sensory nerves. *Front Cell Neurosci.* (2020) 14:598678. doi: 10.3389/fncel.2020.598678
41. Li F, Yang W, Jiang H, Guo C, Huang AJW, Hu H, et al. TRPV1 activity and substance P release are required for corneal cold nociception. *Nat Commun.* (2019) 10:5678. doi: 10.1038/s41467-019-13536-0
42. Pan Z, Wang Z, Yang H, Zhang F, Reinach PS. TRPV1 activation is required for hypertonicity-stimulated inflammatory cytokine release in human corneal epithelial cells. *Invest Ophthalmol Vis Sci.* (2011) 52:485–93. doi: 10.1167/iovs.10-5801
43. Hua X, Su Z, Deng R, Lin J, Li DQ, Pflugfelder SC. Effects of L-carnitine, erythritol and betaine on pro-inflammatory markers in primary human corneal epithelial cells exposed to hyperosmotic stress. *Curr Eye Res.* (2015) 40:657–667. doi: 10.3109/02713683.2014.957776
44. Fakih D, Guerrero-Moreno A, Baudouin C, Réaux-Le Goazigo A, Parsadaniantz SM. Capsazepine decreases corneal pain syndrome in severe dry eye disease. *J Neuroinflammation.* (2021) 18:111. doi: 10.1186/s12974-021-02162-7
45. Benitez-Del-Castillo JM, Moreno-Montañés J, Jiménez-Alfaro I, Muñoz-Negrete FJ, Turman K, Palumaa K, et al. Safety and efficacy clinical trials for syl1001, a novel short interfering rna for the treatment of dry eye disease. *Invest Ophthalmol Vis Sci.* (2016) 57:6447–6454. doi: 10.1167/iovs.16-20303
46. Bereiter DA, Rahman M, Thompson R, Stephenson P, Saito H. TRPV1 and TRPM8 channels and nocifensive behavior in a rat model for dry eye. *Invest Ophthalmol Vis Sci.* (2018) 59:3739–46. doi: 10.1167/iovs.18-24304
47. Vick JS, Askwith CC. ASICs and neuropeptides. *Neuropharmacology.* (2015) 94:36–41. doi: 10.1016/j.neuropharm.2014.12.012
48. Lee CH, Chen CC. Roles of ASICs in nociception and proprioception. *Adv Exp Med Biol.* (2018) 1099:37–47. doi: 10.1007/978-981-13-1756-9_4
49. Santos PL, Guimarães AG, Barreto RS, Serafini MR, Quintans JS, Quintans-Júnior LJ. A review of recent patents on the ASICs as a key drug target. *Recent Pat Biotechnol.* (2015) 9:30–41. doi: 10.2174/1872208309011511111124125
50. Gründer S, Pusch M. Biophysical properties of acid-sensing ion channels (ASICs). *Neuropharmacology.* (2015) 94:9–18. doi: 10.1016/j.neuropharm.2014.12.016
51. Heusser SA, Pless SA. Acid-sensing ion channels as potential therapeutic targets. *Trends Pharmacol Sci.* (2021) 42:1035–50. doi: 10.1016/j.tips.2021.09.008
52. Dibas A, Millar C, Al-Farra A, Yorio T. Neuroprotective effects of psalmotoxin-1, an acid-sensing ion channel (asic) inhibitor, in ischemia reperfusion in mouse eyes. *Curr Eye Res.* (2018) 43:921–33. doi: 10.1080/02713683.2018.1454478
53. Stankowska DL, Mueller BH 2nd, Oku H, Ikeda T, Dibas A. Neuroprotective effects of inhibitors of Acid-Sensing ion channels (ASICs) in optic nerve crush model in rodents. *Curr Eye Res.* (2018) 43:84–95. doi: 10.1080/02713683.2017.1383442
54. Callejo G, Castellanos A, Castany M, Gual A, Luna C, Acosta MC, et al. Acid-sensing ion channels detect moderate acidifications to induce ocular pain. *Pain.* (2015) 156:483–95. doi: 10.1097/01.j.pain.0000460335.49525.17
55. Bron R, Wood RJ, Brock JA, Ivanusic JJ. Piezo2 expression in corneal afferent neurons. *J Comp Neurol.* (2014) 522:2967–79. doi: 10.1002/cne.23560
56. Fang XZ, Zhou T, Xu JQ, Wang YX, Sun MM, He YJ, et al. Structure, kinetic properties and biological function of mechanosensitive Piezo channels. *Cell Biosci.* (2021) 11:13. doi: 10.1186/s13578-020-00522-z
57. Morozumi W, Inagaki S, Iwata Y, Nakamura S, Hara H, Shimazawa M. Piezo channel plays a part in retinal ganglion cell damage. *Exp Eye Res.* (2020) 191:107900. doi: 10.1016/j.exer.2019.107900
58. Fernández-Trillo J, Florez-Paz D, Íñigo-Portugués A, González-González O, Del Campo AG, González A, et al. Piezo2 mediates low-threshold mechanically evoked pain in the cornea. *J Neurosci.* (2020) 40:8976–93. doi: 10.1523/JNEUROSCI.0247-20.2020
59. Iftinca M, Altier C. The cool things to know about TRPM8!. *Channels (Austin).* (2020) 14:413–420. doi: 10.1080/19336950.2020.1841419
60. Fakih D, Baudouin C, Réaux-Le Goazigo A, Mélik Parsadaniantz S. TRPM8: a therapeutic target for neuroinflammatory symptoms induced by severe dry eye disease. *Int J Mol Sci.* (2020) 21:8756. doi: 10.3390/ijms21228756
61. Parra A, Madrid R, Echevarria D, del Olmo S, Morenilla-Palao C, Acosta MC, et al. Ocular surface wetness is regulated by TRPM8-dependent cold thermoreceptors of the cornea. *Nat Med.* (2010) 16:1396–399. doi: 10.1038/nm.2264
62. Piña R, Ugarte G, Campos M, Íñigo-Portugués A, Olivares E, Orio P, et al. Role of TRPM8 channels in altered cold sensitivity of corneal primary

sensory neurons induced by axonal damage. *J Neurosci.* (2019) 39:8177–92. doi: 10.1523/JNEUROSCI.0654-19.2019
63. Kurose M, Meng ID. Dry eye modifies the thermal and menthol responses in rat corneal primary afferent cool cells. *J Neurophysiol.* (2013) 110:495–504. doi: 10.1152/jn.00222.2013
64. Khajavi N, Mergler S, Biebermann H. 3-Iodothyronamine, a Novel Endogenous Modulator of Transient Receptor Potential Melastatin 8?. *Front Endocrinol (Lausanne).* (2017) 8:198. doi: 10.3389/fendo.2017.00198
65. Arcas JM, González A, Gers-Barlag K, González-González O, Bech F, Demirkhanyan L, et al. The immunosuppressant macrolide tacrolimus activates cold-sensing trpm8 channels. *J Neurosci.* (2019) 39:949–69. doi: 10.1523/JNEUROSCI.1726-18.2018
66. Yang JM, Li F, Liu Q, Rüedi M, Wei ET, Lentsman M, et al. A novel TRPM8 agonist relieves dry eye discomfort. *BMC Ophthalmol.* (2017) 17:101. doi: 10.1186/s12886-017-0495-2
67. Yoon HJ, Kim J, Yang JM, Wei ET, Kim SJ, Yoon KC. Topical TRPM8 agonist for relieving neuropathic ocular pain in patients with dry eye: a pilot study. *J Clin Med.* (2021) 10:250. doi: 10.3390/jcm10020250
68. Arita R, Morishige N, Sakamoto I, Imai N, Shimada Y, Igaki M, et al. Effects of a warm compress containing menthol on the tear film in healthy subjects and dry eye patients. *Sci Rep.* (2017) 7:45848. doi: 10.1038/srep45848
69. Corcoran P, Hollander DA, Ousler GW 3rd, Angjeli E, Rimmer D, Lane K, et al. Dynamic sensitivity of corneal trpm8 receptors to menthol instillation in dry eye versus normal subjects. *J Ocul Pharmacol Ther.* (2017) 33:686–692. doi: 10.1089/jop.2017.0050
70. Kaido M, Inoue S, Kawashima M, Ishida R, Nakamura S, Tsubota K. Role of transient receptor potential melastatin 8 activity in menthol-induced cold sensitivity and its qualitative perception in dry eye. *Ocul Surf.* (2021) 19:307–312. doi: 10.1016/j.jtos.2020.10.008
71. Moran O. The gating of the CFTR channel. *Cell Mol Life Sci.* (2017) 74:85–92. doi: 10.1007/s00018-016-2390-z
72. Levin MH, Verkman AS. Aquaporins and CFTR in ocular epithelial fluid transport. *J Membr Biol.* (2006) 210:105–115. doi: 10.1007/s00232-005-0849-1
73. Nandoskar P, Wang Y, Wei R, Liu Y, Zhao P, Lu M, et al. Changes of chloride channels in the lacrimal glands of a rabbit model of Sjögren syndrome. *Cornea.* (2012) 31:273–9. doi: 10.1097/ICO.0b013e3182254b42
74. Panigrahi T, D'Souza S, Shetty R, Padmanabhan Nair A, Ghosh A, Jacob Remington Nelson E, et al. Genistein-Calcitriol mitigates hyperosmotic stress-induced tonebp, cftr dysfunction, vdr degradation and inflammation in dry eye disease. *Clin Transl Sci.* (2021) 14:288–98. doi: 10.1111/cts.12858
75. Chen X, Lee S, Zhang T, Duan T, Pasricha ND, Schallhorn JM, et al. Nanomolar potency aminophenyltriazine cftr activator reverses corneal epithelial injury in a mouse model of dry eye. *J Ocul Pharmacol Ther.* (2020) 36:147–53. doi: 10.1089/jop.2019.0087
76. Lee HK, Park J, Kim BR, Jun I, Kim TI, Namkung W. Isorhamnetin ameliorates dry eye disease via cftr activation in mice. *Int J Mol Sci.* (2021) 22:3954. doi: 10.3390/ijms22083954
77. Flores AM, Casey SD, Felix CM, Phuan PW, Verkman AS, Levin MH. Small-molecule CFTR activators increase tear secretion and prevent experimental dry eye disease. *FASEB J.* (2016) 30:1789–97. doi: 10.1096/fj.201500180
78. Felix CM, Lee S, Levin MH, Verkman AS. Pro-Secretory activity and pharmacology in rabbits of an aminophenyl-1,3,5-Triazine CFTR Activator for dry eye disorders. *Invest Ophthalmol Vis Sci.* (2017) 58:4506–13. doi: 10.1167/iovs.17-22525
79. Nesverova V, Törnroth-Horsefield S. Phosphorylation-dependent regulation of mammalian aquaporins. *Cells.* (2019) 8:82. doi: 10.3390/cells8020082
80. Tran TL, Hamann S, Heegaard S. Aquaporins in the Eye. *Adv Exp Med Biol.* (2017) 969:193–8. doi: 10.1007/978-94-024-1057-0_12
81. Verkman AS, Ruiz-Ederra J, Levin MH. Functions of aquaporins in the eye. *Prog Retin Eye Res.* (2008) 27:420–33. doi: 10.1016/j.preteyeres.2008.04.001
82. Yu D, Thelin WR, Randell SH, Boucher RC. Expression profiles of aquaporins in rat conjunctiva, cornea, lacrimal gland and Meibomian gland. *Exp Eye Res.* (2012) 103:22–32. doi: 10.1016/j.exer.2012.07.005
83. Soyfoo MS, Chivasso C, Perret J, Delporte C. Involvement of aquaporins in the pathogenesis, diagnosis and treatment of Sjögren's Syndrome. *Int J Mol Sci.* (2018) 19:3392. doi: 10.3390/ijms19113392
84. Liu Y, Di G, Hu S, Zhao T, Xu X, Wang X, et al. Expression profiles of Circrna and mRNA in lacrimal glands of aqp5-/- mice with primary dry eye. *Front Physiol.* (2020) 11:1010. doi: 10.3389/fphys.2020.01010
85. Bhattacharya D, Yu L, Wang M. Expression patterns of conjunctival mucin 5AC and aquaporin 5 in response to acute dry eye stress. *PLoS ONE.* (2017) 12:e0187188. doi: 10.1371/journal.pone.0187188
86. Nakamachi T, Ohtaki H, Seki T, Yofu S, Kagami N, Hashimoto H, et al. PACAP suppresses dry eye signs by stimulating tear secretion. *Nat Commun.* (2016) 7:12034. doi: 10.1038/ncomms12034
87. Yu L, Bhattacharya D, Wang Z, Wang M. Topical administration of ambroxol eye drops augments tear secretion in rabbits. *Graefes Arch Clin Exp Ophthalmol.* (2021) 259:1529–1538. doi: 10.1007/s00417-020-05043-6
88. Mani R, Shobha PS, Thilagavathi S, Prema P, Viswanathan N, Vineet R, et al. Altered mucins and aquaporins indicate dry eye outcome in patients undergoing Vitreo-retinal surgery. *PLoS ONE.* (2020) 15:e0233517. doi: 10.1371/journal.pone.0233517
89. Ren Y, Lu H, Reinach PS, Zheng Q, Li J, Tan Q, et al. Hyperosmolarity-induced AQP5 upregulation promotes inflammation and cell death via JNK1/2 Activation in human corneal epithelial cells. *Sci Rep.* (2017) 7:4727. doi: 10.1038/s41598-017-05145-y
90. Burnstock G. Purine and purinergic receptors. *Brain Neurosci Adv.* (2018) 2:2398212818817494. doi: 10.1177/2398212818817494
91. Burnstock G. Purinergic signalling: therapeutic developments. *Front Pharmacol.* (2017) 8:661. doi: 10.3389/fphar.2017.00661
92. von Kügelgen I. Molecular pharmacology of P2Y receptor subtypes. *Biochem Pharmacol.* (2021) 187:114361. doi: 10.1016/j.bcp.2020.114361
93. Jacobson KA, Delicado EG, Gachet C, Kennedy C, von Kügelgen I, Li B, et al. Update of P2Y receptor pharmacology: IUPHAR Review 27. *Br J Pharmacol.* (2020) 177:2413–2433. doi: 10.1111/bph.15005
94. García-Posadas L, Hodges RR, Utheim TP, Olstad OK, Delcroix V, Makarenkova HP, et al. Lacrimal gland myoepithelial cells are altered in a mouse model of dry eye disease. *Am J Pathol.* (2020) 190:2067–79. doi: 10.1016/j.ajpath.2020.06.013
95. Dogru M, Shinzawa M, Kojima T, Shimizu T, Tsubota K. Age-Related conjunctival P2Y2 receptor alterations in the Cu, Zn-Superoxide Dismutase-1 (Sod1)-Knockout dry eye model mice. *Eye Contact Lens.* (2019) 45:405–9. doi: 10.1097/ICL.0000000000000581
96. Endo KI, Sakamoto A, Fujisawa K. Diquafosol tetrasodium elicits total cholesterol release from rabbit meibomian gland cells via P2Y2 purinergic receptor signalling. *Sci Rep.* (2021) 11:6989. doi: 10.1038/s41598-021-86433-6
97. Park JH, Moon SH, Kang DH, Um HJ, Kang SS, Kim JY, et al. Diquafosol sodium inhibits apoptosis and inflammation of corneal epithelial cells via activation of Erk1/2 and Rsk: *in vitro* and *in vivo* dry eye model. *Invest Ophthalmol Vis Sci.* (2018) 59:5108–5115. doi: 10.1167/iovs.17-22925
98. Ohashi Y, Munesue M, Shimazaki J, Takamura E, Yokoi N, Watanabe H, et al. Long-term safety and effectiveness of diquafosol for the treatment of dry eye in a real-world setting: a prospective observational study. *Adv Ther.* (2020) 37:707–17. doi: 10.1007/s12325-019-01188-x
99. Utsunomiya T, Kawahara A, Hanada K, Yoshida A. Effects of diquafosol ophthalmic solution on quality of life in dry eye assessed using the dry eye-related quality-of-life score questionnaire: effectiveness in patients while reading and using visual display terminals. *Cornea.* (2017) 36:908–14. doi: 10.1097/ICO.0000000000001241
100. Song F, Hao S, Gu Y, Yao K, Fu Q. Research advances in pathogenic mechanisms underlying air pollution-induced ocular surface diseases. *Adv Ophthalmol Pract Res.* (2021) 1:100001. doi: 10.1016/j.aopr.2021.100001
101. Gong L, Sun X, Ma Z, Wang Q, Xu X, Chen X, et al. A randomised, parallel-group comparison study of diquafosol ophthalmic solution in patients with dry eye in China and Singapore. *Br J Ophthalmol.* (2015) 99:903–8. doi: 10.1136/bjophthalmol-2014-306084

8

Application of Animal Models in Interpreting Dry Eye Disease

Jun Zhu[1,2], Takenori Inomata[1,3,4], Kendrick Co Shih[5], Yuichi Okumura[1,3], Kenta Fujio[1,3], Tianxiang Huang[1,3], Ken Nagino[3,4], Yasutsugu Akasaki[1,3], Keiichi Fujimoto[1], Ai Yanagawa[3], Maria Miura[1,3], Akie Midorikawa-Inomata[4], Kunihiko Hirosawa[1,3], Mizu Kuwahara[1,3], Hurramhon Shokirova[1], Atsuko Eguchi[4], Yuki Morooka[1,3], Fang Chen[2] and Akira Murakami[1,3]*

[1] Department of Ophthalmology, Juntendo University Graduate School of Medicine, Tokyo, Japan, [2] Department of Ophthalmology, Northern Jiangsu People's Hospital, Yangzhou, China, [3] Department of Digital Medicine, Juntendo University Graduate School of Medicine, Tokyo, Japan, [4] Department of Hospital Administration, Juntendo University Graduate School of Medicine, Tokyo, Japan, [5] Department of Ophthalmology, Li Ka Shing Faculty of Medicine, The University of Hong Kong, Pokfulam, Hong Kong SAR, China

***Correspondence:**
Takenori Inomata
tinoma@juntendo.ac.jp

Different pathophysiologic mechanisms are involved in the initiation, development, and outcome of dry eye disease (DED). Animal models have proven valuable and efficient in establishing ocular surface microenvironments that mimic humans, thus enabling better understanding of the pathogenesis. Several dry eye animal models, including lacrimal secretion insufficiency, evaporation, neuronal dysfunction, and environmental stress models, are related to different etiological factors. Other models may be categorized as having a multifactorial DED. In addition, there are variations in the methodological classification, including surgical lacrimal gland removal, drug-induced models, irradiation impairment, autoimmune antibody-induced models, and transgenic animals. The aforementioned models may manifest varying degrees of severity or specific pathophysiological mechanisms that contribute to the complexity of DED. This review aimed to summarize various dry eye animal models and evaluate their respective characteristics to improve our understanding of the underlying mechanism and identify therapeutic prospects for clinical purposes.

Keywords: dry eye, animal model, lacrimal gland, tear deficiency, evaporative, environmental stress, translational research, DED

INTRODUCTION

Dry eye disease (DED) is one of the most common ocular surface disorders affecting millions of people worldwide (1–3). Its symptoms range from irritation and light sensitivity to blindness in severe cases (4–6). The tear film is the most important component of the ocular surface in maintaining microenvironment stability and providing lubrication to the cornea, thus maintaining its refractive function (7–9). Factors that affect the production or quality of tear film may lead to DED; these include but are not limited to lacrimal gland impairment, inflammation, infection, systemic autoimmune conditions, and environmental stress (10–14). The pathogenesis of DED is complicated, and much remains unknown. Animal models of DED are essential to better investigate the mechanisms underlying this multifactorial condition, explore potential therapeutic targets, and identify factors that can accurately predict prognosis. Conventionally, DED is classified into two categories, namely tear-deficient and evaporative (15). Recent evidence from a translational research using animal models demonstrated that tear film dysfunction involves multiple risk factors, with ocular surface inflammation an important component, where the resident immune cells initiate and propagate alterations in the ocular surface microenvironment (16, 17). Herein, we reviewed various dry eye animal models from published literature according to different modeling methods. We will discuss their therapeutic targets and relative advantages and disadvantages in this translational research.

AQUEOUS DEFICIENT DRY EYE TYPES

Lacrimal Gland Excision/Radiation Models

The surgical removal of the lacrimal gland in mice and rats is the most commonly reported model in DED research. Generally, the main procedures for mice lacrimal gland excision are as follows: after anesthetic administration, an incision is made to expose the extraorbital and/or intraorbital lacrimal gland with the aid of stereoscopic microscopy, and glands are generally excised and removed using micro-forceps and Vannas scissors without injuring surrounding blood vessels and nerves. All excisions are made ipsilaterally, usually on the right side, and only a sham surgery with cutaneous incision is performed on the contralateral side simultaneously (18, 19).

Principally, the excision of the primary lacrimal gland immediately reduces aqueous tear secretion. Compromised tear production manifesting with a reduced Schirmer's test score is the major outcome (20). This model can also be applied to other animals, such as dogs, rabbits, cats, and monkeys (21–24). The aforementioned models have demonstrated reduced Schirmer's test values and decreased basal tear production. However, vast differences in ocular surface anatomy and physiology between these models lead to inconsistency in the extent of affecting tear production, the duration of ocular surface complications, and reversibility. This warrants the selection of an appropriate animal specific to the needs of each study. For example, according to studies on the rat and mouse dry eye model (19, 25), the excision of the extra-orbital lacrimal gland reduces the tear volume and results in significant corneal epitheliopathy. However, decreased tear production does not necessarily manifest signs of ocular surface disease (26). Contrarily, the severity of dry eye symptoms may vary between genders. Mecum et al. (18) reported on a gender predilection that female mice were more susceptible to lacrimal gland excision-induced corneal damage. Regarding conjunctival changes resulting from the lacrimal gland removal, the evidence seems to vary among different animal modes. Stevenson et al. (19) reported increased T helper 17-cell frequencies in the conjunctiva and draining lymph nodes after extraorbital lacrimal gland removal in female C57BL/6 mice over 14 days. In contrast, Maitchouk et al. (21) concluded that the main lacrimal gland removal is not related to keratoconjunctivitis sicca.

External beam radiation therapy is a risk factor for DED following the treatment of head and neck cancers (27–29). Thus, it can be used to induce DED in animals. Hakim et al. (30) reported on a rabbit dry eye model using 15 Gy external beam radiation, which resulted in the functional impairment of the lacrimal gland and reduced tear production. Rocha et al. (31) introduced serial radiation doses at 8 or 6 Gy, delivered over 5 consecutive days, and successfully induced dry eye syndrome in mice. They observed a considerably lower production of tear secretion in the radiation group as well as a reduction in the epithelial thickness of the cornea, the absence of basal epithelium, and the thickening of corneal stroma at 10 days. However, these additional differences were transient and disappeared at 56 days post-radiation. Thus, radiation-induced dry eye models are reproducible and involve reversible alterations that provide a platform for mechanistic research into the treatment and prognosis of DED (32). The nuclear factor of activated T cells 5 plays a potential role, whereas α-lipoic acid exerts a protective effect on this radiation-induced model (33). However, compared with the previous simple lacrimal gland removal method, this method requires special radioactive equipment and poses certain risks and collateral damage.

Blockage of Lacrimal Gland-Associated Nerve Pathways

The lacrimal nerve displays extensive sympathetic innervation, thus influencing tear production and composition (34). Therefore, researchers can develop aqueous-deficient models by blocking the afferent or efferent nerves associated with the lacrimal gland. Parasympathetic blockers are the first and foremost drugs. As a competitive antagonist of muscarinic acetylcholine receptors, atropine blocks the action of acetylcholine, thereby suppressing the function of the parasympathetic nervous system. In an albino rabbit dry eye model (35), atropine eye drops considerably reduced tear production and Schirmer's test scores within 2 days of onset. Aicher et al. (36) subcutaneously injected male Sprague-Dawley rats with 0.1% methyl atropine (1 mg/kg) twice daily for 2 days. Methyl atropine considerably reduced basal tear production compared with pretreatment baselines. This dry eye model can be implemented rapidly and easily; however, it is relatively simple and does not represent complicated pathophysiological processes in human dry eye syndrome.

Another method involves the use of neurturin-deficient ($NRTN^{-/-}$) transgenic mice. Neurturin is a neurotrophic factor that regulates neuronal survival and function (37). Neurturin-deficient mice develop ocular surface inflammation similar to that observed in human DED. This transgenic mouse model substantially decreased aqueous tear production, tear fluorescein clearance, and corneal sensation (38). Moreover, it provided researchers with a method for better understanding the association between lacrimal gland denervation and ocular surface inflammation in DED. Nonetheless, its disadvantages are that the use and verification of this model are time-consuming.

Autoimmune Disease-Associated Dry Eye Models

A specific class of mice shares common characteristics with autoimmune DED, owing to the presence of a specific mutation or gene-editing technique. They release autoreactive lymphocytes to attack their lacrimal glands, consequently resulting in tear secretion deficiency. They can be categorized as experimental autoimmune disease-associated dry eye models (**Table 1**).

Sjögren's syndrome is a systemic autoimmune disease that causes secretory gland dysfunction (53). Several genetically modified mice have been used to mimic Sjögren's syndrome in dry eye studies. The non-obese diabetic (NOD) mouse model is mostly used for type 1 diabetes mellitus (54). NOD mice are susceptible to the spontaneous development of autoimmune insulin-dependent diabetes mellitus (55). Moreover, it facilitates investigating the influence of autoimmune processes on dry eye syndrome (56, 57). Lymphocytic infiltration leads to the degradation of extracellular matrix structures in the lacrimal gland of NOD mice (58). Ju et al. (39) reported that NOD mouse lacrimal glands displayed increased lymphocytic infiltration. Furthermore, they demonstrated substantially increased expression of major histocompatibility (MHC) II and interferon-γ in the lacrimal gland at 12 and 20 weeks. However, this model demonstrated a higher incidence of dacryoadenitis in male NOD mice than in females (59), thus suggesting the spontaneous autoimmune response may be modulated by sex steroids, particularly testosterone. Autoimmune lesions in this model involve autoreactive Th1 cell secretions, including interleukin (IL)-10 and IL-12. Sjögren's syndrome in the NOD mouse model is an interleukin-4, time-dependent, antibody isotype-specific autoimmune disease (60). Recently, Robinson et al. reported on a NOD-derived murine model (40), where NOD.B10.H2b mice, comprising MHC congenic to NOD, exhibited exocrine gland lymphocytic infiltration typical of Sjögren's syndrome-like disease and dysfunction observed in NOD mice, but without diabetes. Thus, the NOD.B10.H2b mouse model is considered interesting for studying primary Sjögren's syndrome.

The MRL/*1pr* mouse is a model of autoimmune arteritis, antiphospholipid syndrome, and systemic lupus erythematosus-like autoimmune syndromes (61–63). The *lpr* gene is a mutated *Fas* antigen that leads to lymphoproliferative disease (64). This model demonstrates anti-Ro/Sjögren's-syndrome type A and anti-La/Sjögren's syndrome type B autoantibody production, a characteristic manifestation of Sjögren's syndrome, besides exhibiting lacrimal gland infiltration, predominantly by $CD4^+$ T cells (41). Unlike the NOD mouse model, the extent of inflammation is considerably greater in the lacrimal glands of female MRL/*lpr* mice than that in males (65). Furthermore, MRL/*lpr* mice develop glomerulonephritis, which is classic in systemic lupus erythematosus but rare in Sjögren's syndrome (66). Therefore, the MRL /*1pr* mouse model is usually considered for secondary Sjögren's syndrome.

The inhibitor of DNA binding 3 (Id3) is an immediate early response gene involved in growth regulation and T-cell receptor-mediated T cell selection during its development (42). Id3-deficient mice develop lymphocyte infiltration in the lacrimal and salivary glands, reducing tear and saliva secretion and detectable anti-Ro and anti-La antibodies in the mouse serum. Similar to the clinical manifestations of primary Sjogren's syndrome, Id3-deficient mice serve as useful dry eye models for primary Sjogren's syndrome.

Conjunctival changes were also observed in autoimmune disease-related dry eye models. Using an autoimmune disease model mouse, BXSB/MpJ-Yaa, Hiraishi et al. (67) observed that goblet cell density in the conjunctiva epithelium decreased at 20 and 28 weeks compared to at 8 weeks. Wang et al. (68) reported spontaneous Sjögren-Like lacrimal keratoconjunctivitis in germ-free C57BL/6 mice, with significant goblet cell loss compared to conventional mice.

Researchers have reported other models, including the New Zealand Black and New Zealand White mouse (30, 35), the NFS/sld mouse (44), the IQI/Jic mouse (48, 69), the CD25 knockout mouse (45, 46), and the transforming growth factor $\beta 1$ knockout mouse (51, 52). These autoimmune models affect the function of the lacrimal gland, eventually resulting in inadequate tear production. Depending on the characteristics of the specific model, they can be applied to different scenarios. Of all autoimmune dry eye models, the NOD mouse (39, 40) and the MRL-1 *pr/1pr* mouse model (41) are most commonly reported in scientific literature.

EVAPORATIVE DRY EYE MODELS

Environmental Stress-Induced Dry Eye Models

In addition to decreased tear production, DED can occur despite normal tear secretion in the context of significant environmental stressors. Numerous models utilize changes in the external environment, ventilation, humidity, or the forced exposure of the ocular surface to simulate evaporative DED.

Dursun et al. (70) introduced a desiccating environment by placing mice in a hood with a continuous airflow blower, with a flow rate of 300 ft/min at 7 s for 1 h, thrice per day for 4 days. Mice placed in the blower hood manifested the most severe ocular surface disease. Simsek et al. (71) used a model in which BALB/c male mice were exposed to an air fan inside a small compartment for 5 h per day for 3 days. The external environment considerably decreased the tear volume and increased corneal fluorescein and lissamine green staining scores. Moreover, the corneal subbasal nerve density was substantially damaged following exposure. Contrarily, several studies have introduced dry eye mouse models induced by air pollution particulate matter (PM), such as PM_{10} and urban particulate matter (UPM). PM_{10} impairs tear film function and destructs the structural organization of the ocular surface in mice. The topical administration of PM_{10} in mice induces ocular surface changes, similar to those induced by DED in humans (72). UPM exposure induces apoptosis in the corneal epithelium and decreases the number of goblet cells in the conjunctiva. Moreover, it affects the stability of the tear film by disrupting its mucin-4 layer (73). The advantage of these models, which simulate the real environment, is highly relevant to the development of environmentally-induced ocular surface diseases, including DED.

In another model, researchers introduced a lid retractor to prevent blinking. This model can be used in a short time and is easy to implement. It enables testing preventive and therapeutic strategies for DED (74). However, minimal changes in the ocular

TABLE 1 | Autoimmune disease-associated dry eye models.

Models	Modeling method	Modeling genre	Sex preference	Pathogenesis	Detectable serum antibodies	Pathogenic effects	References
NOD mouse	Spontaneously developed	SS-like	Male	$CD4^+$ Th1 cell infiltration of the lacrimal gland	Anti-thyroid Ab Anti-ss-A/Ro Anti-b adrenergic R Ab Anti-a-fodrin Ab Anti-M3 muscarinic R Ab	Pancreas, submandibular, and thyroid gland	(39)
NOD.B10.H2b mice	NOD mutant with an altered MHC region	SS-like	Male	Did not develop autoimmune diabetes, but displays lacrimal T-cell infiltration	Similar with NOD mouse	Similar to NOD mouse	(40)
MRL-1 pr/1pr mouse	Mutated Fas antigen	2nd-SS.	Female	Serological manifestations characteristic of SS and exhibit lacrimal gland infiltration, predominantly by CD4– T cells	Anti-ds DNA Ab Anti-ss DNA Ab Anti-gp70 Ab Rheumatoid factor Anti-SA/Ro Anti-SS-B/La	Sialadenitis Dacryoadenitis Kidney Joints blood vessels	(41)
Id3-deficient mice	Gene knockout	pSS-like	ND	T-cell-dominant lymphocyte infiltration in both lacrimal and salivary glands	Anti-SSA/Ro Anti-SSB/La antibodies	Reduced abilities to secrete tears and saliva	(42)
NFS/sld mouse	Spontaneous autosomal recessive mutation	pSS-like	Female	Lymphocytic infiltrates in exocrine glands are dominated by $CD4^+$ T cells, with fewer $CD8^+$ T cells and B cells	Anti-a-fodrin Ab	Inflammatory changes in the submandibular, parotid, and lacrimal glands	(43)
3d-Tx NFS/sld mouse	Thymectomy of NFS/sld mice at 3 days of age	pSS-like	Female	Thymectomy impairs the expansion of regulatory T cells	ND	Severe than NFS/sld mouse	(44)
CD25KO mice	Interleukin 2 receptor alpha gene knockout	SS-like disease	ND	Worsening of corneal surface parameters and an increase of CD4+ T cell infiltrating the cornea	Anti-RBC antibody	Age-dependent SS-like autoimmune lacrimal-keratoconjunctivitis, dacryoadenitis, and corneal epithelial disease	(45, 46)
PD knock-in mouse	p65 S276D knock-in mice	KCS or SS-like	ND	Dependent on NF-κB; TNFR1-independent corneal inflammation	ND	Genetic and independent of decreased lacrimal function; Dacryoadenitis	(47)
IQI/Jic mouse	CR-derived inbred strain	2nd-SS disease	Female	Focal lymphocyte infiltration and tissue destruction in the salivary glands (SG) and LG	Antinuclear autoantibodies	Salivary and lacrimal glands, pancreas, and lungs dysfunction	(48, 49)
Aly/aly mouse	Spontaneous autosomal recessive mutation	SS-like disease	No predilection	Chronic inflammatory cell (CD4+ T cell) infiltration in multiple organs	No detectable autoantibodies against nuclear components or salivary gland proteins	Cell infiltration in multiple organs, including the salivary and lacrimal glands, pancreas, skin, bones and lungs	(50)
TGF-b1 Knock out mouse	Gene knockout	SS-like disease	ND	Mainly CD4+ T cells infiltration	ND	Heart, lung, pancreas, lacrimal, salivary, and submandibular gland	(51, 52)

KCS, keratoconjunctivitis sicca; ND, not determined; pSS, primary Sjögren's syndrome; and 2nd-SS, secondary Sjögren's syndrome.

surface during a short preparation time limit its application in studying dry eye syndrome.

Other models exposed animals to low-humidity environments and continuous airflow. Chen et al. (75) established a murine model of DED using an intelligently controlled environmental system that maintained low humidity. Animals exposed to this environment exhibited decreased aqueous tear production, increased corneal fluorescein staining, and marked thinning and accelerated desquamation of the apical corneal epithelium compared with control eyes. The dry eye environment supposedly upregulated apoptosis on the ocular surface. Furthermore, biological and morphological changes in this model were similar to those in human DED. Barabino et al. (76) developed a controlled-environment chamber and confirmed that low humidity could substantially alter tear secretion, goblet cell density, and related ocular surface signs. Moreover, Nakamura et al. (77) combined a low-humidity environment, continuous airflow, and jogging board treatment, which mimicked both mental and physical stress, to induce abnormal tear dynamics and superficial punctate keratopathy, similar to that in humans.

Meibomian Gland Dysfunction Models

Meibomian glands produce lipids, which are important components of the tear film (78). In physiological states, they prevent or lessen tear film evaporation, serve as the superficial protective layer, and stabilize the tear film by lowering surface tension. Lipid deficiency can lead to dryness of the ocular surface, damage to the conjunctiva and corneal epithelium, and an imbalance of the ocular surface microenvironment (79).

Jester et al. (80) introduced a meibomian gland dysfunction (MGD) model in 34 albino rabbits by topically applying 2% epinephrine twice daily, over 6 months to 1 year. Sixty-eight (56%) rabbits developed signs of MGD. The development and progression of MGD in rabbits appeared to correlate with increasing stratification and keratinization of the meibomian gland duct epithelium. Mishima et al. reported another rabbit MGD model by squeezing out meibomian gland contents and cauterizing the lid margin. Thus, a protective oily film layer could not form over the eyes of the treated animals, eventually leading to rapid tear evaporation. In another rabbit MGD model that used light cautery on meibomian gland orifices, researchers observed increased tear osmolarity in the presence of normal lacrimal gland function and ocular surface abnormalities, similar to that in keratoconjunctivitis sicca (81).

Other types of MGD models comprise transgenic mouse models, including X-linked anhidrotic-hypohidrotic ectodermal dysplasia (Tabby), apolipoprotein C1 transgenic mice, and ACAT-1-/- mice (82, 83). The meibomian glands were absent or abnormal in the aforementioned mice (**Table 2**). Tabby mice sequentially developed corneal epithelial defects, central corneal stromal edema, and corneal neovascularization 8–16 weeks following birth (91). Despite reduced tear film breakup time and tear evaporation times, tear secretion remained normal. This model is useful for identifying novel therapeutic agents for evaporative DED.

CHEMICAL-INDUCED DRY EYE MODELS

Researchers have used chemical substances, drugs, or biological agents to develop a class of lacrimal gland injury models. The scopolamine-induced dry eye model is most commonly used. Simsek et al. (92) assessed morphological changes in the corneal subbasal nerve plexus in wild-type mice following exposure to scopolamine. They observed decreased tear volume and shortened tear film breakup time (TFBUT). Confocal microscopy revealed substantially lower mean corneal subbasal nerve fiber density and reflectivity in the scopolamine-treated groups. Furthermore, the mean tortuosity and mean dendritic cell density were considerably higher in this model. Viau et al. (93) induced dry eye symptoms using scopolamine in 6-week-old female Lewis rats. Scopolamine was delivered via subcutaneously implanted osmotic pumps. TNF-α, IL-1β, and IL-6 mRNA levels increased with scopolamine treatment in both the conjunctiva and ex-orbital lacrimal glands. All animals exhibited unilateral or bilateral keratitis after 17 days. The scopolamine-induced dry eye model could serve as a stable model of moderate severity for dry eye studies.

Benzalkonium chloride (BAK) is the most frequently used preservative in eye drops. Researchers have consistently demonstrated its toxic effects on the ocular surface (94–96). It causes tear film instability, the loss of goblet cells, conjunctival squamous metaplasia and apoptosis, the disruption of the corneal epithelium barrier, and damage to deeper ocular tissues (97). In a rabbit BAK toxicity model, researchers demonstrated damage to the conjunctiva-associated lymphoid tissue via the topical application of BAK (98). In addition, Pauly et al. (99) developed a technical model that closely resembled the human ocular surface environment. They used fluorescence techniques conjugated with confocal microscopy on a 3-D reconstructed corneal epithelial model and observed an increase in apoptotic cells from the superficial to the deeper layers.

Botulinum toxin (BTX) is a potent toxin widely used in modern medicine (100) and has been used in various dry eye models. Park et al. (101) developed a mouse tear-deficient dry eye model without lacrimal gland inflammation by injecting BTX-B into the lacrimal gland. This model could effectively induce dry eye in mice 2 and 4 weeks following injection. The lacrimal structures were adequately maintained without significant T lymphocyte infiltration. Moreover, there are reports of a BTX-A-induced DED model in male C57BL/6 mice (102), which has also been demonstrated to be stable.

Researchers have also used other agents to establish different mouse, rat, or rabbit models, such as the injection of human recombinant interleukin-1 and concanavalin A into lacrimal glands and the oral administration of finasteride. **Table 3** summarizes the chemical-, biological agent-, and drug-induced dry eye animal models.

DISCUSSION

DED is a common ocular disorder that threatens the quality of life. Its symptoms vary from mild to severe, which are considered public health issues (113–115). The pathophysiologic

TABLE 2 | Transgenic models of meibomian gland dysfunction.

Models	Effect results	References
ACAT-1–/–	Similar to dry eye syndrome in humans	(83)
TRAF6–/–	Defective development of epidermal appendixes	(84)
K14-Noggin	Replacement of meibomian glands in eyelids with hair	(85)
Smad4CKO	Hair follicles in place of the meibomian glands	(86)
Barx2–/–	Defective lacrimal gland morphogenesis, defects in meibomian gland	(87)
Klf5CN	Defective eyelids with malformed meibomian glands, the abnormal cornea loss of conjunctival goblet cells	(88)
Fatp4–/–	Abnormal development of both sebaceous glands and meibomian glands, specialized sebaceous glands of the eyelids	(89)
Fgfr2CKO	Significant meibomian gland acinar atrophy and clinical manifestations of MGD	(90)

MGD, meibomian gland dysfunction.

TABLE 3 | A summary of chemical-, biological agent-, and drug-induced dry eye animal models.

Models	Modeling method	Demonstrated outcomes	References
C57BL/6 female mice	Subcutaneous injection of scopolamine hydrobromide, an exposure to an air draft, and 30% ambient humidity	Tear-deficiency dry eye	(103)
Male Sprague-Dawley rats	Topically administered 10% N-acetylcysteine	Mucin-deficiency dry eye	(104)
Rabbit	Topically administered 0.1% benzalkonium chloride	Both aqueous tear and mucin deficiency	(105)
Rabbit	Burned with 50% trichloroacetic acid	Conjunctival goblet cells damage	(22)
Rabbit	Trichloroacetic acid-treated and/or the removal of nictitating membrane	Stable KCS model, similar to surgical LG removal	(106)
Rat	Subcutaneous implantation of scopolamine micro-osmotic pumps	Moderate dry eye	(93)
Wistar rats	Bilateral ovariectomy in female rats and oral finasteride; both male and female rats challenged	Tear deficiency Androgen deficiency dry eye	(107)
CBA/J mice	BTX-B injection into the LG	Mimic those in humans with non-SS, KCS	(108)
CBA/J mice	Transconjunctival injection of BTX-B into the lacrimal gland	Dry eye model without significant inflammatory cells infiltration	(109)
Female Wistar rats	Androgen deficiency dry eye model induced by finasteride	Androgen deficiency dry eye	(110)
Female BALB/c mice	A single injection of interleukin-1α into the lacrimal gland	A severe, but reversible inflammatory response in lacrimal gland acinar epithelial cells	(111, 112)

BTX, botulinum toxin; KCS, keratoconjunctivitis sicca; LG, lacrimal gland; and SS, Sjögren's syndrome.

mechanisms of DED comprise multiple factors that not only involve ocular surface inflammatory processes but are also related to systemic conditions (116, 117). Dry eye animal models for interpreting the underlying mechanisms are indispensable. We reviewed articles on such models, assessed their types, principles, and characters (**Figure 1**), and discussed their potential value for DED. A miscellaneous set of dry eye models has been created and provided to researchers. Their manifestations and severities vary according to the specific pathophysiological mechanism. Researchers should consider an appropriate model according to their objective.

The surgical removal of lacrimal glands, chemical- or drug-induced lacrimal damage, and challenging environments are convenient and effective methods for achieving aqueous deficiency and evaporative dry eye models. Generally, aqueous deficiency and evaporative models are the major classifications (15). Researchers have developed models based on these classifications according to different implementation methods (**Table 4**). They share common traits, including rapid symptom occurrence, short implementation time, and reproducibility in different animals. Moreover, they decrease tear secretion production, which is ideal for assessing the efficacy of different therapies. However, these models have different prerequisites. Specifically, a mouse model using lacrimal gland excision could induce severe aqueous deficiency; More dedicated surgical techniques are required.

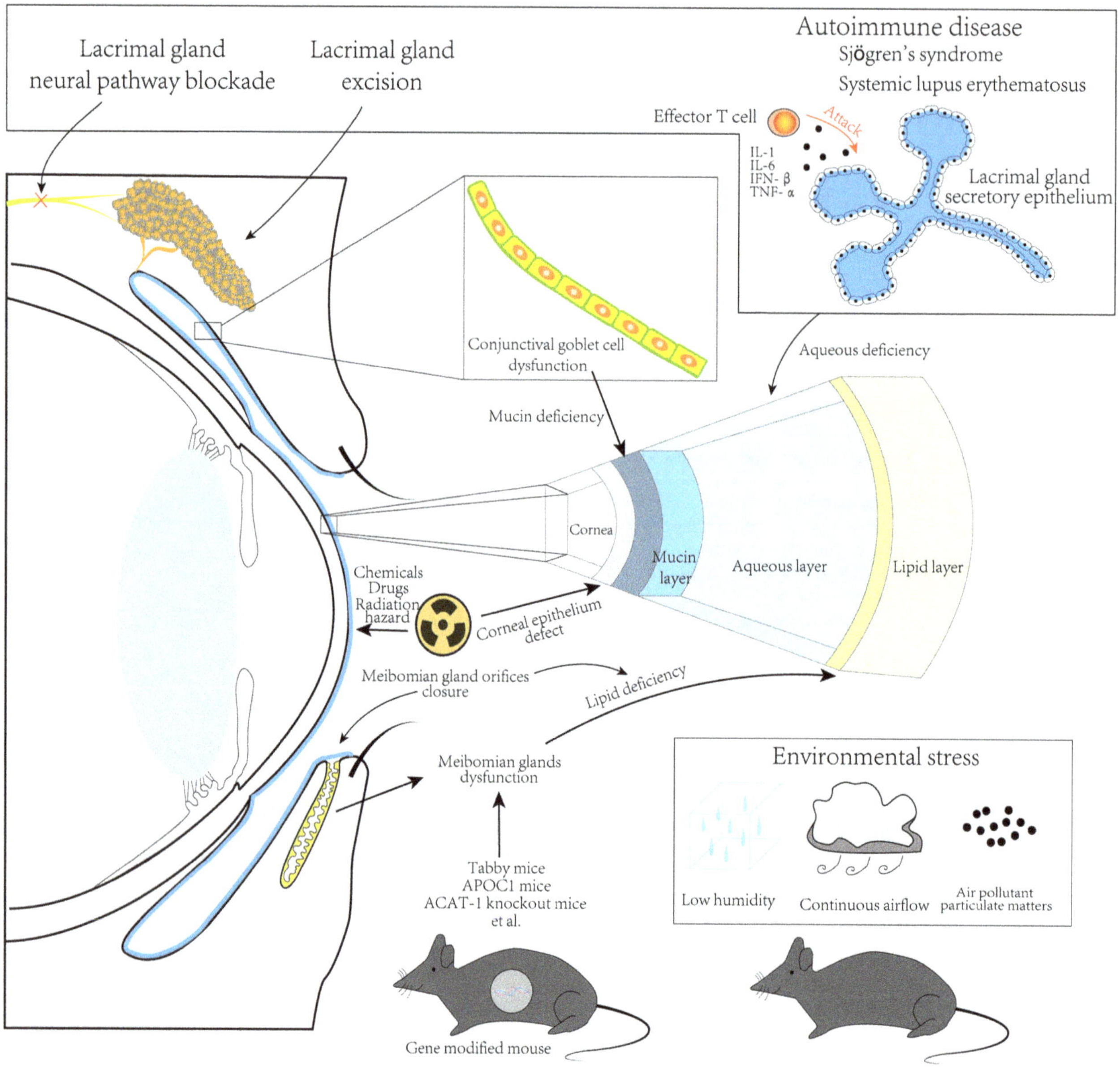

FIGURE 1 | Principles for animal dry eye modeling. A schematic showing approaches to developing animal dry eye models, including major methods used in recently published studies, as described in this review. Lacrimal glands excision, neural pathway blocking, and autoimmune disease models, including Sjögren's syndrome and systemic lupus erythematosus, have been developed by targeting the lacrimal gland. These result in an aqueous deficiency in the tear film. Conjunctival goblet cell damage can result in mucin deficiency in the tear film. Further, chemicals, drugs, and radiation hazards mainly cause corneal epithelium damage. Some gene-modified mice can present with dysfunction or direct damage of the Meibomian glands, resulting in lipid deficiency in the tear film. Environmental stress due to changing humidity, controlling airflow, and/or introduction of air pollution particulate matter, could also be significant in animal dry eye modeling.

In addition, lacrimal gland removal may not fully reproduce the complete clinical dry eye phenotype and systemic diseases associated with DED, including Sjögren's syndrome, rheumatoid arthritis, and systemic lupus erythematosus because it is merely artificial. For chemical-induced models, the use of 1.0% atropine sulfate eye drops in albino rabbits rapidly provided the required symptoms on day 2 of treatment. In addition, Schirmer test scores, corneal fluorescein staining, and Ferning tests confirmed dry eye signs (35). However, the observations were conducted only until day 5, without additional data.

Evaporative DED models were developed by changing the feeding environment or imposing environmental stress on different animals. Animals were kept in a low-humidity environment or continuous airflow chambers for hours or days, which decreased tear film production, shortened the breakup time, and increased corneal fluorescence staining. The aforementioned environmental stress models are economical

TABLE 4 | Dry eye animal models.

Animal models	Type	Species	Procedure	Experimental days	Effects to dry eye examinations			Pros	Cons	References
					Tear secretion volume	Tear film breakup time	CFS			
Lacrimal gland excision	Aqueous deficiency	C57BL/6 WT mice	Exorbital and intraorbital lacrimal gland excision	14 days	↓16.6%	ND	↑↑↑	Inducing severe aqueous deficiency model	More surgically invasive	(118)
Radiation-induced model	Aqueous deficiency	female New Zealand rabbit	Radiation 15 Gy	3 days	↓	ND	ND	Objective surrogate parameters for radiogenic dysfunction	Requires special radioactive equipment	(30)
Drug-induced	Aqueous deficiency	Male New Zealand albino rabbits	1.0% atropine sulfate eye drop	2 days	↓↓	ND	↑	Producing the required symptoms rapidly	Only observed for 5 days, no longer time observation data	(35)
Drug-induced	Lacrimal Gland Denervation	Male Sprague-Dawley rats	192-IgG-saporin was microinjected into the lacrimal gland	3–4 weeks	No changes	ND	ND	Useful for exploring the mechanism underlying corneal hypoalgesia.	Microsurgery requirements; Normal basal tear production	(36)
Autoimmune model	Aqueous deficiency	NOD mice	Derived from the outbred Jcl:ICR line of mice	10–14 weeks	↓↓	61.43% 1~2 second	↑	Ideal model for autoimmune related DED	Discrepancies between preclinical studies and clinical outcomes	(54, 56, 119, 120)
Autoimmune model	Aqueous deficiency	MRL/lpr mice	Derived from the MRL/n mouse strain	16–18 weeks (female) 18–20 (male)	↓	ND	ND	A pivotal model for neurological SLE	Lack of data in the literature	(121, 122)
Autoimmune model	Aqueous deficiency	Id3-deficient mice	Gene knockout	8 weeks	↓	ND	ND	Ideal primary Sjogren's syndrome model	Technical challenges in gene knockout	(42)
Autoimmune model	Aqueous deficiency	IQI/Jic mice	Developed from outbred ICR mice	At least 9 months	ND	ND	ND	Model for secondary Sjogren's syndrome model	The age of onset limited its application	(48, 69)

(Continued)

TABLE 4 | Continued

Animal models	Type	Species	Procedure	Experimental days	Effects to dry eye examinations			Pros	Cons	References
					Tear secretion volume	**Tear film breakup time**	**CFS**			
Environmental stress	Evaporative dry eye model	Balb/c male mice	Exposed to an air fan 5 hours a day for 3 days	3 days	↓↓↓	↓↓↓	↑↑↑	Promising model to study the ocular surface and corneal nerve changes	Only male mice and acute alterations were assessed	(71)
Environmental stress	Evaporative dry eye mode	Rabbit	Eyes were held open with an eye specula	1–3 h	ND	ND	↑↑	Simply and short-term to implement	Not suitable for mechanism research	(74)
Meibomian gland dysfunction	Evaporative dry eye mode	New Zealand rabbit	Meibomian gland orifices were closed by electrical coagulation or light cautery	1–14 days	↓↓↓ (Observed on day 1–3)	↓ (On day 3, 7, 14)	No difference	Suitable for MGD related dry eye research	Biochemistry and biophysics differences between rabbit and human meibum	(81, 123)

CFS, corneal fluorescein staining; DED, dry eye disease; ICR, imprinting control region; MGD, meibomian gland dysfunction; ND, not determined; and SLE, systemic lupus erythematosus.
↑, increased; ↓, decreased.

and easy to implement. Moreover, some studies focused on air pollution particulate matters, such as $PM_{2.5}$, PM_{10} exposure, or simulating office working environments (72, 124, 125). These studies are valuable for investigating environmental factors of DED and the evaluation of related dry eye medicine therapies.

Evaporative dry eye models can be achieved by Meibomian gland dysfunction. One type involves the closure of the Meibomian gland orifices using electrical coagulation or light cautery. Lipid layer deficiency indirectly leads to aqueous layer evaporation. Usually, this type of model is combined with a low-humidity environment or rapid airflow to enhance evaporation. The abovementioned dysfunction of the Meibomian gland could provide tools for evaporative DED research; however, biochemical and biophysical differences between animal and human meibum limit its application. Other MGD models comprise transgenic models, such as ACAT-1, TRAF6, and Barx2 knockout mice, which exhibit the abnormal development of meibomian glands (83, 84, 87). These models are technically challenging, time-consuming, and expensive.

The short TFBUT-type dry eye model, with or without decreased tear secretion, highlights the importance of tear film stability in DED. Tear film stability is considered one of the important factors for understanding DED (126). Zhang Y et al. (127) developed a murine model based on graft-vs.-host disease (GVHD). Shimizu et al. (128) evaluated TFBUT in this GVHD-related model and observed significant differences in TFBUT, tear secretion, and corneal fluorescein scores between the syngeneic and GVHD groups from 9 to 12 weeks of age. Carpena-Torres et al. (129) reported on the topical instillation of 0.2% benzalkonium chloride for 5 consecutive days for establishing a dry eye model. The results demonstrated a significant difference in TFBUT before and after instillation; however, there was no difference in tear secretion. Different dry eye models are essential for understanding short TFBUT-type DED. Researchers have demonstrated a higher incidence of short TFBUT and concomitant keratoconjunctivitis in patients with thyroid eye disease (130, 131). Thus, these models facilitate understanding the etiology of short TBUT-type DED, particularly for patients clinically diagnosed with DED and normal tear secretion.

Dry eye models developed from autoimmune diseases provide insight into the immunopathogenic mechanisms of DED. NOD mice and MRL/*lpr* mice are typical systemic autoimmune disease models of Sjögren's syndrome, presenting multiple organ inflammatory lesions, including lacrimal gland damage that eventually results in aqueous deficiency. Both demonstrated significant lymphocytic infiltration of $CD4^{+}$ T cells in the lacrimal gland. Dacryoadenitis revealed a higher incidence in male NOD mice than female mice. Compared with human Sjögren's syndrome, which is predominantly associated with female predilection, tear secretion was not profound in mouse models (57). MRL/*lpr* mice displayed more severe lacrimal gland inflammation in females than in males (65). Moreover, researchers observed a significant Th2 T cell response in the lacrimal gland of MRL/*lpr* mice, thus suggesting a mechanism different from the NOD mouse model (132). Nevertheless, these two models have been used for decades, with mature technology and sufficient research support, which are ideal dry eye models for DED.

This review summarized several major types of dry eye animal models and discussed their advantages and disadvantages in interpreting DED. This study had several limitations. It involved a limited number of animal species. The results of animal models differ considerably from human clinical manifestations. Moreover, they exhibit anatomical differences in the lacrimal gland system. Despite the variety of dry eye animal models, there are no widely homogeneous criteria for evaluating abnormalities of the ocular surface and the quality of tear film, thus making a model-wise comparison difficult.

CONCLUSION

Researchers have used several dry eye animal models in translational research, each focusing on different pathophysiological mechanisms of DED. Of these models, lacrimal gland excision is the easiest and most practical method, and it is widely used in dry eye research. However, it is relatively simple as it only reflects the aqueous deficiency component of DED. Several dry eye models, such as NOD mice, MRL/*lpr* mice, and specific transgenic models, provide researchers with a better understanding of the underlying mechanisms of DED and ideas for the development of novel biological treatments. Models based on environmental stress and drug toxicity may be more feasible for studies on real-world risk factors for DED. However, DED in humans is usually multifactorial in nature and involves complicated pathophysiological and immune responses. Therefore, no single dry eye animal model can serve as the best tool for research.

AUTHOR CONTRIBUTIONS

TI: conceptualization and funding acquisition. TI and JZ: methodology, validation, and project administration. JZ: data curation and writing—original draft preparation. TI and KS: writing—review and editing. FC and AM: supervision. YO, KFujio, TH, KN, YA, KFujim, AY, MM, AM-I, KH, MK, HS, AE, and YM: review and suggestion. All authors have read and agreed to the publishing of the final version.

ACKNOWLEDGMENTS

The authors wish to thank the staff of the Laboratory of Molecular and Biochemical Research at the Research Support Center of the Juntendo University Graduate School of Medicine for their technical assistance.

REFERENCES

1. Uchino M. What we know about the epidemiology of dry eye disease in Japan. *Invest Ophthalmol Vis Sci.* (2018) 59:DES1-6. doi: 10.1167/iovs.17-23491
2. Osae AE, Gehlsen U, Horstmann J, Siebelmann S, Stern ME, Kumah DB, et al. Epidemiology of dry eye disease in Africa: the sparse information, gaps and opportunities. *Ocul Surf.* (2017) 15:159-68. doi: 10.1016/j.jtos.2017.01.001

3. Donthineni PR, Das AV, Basu S. Dry eye disease in children and adolescents in India. *Ocul Surf.* (2020) 18:777–82. doi: 10.1016/j.jtos.2020.07.019
4. Paulsen AJ, Cruickshanks KJ, Fischer ME, Huang GH, Klein BE, Klein R, et al. Dry eye in the beaver dam offspring study: prevalence, risk factors, and health-related quality of life. *Am J Ophthalmol.* (2014) 157:799–806. doi: 10.1016/j.ajo.2013.12.023
5. Inomata T, Iwagami M, Nakamura M, Shiang T, Yoshimura Y, Fujimoto K, et al. Characteristics and risk factors associated with diagnosed and undiagnosed symptomatic dry eye using a smartphone application. *JAMA Ophthalmol.* (2020) 138:58–68. doi: 10.1001/jamaophthalmol.2019.4815
6. Chhadva P, Alexander A, McClellan AL, McManus KT, Seiden B, Galor A. The impact of conjunctivochalasis on dry eye symptoms and signs. *Invest Ophthalmol Vis Sci.* (2015) 56:2867–71. doi: 10.1167/iovs.14-16337
7. Tsubota K. Tear dynamics and dry eye. *Prog Retin Eye Res.* (1998) 17:565–96. doi: 10.1016/S1350-9462(98)00004-4
8. Johnson ME, Murphy PJ. Changes in the tear film and ocular surface from dry eye syndrome. *Prog Retin Eye Res.* (2004) 23:449–74. doi: 10.1016/j.preteyeres.2004.04.003
9. Willshire C, Bron AJ, Gaffney EA, Pearce EI. Basal tear osmolarity as a metric to estimate body hydration and dry eye severity. *Prog Retin Eye Res.* (2018) 64:56–64. doi: 10.1016/j.preteyeres.2018.02.001
10. Rhee MK, Mah FS. Inflammation in dry eye disease: how do we break the cycle? *Ophthalmology.* (2017) 124:S14–9. doi: 10.1016/j.ophtha.2017.08.029
11. Lopez-Miguel A, Teson M, Martin-Montanez V, Enriquez-de-Salamanca A, Stern ME, Gonzalez-Garcia MJ, et al. Clinical and molecular inflammatory response in sjogren syndrome-associated dry eye patients under desiccating stress. *Am J Ophthalmol.* (2016) 161:133–41. doi: 10.1016/j.ajo.2015.09.039
12. Chen Y, Dana R. Autoimmunity in dry eye disease - an updated review of evidence on effector and memory Th17 cells in disease pathogenicity. *Autoimmun Rev.* (2021) 20:102933. doi: 10.1016/j.autrev.2021.102933
13. Ceribelli A, Cavazzana I, Cattaneo R, Franceschini F. Hepatitis C virus infection and primary sjogren's syndrome: a clinical and serologic description of 9 patients. *Autoimmun Rev.* (2008) 8:92–4. doi: 10.1016/j.autrev.2008.07.003
14. Chhadva P, Goldhardt R, Galor A. Meibomian gland disease: the role of gland dysfunction in dry eye disease. *Ophthalmology.* (2017) 124:S20–6. doi: 10.1016/j.ophtha.2017.05.031
15. The definition and classification of dry eye disease: report of the definition and classification subcommittee of the international dry eye workshop (2007). *Ocul Surf.* (2007) 5:75–92. doi: 10.1016/S1542-0124(12)70081-2
16. Inomata T, Hua J, Nakao T, Shiang T, Chiang H, Amouzegar A, et al. Corneal tissue from dry eye donors leads to enhanced graft rejection. *Cornea.* (2018) 37:95–101. doi: 10.1097/ICO.0000000000001400
17. Hua J, Inomata T, Chen Y, Foulsham W, Stevenson W, Shiang T, et al. Pathological conversion of regulatory T cells is associated with loss of allotolerance. *Sci Rep.* (2018) 8:7059. doi: 10.1038/s41598-018-2 5384-x
18. Mecum NE, Cyr D, Malon J, Demers D, Cao L, Meng ID. Evaluation of corneal damage after lacrimal gland excision in male and female mice. *Invest Ophthalmol Vis Sci.* (2019) 60:3264–74. doi: 10.1167/iovs.18-26457
19. Stevenson W, Chen Y, Lee SM, Lee HS, Hua J, Dohlman T, et al. Extraorbital lacrimal gland excision: a reproducible model of severe aqueous tear-deficient dry eye disease. *Cornea.* (2014) 33:1336–41. doi: 10.1097/ICO.0000000000000264
20. Nemet A, Belkin M, Rosner M. Transplantation of newborn lacrimal gland cells in a rat model of reduced tear secretion. *Isr Med Assoc J.* (2007) 9:94–8.
21. Maitchouk DY, Beuerman RW, Ohta T, Stern M, Varnell RJ. Tear production after unilateral removal of the main lacrimal gland in squirrel monkeys. *Arch Ophthalmol.* (2000) 118:246–52. doi: 10.1001/archopht.118.2.246
22. Li N, Deng X, Gao Y, Zhang S, He M, Zhao D. Establishment of the mild, moderate and severe dry eye models using three methods in rabbits. *BMC Ophthalmol.* (2013) 13:50. doi: 10.1186/1471-2415-13-50
23. Helper LC, Magrane WG, Koehm J, Johnson R. Surgical induction of keratoconjunctivitis sicca in the dog. *J Am Vet Med Assoc.* (1974) 165:172–4.
24. McLaughlin SA, Brightman AH, Helper LC, Primm ND, Brown MG, Greeley S. Effect of removal of lacrimal and third eyelid glands on Schirmer tear test results in cats. *J Am Vet Med Assoc.* (1988) 193:820–2.
25. Skrzypecki J, Tomasz H, Karolina C. Variability of dry eye disease following removal of lacrimal glands in rats. *Adv Exp Med Biol.* (2019) 1153:109–15. doi: 10.1007/5584_2019_348
26. Barabino S, Dana MR. Animal models of dry eye: a critical assessment of opportunities and limitations. *Invest Ophthalmol Vis Sci.* (2004) 45:1641–6. doi: 10.1167/iovs.03-1055
27. Parsons JT, Bova FJ, Fitzgerald CR, Mendenhall WM, Million RR. Severe dry-eye syndrome following external beam irradiation. *Int J Radiat Oncol Biol Phys.* (1994) 30:775–80. doi: 10.1016/0360-3016(94)90348-4
28. Jeganathan VS, Wirth A, MacManus MP. Ocular risks from orbital and periorbital radiation therapy: a critical review. *Int J Radiat Oncol Biol Phys.* (2011) 79:650–9. doi: 10.1016/j.ijrobp.2010.09.056
29. Bhandare N, Moiseenko V, Song WY, Morris CG, Bhatti MT, Mendenhall WM. Severe dry eye syndrome after radiotherapy for head-and-neck tumors. *Int J Radiat Oncol Biol Phys.* (2012) 82:1501–8. doi: 10.1016/j.ijrobp.2011.05.026
30. Hakim SG, Schroder C, Geerling G, Lauer I, Wedel T, Kosmehl H, et al. Early and late immunohistochemical and ultrastructural changes associated with functional impairment of the lachrymal gland following external beam radiation. *Int J Exp Pathol.* (2006) 87:65–71. doi: 10.1111/j.0959-9673.2006.00456.x
31. Rocha EM, Cotrim AP, Zheng C, Riveros PP, Baum BJ, Chiorini JA. Recovery of radiation-induced dry eye and corneal damage by pretreatment with adenoviral vector-mediated transfer of erythropoietin to the salivary glands in mice. *Hum Gene Ther.* (2013) 24:417–23. doi: 10.1089/hum.2012.111
32. Harris DL, Yamaguchi T, Hamrah P. A novel murine model of radiation keratopathy. *Invest Ophthalmol Vis Sci.* (2018) 59:3889–96. doi: 10.1167/iovs.18-24567
33. Kim H, Yoo WS, Jung JH, Jeong BK, Woo SH, Kim JH, et al. Alpha-lipoic acid ameliorates radiation-induced lacrimal gland injury through NFAT5-dependent signaling. *Int J Mol Sci.* (2019) 20:5691. doi: 10.3390/ijms20225691
34. Ding C, Walcott B, Keyser KT. Sympathetic neural control of the mouse lacrimal gland. *Invest Ophthalmol Vis Sci.* (2003) 44:1513–20. doi: 10.1167/iovs.02-0406
35. Burgalassi S, Panichi L, Chetoni P, Saettone MF, Boldrini E. Development of a simple dry eye model in the albino rabbit and evaluation of some tear substitutes. *Ophthalmic Res.* (1999) 31:229–35. doi: 10.1159/000055537
36. Aicher SA, Hermes SM, Hegarty DM. Denervation of the lacrimal gland leads to corneal hypoalgesia in a novel rat model of aqueous dry eye disease. *Invest Ophthalmol Vis Sci.* (2015) 56:6981–9. doi: 10.1167/iovs.15-17497
37. Heuckeroth RO, Enomoto H, Grider JR, Golden JP, Hanke JA, Jackman A, et al. Gene targeting reveals a critical role for neurturin in the development and maintenance of enteric, sensory, and parasympathetic neurons. *Neuron.* (1999) 22:253–63. doi: 10.1016/S0896-6273(00)81087-9
38. Song XJ, Li DQ, Farley W, Luo LH, Heuckeroth RO, Milbrandt J, et al. Neurturin-deficient mice develop dry eye and keratoconjunctivitis sicca. *Invest Ophthalmol Vis Sci.* (2003) 44:4223–9. doi: 10.1167/iovs.02-1319
39. Ju Y, Janga SR, Klinngam W, MacKay JA, Hawley D, Zoukhri D, et al. NOD and NOR mice exhibit comparable development of lacrimal gland secretory dysfunction but NOD mice have more severe autoimmune dacryoadenitis. *Exp Eye Res.* (2018) 176:243–51. doi: 10.1016/j.exer.2018.09.002
40. Robinson CP, Yamachika S, Bounous DI, Brayer J, Jonsson R, Holmdahl R, et al. A novel NOD-derived murine model of primary Sjogren's syndrome. *Arthritis Rheum.* (1998) 41:150–6. doi: 10.1002/1529-0131(199801)41:1<150::AID-ART18>3.0.CO;2-T
41. Schrader S, Mircheff AK, Geerling G. Animal models of dry eye. *Dev Ophthalmol.* (2008) 41:298–312. doi: 10.1159/000131097
42. Li H, Dai M, Zhuang Y, A T. cell intrinsic role of Id3 in a mouse model for primary sjogren's syndrome. *Immunity.* (2004) 21:551–60. doi: 10.1016/j.immuni.2004.08.013
43. Hayashi Y, Kojima A, Hata M, Hirokawa K. A new mutation involving the sublingual gland in NFS/N mice. partially arrested mucous cell differentiation. *Am J Pathol.* (1988) 132:187–91.
44. Haneji N, Hamano H, Yanagi K, Hayashi Y. A new animal model for primary Sjogren's syndrome in NFS/sld mutant mice. *J Immunol.* (1994) 153:2769–77.
45. De Paiva CS, Hwang CS, Pitcher JD3rd, Pangelinan SB, Rahimy E, Chen W, et al. Age-related T-cell cytokine profile parallels corneal disease severity in Sjogren's syndrome-like keratoconjunctivitis sicca in CD25KO mice. *Rheumatology.* (2010) 49:246–58. doi: 10.1093/rheumatology/kep357

46. Rahimy E, Pitcher JD3rd, Pangelinan SB, Chen W, Farley WJ, Niederkorn JY, et al. Spontaneous autoimmune dacryoadenitis in aged CD25KO mice. *Am J Pathol.* (2010) 177:744–53. doi: 10.2353/ajpath.2010.091116
47. Dong J, Jimi E, Zeiss C, Hayden MS, Ghosh S. Constitutively active NF-kappaB triggers systemic TNFalpha-dependent inflammation and localized TNFalpha-independent inflammatory disease. *Genes Dev.* (2010) 24:1709–17. doi: 10.1101/gad.1958410
48. Saegusa J, Kubota H. Sialadenitis in IQI/Jic mice: a new animal model of Sjogren's syndrome. *J Vet Med Sci.* (1997) 59:897–903. doi: 10.1292/jvms.59.897
49. Jung JY, Saegusa J, Nakayama H, Doi K. Comparative study on picryl chloride (PCL)-induced contact dermatitis in female IQI/Jic and BALB/c mice. *Exp Anim.* (2004) 53:89–96. doi: 10.1538/expanim.53.89
50. Miyawaki S, Nakamura Y, Suzuka H, Koba M, Yasumizu R, Ikehara S, et al. A new mutation, aly, that induces a generalized lack of lymph nodes accompanied by immunodeficiency in mice. *Eur J Immunol.* (1994) 24:429–34. doi: 10.1002/eji.1830240224
51. McCartney-Francis NL, Mizel DE, Frazier-Jessen M, Kulkarni AB, McCarthy JB, Wahl SM. Lacrimal gland inflammation is responsible for ocular pathology in TGF-beta 1 null mice. *Am J Pathol.* (1997) 151:1281–8.
52. Shull MM, Ormsby I, Kier AB, Pawlowski S, Diebold RJ, Yin M, et al. Targeted disruption of the mouse transforming growth factor-beta 1 gene results in multifocal inflammatory disease. *Nature.* (1992) 359:693–9. doi: 10.1038/359693a0
53. Ramos-Casals M, Brito-Zeron P, Siso-Almirall A, Bosch X. Primary sjogren syndrome. *BMJ.* (2012) 344:e3821. doi: 10.1136/bmj.e3821
54. Reed JC, Herold KC. Thinking bedside at the bench: the NOD mouse model of T1DM. *Nat Rev Endocrinol.* (2015) 11:308–14. doi: 10.1038/nrendo.2014.236
55. Kikutani H, Makino S. The murine autoimmune diabetes model: NOD and related strains. *Adv Immunol.* (1992) 51:285–322. doi: 10.1016/S0065-2776(08)60490-3
56. Xiao W, Wu Y, Zhang J, Ye W, Xu GT. Selecting highly sensitive non-obese diabetic mice for improving the study of Sjogren's syndrome. *Graefes Arch Clin Exp Ophthalmol.* (2009) 247:59–66. doi: 10.1007/s00417-008-0941-1
57. Humphreys-Beher MG, Hu Y, Nakagawa Y, Wang PL, Purushotham KR. Utilization of the non-obese diabetic (NOD) mouse as an animal model for the study of secondary Sjogren's syndrome. *Adv Exp Med Biol.* (1994) 350:631–6. doi: 10.1007/978-1-4615-2417-5_105
58. Schenke-Layland K, Xie J, Magnusson M, Angelis E, Li X, Wu K, et al. Lymphocytic infiltration leads to degradation of lacrimal gland extracellular matrix structures in NOD mice exhibiting a sjogren's syndrome-like exocrinopathy. *Exp Eye Res.* (2010) 90:223–37. doi: 10.1016/j.exer.2009.10.008
59. Takahashi M, Ishimaru N, Yanagi K, Haneji N, Saito I, Hayashi Y. High incidence of autoimmune dacryoadenitis in male non-obese diabetic (NOD) mice depending on sex steroid. *Clin Exp Immunol.* (1997) 109:555–61. doi: 10.1046/j.1365-2249.1997.4691368.x
60. Gao J, Killedar S, Cornelius JG, Nguyen C, Cha S, Peck AB. Sjogren's syndrome in the NOD mouse model is an interleukin-4 time-dependent, antibody isotype-specific autoimmune disease. *J Autoimmun.* (2006) 26:90–103. doi: 10.1016/j.jaut.2005.11.004
61. Andrews BS, Eisenberg RA, Theofilopoulos AN, Izui S, Wilson CB, McConahey PJ, et al. Spontaneous murine lupus-like syndromes. clinical and immunopathological manifestations in several strains. *J Exp Med.* (1978) 148:1198–215. doi: 10.1084/jem.148.5.1198
62. Smith HR, Hansen CL, Rose R, Canoso RT. Autoimmune MRL-1 pr/1pr mice are an animal model for the secondary antiphospholipid syndrome. *J Rheumatol.* (1990) 17:911–5.
63. Moyer CF, Reinisch CL. Vasculitis in MRL/1 pr mice: model of cell-mediated autoimmunity. *Toxicol Pathol.* (1989) 17:122–8. doi: 10.1177/019262338901700108
64. Watanabe-Fukunaga R, Brannan CI, Copeland NG, Jenkins NA, Nagata S. Lymphoproliferation disorder in mice explained by defects in Fas antigen that mediates apoptosis. *Nature.* (1992) 356:314–7. doi: 10.1038/356314a0
65. Toda I, Sullivan BD, Rocha EM, Da Silveira LA, Wickham LA, Sullivan DA. Impact of gender on exocrine gland inflammation in mouse models of Sjogren's syndrome. *Exp Eye Res.* (1999) 69:355–66. doi: 10.1006/exer.1999.0715
66. Killian M, Batteux F, Paul S. The MRL/lpr mouse model: an important animal model for systemic sjogren syndrome and polyautoimmunity. *J Rheumatol.* (2020) 47:157. doi: 10.3899/jrheum.190820
67. Hiraishi M, Masum MA, Namba T, Otani Y, Elewa YH, Ichii O, et al. Histopathological changes in tear-secreting tissues and cornea in a mouse model of autoimmune disease. *Exp Biol Med.* (2020) 245:999–1008. doi: 10.1177/1535370220928275
68. Wang C, Zaheer M, Bian F, Quach D, Swennes AG, Britton RA, et al. Sjogren-like lacrimal keratoconjunctivitis in germ-free mice. *Int J Mol Sci.* (2018) 19:565. doi: 10.3390/ijms19020565
69. Takada K, Takiguchi M, Konno A, Inaba M. Spontaneous development of multiple glandular and extraglandular lesions in aged IQI/Jic mice: a model for primary sjogren's syndrome. *Rheumatology.* (2004) 43:858–62. doi: 10.1093/rheumatology/keh209
70. Dursun D, Wang M, Monroy D, Li DQ, Lokeshwar BL, Stern ME, et al. A mouse model of keratoconjunctivitis sicca. *Invest Ophthalmol Vis Sci.* (2002) 43:632–8.
71. Simsek C, Kojima T, Dogru M, Tsubota K. Alterations of murine subbasal corneal nerves after environmental dry eye stress. *Invest Ophthalmol Vis Sci.* (2018) 59:1986–95. doi: 10.1167/iovs.17-23743
72. Li J, Tan G, Ding X, Wang Y, Wu A, Yang Q, et al. A mouse dry eye model induced by topical administration of the air pollutant particulate matter 10. *Biomed Pharmacother.* (2017) 96:524–34. doi: 10.1016/j.biopha.2017.10.032
73. Song SJ, Hyun SW, Lee TG, Park B, Jo K, Kim CS. New application for assessment of dry eye syndrome induced by particulate matter exposure. *Ecotoxicol Environ Saf.* (2020) 205:111125. doi: 10.1016/j.ecoenv.2020.111125
74. Fujihara T, Nagano T, Nakamura M, Shirasawa E. Establishment of a rabbit short-term dry eye model. *J Ocul Pharmacol Ther.* (1995) 11:503–8. doi: 10.1089/jop.1995.11.503
75. Chen W, Zhang X, Zhang J, Chen J, Wang S, Wang Q, et al. A murine model of dry eye induced by an intelligently controlled environmental system. *Invest Ophthalmol Vis Sci.* (2008) 49:1386–91. doi: 10.1167/iovs.07-0744
76. Barabino S, Shen L, Chen L, Rashid S, Rolando M, Dana MR. The controlled-environment chamber: a new mouse model of dry eye. *Invest Ophthalmol Vis Sci.* (2005) 46:2766–71. doi: 10.1167/iovs.04-1326
77. Nakamura S, Shibuya M, Nakashima H, Imagawa T, Uehara M, Tsubota K. D-beta-hydroxybutyrate protects against corneal epithelial disorders in a rat dry eye model with jogging board. *Invest Ophthalmol Vis Sci.* (2005) 46:2379–87. doi: 10.1167/iovs.04-1344
78. Butovich IA. Lipidomics of human Meibomian gland secretions: chemistry, biophysics, and physiological role of meibomian lipids. *Prog Lipid Res.* (2011) 50:278–301. doi: 10.1016/j.plipres.2011.03.003
79. Bron AJ, Tiffany JM. The contribution of meibomian disease to dry eye. *Ocul Surf.* (2004) 2:149–65. doi: 10.1016/S1542-0124(12)70150-7
80. Jester JV, Nicolaides N, Kiss-Palvolgyi I, Smith RE. Meibomian gland dysfunction. II the role of keratinization in a rabbit model of MGD. *Invest Ophthalmol Vis Sci.* (1989) 30:936–45.
81. Gilbard JP, Rossi SR, Heyda KG. Tear film and ocular surface changes after closure of the meibomian gland orifices in the rabbit. *Ophthalmology.* (1989) 96:1180–6. doi: 10.1016/S0161-6420(89)32753-9
82. Jong MC, Gijbels MJ, Dahlmans VE, Gorp PJ, Koopman SJ, Ponec M, et al. Hyperlipidemia and cutaneous abnormalities in transgenic mice overexpressing human apolipoprotein C1. *J Clin Invest.* (1998) 101:145–52. doi: 10.1172/JCI791
83. Yagyu H, Kitamine T, Osuga J, Tozawa R, Chen Z, Kaji Y, et al. Absence of ACAT-1 attenuates atherosclerosis but causes dry eye and cutaneous xanthomatosis in mice with congenital hyperlipidemia. *J Biol Chem.* (2000) 275:21324–30. doi: 10.1074/jbc.M002541200
84. Naito A, Yoshida H, Nishioka E, Satoh M, Azuma S, Yamamoto T, et al. TRAF6-deficient mice display hypohidrotic ectodermal dysplasia. *Proc Natl Acad Sci U S A.* (2002) 99:8766–71. doi: 10.1073/pnas.132636999
85. Plikus M, Wang WP, Liu J, Wang X, Jiang TX, Chuong CM. Morpho-regulation of ectodermal organs: integument pathology and phenotypic variations in K14-Noggin engineered mice through modulation of bone morphogenic protein pathway. *Am J Pathol.* (2004) 164:1099–114. doi: 10.1016/S0002-9440(10)63197-5

86. Huang J, Dattilo LK, Rajagopal R, Liu Y, Kaartinen V, Mishina Y et al. FGF-regulated BMP signaling is required for eyelid closure and t specify conjunctival epithelial cell fate. *Development.* (2009) 136:1741–50. doi: 10.1242/dev.034082
87. Tsau C, Ito M, Gromova A, Hoffman MP, Meech R, Makarenkova HP. Barx2 and Fgf10 regulate ocular glands branching morphogenesis by controlling extracellular matrix remodeling. *Development.* (2011) 138:3307–17. doi: 10.1242/dev.066241
88. Kenchegowda D, Swamynathan S, Gupta D, Wan H, Whitsett J, Swamynathan SK. Conditional disruption of mouse Klf5 results in defective eyelids with malformed meibomian glands, abnormal cornea and loss of conjunctival goblet cells. *Dev Biol.* (2011) 356:5–18. doi: 10.1016/j.ydbio.2011.05.005
89. Lin MH, Hsu FF, Miner JH. Requirement of fatty acid transport protein 4 for development, maturation, and function of sebaceous glands in a mouse model of ichthyosis prematurity syndrome. *J Biol Chem.* (2013) 288:3964–76. doi: 10.1074/jbc.M112.416990
90. Reneker LW, Wang L, Irlmeier RT, Huang AJW. Fibroblast growth factor receptor 2 (FGFR2) is required for meibomian gland homeostasi in the adult mouse. *Invest Ophthalmol Vis Sci.* (2017) 58:2638–46. doi: 10.1167/iovs.16-21204
91. Wang YC, Li S, Chen X, Ma B, He H, Liu T, et al. Meibomian gland absence related dry eye in ectodysplasin a mutant mice. *Am J Pathol.* (2016) 186:32–42. doi: 10.1016/j.ajpath.2015.09.019
92. Simsek C, Kojima T, Nagata T, Dogru M, Tsubota K. Changes in murine subbasal corneal nerves after scopolamine-induced dry eye stress exposure. *Invest Ophthalmol Vis Sci.* (2019) 60:615–23. doi: 10.1167/iovs.18-26318
93. Viau S, Maire MA, Pasquis B, Gregoire S, Fourgeux C, Acar N, et al. Time course of ocular surface and lacrimal gland changes in a new scopolamine-induced dry eye model. *Graefes Arch Clin Exp Ophthalmol.* (2008) 246:857–67. doi: 10.1007/s00417-008-0784-9
94. Jaenen N, Baudouin C, Pouliquen P, Manni G, Figueiredo A, Zeyen T. Ocular symptoms and signs with preserved and preservative-free glaucoma medications. *Eur J Ophthalmol.* (2007) 17:341–9. doi: 10.1177/112067210701700311
95. Pisella PJ, Pouliquen P, Baudouin C. Prevalence of ocular symptoms and signs with preserved and preservative free glaucoma medication. *Br J Ophthalmol.* (2002) 86:418–23. doi: 10.1136/bjo.86.4.418
96. Galletti JG, Gabelloni ML, Morande PE, Sabbione F, Vermeulen ME, Trevani AS, et al. Benzalkonium chloride breaks down conjunctival immunological tolerance in a murine model. *Mucosal Immunol.* (2013) 6:24–34. doi: 10.1038/mi.2012.44
97. Baudouin C, Labbe A, Liang H, Pauly A, Brignole-Baudouin F. Preservatives in eyedrops: the good, the bad and the ugly. *Prog Retin Eye Res.* (2010) 29:312–34. doi: 10.1016/j.preteyeres.2010.03.001
98. Liang H, Baudouin C, Labbe A, Riancho L, Brignole-Baudouin F Conjunctiva-associated lymphoid tissue (CALT) reactions to antiglaucoma prostaglandins with or without BAK-preservative in rabbit acute toxicity study. *PLoS ONE.* (2012) 7:e33913. doi: 10.1371/journal.pone.0033913
99. Pauly A, Meloni M, Brignole-Baudouin F, Warnet JM, Baudouin C. Multiple endpoint analysis of the 3D-reconstituted corneal epithelium after treatment with benzalkonium chloride: early detection of toxic damage. *Invest Ophthalmol Vis Sci.* (2009) 50:1644–52. doi: 10.1167/iovs.08-2992
100. Jankovic J. Botulinum toxin: state of the art. *Mov Disord.* (2017) 32:1131–8. doi: 10.1002/mds.27072
101. Park CY, Zhuang W, Lekhanont K, Zhang C, Cano M, Lee WS, et al. Lacrimal gland inflammatory cytokine gene expression in the botulinum toxin B-induced murine dry eye model. *Mol Vis.* (2007) 13:2222–32.
102. Kim DW, Lee SH, Ku SK, Cho SH, Cho SW, Yoon GH, et al. Transduced PEP-1-FK506BP ameliorates corneal injury in Botulinum toxin A-induced dry eye mouse model. *BMB Rep.* (2013) 46:124–9. doi: 10.5483/BMBRep.2013.46.2.272
103. Choi W, Lee JB, Cui L, Li Y, Li Z, Choi JS, et al. Therapeutic efficacy of topically applied antioxidant medicinal plant extracts in a mouse model of experimental dry eye. *Oxid Med Cell Longev.* (2016) 2016:4727415. doi: 10.1155/2016/4727415
104. Li X, Kang B, Woo IH, Eom Y, Lee HK, Kim HM, et al. Effects of topical mucolytic agents on the tears and ocular surface: a plausible animal model of mucin-deficient dry eye. *Invest Ophthalmol Vis Sci.* (2018) 59:3104–14. doi: 10.1167/iovs.18-23860
105. Xiong C, Chen D, Liu J, Liu B, Li N, Zhou Y, et al. A rabbit dry eye model induced by topical medication of a preservative benzalkonium chloride. *Invest Ophthalmol Vis Sci.* (2008) 49:1850–6. doi: 10.1167/iovs.07-0720
106. Chen ZY, Liang QF, Yu GY. Establishment of a rabbit model for keratoconjunctivitis sicca. *Cornea.* (2011) 30:1024–9. doi: 10.1097/ICO.0b013e3181f1b0fc
107. Singh S, Moksha L, Sharma N, Titiyal JS, Biswas NR, Velpandian T. Development and evaluation of animal models for sex steroid deficient dry eye. *J Pharmacol Toxicol Methods.* (2014) 70:29–34. doi: 10.1016/j.vascn.2014.03.004
108. Zhu L, Shen J, Zhang C, Park CY, Kohanim S, Yew M, et al. Inflammatory cytokine expression on the ocular surface in the botulium toxin B induced murine dry eye model. *Mol Vis.* (2009) 15:250–8.
109. Suwan-apichon O, Rizen M, Rangsin R, Herretes S, Reyes JM, Lekhanont K, et al. Botulinum toxin B-induced mouse model of keratoconjunctivitis sicca. *Invest Ophthalmol Vis Sci.* (2006) 47:133–9. doi: 10.1167/iovs.05-0380
110. Li K, Zhang C, Yang Z, Wang Y, Si H. Evaluation of a novel dry eye model induced by oral administration of finasteride. *Mol Med Rep.* (2017) 16:8763–70. doi: 10.3892/mmr.2017.7754
111. Zoukhri D, Fix A, Alroy J, Kublin CL. Mechanisms of murine lacrimal gland repair after experimentally induced inflammation. *Invest Ophthalmol Vis Sci.* (2008) 49:4399–406. doi: 10.1167/iovs.08-1730
112. Zoukhri D, Macari E, Kublin CL. A single injection of interleukin-1 induces reversible aqueous-tear deficiency, lacrimal gland inflammation, and acinar and ductal cell proliferation. *Exp Eye Res.* (2007) 84:894–904. doi: 10.1016/j.exer.2007.01.015
113. Clayton JA. Dry eye. *N Engl J Med.* (2018) 378:2212–23. doi: 10.1056/NEJMra1407936
114. Stapleton F, Alves M, Bunya VY, Jalbert I, Lekhanont K, Malet F, et al. TFOS DEWS II epidemiology report. *Ocul Surf.* (2017) 15:334–65. doi: 10.1016/j.jtos.2017.05.003
115. Inomata T, Shiang T, Iwagami M, Sakemi F, Fujimoto K, Okumura Y, et al. Changes in distribution of dry eye disease by the new 2016 diagnostic criteria from the Asia dry eye society. *Sci Rep.* (2018) 8:1918. doi: 10.1038/s41598-018-19775-3
116. Barabino S, Chen Y, Chauhan S, Dana R. Ocular surface immunity: homeostatic mechanisms and their disruption in dry eye disease. *Prog Retin Eye Res.* (2012) 31:271–85. doi: 10.1016/j.preteyeres.2012.02.003
117. Inomata T, Nakamura M, Iwagami M, Shiang T, Yoshimura Y, Fujimoto K, et al. Risk factors for severe dry eye disease: crowdsourced research using dryeyerhythm. *Ophthalmology.* (2019) 126:766–8. doi: 10.1016/j.ophtha.2018.12.013
118. Shinomiya K, Ueta M, Kinoshita S. A new dry eye mouse model produced by exorbital and intraorbital lacrimal gland excision. *Sci Rep.* (2018) 8:1483. doi: 10.1038/s41598-018-19578-6
119. Anderson MS, Bluestone JA. The NOD mouse: a model of immune dysregulation. *Annu Rev Immunol.* (2005) 23:447–85. doi: 10.1146/annurev.immunol.23.021704.115643
120. Yoon KC, De Paiva CS, Qi H, Chen Z, Farley WJ, Li DQ, et al. Desiccating environmental stress exacerbates autoimmune lacrimal keratoconjunctivitis in non-obese diabetic mice. *J Autoimmun.* (2008) 30:212–21. doi: 10.1016/j.jaut.2007.09.003
121. Verhagen C, Rowshani T, Willekens B, van Haeringen NJ. Spontaneous development of corneal crystalline deposits in MRL/Mp mice. *Invest Ophthalmol Vis Sci.* (1995) 36:454–61.
122. Jeltsch-David H, Muller S. Neuropsychiatric systemic lupus erythematosus and cognitive dysfunction: the MRL-lpr mouse strain as a model. *Autoimmun Rev.* (2014) 13:963–73. doi: 10.1016/j.autrev.2014.08.015
123. Eom Y, Han JY, Kang B, Hwang HS, Lee HK, Kim HM, et al. Meibomian glands and ocular surface changes after closure of meibomian gland orifices in rabbits. *Cornea.* (2018) 37:218–26. doi: 10.1097/ICO.0000000000001460
124. Tan G, Li J, Yang Q, Wu A, Qu DY, Wang Y, et al. Air pollutant particulate matter 2. 5 induces dry eye syndrome in mice. *Sci Rep.* (2018) 8:17828. doi: 10.1038/s41598-018-36181-x

125. Kim Y, Choi YH, Kim MK, Paik HJ, Kim DH. Different adverse effects of air pollutants on dry eye disease: Ozone, PM2.5, and PM10. *Environ Pollut.* (2020) 265:115039. doi: 10.1016/j.envpol.2020.115039
126. Pflugfelder SC, de Paiva CS. The pathophysiology of dry eye disease: what we know and future directions for research. *Ophthalmology.* (2017) 124:S4–13. doi: 10.1016/j.ophtha.2017.07.010
127. Zhang Y, McCormick LL, Desai SR, Wu C, Gilliam AC. Murine sclerodermatous graft-versus-host disease, a model for human scleroderma: cutaneous cytokines, chemokines, and immune cell activation. *J Immunol.* (2002) 168:3088–98. doi: 10.4049/jimmunol.168.6.3088
128. Shimizu E, Ogawa Y, Yazu H, Aketa N, Yang F, Yamane M, et al. "Smart Eye Camera": An innovative technique to evaluate tear film breakup time in a murine dry eye disease model. *PLoS ONE.* (2019) 14:e0215130. doi: 10.1371/journal.pone.0215130
129. Carpena-Torres C, Pintor J, Huete-Toral F, Martin-Gil A, Rodriguez-Pomar C, Martinez-Aguila A, et al. Efficacy of artificial tears based on an extract of artemia salina containing dinucleotides in a rabbit dry eye model. *Int J Mol Sci.* (2021) 22:11999. doi: 10.3390/ijms222111999
130. Alanazi SA, Alomran AA, Abusharha A, Fagehi R, Al-Johani NJ, El-Hiti GA, et al. An assessment of the ocular tear film in patients with thyroid disorders. *Clin ophthalmol.* (2019) 13:1019–26. doi: 10.2147/OPTH.S210044
131. Takahashi Y, Lee PAL, Vaidya A, Kono S, Kakizaki H. Tear film break-up patterns in thyroid eye disease. *Sci Rep.* (2021) 11:5288. doi: 10.1038/s41598-021-84661-4
132. Jabs DA, Lee B, Whittum-Hudson JA, Prendergast RA. Th1 versus Th2 immune responses in autoimmune lacrimal gland disease in MRL/Mp mice. *Invest Ophthalmol Vis Sci.* (2000) 41:826–31. doi: 10.1097/00003226-200011002-00086

9

Therapeutic Effects of Topical Application of *Lycium barbarum* Polysaccharide in a Murine Model of Dry Eye

Danyi Qin, Yingping Deng, Lixiang Wang and Hongbo Yin*

Department of Ophthalmology, West China Hospital of Sichuan University, Chengdu, China

***Correspondence:**
Hongbo Yin
hongbo_yin@163.com

Purpose: To evaluate the safety and efficacy of *Lycium barbarum* polysaccharide (LBP) eye drops in a murine model of dry eye disease (DED).

Methods: Six- to eight-week-old female C57BL/6 mice were subjected to a combination of desiccating stress (DS) and topical benzalkonium chloride (BAC) to induce DED. Five microliters of LBP eye drops (0.625, 2.5, or 12.5 mg/ml) or PBS was applied topically 3 times per day for 10 days to subsequently test their efficacy. Tear secretion, tear breakup time (TBUT), corneal irregularity, and corneal fluorescein staining scores were measured on days 3 and 10 after treatment. The expression of tumor necrosis factor-alpha (TNF-α) in the cornea was assessed by quantitative (q) RT–PCR on days 10. The ocular irritation of LBP eye drops of corresponding concentrations was evaluated on 10- to 12-week-old female Sprague–Dawley rats.

Results: Compared with PBS-treated groups, mice treated with 0.625, 2.5, and 12.5 mg/ml LBP showed a significant improvement in the clinical signs of DED in a dose-dependent manner, including corneal epithelial integrity, corneal regularity, and tear production, as well as significant inhibition of inflammatory cell infiltration and TNF-α expression levels in the cornea. All corresponding concentrations of LBP eye drops revealed no obvious ocular irritation.

Conclusion: Topical application of LBP could ameliorate dry eye in a murine model of DED without obvious ocular irritation.

Keywords: *Lycium barbarum* polysaccharide, dry eye disease, inflammation, ocular surface, cornea

INTRODUCTION

Dry eye disease (DED) is a chronic multifactorial ocular surface disease characterized by the loss of homeostasis of the tear film (1), affecting 5–50% of the population on a global scale (2). Ocular manifestations of DED include ocular discomfort, vision fluctuation, and potential damage to the ocular surface. The fundamental mechanism of DED is the vicious cycle caused by tear film hyperosmolarity and ocular surface inflammation, in which mitogen-activated protein kinase (MAPK) and nuclear factor kappa B (NF-κB) are the main signaling pathways (3). Glucocorticoids, non-steroidal anti-inflammatory drugs (NSAIDs), and immunosuppressive agents are the most popular topical anti-inflammatory agents for DED (4). However, local and systemic side effects are relatively common and restrict their application in some cases (5–7). Thus, safe and effective DED treatments are under active exploration.

Wolfberry (*Lycium barbarum* or goji berry) has been used as a valuable traditional Chinese medicine for more than 2,000 years, whose main active ingredient is Lycium barbarum polysaccharide (LBP) (8). Versatile functions of LBP, including immune-regulatory, anti-oxidative, anti-aging, and anti-inflammatory effects, have been revealed in several animal models of systemic diseases (9–11), as well as ocular fundus diseases (12–14). However, there is no relevant study about its anti-inflammatory effect on the ocular surface, especially with the drug delivery route of topical administration. Since inflammation plays a vital role in the progression of DED, LBP is likely to take effect.

In the current study, we investigated the safety and efficacy of LBP eye drops in a murine model of DED and explored their potential mechanisms to provide primary data for LBP ophthalmic preparations.

MATERIALS AND METHODS

Preparation of *Lycium barbarum* Polysaccharide Eye Drops

Lycium barbarum polysaccharide (Catalog No. SP9311; Solarbio, Beijing, China) was diluted in sterile phosphate-buffered saline (PBS) to final concentrations of 0.625, 2.5, and 12.5 mg/ml. The eye drops were all freshly prepared and stored at 4°C prior to their use.

Animals

Ten- to twelve-week-old female Sprague–Dawley (SD) rats and six- to eight-week-old female C57BL/6 (B6) mice were obtained from SPF (Beijing) Biotechnology Co., Ltd. All animals were kept under standard laboratory conditions with 12-h/12-h light-dark cycles, with food and water *ad libitum*. All animals were acclimated to the experimental environment for at least 1 week before the beginning of the study. Efforts were made to minimize the number of experimental animals and their suffering. All procedures conformed to the Association for Research in Vision and Ophthalmology Statement for the Use of Animals in Ophthalmic and Vision Research, and the present study was approved by the Animal Care and Use Committee (IACUC) of National Chengdu New Drug Safety Evaluation Center (approval number S2019022-P015-04).

Mouse Model of Dry Eye

Desiccating stress (DS) was created by subcutaneous injection of 0.025 g/kg scopolamine hydrobromide (Chengdu YiRui Bio-Technology, Co., Ltd, Chengdu, batch number YRQ098-200901) 3 times daily (10 a.m., 1 p.m., and 4 p.m.) and exposure to a mini fan in a controlled dry environment (airflow rate of 15 L/min, relative humidity of 30–40%) 8 h per day for 7 days. This approach has been demonstrated to successfully induce the dry eye condition in mice (15). To enhance the ocular surface inflammation, 0.3% benzalkonium chloride (BAC) (Sigma–Aldrich, St. Louis, MO, United States, B6295) was topically applied on the ocular surface 3 times daily (10 a.m., 1 p.m., and 4 p.m.) simultaneously, as described by Zhang (16). A group of age-matched mice that did not receive any treatment served as non-stressed (NS) controls.

Efficacy of *Lycium barbarum* Polysaccharide Eye Drops on B6 Mice

To evaluate the efficacy of LBP on the ocular surface of dry eye, 5 μl topical LBP was applied to B6 mice subjected to DS and BAC at low doses (LLBP, 0.625 mg/ml), medium doses (MLBP, 2.5 mg/ml), or high doses (HLBP, 12.5 mg/ml) 3 times daily (10 a.m., 1 p.m., and 4 p.m.) for 10 days. Animals in the vehicle control group and NS control group were given topical PBS with the same dosing regimen. The effects were evaluated with the tear secretion test, tear breakup time (TBUT), corneal fluorescein staining, and corneal irregularity test on days 3 and days 10 after treatment. Mice were then euthanized, and the globes were collected for histology study at the end of the study.

Tear production was measured with phenol red cotton threads (Tianjin Jingming Technological Development Co., Ltd., Tianjin, China). The thread was placed at the lateral 1/3 of the lower eyelid margin for 1 min, and the length of the wet part was measured.

To measure the TBUT, 2 μl of 0.1% sodium fluorescein was applied to the conjunctival sac. Mice were manually allowed to blink three times, and the time from the last blink to the first onset of breaking spots on the ocular surface was observed with the cobalt blue filter of a slit-lamp microscope (66 Vision Tech Co., Ltd., Hangzhou, China). In addition, corneal staining with fluorescein was observed and graded following the standard by the Chinese consensus of DED (17). Briefly, the cornea was equally divided into four quadrants and scored individually: Absent, 0; punctate staining $\leq$ 30 spots, 1; punctate staining > 30 spots but not diffuse, 2; diffuse staining, 3. The scores of each quadrant were summed (maximum, 12 points).

Corneal irregularity scores were evaluated by reflecting a ring light on the ocular surface to assess corneal smoothness (18). Corneal irregularity was scored as follows: no distortion, 0; distortion in one quadrant, 1; distortion in two quadrants, 2; distortion in three quadrants, 3; distortion in all four quadrants, 4; severe distortion and no ring shape recognizable, 5.

Safety Evaluation

To evaluate the safety of LBP eye drops on the ocular surface, LBP treatment was performed on SD rats by topical application of 10 μl LBP (0.625, 2.5, or 12.5 mg/ml) or vehicle (PBS) eye drops 3 times daily (10 a.m., 1 p.m., and 4 p.m.) for 7 days. Blank eyes with no treatment were used as a non-treatment control. Ocular irritation was observed on days 1, 2, 3, and 7 after treatment. Irritation of the cornea, iris, and conjunctiva was separately

TABLE 1 | The primers sequence.

Gene	Primer	The primers sequence
TNF-α	Forward	5′-CTGAACTTCGGGGTGATCGG-3′
	Reverse	5′-GGCTTGTCACTCGAATTTTGAGA-3′
β-actin	Forward	5′-GTCCCTCACCCTCCCAAAAG-3′
	Reverse	5′-GCTGCCTCAACACCTCAACCC-3′

scored on a 0–4 scale and summed to a total grade following the standard of the Draize scale scoring system (maximum 100 points) (19).

Histology Study

Both the eyes and adnexa of SD rats and the right eyes and adnexa of B6 mice from each group were surgically excised after euthanasia at the end of the study. The tissues were fixed in 10% formalin solution, trimmed, embedded in paraffin, cut into serial sagittal sections (5 μm thick), and stained with hematoxylin and eosin (H&E) following standard protocols. The slides were imaged using a DP72 digital camera (Olympus, Tokyo, Japan). The cell types were identified by the morphology. The density of inflammatory cells (polymorphonuclear and monocytes) in the cornea was manually counted in 10 cross-sectional high-power fields (HPFs) at 40× magnification that evenly distribute from the nasal to the temporal limbus.

Corneal TNF-α Level

The relative mRNA expression level of TNF-α in the cornea of the left eyes of B6 mice was examined with quantitative reverse-transcription polymerase chain reaction (qRT–PCR). The cornea was carefully excised from the globe, immediately frozen with liquid nitrogen, and transferred to a -70°C refrigerator for storage before the test. Total RNA was extracted using a total RNA isolation kit (Catalog no. R1200; Solarbio, Beijing, China). First-strand cDNA was synthesized using a reverse transcription kit (Catalog no. FP205; TIANGEN, Beijing, China). Real-time PCR was performed on a real-time PCR system (Q2000A Biosystems, LongGene, Hangzhou, China). The primers are provided in **Table 1**. The parameters were predenaturation at 95°C for 15 min, followed by 40 cycles of denaturation at 95°C for 10 s, annealing for 20 s, and final extension at 72°C for 30 s. A melting curve analysis was conducted to check the amplification specificity. Samples and standards were assessed in duplicate. The $2^{-\Delta\Delta Ct}$ method was employed to calculate the relative TNF-α expression levels using β-actin as a reference gene (20, 21).

Statistical Analysis

Continuous data following a normal distribution are represented as the mean ± standard deviation (SD); otherwise, they are represented as the median (interquartile range) (IQR). Statistical significance was evaluated by multiway ANOVA with Tukey's *post-hoc* test or by Kruskal–Wallis test when appropriate using SPSS Statistics 26.0 (IBM, Armonk, NY, United States) and GraphPad Prism 5.0 software (GraphPad Software; San Diego, CA, United States). $P < 0.05$ was considered statistically significant.

RESULTS

Topical Application of *Lycium barbarum* Polysaccharide Improved Corneal Epithelial Integrity and Regularity

The corneal fluorescein staining scores significantly increased in the DS + PBS group compared to the NS group 7 days after modeling [**Figure 1B**; NS vs. DS + PBS, 1.5 (2.25) vs. 12 (0.75), $P < 0.0001$]. As shown in **Figures 1A,B**, compared with PBS treatment, topical application of HLBP significantly decreased corneal fluorescein staining on both days 3 [**Figure 1B**; DS + PBS vs. DS + HLBP, 8 (3.25) vs. 6 (2); $P < 0.05$] and days 10 [**Figure 1B**; DS + PBS vs. DS + HLBP, 9.5 (4) vs. 5 (2.25); $P < 0.05$]. The corneal irregularity scores were significantly increased in the DS + PBS group compared with the NS group [**Figure 1D**; NS vs. DS + PBS, 0 (0) vs. 2 (2), $P < 0.0001$]. As shown in **Figures 1C,D**, topical application of HLBP significantly improved corneal surface regularity compared with the DS + PBS group on days 10 [**Figure 1D**; DS + PBS vs. DS + HLBP, 2 (2.25) vs. 1 (1); $P < 0.05$].

Topical Application of *Lycium barbarum* Polysaccharide Improved the Tear Secretion Rate and Tear Film Stability

Compared to the NS group, the DS + PBS group showed a significantly decreased tear secretion rate (**Figure 2A**; NS vs. DS + PBS, 10.400 ± 2.836 mm/min vs. 1.825 ± 1.107 mm/min, $P < 0.0001$). Topical application of HLBP significantly increased the tear secretion rate on days 3 (**Figure 2A**; DS + PBS vs. DS + HLBP, 4.200 ± 1.229 mm vs. 6.700 ± 0.6749 mm; $P < 0.05$), and topical application of LLBP, MLBP, and HLBP all significantly increased the tear secretion rate on days 10 (**Figure 2A**; DS + PBS vs. DS + LLBP, 4.900 ± 1.912 mm vs. 7.700 ± 2.214 mm; $P < 0.05$; DS + PBS vs. DS + MLBP, 4.900 ± 1.912 mm vs. 8.100 ± 2.601 mm; $P < 0.05$; DS + PBS vs. DS + HLBP, 4.900 ± 1.912 mm vs. 8.600 ± 1.897 mm; $P < 0.01$). These results suggested that topical application of LBP could improve tear production during DS.

TBUTs significantly decreased in the DS + PBS group compared with the NS group [**Figure 2B**; NS vs. DS + PBS, 4.5 (2.25) s vs. 0 (0) s, $P < 0.0001$]. After 10 days of topical treatment with HLBP, the TBUTs significantly improved compared with PBS treatment [**Figure 2B**; DS + PBS vs. DS + HLBP, 1 (0.25) s vs. 2 (1) s; $P < 0.05$].

Topical Application of *Lycium barbarum* Polysaccharide Inhibited Ocular Surface Inflammation

Compared with the NS group, the DS + PBS group showed obvious inflammatory cell infiltration on the ocular surface (**Figure 3A**; NS vs. DS + PBS, 12.700 ± 3.199/HPF vs.

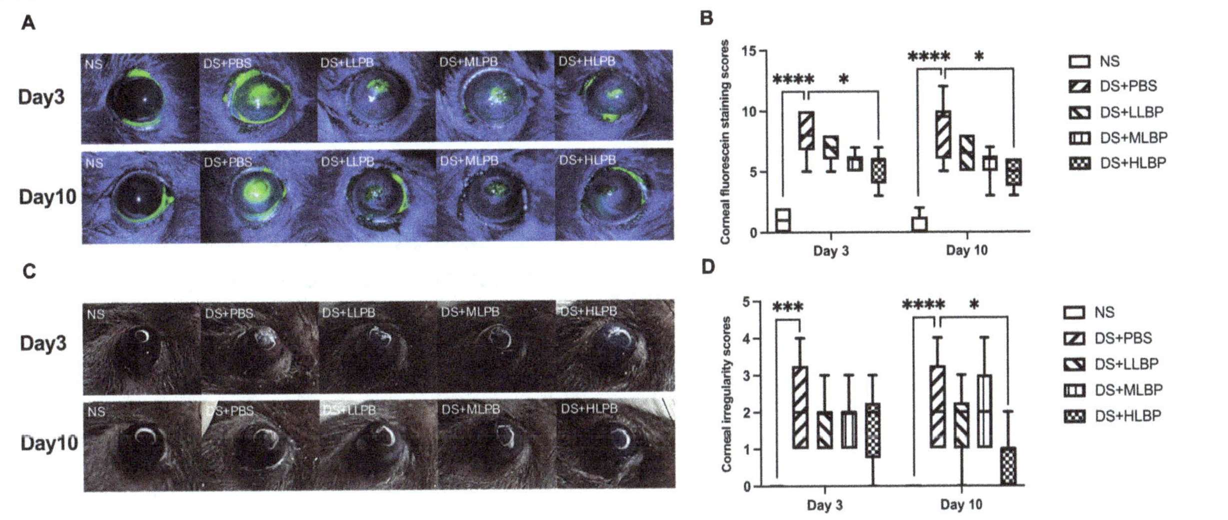

FIGURE 1 | The effects of topical application of LBP on corneal epithelial integrity and regularity in a mouse DED model. **(A)** Representative images of corneal fluorescein staining in different groups on days 3 and 10 after treatment. **(B)** The results of corneal fluorescein staining scores of different groups on days 3 and 10 after treatment. **(C)** Representative images of corneal irregularity in different groups on days 3 and 10 after treatment. **(D)** The comprehensive results of corneal irregularity scores of different groups on days 3 and 10 after treatment. Data were shown as median (IQR). $^{*}P < 0.05$, $^{***}P < 0.001$, $^{****}P < 0.0001$.

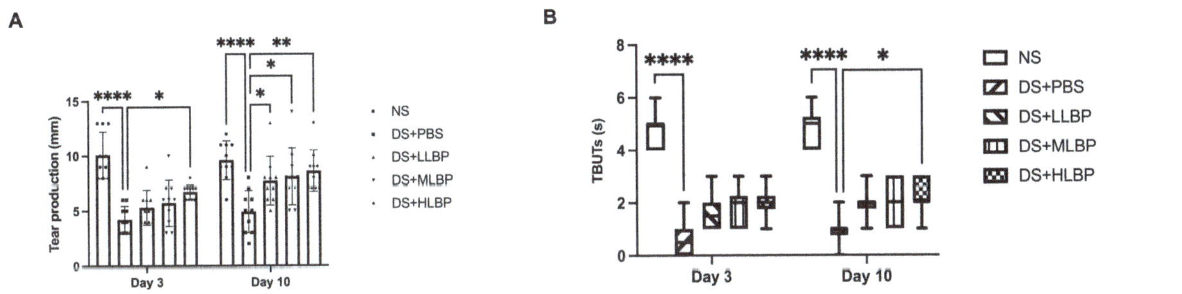

FIGURE 2 | **(A)** The effects of topical application of LBP on the tear secretion rate on days 3 and 10 after treatment. **(B)** The effects of topical application of LBP on TBUTs on days 3 and 10 after treatment. Data of tear secretion rate were shown as the mean ± SD. Data of TBUTs were shown as median (IQR). $^{*}P < 0.05$, $^{**}P < 0.01$, $^{****}P < 0.0001$.

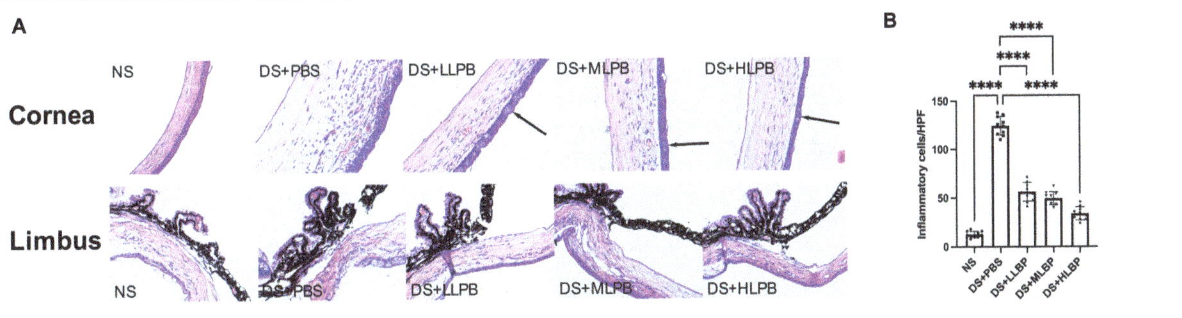

FIGURE 3 | **(A)** Representative images of H&E staining in the cornea and limbus of different groups on days 10 after treatment. The arrows showed corneal conjunctivization (magnification: 40×). **(B)** The inflammatory cell count in the cornea and limbus of different groups on days 10 after treatment. $^{****}P < 0.0001$.

124.400 ± 9.743/HPF, $P < 0.0001$), accompanied by corneal edema and neovascularization. In addition, corneal conjunctivization could be observed in some cases in the DS groups. Topical application of LBP effectively suppressed the DS-induced infiltration of inflammatory cells on the ocular surface in a dose-dependent manner (**Figure 3B**; DS + PBS vs. DS + LLBP, 124.400 ± 9.743/HPF vs. 56.300 ± 9.581/HPF; $P < 0.0001$; DS + PBS vs. DS + MLBP, 124.400 ± 9.743/HPF vs. 49.600 ± 6.637/HPF; $P < 0.0001$; DS + PBS vs. DS + HLBP, 124.400 ± 9.743/HPF vs. 33.900 ± 6.839/HPF; $P < 0.0001$).

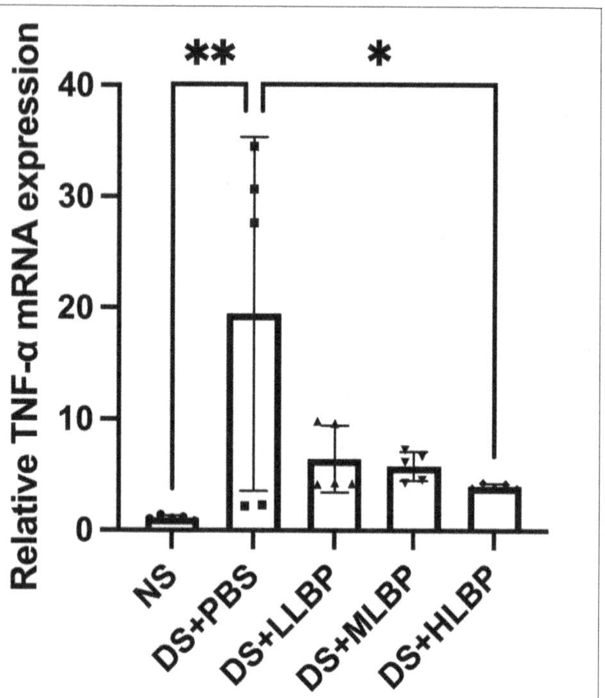

FIGURE 4 | The effects of topical application of LBP on the relative expression level of TNF-α mRNA in the cornea. Data were shown as the mean ± SD. *$P < 0.05$, **$P < 0.01$.

Edema and neovascularization in the cornea, limbus, and iris were also alleviated after treatment.

Topical Application of *Lycium barbarum* Polysaccharide Reduced TNF-α Production in the Cornea of B6 Mice

The relative expression level of TNF-α mRNA in the cornea significantly increased in the DS + PBS group compared to the NS group (**Figure 4**; NS vs. DS + PBS, 1.100 ± 0.213 vs. 19.470 ± 15.920; $P < 0.01$). Topical application of HLBP for 10 days significantly decreased the relative TNF-α expression level in the cornea (**Figure 4**; DS + PBS vs. DS + HLBP, 19.470 ± 15.920 vs. 3.989 ± 0.236; $P < 0.05$).

Topical Application of *Lycium barbarum* Polysaccharide Did Not Induce Irritations or Pathological Changes on the Ocular Surface in Sprague–Dawley Rats

Tables 2, 3 demonstrate the results of the safety test evaluated by the Draize scale scoring system and corneal fluorescein staining, respectively. For all time points and tissues, the scores of each group remained nearly constant. There were no significant differences in the Draize or fluorescence scores among all groups at any time point. **Figure 5** shows the results of H&E staining of the ocular surface from the HLBP group on days 7. There was no congestion or edema in the conjunctiva. The structure of the iris and each layer of the cornea remained normal. No obvious inflammatory cell infiltration or other histopathological changes were observed.

DISCUSSION

Dry eye disease is one of the most common chronic inflammatory ocular surface diseases with an increasingly high prevalence. Safe and effective anti-inflammatory therapies are always needed. LBP, a water-soluble polysaccharide, possesses an effect of anti-inflammation. However, very few studies concentrate on its effects on ocular surface diseases. Moreover, the methods of LBP administration in almost all the studies are oral administration or gavage, rather than topical application *via* eye drops. Therefore, this study evaluated the ocular surface irritation and the effects of LBP eye drops on DED.

Our findings demonstrated that topical application of LBP could effectively improve corneal epithelial integrity, corneal regularity, and tear production in a murine DED model induced

TABLE 2 | The comprehensive results of ocular surface irritation scored following the Draize scale scoring system.

Draize scores [median (IQR)]	NT	PBS	LLBP	MLBP	HLBP	*P*-value
Day 0	0 (0)	0 (0)	0 (0)	0 (0)	0 (0)	1.000
Day 1	0 (0)	1 (2)	1 (2)	3 (2)	0 (0)	0.213
Day 2	0 (0)	0 (0)	1 (2)	1 (2)	0 (0)	0.497
Day 3	0 (0)	0 (0)	0 (0)	2 (2)	0 (0)	0.061
Day 7	0 (0)	0 (0)	0 (0)	1 (2)	0 (0)	0.406

TABLE 3 | The results of corneal fluorescein staining scores in the safety test.

Corneal fluorescein scores [median (IQR)]	NT	PBS	LLBP	MLBP	HLBP	*P*-value
Day 0	0 (0)	0 (2)	0 (0)	0 (0)	0 (0)	0.406
Day 1	0 (0)	0 (0)	0 (0)	0 (0)	0 (0)	1.000
Day 2	0 (0)	0 (0)	0 (0)	0 (0)	0 (0)	1.000
Day 3	0 (0)	0 (0)	0 (0)	0 (0)	0 (0)	1.000
Day 7	0 (0)	0 (0)	0 (0)	0 (0)	0 (0)	1.000

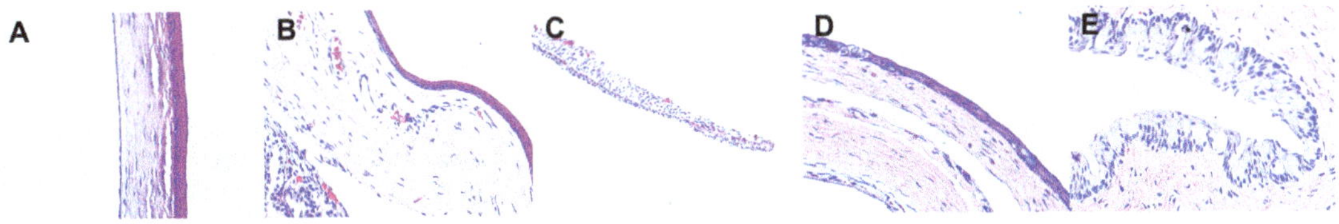

FIGURE 5 | Representative images of H&E staining of ocular tissues on days 7. **(A)** the cornea; **(B)** the limbus; **(C)** the iris; **(D)** the bulbar conjunctiva; **(E)** the fornix conjunctiva (magnification: 40×).

by DS and BAC. It could also decrease inflammatory cell infiltration, alleviate edema of the ocular tissues, and reduce the expression of TNF-α in the cornea. It showed little irritation or toxicity to the ocular surface. These results are consistent with our hypothesis.

Subcutaneous injection of scopolamine hydrobromide combined with DES is commonly used to establish DED models in mice (15). However, the dry eye symptoms are self-limited and begin to subside once DS is eliminated in our previous work, which is consistent with Yoon's study (22). Topical administration of BAC drops is another valid approach to induce dry eye (16). Therefore, we combined DS and BAC to acquire a stable and reliable murine DED model, whose severe manifestations of dry eye persisted through the end of our study and could be ameliorated by topical treatment with LBP.

Ocular surface inflammation induced by tear film instability and tear hyperosmolarity plays a vital role in the pathogenesis and progression of chronic DED (1). Inflammatory cytokines, such as interferon-1 (IL-1) produced mainly by Th1 cells and TNF-α produced mainly by Th17 cells, are elevated in the cornea and conjunctiva of dry eye (3). TNF-α is significantly increased in the tears of dry eye patients as one of the most common pro-inflammatory cytokines. TNF-α triggers several signal transduction pathways, such as NF-κB, p38 MAPK, extracellular signal-regulated kinase (ERK), and c-Jun N-terminal kinase (JNK), by interacting with TNF receptor 1 (TNFR1) and TNF receptor 2 (TNFR2) on the ocular surface (23, 24). TNF-α is considered to be correlated with disease severity, including OSDI score and tear secretion. It can stimulate matrix metalloproteinase (MMP) activation, promote mononuclear cell infiltration into glands, and enhance the apoptosis of glandular epithelial cells (25, 26). In addition, numerous attempts have been made to develop TNF-α blockers as potential therapeutic agents for the treatment of inflammatory diseases (27). Thus, TNF-α could serve as an inflammatory biomarker of DED. Meanwhile, the mechanism of the anti-inflammatory effects of LBP in many systemic diseases was found to be related to TNF-α and its upstream and downstream pathways (9, 10, 28, 29). In our study, the expression of TNF-α in the cornea significantly increased in the murine DED model, and decreased after the treatment of HLBP. Accordingly, we speculated that LBP eye drops inhibited the inflammation on the ocular surface by decreasing TNF-α, which needs to be further evaluated in the future studies.

This is the first study to investigate the safety and efficacy of LBP eye drops in treating DED. Our study uncovered that topical application of LBP alleviated dry eye symptoms and inhibited ocular surface inflammation in a murine DED model, providing the primary data for LBP ophthalmic preparations. Additionally, LBP has an advantage over other anti-inflammatory drugs due to its easy availability in natural plants and low price, without toxicity or short-term side effects. However, there are several limitations in our study. The underlying mechanism is still unclear. Further studies are needed to explore the specific anti-inflammatory pathways of LBP in DED treatment. The long-term efficacy and safety remain to be determined.

ETHICS STATEMENT

The animal study was reviewed and approved by the Animal Care and Use Committee (IACUC) of National Chengdu New Drug Safety Evaluation Center (approval number S2019022-P015-04).

AUTHOR CONTRIBUTIONS

DQ, YD, LW, and HY performed the material preparation and data collection and analysis. DQ wrote the first draft of the manuscript. All authors contributed to the study conception and design, commented on previous versions of the manuscript, and read and approved the final manuscript.

REFERENCES

1. Craig JP, Nichols KK, Akpek EK, Caffery B, Dua HS, Joo CK, et al. TFOS DEWS II definition and classification report. *Ocul Surf.* (2017) 15:276–83. doi: 10.1016/j.jtos.2017.05.008
2. Stapleton F, Alves M, Bunya VY, Jalbert I, Lekhanont K, Malet F, et al. TFOS DEWS II epidemiology report. *Ocul Surf.* (2017) 15:334–65. doi: 10.1016/j.jtos.2017.05.003
3. Bron AJ, de Paiva CS, Chauhan SK, Bonini S, Gabison EE, Jain S, et al. TFOS DEWS II pathophysiology report. *Ocul Surf.* (2017) 15:438–510. doi: 10.1016/j.jtos.2017.05.011
4. Hessen M, Akpek EK. Dry eye: an inflammatory ocular disease. *J Ophthalmic Vis Res.* (2014) 9:240–50.
5. Cutolo CA, Barabino S, Bonzano C, Traverso CE. The use of topical corticosteroids for treatment of dry eye syndrome. *Ocul Immunol Inflamm.* (2019) 27:266–75. doi: 10.1080/09273948.2017.1341988
6. Rigas B, Huang W, Honkanen R. NSAID-induced corneal melt: clinical importance, pathogenesis, and risk mitigation. *Surv Ophthalmol.* (2020) 65:1–11. doi: 10.1016/j.survophthal.2019.07.001
7. Hornbeak DM, Thorne JE. Immunosuppressive therapy for eye diseases: effectiveness, safety, side effects and their prevention. *Taiwan J Ophthalmol.* (2015) 5:156–63. doi: 10.1016/j.tjo.2015.03.004

8. Xiao Z, Deng Q, Zhou W, Zhang Y. Immune activities of polysaccharides isolated from *Lycium barbarum* L. What do we know so far? *Pharmacol Ther.* (2021) 229:107921. doi: 10.1016/j.pharmthera.2021.107921
9. Chen L, Li W, Qi D, Wang D. *Lycium barbarum* polysaccharide protects against LPS-induced ARDS by inhibiting apoptosis, oxidative stress, and inflammation in pulmonary endothelial cells. *Free Radic Res.* (2018) 52:480–90. doi: 10.1080/10715762.2018.1447105
10. Xiong GF, Li DW, Zheng MB, Liu SC. The effects of *Lycium barbarum* polysaccharide (LBP) in a mouse model of cerulein-induced acute pancreatitis. *Med Sci Monit.* (2019) 25:3880–6. doi: 10.12659/MSM.913820
11. Wang Y, Xiao J, Duan Y, Miao M, Huang B, Chen J, et al. *Lycium barbarum* polysaccharide ameliorates Sjogren's syndrome in a murine model. *Mol Nutr Food Res.* (2021) 65:e2001118. doi: 10.1002/mnfr.202001118
12. Yang D, So KF, Lo AC. *Lycium barbarum* polysaccharide extracts preserve retinal function and attenuate inner retinal neuronal damage in a mouse model of transient retinal ischaemia. *Clin Exp Ophthalmol.* (2017) 45:717–29. doi: 10.1111/ceo.12950
13. Tang L, Bao S, Du Y, Jiang Z, Wuliji AO, Ren X, et al. Antioxidant effects of *Lycium barbarum* polysaccharides on photoreceptor degeneration in the light-exposed mouse retina. *Biomed Pharmacother.* (2018) 103:829–37. doi: 10.1016/j.biopha.2018.04.104
14. Lakshmanan Y, Wong FSY, Zuo B, So KF, Bui BV, Chan HH. Posttreatment intervention with *Lycium barbarum* polysaccharides is neuroprotective in a rat model of chronic ocular hypertension. *Invest Ophthalmol Vis Sci.* (2019) 60:4606–18. doi: 10.1167/iovs.19-27886
15. Chen Y, Chauhan SK, Lee HS, Stevenson W, Schaumburg CS, Sadrai Z, et al. Effect of desiccating environmental stress versus systemic muscarinic AChR blockade on dry eye immunopathogenesis. *Invest Ophthalmol Vis Sci.* (2013) 54:2457–64. doi: 10.1167/iovs.12-11121
16. Zhang R, Park M, Richardson A, Tedla N, Pandzic E, de Paiva CS, et al. Dose-dependent benzalkonium chloride toxicity imparts ocular surface epithelial changes with features of dry eye disease. *Ocul Surf.* (2020) 18:158–69. doi: 10.1016/j.jtos.2019.11.006
17. Corneal Disease Group of Ophthalmological Society CMA. Experts'consensus about clinical diagnosis and treatment of dry eye (2013). *Chin J Ophthalmol.* (2013) 49:73–5.
18. De Paiva CS, Corrales RM, Villarreal AL, Farley W, Li DQ, Stern ME, et al. Apical corneal barrier disruption in experimental murine dry eye is abrogated by methylprednisolone and doxycycline. *Invest Ophthalmol Vis Sci.* (2006) 47:2847–56. doi: 10.1167/iovs.05-1281
19. Wilhelmus KR. The Draize eye test. *Surv Ophthalmol.* (2001) 45:493–515. doi: 10.1016/s0039-6257(01)00211-9
20. Livak KJ, Schmittgen TD. Analysis of relative gene expression data using real-time quantitative PCR and the 2(-Delta Delta C(T)) Method. *Methods.* (2001) 25:402–8. doi: 10.1006/meth.2001.1262
21. Schmittgen TD, Livak KJ. Analyzing real-time PCR data by the comparative C(T) method. *Nat Protoc.* (2008) 3:1101–8. doi: 10.1038/nprot.2008.73
22. Yoon KC, Ahn KY, Choi W, Li Z, Choi JS, Lee SH, et al. Tear production and ocular surface changes in experimental dry eye after elimination of desiccating stress. *Invest Ophthalmol Vis Sci.* (2011) 52:7267–73. doi: 10.1167/iovs.11-7231
23. Zhao H, Li Q, Ye M, Yu J. Tear luminex analysis in dry eye patients. *Med Sci Monit.* (2018) 24:7595–602. doi: 10.12659/MSM.912010
24. Luo L, Li DQ, Doshi A, Farley W, Corrales RM, Pflugfelder SC. Experimental dry eye stimulates production of inflammatory cytokines and MMP-9 and activates MAPK signaling pathways on the ocular surface. *Invest Ophthalmol Vis Sci.* (2004) 45:4293–301. doi: 10.1167/iovs.03-1145
25. Fong PY, Shih KC, Lam PY, Chan TCY, Jhanji V, Tong L. Role of tear film biomarkers in the diagnosis and management of dry eye disease. *Taiwan J Ophthalmol.* (2019) 9:150–9. doi: 10.4103/tjo.tjo_56_19
26. Jamerson EC, Elhusseiny AM, ElSheikh RH, Eleiwa TK, El Sayed YM. Role of matrix metalloproteinase 9 in ocular surface disorders. *Eye Contact Lens.* (2020) 46(Suppl. 2):S57–63. doi: 10.1097/ICL.0000000000000668
27. Choi W, Noh H, Yeo A, Jang H, Ahn HK, Song YJ, et al. The effect of TNF-alpha blocker HL036337 and its best concentration to inhibit dry eye inflammation. *Korean J Ophthalmol.* (2016) 30:302–8. doi: 10.3341/kjo.2016.30.4.302
28. Liu Q, Han Q, Lu M, Wang H, Tang F. *Lycium barbarum* polysaccharide attenuates cardiac hypertrophy, inhibits calpain-1 expression and inhibits NF-kappaB activation in streptozotocin-induced diabetic rats. *Exp Ther Med.* (2019) 18:509–16. doi: 10.3892/etm.2019.7612
29. Cui F, Shi CL, Zhou XJ, Gao XP, Wang LY, He B, et al. *Lycium barbarum* polysaccharide extracted from *Lycium barbarum* leaves ameliorates asthma in mice by reducing inflammation and modulating gut microbiota. *J Med Food.* (2020) 23:699–710. doi: 10.1089/jmf.2019

10

Advances in Dry Eye Disease Examination Techniques

*Yaying Wu, Chunyang Wang, Xin Wang, Yujie Mou, Kelan Yuan, Xiaodan Huang and Xiuming Jin**

Eye Center, School of Medicine, 2nd Affiliated Hospital, Zhejiang University, Hangzhou, China

***Correspondence:**
Xiuming Jin
lzyjxm@zju.edu.cn

Dry eye-related ocular surface examination is very important in the diagnosis and treatment of dry eye disease. With the recent advances in science and technology, dry eye examination techniques have progressed rapidly, which has greatly improved dry eye diagnoses and treatment. However, clinically, confusion remains about which examination to choose, how to ensure the repeatability of the examination, and how to accurately interpret the examination results. In this review, we systematically evaluate previous examinations of dry eye, analyze the latest views and research hotspots, and provide a reference for the diagnosis and management of dry eye.

Keywords: dry eye, examination, tear, meibomian gland, demodex mites

INTRODUCTION

Dry eye is a multifactor disease defined as "the loss of tear film homeostasis accompanied by ocular symptoms, caused by tear film instability and hyperosmolar, ocular surface inflammation and damage, and neuroparesthesia" (1). The global prevalence of dry eye disease is 5–50% depending on the population and disease definition, whereas in the United States, over 16 million adults have been diagnosed with the disease (2). Traditionally, dry eye has been classified as aqueous deficiency, evaporative, or mixed mode. This classification has been extended to take into account anatomical contributions to signs and symptoms, including neurological abnormalities (1). Common diagnostic methods include consideration of the chief complaint, a questionnaire, a physical examination, a tear film rupture test, corneal punctate staining, and a tear secretion test (3–5). Others include tear osmotic pressure and the tear ferning test (6–8). However, to an extent, the pathogenic factors and disease development of dry eye are complicated, and the separation of subjective feeling and objective signs is often encountered in clinical practice, which brings certain challenges to the diagnosis and treatment of the condition (9–14). With the advent of the technological era and prolific screen reading, the incidence of dry eye has increased (15, 16). As a result, greater attention is being paid to dry eye, so clinics have in turn developed more sophisticated means of checking for the condition through more targeted point-of-care tests and imaging technologies to help clinical doctors diagnose the type and severity of dry eye more effectively (17). In view of the importance of the systematic examination and evaluation of dry eye, in this paper, we summarize the relevant examination methods currently known, evaluate the new technologies available, and explore the progress of dry eye diagnostic methods, which may be helpful in the clinical diagnosis and treatment of dry eye.

A worker must first sharpen their tools if they want to do well. The examination of dry eye is very important for the diagnosis and treatment of dry eye. With recent advances in science and technology, the examination of dry eye has progressed rapidly, which has greatly improved dry eye diagnosis and treatment. In this paper, we summarize and analyze the latest progress in dry eye examination, which may be helpful in the clinical diagnosis and treatment of dry eye.

TEAR EXAMINATION

The normal tear film is made up of three layers: the lipid layer, the aqueous layer, and the mucin layer. Tears play an important role in maintaining the stability of the ocular surface microenvironment. Changes in the quality or quantity of tears will lead to the occurrence of dry eyes, and tear supplementation is an important part of dry eye treatment. The examination of the quality and quantity of tears is therefore an important indicator for the diagnosis of dry eye. In addition to the traditional tear secretion test and tear river height [tear meniscus height (TMH)] measurement, tear osmotic pressure, tear inflammatory factors, and the tear ferning test play important roles in the diagnosis of dry eye (18).

Tear Examination

Schirmer's Test

Schirmer's test has been used as a diagnostic test for dry eye disease since 1903 and can help to evaluate tear volumes (19). The test is based on the physical tendency of a fluid to travel along a strip of porous material by capillary action due to surface tension (20–22). No consensus exists on the diagnostic criteria of dry eye in Schirmer's test. A reading of <5 mm is considered to indicate dry eyes and <10 mm marginally dry eyes. Schirmer's test measures total tear secretion, including reflex, and basal tears. The test is known to measure reflex tears without anesthesia and basal tears with anesthesia (23–25). However, the concept of basal tears is uncertain. It may not be necessary to measure true basal tears with anesthesia because even light stimulation can change tear secretion (26–28).

Schirmer's test is popular for diagnosing dry eye because of its simple operation and the absence of a requirement for equipment. However, the disadvantages include poor repeatability, low sensitivity and specificity, and sharp patient discomfort (29). The change in light, room humidity, and temperature and patient's anxiety may explain the poor repeatability. Furthermore, the variability in Schirmer's test results may be caused by reflex tearing (23). To increase the reliability of Schirmer's test, many variations in Schirmer's test have been proposed. In a comparative study of Schirmer's test with and without anesthesia, Kashkouli et al. found that the value of Schirmer's test with anesthesia may be more objective and reliable than that without anesthesia (30), and they discovered that a shorter 1-min test with anesthesia not only decreased patient's discomfort but also saved time. Hamano et al. modified Schirmer's test using a cotton thread impregnated with phenol red dye instead of uncomfortable filter paper (31). In this test, which is called the phenol red thread (PRT) test, the color of the dye changes from yellow to red depending on the pH of the tears (21). However, the relationship between the PRT and Schirmer's test in the measurement of tear secretion is not clear (27). Although Schirmer's test without anesthesia may not be acceptable given its shortcomings, it can be considered a valid option for diagnosing severe dry eye because of its reproducibility (32–34).

In view of the shortcomings of the tear secretion test, nonimmersive and improved tear detection, tear composition, physical and chemical properties, and other aspects of inspection and evaluation may be new directions for exploration.

Tear Meniscus Volume

The tear menisci provide a reservoir that contributes to the formation of the preocular tear film with each blink and accommodates excess tears during reflex tearing, lacrimal obstruction, and after topical drop instillation (35). It has been reported that the tear meniscus contains 75–90% of the aqueous tear volume, which is positively correlated with the lacrimal secretory rate (36). The meniscus volume is also reported to be reduced in tear-deficient dry eye (37, 38). Thus, the quantitative assessment of tear meniscus parameters may be useful in the diagnosis of dry eye disease. Tear meniscus variables, such as height, width, cross-sectional area, and meniscus curvature, have been reported to be of value in the diagnosis of dry eye (39, 40). TMH and strip meniscometry (SM) can be used to evaluate tear meniscus volume.

Tear Meniscus Height

Tear meniscus height has been confirmed to have good reliability and accuracy in detecting tear meniscus volume (41, 42). Invasive and noninvasive techniques can be used to measure TMH (see **Figure 1**). TMH can be viewed under cobalt blue light using a slit lamp and fluorescein instillation (43, 44). However, invasive TMH assessments are challenging as a result of their limitations. Frequent blinking, drug stimulation, time intervals, humidity, and temperature have been reported to influence invasive TMH results (45–47). Noninvasive TMH was therefore introduced, and optical coherence tomography (OCT) measurement of the tear menisci was found to be more reliable and was validated. Noninvasive TMH can be used together with noninvasive tear breakup time (NIBUT) on the same instrument, and they have been shown to be positively correlated (48, 49).

Strip Meniscometry

Strip meniscometry (39, 40, 50–52) involves using an SMTube, which is a thin strip (length: 85 mm, width: 7 mm, and height: 0.3 mm) with a capillary absorber in the center and two columns of scale on both sides, to measure tear meniscus volume. The examiner holds the center part of the strip and immerses the tip into the tear meniscus of the lower eyelid for 5 s to absorb tears. The SMTube attached to the tear meniscus absorbs the tears into the ditch, and the strip color turns blue, indicating the volume. At the end of 5 s, the strip is taken out, and the blue-stained column length is measured. The length of the stained column for normal people is equal to or >5 mm, whereas it is <5 mm for patients with dry eye (see **Figure 2**). Dogru et al. (39) and Miyasaka et al. (53) demonstrated that SM results correlate with those of Schirmer's test. A good correlation between TBUT and SMTube measurements has also been reported (52). The SMTube is useful for the diagnosis of dry eye, and its validity can be evaluated effectively using the CASIA SS-1000 AS-OCT TM parameters. Lee et al. (50) compared

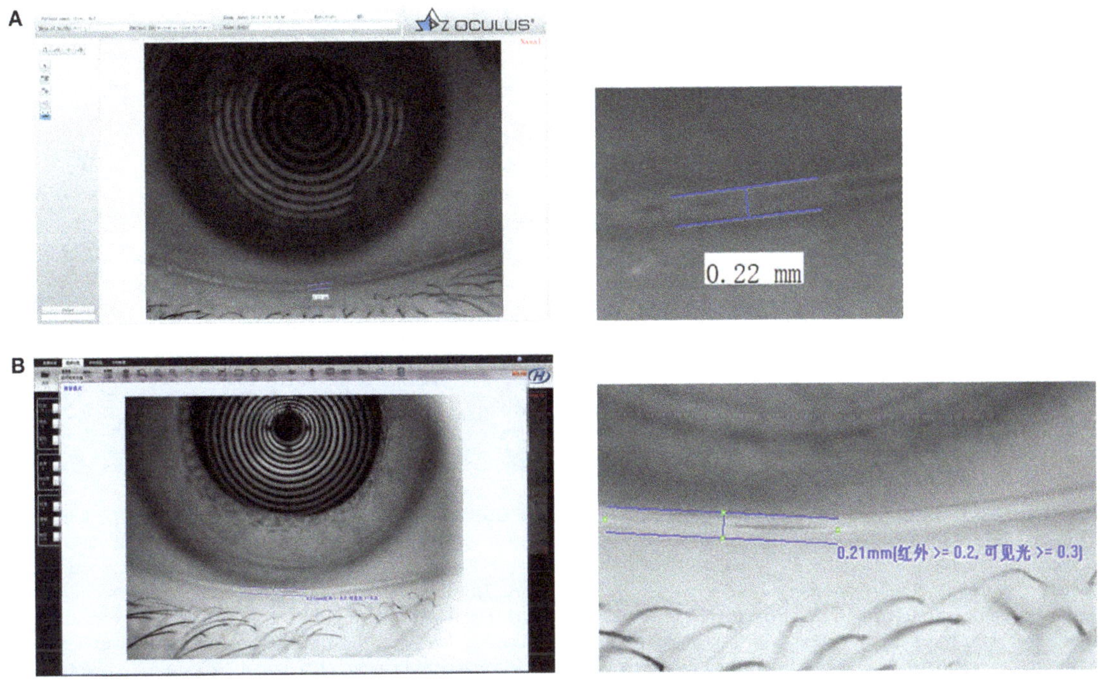

FIGURE 1 | Tear film thickness. **(A)** An example of tear film thickness from OCULUS Keratograph 5M. **(B)** An example of tear film thickness from Kanghua dry eye analyzer.

tear meniscus measurements using SM and the Keratograph 5M between 3 patient groups with subtypes of dry eye disease and found that tear meniscus measurements using SM and the Keratograph 5M can compensate for the detection of aqueous-deficient components of dry eye (53). The SMTube is useful for evaluating tear volume and therapeutic effects in patients with lacrimal passage obstruction. Hao et al. (40) showed that the SMTube has acceptable repeatability and reproducibility and specific correlations with TMH, BUT, and Schirmer's test. SM can provide clinical staff in busy outpatient services with a swift and convenient inspection method.

Tear Ferning Test

The tear ferning test is a simple tear detection method that can reflect some biochemical characteristics of tear film relatively quickly and cheaply (see **Figure 3**) (44, 54). Golding et al. (55) pointed out that the salts and polymers in tears are the important factors affecting the crystallization of tear ferns in the microscopic photographic study of tear crystal patterns in the tear ferning test. In their analysis of normal tears, they found that the fern-like crystals are mainly composed of sodium chloride, potassium chloride, and trace ions, and the surface of the crystals is covered by mucins and high molecular proteins, which indirectly control the formation of the crystals. Kogbe et al. (56) found that fern-like crystal patterns and branching patterns are particularly dependent on the ratios of monovalent sodium and iron ions to divalent calcium and magnesium ions. The tear fern crystal map in the tear ferning test is a relatively inexpensive and quick test of the total biochemical level of tear samples. Traipe-Castro et al. (57) studied the dynamics of tear evaporation and found that the crystalline pattern of dry healthy tears can be divided into four structural regions, namely zone 1 (outermost), a transition zone, zone 2 (near central region crystal), and zone 3 (central main crystal). The crystal pattern of ferns produced by a single tear sample depends not only on the composition of the tear, but also on the environmental conditions of the dry tear. Reducing the pressure and humidity or increasing the temperature to speed up the drying speed of the tear results in a smaller crystal morphology and different proportions of the four structural regions in the crystal pattern. In addition to diagnosing dry eye, the tear ferning test can be used to diagnose keratoconjunctivitis and cystic fibrosis disease and for soft contact lens tolerance prediction in clinical practice (58–60). The tear ferning test has good clinical guiding significance. However, the current method has disadvantages, such as the difficulty in controlling environmental conditions and the slow speed of the experimental results. If a method for rapid crystallization could be found, this examination method may have more clinical value.

Tear Osmotic Pressure

The measurement of tear osmotic pressure indicates the balance among tear secretion, evaporation, absorption, and drainage (61). Vapor pressure osmometry and freezing point depression have been used to measure tear osmotic pressure in the past (62, 63). The tear osmolarity test is considered as one of the most accurate dry eye diagnosis methods (64). Most recent techniques to measure tear osmotic pressure involve the use of

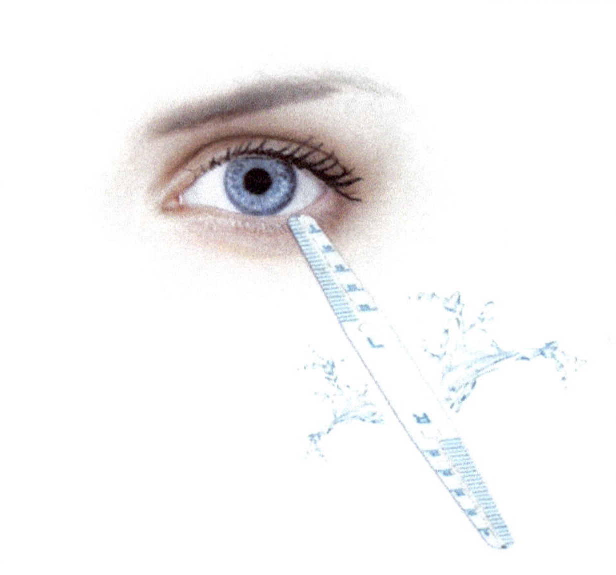

FIGURE 2 | SMTube. The method of strip meniscometry (SM) is using SMTube which is a thin strip (length: 85 mm, width: 7 mm, and height: 0.3 mm) with a capillary absorber in the center and two columns of scale on both sides to measure the tear meniscus volume. The examiner held the center part of the strip and immersed the tip into the tear meniscus of the lower eyelid for 5 s to absorb tears. The SMTube attached to the tear meniscus absorbed the tears into the ditch and the strip color turned blue, indicating the volume. At the end of 5 s, the strip was taken out and the blue stained column length was measured. The length of the stained column for normal people was equal to or >5 mm, whereas it was <5 mm for DED patients.

the TearLab (TearLab Corporation, Escondido, CA) and I-PEN (I-MED Pharma Inc., Dollard-des-Ormeaux, Canada) osmolarity systems (65, 66).

TearLab Osmometer

The TearLab osmometer (TearLab, San Diego, CA) was approved by the US Food and Drug Administration in 2008 for the measurement of tear osmolarity *in vivo* by clinical practitioners. Since then, several studies have demonstrated that it is a reliable test with good performance and complements for the diagnosis of dry eye (67–69). Some studies have concluded that the TearLab osmometer is the best single marker for diagnosing and classifying dry eye levels of severity and for distinguishing between different dry eye severity levels (70, 71). On the other hand, several clinical studies have raised questions about the diagnostic ability of tear osmolarity in dry eyes measured with the TearLab osmometer (72–77).

I-PEN Tear Osmolarity Test

Tear osmolarity is performed using the I-PEN osmolarity system 5 min after a PRT test. The I-PEN osmolarity system is used a distance away from electronic devices to ensure the accuracy of the readings. Each subject is asked to close their eyelids gently for 30 s, and the disposable single-use sensor then softly makes contact with the palpebral conjunctiva from the lower eyelid at a 30° angle. By design, the I-PEN beeps after a few seconds and displays an osmolarity reading on the screen (78, 79). Tear

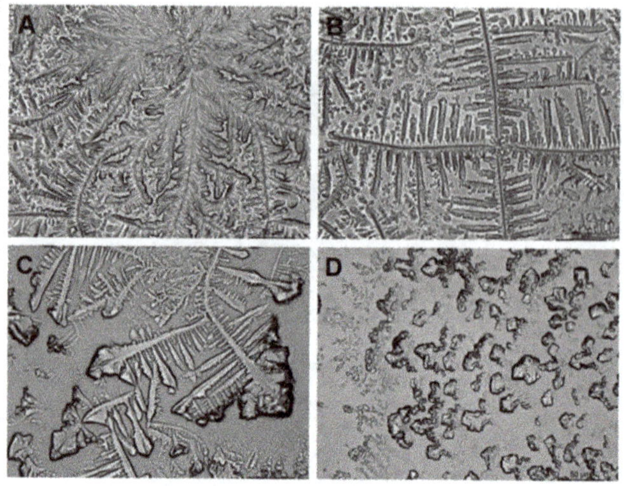

FIGURE 3 | Tear ferning test classification descriptions (Rolando's classification). Type 1: uniform arborization in the entire field of observation without spaces between the ferns. Single ferns are big and closely branched **(A)**. Type 2: Arborization is abundant, but the single ferns are smaller and have a lower frequency of branching than in grade 1; empty spaces appear between the ferns **(B)**. Type 3: Single ferns are little and incompletely formed with rare or no branching **(C)**. Type 4: No ferning is present; mucus may appear in clusters and threads **(D)**.

osmolarity is measured three times in the right eye of each subject with 5-min intervals between measurements. Based on the I-PEN tear osmolarity measurements, subjects are classified as having a healthy eye (<290 mOsm/L), minor dry eye (290–310 mOsm/L), mild dry eye (310–330 mOsm/L), and moderate dry eye (330–350 mOsm/L).

Shimazaki et al. (78) studied the efficacy and safety of the handheld I-PEN in Japanese patients with dry eye disease and those without dry eye disease and found no correlations between the tear film osmolarity values obtained with the I-PEN system and any subjective or objective parameters of dry eye. Meanwhile, in the study of Fagehi et al. (79), the mean measurement of I-PEN tear osmolarity was 303.8 ± 4.8 mOsm/L, which is in agreement with the range reported for healthy subjects. The I-PEN is reliable and has the advantage of portability compared to other osmolarity systems (79). Park et al. (80) obtained similar results, indicating that the I-PEN osmometer can be considered suitable for the use in clinical settings, with good performance in the diagnosis of dry eye. König et al. (81) found that the I-PEN osmometer provided significantly higher tear film osmolarities than those measured using the TearLab osmometer. In one study, tear osmotic pressure measured using the I-PEN osmometer has shown a significant decrease after treatment with a botulinum toxin A injection in patients with intractable dry eye disease (82). Tavakoli et al. found that, *in vivo*, both instruments displayed poor repeatability (83). Some studies have found that after treatment, the osmotic pressure of tears in patients with dry eye is significantly reduced (74–86). However, other studies have found that the osmotic pressure of tears does not change significantly after treatment (84–88). This may be related to the duration of the treatment, the severity of the disease, and the efficacy of the different treatments. The key elements in the diagnosis of dry eye are increased osmolarity of the tear film and inflammation of the ocular surface, which are accompanied by ocular symptoms. In terms of clinical treatment, we can select different artificial tears based on the osmotic pressure of patients with dry eye.

Tear Inflammatory Factor

There is very strong and valid evidence that inflammation constitutes an important pillar in the pathophysiology of dry eye. Increased inflammatory cells, increased expression of immune activation and adhesion molecules, T-helper type 1 (Th-1) and Th-17 attracting immune pathways, cytokines, and chemokines are all evidence supporting the inflammatory pathology of dry eye (89, 90).

Currently, the only commercial options to investigate tear film biomarkers are InflammaDry® (matrix metalloproteinase 9, MMP-9) and the TearScan™ Lactoferrin Diagnostic Test Kit (91). MMP-9 is an endopeptidase that helps remodel the extracellular matrix and plays a crucial role in dry eye. The point-of-care test InflammaDry (Quidel, San Diego, CA) can detect this biomarker in tear film with a low limit of detection of 40 ng/mL (91). This test should be carried out prior to the use of anesthetics, corneal staining, or Schirmer's test. A fleece placed at the tip of a sample collector is inserted multiple times along the patient's palpebral conjunctiva. The sample collector is then placed into the supplied test cassette and secured prior to immersing it in the buffer. Once 10 min has passed, the test cassette may display a blue line, which represents a valid test. If the blue line does not appear, the test is considered as invalid and must be repeated. A positive result is indicated by the presence of pink and blue lines, thus providing a qualitative (yes or no) response. To carry out this test accurately, a sufficient sample (5 μL) needs to be collected to avoid a false-negative result. In some studies, the InflammaDry test has demonstrated high positive and negative agreement for confirming suspected dry eye disease (92, 93). These studies have further shown that tear MMP-9 positivity may serve as a reliable response predictor of topical corticosteroid treatment in dry eye. Kim et al. (94) found that the subjective 5-scale grading system in the point-of-care MMP-9 immunoassay is an easy and reliable method with acceptable accuracy. Whereas, inflammation is known to play a role in dry eye, it is not always present in those with symptoms. Lanza et al. (95) suggested that a clinical examination alone cannot identify patients with clinically significant inflammation. In their study, there was no difference in the dry eye profiles of patients when evaluating symptoms and signs and those who tested positive vs. negative for MMP-9 on the ocular surface. A randomized, double-blind, placebo-controlled dry eye study in humans reported that lactoferrin supplementation can increase tearing, whereas a randomized controlled study of cataract surgery-induced dry eye found that it can restore tearing and TBUT (96, 97).

Tear Film Examination

The most superficial layer of tear film is the lipid layer secreted by the meibomian glands. When this layer is deficient, it may result in an evaporative dry eye (18). The main methods of tear film examination are TBUT and tear film thickness, but the correlation between these two examinations needs further investigation.

Tear Breakup Time

Tear breakup time has been the most frequently adopted dry eye examination method over the past two decades (98). TBUT was first introduced by Norn (99) to assess the stability of tear film. It is traditionally defined as "the interval between the last complete blink and the first appearance of a dry spot or disruption in the tear film" (99). According to current perspectives, measurements of TBUT can be divided into two distinct patterns: invasive and noninvasive.

Invasive Tear Breakup Time

The most common clinical method of measuring invasive TBUT is sodium fluorescein (100). The general process involved in examining TBUT with fluorescein is convenient and accessible. Liquid containing light fluorescence or a sterile fluorescein paper strip infiltrated with normal saline is presented to the superior bulbar conjunctiva for 1–2 s so that the fluorescein is uniformly distributed on the precorneal ocular surface (101, 102). This study has shown that the volume of fluorescent liquid used can significantly affect TBUT results, so a micropipette can be used to control the volume (102). The use of a dry fluorescein applicator is also an effective way to minimize the influence of liquid volume (46, 103). After the patient blinks several times, the time from the last blink of the eye to the first dry spot on the tear film is measured under a cobalt blue filter. Two or three consecutive measurements are recorded. The average value provides a more reliable result (104). A recent study showed that the maximum TBUT may also be considered to diagnose dry eye (105). The sensitivity and specificity of the TBUT test are 72 and 61%, respectively. The diagnostic criteria for fluorescein TBUT in diagnosing dry eye are <10 s (105). Generally, fluorescein TBUT values can be expected to be shorter than the values of noninvasive TBUT. A fluorescein TBUT of <5 s has also been reported to contribute to the diagnosis of dry eye (106).

Noninvasive Tear Breakup Time

In recent years, due to the weak points of invasive TBUT, NIBUT, which relies on technical apparatus, has become more popular (107). Invasive TBUT may be affected by volume, the concentration and types of fluorescence used, and the experience of the examiner (108, 109). NIBUT does not involve the instillation of any substances nor is there any direct physical contact with the tear film and conjunctiva. NIBUT is measured by the automated capture of Placido disk images, which are obtained from the anterior ocular surface using a corneal topography system (110–113). Computer software is used to identify irregularities and the breakup of the precorneal tear film, and the first and average time is calculated (114, 115). These several studies have reported better sensitivity and specificity for NIBUT than invasive TBUT. NIBUT has 82–84% sensitivity and 76–94% specificity (116). In addition, 10 s has been proposed as the cutoff value, and <10 s can indicate a diagnosis of dry eye (117). The disadvantage of NIBUT using technical apparatus is that, instead of repeating the test three times, a random time is checked once, so there is room for error, and this method therefore needs to be improved in the future.

Tear Film Thickness

A stable eye tear film is a sign of good eye health, mainly because it forms the main refractor through which light enters the visual system and protects and moistens the cornea. Wolff (118) proposed a three-layer model of tear film: the mucin layer covering the eye surface reduces the hydrophobicity of epithelial cells; care of the water layer of exposed ocular epithelium by providing lubricity, some nutrients, antimicrobial proteins, and appropriate osmotic pressure; Additionally, the lipid layer prevents the water layer from being lost through overfilling and evaporation. When the eyes are open, the tears are distributed in three compartments, which are the fornical compartment, the tear menisci, and the preocular tear film (118). The preocular tear film overlies the exposed conjunctiva and cornea (119, 120).

Measurement of the lipid layer thickness (LLT) could serve as an useful examination method in clinical practice diagnosing MGD. In previous clinical routine, the LLT is usually measured indirectly by the determination of the TBUT. Nowadays, various technologies and new devices are currently being utilized to assess LLT. It is 2–5.5 μm thick in the corneal region. A suitable method for the direct quantification of the LLT is interferometry techniques (120–122). LipiView II interferometer (TearScience Inc, Morrisville, NC) could provide the clinician with the important output parameter, such as average LLT of the tear film and be capable of quantifying LLT (123). On the other hand, LipiView II could automatically detect and analyze blink rate and blinking quality through the videos recorded. It displays the number of complete blinks and incomplete blinks and blink frequency numerically to help clinician analyze blinking pattern and take images of MG for visualizing the morphology of the MGs (see **Figure 4**). Compelling visuals and video captures provide an opportunity to educate patients about their personal ocular health and how healthy meibomian gland function protects the ocular surface, keeping their eyes moist to ensure clear, comfortable, healthy, and stable vision (124). Willcox MDP et al. pointed that abnormal blinking habits such as partial blinking are strongly associated with MGD (125). Using meibography, the grading of dropout at baseline and subsequent examinations can be used to track long-term progression of MGD (62). A study compared the Subjective Keeler Tearscope-Plus™ with the Objective Oculus® Keratograph 5M and LipiView® and found that the results of tear stability or lipid thickness were interchangeable (126). Another study compared the LipiView® II with IDRA® for ocular surface analysis and found no significant difference in LLT, but these devices should not be used interchangeably for the evaluation of meibomian gland dropout and partial blink rates (127).

Examination of the Eyelid Margin and Meibomian Glands

Meibomian gland dysfunction (MGD) is the main cause of dry eye, with 86% of dry eye cases being caused by MGD. Meibomian gland dropout is significantly correlated with the other clinical features of MGD, such as the quality of the expressed meibum, altered tear film lipid layer stability, and ocular surface damage. Meibomian gland morphology and function are routinely examined to diagnose MGD (128). Using meibography, the grading of the dropout at baseline and subsequent examinations can be used to track the long-term progression of MGD (129–131). Evaluating changes in the eyelids, eyelid margins, and meibomian glands is of great value in the diagnosis of MGD. These can be assessed by observing the opening state of the meibomian glands, squeezing the meibomian glands on the eyelid skin, and observing the difficulties and character of eyelid ester excretion. Specific scoring criteria were established following the consensus of experts on the diagnosis and treatment of MGD in China in 2017 (129).

Eyelid Margin Examination

Patients with MGD are prone to eyelid margin abnormalities. Abnormal eyelid margins can be valuable in diagnosing MGD. For example, MGD patients may have a thickened, blunt eyelid margin, an irregular shape, a Marx line (the junction of the skin and mucosa), a receded opening of the meibomian glands, hyperemia of the eyelid margin, and neovascularization. Slit lamp examination of the entire area of the upper and lower eyelids may reveal abnormal signs, including irregular eyelid margins (with notching along the eyelid margins), telangiectasis, and a shift of the mucocutaneous junction (130–132). Amano examined total MGD patients and noted that the slit lamp findings of lid margin abnormalities, a shift of the mucocutaneous junction, telangiectasia, and plugging were more frequent (133).

Meibomian Gland Infrared Meibography

Several modalities of meibomian gland imaging are used in MG examinations, including contact meibography (not currently popular), noncontact infrared meibography (e.g., IR meibography and the mobile pen-shaped meibography system), keratography (Keratograph 5M, OCULUS, Wetzlar, Germany), Kanghua Dry Eye Analyzer (DED-1L, Kanghua, Chongqing, China) and LipiView II (TearScience, Morrisville, NC) (see **Figure 5**), *in vivo* confocal microscopy (IVCM, see Section Other Examinations), and OCT meibography (134). The MG area ratio, diameter deformation, tortuosity, and signal intensity could be considered as promising biomarkers for MGD diagnosis and objective grading (131). Meibomian gland infrared meibography may provide a reference for clinical treatment of MGD, especially nondrug treatment, such as Lipiflow, IPL, and meibomian gland massage.

Lid Wiper Examination

The lid wiper is a component of the conjunctival margin of the upper and lower eyelids (135). Shiraishi et al. noted that lissamine green staining was detected in more than 10% of lid wiper epitheliopathy patients with dry eye symptoms (136). Studies have suggested that the best staining method is as follows: lissamine green or fluorescein sodium test paper is soaked and used to make contact with the conjunctiva of the lower eyelid. After more than 1 min, the conjunctiva is restained once. The degree and range of staining of the lid margin epithelial cells are

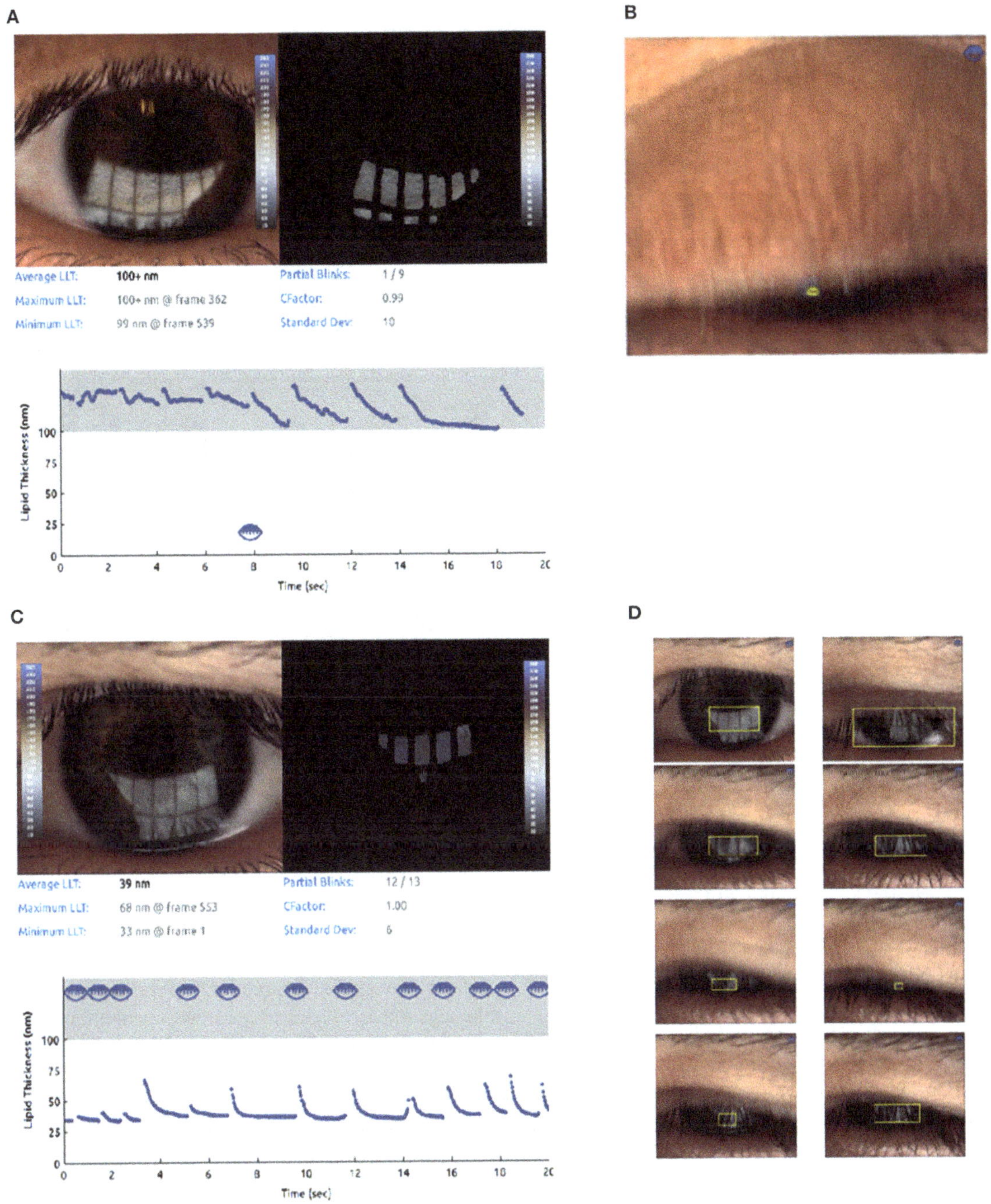

FIGURE 4 | Lipid imagine report and incomplete blinking (an example from LipiView II ocular surface interferometer). The computer system captures a video image file that is recorded over time since the interference pattern changes as the tear film is distributed across the cornea during blinking. **(A)** Lipid imagine report and incomplete blinking. **(B)** Partial blink imagines. **(C)** Another for lipid imagine report and incomplete blinking. **(D)** Another for partial blink imagines.

then examined under a slit lamp microscope with a cobalt blue light. A staining length of ≥2 mm and/or ≥25% of the eyelid margin width are considered positive in the diagnosis of lid wiper epitheliopathy (137).

To date, studies have found that the incidence of lid wiper epitheliopathy in patients with dry eye symptoms increases, and lid margin staining can be combined with traditional dry eye diagnosis methods to improve diagnosis rates.

Inspection of the Eyelid for Demodex Mites

Ocular mite infection is significantly correlated with dry eye, MGD, and age. When Demodex mites infect the margin of the eyelid, the skin of the margin of the eyelid, the hair follicles and

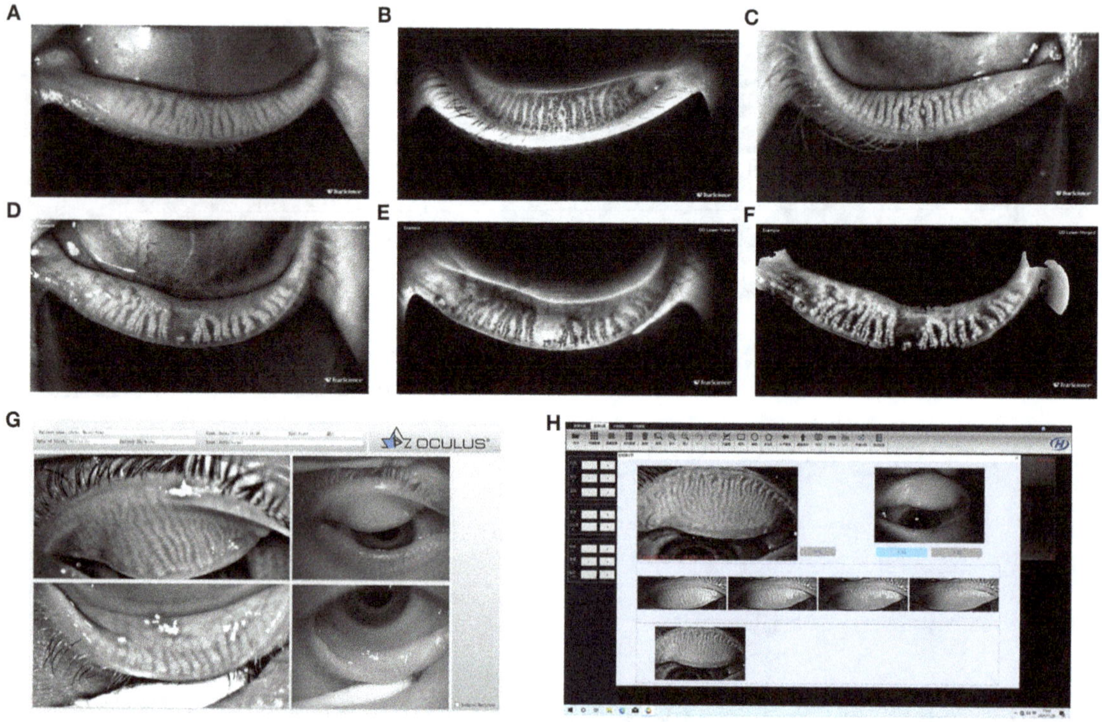

FIGURE 5 | Meibomian gland morphology. Ocular surface interferometer—LipiView II interferometer **(A–C)**; Dynamic Meibomian Imager—LipiScan **(D–F)**; OCULUS Keratograph 5M **(G)**; Kanghua Dry Eye Analyzer **(H)**. Examples for LipiView II and LipiScan: The images of the glands may be viewed on the computer screen display and in a printed report. Three modes of gland images are provided: Reflected infrared view is shown for both upper and lower eyelid gland images. **(A,D)** Show only lower eyelid gland images. Transillumination infrared view is shown only for lower eyelid gland images, if images were captured using handheld near-infrared lid everter **(B,E)**. Merged view is the combination of the reflected infrared and trans infrared views and is shown only for the lower eyelid gland images **(C,F)**.

glands of the eyelid, and the meibomian glands will accumulate mites, and symptoms related to dry eye will occur (138). In addition, a typical clinical manifestation of Demodex blepharitis is cylindrical dandruff at the root of the eyelash, and this is considered pathognomonic for Demodex blepharitis (139). To detect Demodex mites, an optical microscope is used to examine eyelashes with typical cylindrical dandruff characteristics. These lashes are then removed and placed on a slide to observe the number and morphology of the Demodex mites. The use of IVCM (see Section Other Examinations) could be an easy way to improve this diagnosis. The advantage of IVCM is that it can be used to quickly and simultaneously detect microorganisms and eyelid structure. It is noninvasive and does not require the removal of eyelashes. It can be used repeatedly to determine a prognosis in patients, but it cannot be used to accurately to identify the type of mite.

Ocular Surface Staining

Ocular surface cell staining can evaluate the barrier function and integrity of epithelial cells as one of the evaluation indexes of the severity of dry eye (140). When the integrity of ocular surface cells has been damaged, they can be stained with specific dyeing agents to display the defects. The degree and area of staining are related to the severity of the ocular surface damage. Ocular surface cell staining can therefore be used to evaluate the barrier function and integrity of epithelial cells. Fluorescein sodium staining is commonly used in clinics although lissamine green staining and rose bengal staining are sometimes also used.

Fluorescein Staining

The mechanism of fluorescein staining involves dyeing corneal defects through the diffusion of the fluorescein between cells into the adjacent intercellular space with penetration into the lower stroma. Healthy corneal epithelial cells are therefore not stained unless they have defects. This method is mainly used to assist in the diagnosis of epithelial defect-related diseases, such as corneal abrasions, keratitis, and corneal erosion. It can also be used to evaluate the therapeutic effects of epithelial injury (140). Sodium fluorescein staining is not a specific index of dry eye but plays an auxiliary role in its diagnosis.

Sodium fluorescein is available in two forms: eye drops and impregnated paper strips. For both the eye drops and paper strip methods of instillation, the aim is to achieve highly fluorescent staining of the areas with loss of epithelial integrity (141). Studies have shown that high concentrations of sodium fluorescein are nonfluorescent and fluorescent at a concentration of <0.1% (142). It is therefore general practice for doctors to deliver 2 μL of 2% sodium fluorescein eye drops or fluorescein sodium strips soaked in physiological saline or other eye drops into the conjunctival sac using a micropipette. The whole tear film is then filled by the patient blinking their eyes. Ocular surface staining can then be observed using a blue exciter filter over the white light source and a complementary yellow or orange barrier filter over the slit lamp objective (142).

Rose Bengal Staining

A derivative of fluorescein, rose bengal is believed to not stain healthy epithelial cells. According to Roberts et al.'s study (143), the reason that the normal ocular surface does not stain with rose bengal is the obstruction of a healthy and intact ocular tear film. Accordingly, as long as the tear film protection is insufficient, there will be rose red staining. This feature can be used to assist in the diagnosis of dry eye. In a study by Korb (144), rose bengal was found to be the preferred dye for bulb conjunctival staining, whereas sodium fluorescein was the preferred dye for corneal staining, with an optimal concentration of 1%. Due to the cytotoxic effect of rose bengal, patients will feel tingling if anesthetic eye drops are not used. Furthermore, the sensitivity and specificity of rose bengal are not as good as those of sodium fluorescein, so it is not widely used and can only be used as a reference (137, 144, 145).

Lissamine Green Staining

Lissamine green staining has similar characteristics to rose bengal, but its cytotoxicity is much less than rose bengal, so lissamine green staining is commonly used as a substitute in conjunctiva staining in clinical practice (146, 147). These two dyes do not spread throughout the conjunctiva due to the blocking effect of the mucins in tear film, so their staining areas last longer than sodium fluorescein. Yoon found that a mixed solution of 1% fluorescein and 1% lissamine green can simultaneously stain the cornea and conjunctiva while maintaining the unique staining characteristics of each dye (147).

Notwithstanding, the use of mixed dyes may necessitate a long waiting time. The use of different dyes on the corneal and conjunctival epithelial cells may also have subtle effects on the damaged areas. Fluorescein sodium strips are therefore commonly used in clinical practice. Although reactive dyes have been used to stain the cornea and conjunctiva to assess ocular surface disease in dry eye for a long time, there is no uniform or clear ocular surface stain rating scale due to the different concentrations and methods of staining used in different regions. The general content is to classify the dyeing area, density, area, and type. Most studies use the Oxford scale, but the type of scale used depends on the researchers' requirements (148). Dyes are therefore an effective adjunct to the diagnosis of dry eye and to determine the type and severity of dry eye.

Dry Eye Analyzer

The dry eye analyzer is a device that integrates a variety of dry eye examinations. The dry eye analyzer can provide fast, convenient, and efficient dry eye examinations, but its relationship with traditional examinations needs to be clarified. Dry eye analyzer examinations may include tear river height (TMH) (see Section Tear Breakup Time), NIBUT (see Section Tear Breakup Time), tear film thickness (see Section Tear Film Thickness), infrared photography of the meibomian glands (see Section Eyelid Margin Examination), and conjunctival hyperemia analysis (see **Figures 6**, 7).

Conjunctival Hyperemia Analysis

Bulbar hyperemia is a common clinical sign and important indicator of ocular disease (149). It is one of the most common contributors of ocular complaints that prompt visits to medical centers. The translucent appearance of the conjunctiva allows immediate observation of changes in microvascular circulation. Conjunctival congestion is caused by dilation of blood vessels in microangiopathic degeneration caused by an inflammatory response. Our understanding of these neurogenic and immune-mediated pathways has progressed over time, and they are now known to play a critical role in the development of targeted novel therapies. Due to a multitude of underlying etiologies, patients must be accurately diagnosed for the efficacious management of conjunctival hyperemia. The diagnostic techniques used for the grading of conjunctival hyperemia have also evolved from descriptive and subjective grading scales to more reliable computer-based objective grading scales (150).

In 1996, Owen et al. (151) developed a novel computer software method to quantify the conjunctival plexus on the scleral background to measure its vascular surface area from photographs. Huntjens et al. employed Advanced Ophthalmic Systems software, which uses an objective approach to grading conjunctival hyperemia, and found excellent repeatability and improved agreement between experienced and novice observers (152).

Research has begun to focus on the relationship between red eyes and dry eye, but the consistency between objective and subjective tests needs to be further strengthened. Schulze et al. quantified bulbar redness using the validated bulbar redness grading scale and an automated objective method (OCULUS Keratograph 5M) in participants with dry eye disease and nondry eye disease controls, but statistically significant differences in redness between the dry eye disease and control groups were only found using the validated bulbar redness scale (153).

Other Examinations

Confocal Microscope

Confocal microscopy is a new technology that can aid in the *in vivo* assessment of structural changes in several ocular surface diseases on a cellular level. The application of IVCM in dry eye disease will be a powerful method to evaluate morphological changes in the ocular surface globally in the future (154). In the dry eye field, IVCM has been applied in the examination of the cornea, bulbar and palpebral conjunctiva, meibomian glands, and lacrimal glands (155–169).

First-generation confocal microscopy with an *in vivo* white-light through-focusing confocal microscope (Tandem Scanning Corp., Reston, VA) was developed and has advanced to an *in vivo* white-light slit-scanning confocal microscope (ConfoScan, Nidek Technologies, Vigonza, Veneto, Italy) (second generation). A new-generation *in vivo* laser-scanning confocal microscope (Heidelberg Retina Tomograph, Rostock Corneal Module; Heidelberg Engineering GmgH, Heidelberg, Baden-Württemberg, Germany) for corneal examination was recently reported to yield impressive, high-quality images in many corneal pathologies (169).

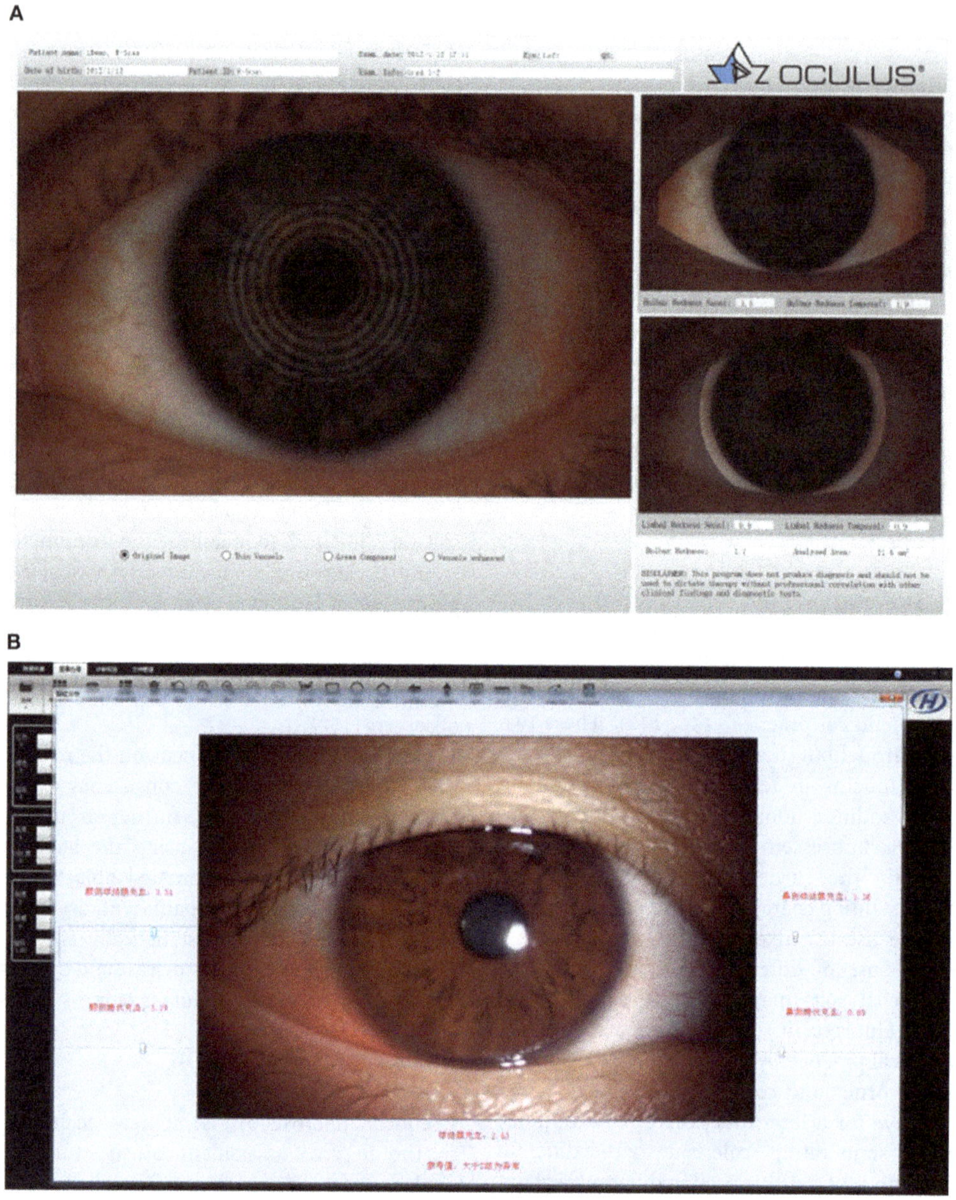

FIGURE 6 | Bulbar redness. **(A)** OCULUS Keratograph 5M for bulbar redness grading scale. **(B)** Kanghua dry eye analyzer for bulbar redness grading scale.

Confocal microscopy requires trained operators to acquire good quality scans but lacks built-in software to analyze nerves and inflammatory cells. As such, it is not used as often in clinical settings to diagnose dry eye. The relationship between corneal sensation and subbasal nerve morphology, as evaluated with IVCM, depends on the pathophysiological mechanism of ocular surface disease. In a recent review of the use of IVCM in dry eye, corneal subbasal nerves were implicated in the pathogenesis of the condition. There are many reports suggesting that corneal subbasal nerve density may decrease in dry eyes with Sjogren's syndrome (SS) (156, 158, 161). Ma et al. (165) found that a higher aggregated measure of tortuosity may be linked to ocular discomfort, visual function disturbance, and tear film instability. At the same time, Ma et al. (166) determined that objective visual quality is correlated with clinical symptoms and signs in patients with dry eye, which suggests that nerve changes may be a factor related to poor visual quality in these patients. Lin et al.'s study (167) showed that inflammatory dendritic cell density increases dramatically in the corneal epithelium of dry eye patients with non-SS and SS. Nerve fibers have an important influence on corneal tropism and contribute to the maintenance of healthy corneas. It has been postulated that inflammatory cells may induce a diminution of nerve fibers in the subbasal nerve plexus in dry eye patients with SS. The migration and maturation of dendritic cells are activated in response to proinflammatory stimulation. Dramatic increases in the number of dendritic cells in the corneal epithelium are thought to play a role in dry eye pathophysiology. Furthermore, some studies have determined

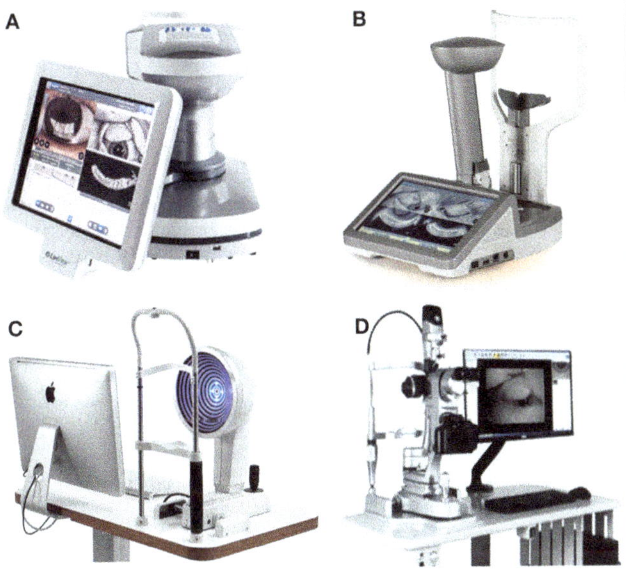

FIGURE 7 | Dry eye analyzers. **(A)** LipiView II ocular surface interferometer. **(B)** LipiScan dynamic meibomian imager. **(C)** OCULUS Keratograph 5M. **(D)** Kanghua dry eye analyzer.

that ocular Demodex mite infestation may be involved in ocular surface discomfort, inflammation, and meibomian gland dropout in patients with MGD (139, 168).

Incomplete Blinking

Incomplete blinking is an important parameters of dry eye disease. Spontaneous blinking can be divided into complete blinking and incomplete blinking. Incomplete blinking was associated with a higher ocular surface disease index (OSDI) score, more meibomian gland dropout (MGD), and reduced tear film stability. LipiView II automatically detects and analyzes blink rate and blinking quality through the videos recorded. It displays the number of complete blinks and incomplete blinks and blink frequency numerically to help clinician to analyze blinking pattern (124).

OUTLOOK

The rapid progress in the development of dry eye diagnosis technologies has greatly promoted the level of diagnosis and treatment of dry eye and made dry eye a hot spot in the field of clinical ocular surfaces. In particular, the recent construction of a dry eye diagnosis and treatment center in China has received increased attention and developed rapidly (170). However, many areas worthy of exploration in the diagnosis of dry eye remained. These include the detection of the mechanism of dry eye-related neuropathy, *in vivo* functional examination of the meibomian glands, the correlation between tear film thickness, BUT, and noninvasive BUT, more accurate, and reliable tear and tear film examination methods. It is hoped that improvements in dry eye examination methods will promote all-round progress in the understanding, diagnosis, and treatment of dry eye and related researches (171).

AUTHOR CONTRIBUTIONS

XJ: conceptualization, writing—reviewing and editing, and supervision. YW: data curation, writing—original draft preparation, reviewing and editing, and visualization. CW: writing—original draft preparation. XW, KY, and YM: writing—original draft preparation. XH: writing—reviewing and editing. All authors contributed to the article and approved the submitted version.

REFERENCES

1. Craig JP, Nichols KK, Akpek EK, Caffery B, Dua HS, Joo CK, et al. TFOS DEWS II definition and classification report. *Ocul Surf.* (2017) 15:276–83. doi: 10.1016/j.jtos.2017.05.008
2. Tchegnon E, Liao CP, Ghotbi E, Shipman T, Wang Y, McKay RM, et al. Epithelial stem cell homeostasis in Meibomian gland development, dysfunction, and dry eye disease. *JCI Insight.* (2021) 6:e151078. doi: 10.1172/jci.insight.151078
3. Eom Y, Lee JS, Keun Lee H, Myung Kim H, Suk Song J. Comparison of conjunctival staining between lissamine green and yellow filtered fluorescein sodium. *Can J Ophthalmol.* (2015) 50:273–7. doi: 10.1016/j.jcjo.2015.05.007
4. Chen M, Miki M, Lin S, Yung Choi S. Sodium Fluorescein staining of the cornea for the diagnosis of dry eye: a comparison of three eye solutions. *Med Hypothesis Discov Innov Ophthalmol.* (2017) 6:105–9.
5. Ding JE, Kim YH Yi SM, Graham AD Li W, Lin MC. Ocular surface cooling rate associated with tear film characteristics and the maximum interblink period. *Sci Rep.* (2021) 11:15030. doi: 10.1038/s41598-021-94568-9
6. Alishahi M, Kamali R. Forced diffusion of water molecules through aquaporin-5 biomembr a molecular dynamics study. *Biophys Physicobiol.* (2018) 15:255–62. doi: 10.2142/biophysico.15.0_255
7. van Setten GB. Osmokinetics: A new dynamic concept in dry eye disease. *J Fr Ophtalmol.* (2019) 42:221–5. doi: 10.1016/j.jfo.2018.11.001
8. Fagehi R, El-Hiti GA, Alqarni BM, Alanazi MA, Masmali AM, Almubrad T. Improvement in tear ferning patterns of sheep tears after addition of various electrolyte solutions. *Front Med.* (2021) 8:721969. doi: 10.3389/fmed.2021.721969
9. van Setten GB. Impact of attrition, intercellular shear in dry eye disease: when cells are challenged and neurons are triggered. *Int J Mol Sci.* (2020) 21:4333. doi: 10.3390/ijms21124333
10. Guzmán M, Miglio M, Keitelman I, Shiromizu CM, Sabbione F, Fuentes F, et al. Transient tear hyperosmolarity disrupts the neuroimmune homeostasis of the ocular surface and facilitates dry eye onset. *Immunology.* (2020) 161:148–61. doi: 10.1111/imm.13243
11. Hori J, Kunishige T, Nakano Y. Immune checkpoints contribute corneal immune privilege: implications for dry eye associated with checkpoint inhibitors. *Int J Mol Sci.* (2020) 21:3962. doi: 10.3390/ijms 21113962
12. Aragona P, Giannaccare G, Mencucci R, Rubino P, Cantera E. Rolando M. Modern approach to the treatment of dry eye, a complex multifactorial disease: a PICASSO board review. *Br J Ophthalmol.* (2021) 105:446-53. doi: 10.1136/bjophthalmol-2019-315747
13. Chinese Branch of the Asian Dry Eye Soci Ocular Surface and Tear Film Diseases Group of Ophthalmology Committee of Cross-Straits Medicine

Exchange Associate Ocular Surface and Dry Eye Group of Chinese Ophthalmologist Association. [Chinese expert consensus on dry eye: dry eye related to immunologic diseases (2021)]. *Zhonghua Yan Ke Za Zhi.* (2021) 57:898–907. doi: 10.3760/cma.j.cn112142-20210726-00350

14. Chinese Optometric Association of Chinese Ophthalmological Soci Optometry Group of Chinese Ophthalmologist Associate Refractive Surgery Group of Chinese Ophthalmologist Association. [Expert consensus on the diagnosis and treatment of dry eye during perioperative period of corneal refractive surgery in China (2021)]. *Zhonghua Yan Ke Za Zhi.* (2021) 57:644–50. doi: 10.3760/cma.j.cn112142-20210312-00124
15. Saldanha IJ, Petris R, Makara M, Channa P, Akpek EK. Impact of the COVID-19 pandemic on eye strain and dry eye symptoms. *Ocul Surf.* (2021) 22:38–46. doi: 10.1016/j.jtos.2021.06.004
16. Starr CE, Dana R, Pflugfelder SC, Holland EJ, Zhang S. Owen D, et al. Dry eye disease flares: a rapid evidence assessment. *Ocul Surf.* (2021) 22:51–9. doi: 10.1016/j.jtos.2021.07.001
17. Shen Lee B, Kabat AG, Bacharach J, Karpecki P, Luchs J. Managing dry eye disease and facilitating realistic patient expectations: a review and appraisal of current therapies. *Clin Ophthalmol.* (2020) 14:119–26. doi: 10.2147/OPTH.S228838
18. Tiffany JM. The normal tear film. *Dev Ophthalmol.* (2008) 41:1–20. doi: 10.1159/000131066
19. Schirmer O. Studien zur physiologie und pathologie der tranen-absonderung und tranenabfuhr. *Graefes Arch Clin Exp Ophthalmol.* (1903) 56:197–291. doi: 10.1007/BF01946264
20. Rodney WM, Louie J, Puffer JC. Schirmer's test of lacrimation. *Am Fam Physician.* (1981) 24:161–4.
21. Savini G, Prabhawasat P, Kojima T, Grueterich M, Espana E, Goto E. The challenge of dry eye diagnosis. *Clin Ophthalmol.* (2008) 2:31–55. doi: 10.2147/OPTH.S1496
22. Shapiro A, Merin S. Schirmer test and break-up time of tear film in normal subjects. *Am J Ophthalmol.* (1979) 88:752–7. doi: 10.1016/0002-9394(79)90678-0
23. JordanA, BaumJ. Basic tear flow. Does it exist? *Ophthalmology.*1980 87:920–930. doi: 10.1016/S0161-6420(80)35143-9
24. Lamberts DW, Foster CS, Perry HD. Schirmer test after topical anesthesia and the tear meniscus height in normal eyes. *Arch Ophthalmol.* (1979) 97:1082–5. doi: 10.1001/archopht.1979.01020010536004
25. Jones LT. The lacrimal secretory system and its treatment. *Am J Ophthalmol.* (1966) 62:47–60. doi: 10.1016/0002-9394(66)91676-X
26. Tabak S. A short Schirmer tear test. *Contacto.* (1972) 16:38–42.
27. Clinch TE, Benedetto DA, Felberg NT, Laibson PR. Schirmer's test. A closer look. *Arch Ophthalmol.* (1983) 101:1383–6. doi: 10.1001/archopht.1983.01040020385009
28. Saleh TA, McDermott B, Bates AK, Ewings P. Phenol red thread test vs Schirmer's test: a comparative study. *Eye.* (2006) 20:913–5. doi: 10.1038/sj.eye.6702052
29. Li N, Deng XG, He MF. Comparison of the Schirmer I test with and without topical anesthesia for diagnosing dry eye. *Int J Ophthalmol.* (2012) 5:478–81. doi: 10.3980/j.issn.2222-3959.2012.04.14
30. Kashkouli MB, Pakdel F, Amani A, Asefi M, Aghai GH, Falavarjani KG, et al. modified Schirmer test in dry eye and normal subjects: open versus closed eye and 1-minute versus 5-minute tests. *Cornea.* (2010) 29:384–7. doi: 10.1097/ICO.0b013e3181ba6ef3
31. Hamano H, Hori M, Hamano T, Mitsunaga S, Maeshima J, Kojima S, et al. A new method for measuring tears. *CLAO J.* (1983) 9:281–9
32. Tsubota K, Xu KP, Fujihara T, Katagiri S, Takeuchi T. Decreased reflex tearing is associated with lymphocytic infiltration in lacrimal glands. *J Rheumatol.* (1996) 23:313–20.
33. Nichols KK, Mitchell GL, Zadnik K. The repeatability of clinical measurements of dry eye. *Cornea.* (2004) 23:272–85. doi: 10.1097/00003226-200404000-00010
34. Lilley J, O'Neil EC, Bunya VY, Johnson K, Ying GS, Hua P, et al. Efficacy of an Intranasal Tear Neurostimulator in Sjögren Syndrome Patients. *Clin Ophthalmol.* (2021) 15:4291–6. doi: 10.2147/OPTH.S312108
35. Guillon JP. Current clinical techniques to study the tear film and tear secretions. In: Korb D, Craig J, Doughty M, Guillon JP, Smith G, Tomlinson A, editors. *The Tear Film.* London: Butterworth Heinem (2002). p. 51–83. doi: 10.1016/B978-0-7506-4196-8.50006-7
36. Holly FJ. Physical chemistry of the normal and disordered tear film. *Trans Ophthalmol Soc UK.* (1985) 104:374–80.
37. Mainstone JC, Bruce AS, Golding TR. Tear meniscus measurement in the diagnosis of dry eye. *Curr Eye Res.* (1996) 15:653–61. doi: 10.3109/02713689609008906
38. Oguz H, Yokoi N, Kinoshita S. The height and radius of the tear meniscus and methods for examining these parameters. *Cornea.* (2000) 19:497–500. doi: 10.1097/00003226-200007000-00019
39. Dogru M, Ishida K, Matsumoto Y, Goto E, Ishioka M, Kojima T, et al. Strip meniscometry: a new and simple method of tear meniscus evaluation. *Invest Ophthalmol Vis Sci.* (2006) 47:1895–901. doi: 10.1167/iovs.05-0802
40. Hao Y, Tian L, Cao K, Jie Y. Repeatability and reproducibility of SMTube measurement in dry eye disease patients. *J Ophthalmol.* (2021) 2021:1589378. doi: 10.1155/2021/1589378
41. Vigo L, Pellegrini M, Bernabei F, Carones F, Scorcia V, Giannaccare G. Diagnostic performance of a novel noninvasive workup in the setting of dry eye disease. *J Ophthalmol.* (2020) 2020:5804123. doi: 10.1155/2020/5804123
42. Chang AY, Purt B. Biochemistry, tear film. In: *StatPearls.* Treasure Island (FL): StatPearls Publish (accessed on Jun 15, 2021).
43. Golding TR, Bruce AS, Mainstone JC. Relationship between tear-meniscus parameters and tear-film breakup. *Cornea.* (1997) 16:649–61. doi: 10.1097/00003226-199711000-00009
44. Shah AM, Galor A. Impact of ocular surface temperature on tear characteristics: current insights. *Clin Optom.* (2021) 13:51–62. doi: 10.2147/OPTO.S281601
45. Yokoi N, Bron A, Tiffany J, Brown N, Hsuan J, Fowler C. Reflective meniscometry: a non-invasive method to measure tear meniscus curvature. *Br J Ophthalmol.* (1999) 83:92–7. doi: 10.1136/bjo.83.1.92
46. Johnson ME, Murphy PJ. Measurement of ocular surface irritation on a linear interval scale with the ocular comfort index. *Invest Ophthalmol Vis Sci.* (2007) 48:4451–8. doi: 10.1167/iovs.06-1253
47. Bandlitz S, Purslow C, Murphy PJ, Pult H. The relationship between tear meniscus regularity and conjunctival folds. *Optom Vis Sci.* (2014) 91:1037–44. doi: 10.1097/OPX.0000000000000358
48. Li J, Ma J, Hu M, Yu J, Zhao Y. Assessment of tear film lipid layer thickness in patients with Meibomian gland dysfunction at different ages. *BMC Ophthalmol.* (2020) 20:394. doi: 10.1186/s12886-020-01667-8
49. Koh S, Ikeda C, Watanabe S, Oie Y, Soma T, Watanabe H, et al. Effect of non-invasive tear stability assessment on tear meniscus height. *Acta Ophthalmol.* (2015) 93:e135–9. doi: 10.1111/aos.12516
50. Lee KW, Kim JY, Chin HS, Seo KY, Kim TI, Jung JW. Assessment of the tear meniscus by strip meniscometry and keratograph in patients with dry eye disease according to the presence of meibomian gland dysfunction. *Cornea.* (2017) 36:189–95. doi: 10.1097/ICO.0000000000001033
51. Shinzawa M, Dogru M, Miyasaka K, Shimazaki J, Sekiryu T. Application of CASIA SS-1000 Optical Coherence Tomography Tear Meniscus Imaging in Testing the Efficacy of New Strip Meniscometry in Dry Eye Diagnosis. *Eye Contact Lens.* (2018) 44 Suppl 1:S44–9. doi: 10.1097/ICL.0000000000000312
52. Ishikawa S, Takeuchi M, Kato N. The combination of strip meniscometry and dry eye-related quality-of-life score is useful for dry eye screening during health checkup: Cross-sectional study. *Medicine.* (2018) 97:e12969. doi: 10.1097/MD.0000000000012969
53. Miyasaka K, Kazama Y, Iwashita H, Wakaiki S, Saito A, A. novel strip meniscometry method for measuring aqueous tear volume in dogs: clinical correlations with the Schirmer tear and phenol red thread tests. *Vet Ophthalmol.* (2019) 22:864–71. doi: 10.1111/vop.12664
54. Rolando M. Tear mucus ferning test in normal and keratoconjunctivitis sicca eyes. *Chibret Int J Ophthalmol.* (1984) 2:32–41.
55. Golding TR, Baker AT, Rechberger J. Brennan NA. X-ray and scanning electron microscopic analysis of the structural composition of tear ferns. *Cornea.* (1994) 13:58–66. doi: 10.1097/00003226-199401000-00010
56. Kogbe O. Liotet S. An interesting use of the study of tear ferning patterns in contactology. *Ophthalmologica.* (1987) 194:150–3. doi: 10.1159/000309753
57. Traipe-Castro L, Salinas-Toro D, López D, Zanolli M, Srur M, Valenzuela F, et al. Dynamics of tear fluid desiccation on a glass surface: a contribution to tear quality assessment. *Biol Res.* (2014) 47:25. doi: 10.1186/0717-6287-47-25
58. Nebbioso M, Sacchetti M, Bianchi G, Zicari AM, Duse M, Del Regno P, et al. Tear ferning test and pathological effects on ocular surface before and after

topical cyclosporine in vernal keratoconjunctivitis patients. *J Ophthalmol.* (2018) 2018:1061276. doi: 10.1155/2018/1061276

59. Rolando M, Baldi F, Calabria G. Tear mucus crystallization in children with cystic fibrosis. *Ophthalmologica.* (1988) 197:202–6. doi: 10.1159/000309944
60. Ravazzoni L, Ghini C, Macrí A. Rolando M. Forecasting of hydrophilic contact lens tolerance by means of tear ferning test. *Graefes Arch Clin Exp Ophthalmol.* (1998) 236:354–8. doi: 10.1007/s004170050090
61. Tomlinson A, Khanal S. Assessment of tear film dynamics: quantification approach. *Ocul Surf.* (2005) 3:81–95. doi: 10.1016/S1542-0124(12)70157-X
62. Tomlinson A, Bron AJ, Korb DR, Amano S, Paugh JR, Pearce EI, et al. The international workshop on meibomian gland dysfunction: report of the diagnosis subcommittee. *Invest Ophthalmol Vis Sci.* (2011) 52:2006–49. doi: 10.1167/iovs.10-6997f
63. Srinivasan S, Nichols KK. Collecting tear osmolarity measurements in the diagnosis of dry eye. *Expert Rev Ophthalmol.* (2009) 4:451–3. doi: 10.1586/eop.09.43
64. Khanal S, Tomlinson A, McFadyen A, Diaper C, Ramaesh K. Dry eye diagnosis. *Invest Ophthalmol Vis Sci.* (2008) 49:1407–14. doi: 10.1167/iovs.07-0635
65. Masmali AM, Murphy PJ, Purslow C. Development of a new grading scale for tear ferning. *Cont Lens Anterior Eye.* (2014) 37:178–84. doi: 10.1016/j.clae.2013.09.011
66. Benelli U, Nardi M, Posarelli C, Albert TG. Tear osmolarity measurement using the TearLab Osmolarity System in the assessment of dry eye treatment effectiveness. *Cont Lens Anterior Eye.* (2010) 33:61–7. doi: 10.1016/j.clae.2010.01.003
67. Versura P, Profazio V, Campos E. Performance of tear osmolarity compared to previous diagnostic tests for dry eye diseases. *J Curr Eye Res.* (2010) 35:553–64. doi: 10.3109/02713683.2010.484557
68. Jacobi C, Jacobi A, Kruse FE, Cursiefen C. Tear film osmolarity measurements in dry eye disease using electrical impedance technology. *Cornea.* (2011) 30:1289–92. doi: 10.1097/ICO.0b013e31821de383
69. Masmali A, Alrabiah S, Alharbi A, El-Hiti GA, Almubrad T. Investigation of tear osmolarity using the TearLab Osmolarity System in normal adults in Saudi Arabia. *J Eye contact lens.* (2014) 40:74–8. doi: 10.1097/ICL.0000000000000002
70. Lemp MA, Bron AJ, Baudouin C, Benítez Del Castillo JM, Geffen D, Tauber J, et al. Tear osmolarity in the diagnosis and management of dry eye disease. *Am J Ophthalmol.* (2011) 151:792–8.e1. doi: 10.1016/j.ajo.2010.10.032
71. Sullivan BD, Whitmer D, Nichols KK, Tomlinson A, Foulks GN, Geerling G, et al. An objective approach to dry eye disease severity. *Invest Ophthalmol Vis Sci.* (2010) 51:6125–30. doi: 10.1167/iovs.10-5390
72. Messmer EM, Bulgen M, Kampik, A. *In Research Projects in Dry Eye Syndrome.* Germany: Karger Publishers (2010). vol. 45. p. 129–138. doi: 10.1159/000315026
73. Bunya VY, Fuerst NM, Pistilli M, McCabe BE, Salvo R, Macchi I, et al. Variability of Tear Osmolarity in Patients With Dry Eye. *JAMA Ophthalmol.* (2015) 133:662–7. doi: 10.1001/jamaophthalmol.2015.0429
74. Szalai E, Berta A, Szekanecz Z, Szûcs G, Módis L. Evaluation of tear osmolarity in non-Sjögren and Sjögren syndrome dry eye patients with the TearLab system. *J Cornea.* (2012) 31:867–71. doi: 10.1097/ICO.0b013e3182532047
75. Baenninger PB, Voegeli S, Bachmann LM, Faes L, Iselin K, Kaufmann C, et al. Variability of tear osmolarity measurements with a point-of-care system in healthy subjects-systematic review. *Cornea.* (2018) 37:938–45. doi: 10.1097/ICO.0000000000001562
76. Tashbayev B, Utheim TP, Utheim ØA, Ræder S, Jensen JL, Yazdani M, et al. Utility of tear osmolarity measurement in diagnosis of dry eye disease. *Sci Rep.* (2020) 10:5542. doi: 10.1038/s41598-020-62583-x
77. Chan CC, Borovik A, Hofmann I, Gulliver E, Rocha G. Validity and reliability of a novel handheld osmolarity system for measurement of a national institute of standards traceable solution. *Cornea.* (2018) 37:1169–74. doi: 10.1097/ICO.0000000000001653
78. Shimazaki J, Sakata M, Den S, Iwasaki M, Toda I. Tear film osmolarity measurement in japanese dry eye patients using a handheld osmolarity system. *Diagnostics.* (2020) 10:789. doi: 10.3390/diagnostics10100789
79. Fagehi R, Al-Bishry AB, Alanazi MA, Abusharha A, El-Hiti GA, Masmali AM. Investigation of the repeatability of tear osmolarity using an I-PEN osmolarity device. *Taiwan J Ophthalmol.* (2020) 11:168–74. doi: 10.4103/tjo.tjo_65_20
80. Park J, Choi Y, Han G, Shin E, Han J, Chung TY, et al. Evaluation of tear osmolarity measured by I-Pen osmolarity system in patients with dry eye. *Sci Rep.* 2021 11:7726. doi: 10.1038/s41598-021-87336-2
81. König S, Priglinger S, Schaumberger M, Messmer EM. Tränenfilmosmolarität gesunder Probanden: Vergleichbarkeit zweier Osmometer [Tear Film Osmolarity in Normal Individuals: Comparison of Two Osmometers]. *Klin Monbl Augenheilkd.* (2020) 237:649–54. doi: 10.1055/a-1155-6468
82. Choi EW, Yeom DJ, Jang SY. Botulinum toxin a injection for the treatment of intractable dry eye disease. *Medicina.* (2021) 57:247. doi: 10.3390/medicina57030247
83. Tavakoli A, Markoulli M, Flanagan J, Papas E. The validity of point of care tear film osmometers in the diagnosis of dry eye. *Ophthalmic Physiol Opt.* (2021) doi: 10.1111/opo.12901
84. Ibrahim OM, Dogru M, Ward SK, Matsumoto Y, Wakamatsu TH, Ishida K, et al. The efficacy, sensitivity, and specificity of strip meniscometry in conjunction with tear function tests in the assessment of tear meniscus. *Invest Ophthalmol Vis Sci.* (2011) 52:2194–8. doi: 10.1167/iovs.10-5986
85. Shen Z, Zhu Y, Song X, Yan J, Yao K. Dry eye after small incision lenticule extraction (SMILE) versus femtosecond laser-assisted *in situ* keratomileusis (FS-LASIK) for Myopia: a meta-analysis. *PLoS ONE.* (2016) 11:e0168081. doi: 10.1371/journal.pone.0168081
86. Kim MJ, Stinnett SS, Gupta PK. Effect of thermal pulsation treatment on tear film parameters in dry eye disease patients. *Clin Ophthalmol.* (2017) 11:883–6. doi: 10.2147/OPTH.S136203
87. Downie LE, Ng SM, Lindsley KB, Akpek EK. Omega-3 and omega-6 polyunsaturated fatty acids for dry eye disease. *Cochrane Database Syst Rev.* (2019) 12:CD011016. doi: 10.1002/14651858.CD011016.pub2
88. García-Conca V, Abad-Collado M, Hueso-Abancens JR, Mengual-Verdú E, Piñero DP, Aguirre-Balsalobre F, et al. Efficacy and safety of treatment of hyposecretory dry eye with platelet-rich plasma. *Acta Ophthalmol.* (2019) 97:e170–8. doi: 10.1111/aos.13907
89. Pflugfelder SC, Jones D, Ji Z, Afonso A, Monroy D. Altered cytokine balance in the tear fluid and conjunctiva of patients with Sjögren's syndrome keratoconjunctivitis sicca. *Curr Eye Res.* (1999) 19:201–11. doi: 10.1076/ceyr.19.3.201.5309
90. Willcox MDP, Argüeso P, Georgiev GA, Holopainen JM, Laurie GW, Millar TJ, et al. TFOS DEWS II Tear Film Report. *Ocul Surf.* (2017) 15:366–403. doi: 10.1016/j.jtos.2017.03.006
91. Sambursky R, Davitt WF, Latkany R, Tauber S, Starr C, Friedberg M, et al. Sensitivity and specificity of a point-of-care matrix metalloproteinase 9 immunoassay for diagnosing inflammation related to dry eye. *JAMA Ophthalmol.* (2013) 131:24–8. doi: 10.1001/jamaophthalmol.2013.561
92. Sambursky R, Davitt WF, Friedberg M, Tauber S. Prospective, multicenter, clinical evaluation of point-of-care matrix metalloproteinase-9 test for confirming dry eye disease. *Cornea.* (2014) 33:812–8. doi: 10.1097/ICO.0000000000000175
93. Ryu KJ, Kim S, Kim MK, Paik HJ, Kim DH. Short-term therapeutic effects of topical corticosteroids on refractory dry eye disease: clinical usefulness of matrix metalloproteinase 9 testing as a response prediction marker. *Clin Ophthalmol.* (2021) 15:759–67. doi: 10.2147/OPTH.S300047
94. Kim M, Oh JY, Bae SH, Lee SH, Lee WJ, Chun YS, et al. Assessment of reliability and validity of the 5-scale grading system of the point-of-care immunoassay for tear matrix metalloproteinase-9. *Sci Rep.* (2021) 11:12394. doi: 10.1038/s41598-021-92020-6
95. Lanza NL, Valenzuela F, Perez VL, Galor A. The Matrix Metalloproteinase 9 Point-of-Care Test in Dry Eye. *Ocul Surf.* (2016) 14:189–95. doi: 10.1016/j.jtos.2015.10.004
96. Kawashima M, Nakamura S, Izuta Y, Inoue S, Tsubota K. Dietary supplementation with a combination of Lactoferrin, Fish Oil, and *Enterococcus faecium* WB2000 for treating dry eye: a rat model and human clinical study. *Ocul Surf.* (2016) 14:255–63. doi: 10.1016/j.jtos.2015.12.005
97. Devendra J, Singh S. Effect of oral lactoferrin on cataract surgery induced dry eye: a randomised controlled trial. *J Clin Diagn Res.* (2015) 9:NC06–9. doi: 10.7860/JCDR/2015/15797.6670
98. Tsubota K, Pflugfelder SC, Liu Z, Baudouin C, Kim HM, Messmer EM, et al. Defining dry eye from a clinical perspective. *Int J Mol Sci.* (2020) 21:9271. doi: 10.3390/ijms21239271

99. Norn MS. Desiccation of the precorneal film. I corneal wetting-time. *Acta Ophthalmol.* (1969) 47:865–80. doi: 10.1111/j.1755-3768.1969.tb03711.x
100. Cox SM, Nichols KK, Nichols JJ. Agreement between automated and traditional measures of tear film breakup. *Optom Vis Sci.* (2015) 92:257–63. doi: 10.1097/OPX.0000000000000648
101. Mengher LSB. A J, Tonge SR, Gilbert DJ. Effect of fluorescein instillation on the pre-corneal tear fifilm stability *Curr Eye Res.* (1985) 4:9–12. doi: 10.3109/02713688508999961
102. Mooi JK, Wang MTM, Lim J, Müller A, Craig JP. Minimising instilled volume reduces the impact of fluorescein on clinical measurements of tear film stability. *Cont Lens Anterior Eye.* (2017) 40:170–4.
103. Pult H, Riede-Pult BH, A. new modified fluorescein strip: Its repeatability and usefulness in tear film break-up time analysis. *Cont Lens Anterior Eye.* (2012) 35:35–8. doi: 10.1016/j.clae.2011.07.005
104. Kallarackal GU, Ansari EA, Amos N, Martin JC, Lane C, Camilleri JP, et al. comparative study to assess the clinical use of Fluorescein Meniscus Time (FMT) with Tear Break up Time (TBUT) and Schirmer's tests (ST) in the diagnosis of dry eyes. *Eye (Lond).* (2002) 16:594–600. doi: 10.1038/sj.eye.6700177
105. Mou Y, Xiang H, Lin L, Yuan K, Wang X, Wu Y, Min J, Jin X. Reliability and efficacy of maximum fluorescein tear break-up time in diagnosing dry eye disease. *Sci Rep.* (2021) 11:11517. doi: 10.1038/s41598-021-91110-9
106. Vitali C, Moutsopoulos HM, Bombardieri S. The European Community Study Group on diagnostic criteria for Sjögren's Syndrome. Sensitivity and specificity of tests for ocular and oral involvement in Sjögren's syndrome. *Annl Rheum Dis.* (1994) 53:637–47. doi: 10.1136/ard.53.10.637
107. Wolffsohn JS, Arita R, Chalmers R, Djalilian A, Dogru M, Dumbleton K, et al. TFOS DEWS II diagnostic methodology report. *Ocul Surf.* (2017) 15:539–74. doi: 10.1016/j.jtos.2017.05.001
108. Tsubota K. Short tear film breakup time-type dry eye. *Invest Ophthalmol Vis Sci.* (2018) 59:DES64-DES70. doi: 10.1167/iovs.17-23746
109. Kojima T, Dogru M, Kawashima M, Nakamura S, Tsubota K. Advances in the diagnosis and treatment of dry eye. *Prog Retin Eye Res.* (2020) 29:100842. doi: 10.1016/j.preteyeres.2020.100842
110. Mcmonnies CW. Tear instability importance, mechanisms, validity and reliability of assessment. *J Optom.* (2018) 11:203-210. doi: 10.1016/j.optom.2017.11.004
111. Braun RJ, Gewecke NR, Begley CG, King-Smith PE, Siddique JI, A. model for tear film thinning with osmolarity and fluorescein. *Invest Ophthalmol Vis Sci.* (2014) 55:1133–42. doi: 10.1167/iovs.13-12773
112. King-Smith PE, Ramamoorthy P, Braun RJ, Nichols JJ. Tear film images and breakup analyzed using fluorescent quenching. *Invest Ophthalmol Vis Sci.* (2013) 54:6003–11. doi: 10.1167/iovs.13-12628
113. Wang MT, Murphy PJ, Blades KJ, Craig JP. Comparison of non-invasive tear film stability measurement techniques. *Clin Exp Optom.* (2018) 101:13–7. doi: 10.1111/cxo.12546
114. Mengher LS, Bron AJ, Tonge SR, Gilbert DJ, A. non-invasive instrument for clinical assessment of the pre-corneal tear film stability. *Curr Eye Res.* (1985) 4:1–7. doi: 10.3109/02713688508999960
115. Hirji N, Patel S, Callander M. Human tear film pre-rupture phase time (TPRPT) - a non-invasive technique for evaluating the pre-corneal tear film using a novel keratometer mire. *Ophthal Physiol Opt.* (1989) 9:139–42. doi: 10.1111/j.1475-1313.1989.tb00833.x
116. Goto T, Zheng X, Klyce SD, Kataoka H, Uno T, Karon M, et al. A new method for tear film stability analysis using video keratography. *Am J Ophthalmol.* (2003) 135:607–12. doi: 10.1016/S0002-9394(02)02221-3
117. Kojima T, Ishida R, Dogru M, Goto E, Takano Y, Matsumoto Y, et al. A new noninvasive tear stability analysis system for the assessment of dry eyes. *Invest Ophthalmol Vis Sci.* (2004) 45:1369–74. doi: 10.1167/iovs.03-0712
118. Wolff E. The muco-cutaneous junction of the lid margin and the distribution of the tear fluid. *Trans Ophthalmol Soc U K.* (1946) 66:291–308.
119. Holly FJ, Lemp MA. Tear physiology and dry eyes. *Surv Ophthalmol.* (1977) 22:69–87. doi: 10.1016/0039-6257(77)90087-X
120. King-Smith PE, Fink BA, Hill RM, Koelling KW, Tiffany JM. The thickness of the tear film. *Curr Eye Res.* (2004) 29:357–68. doi: 10.1080/02713680490516099
121. King-Smith PE, Fink BA, Fogt N, Nichols KK, Hill RM, Wilson GS. The thickness of the human precorneal tear film: evidence from reflection spectra. *Invest Ophthalmol Vis Sci.* (2000) 41:3348–59.
122. Chen Q, Wang J, Tao A, Shen M, Jiao S, Lu F. Ultrahigh-resolution measurement by optical coherence tomography of dynamic tear film changes on contact lenses. *Invest Ophthalmol Vis Sci.* (2010) 51:1988–93. doi: 10.1167/iovs.09-4389
123. Zhao Y, Tan CL, Tong L. Intra-observer and inter-observer repeatability of ocular surface interferometer in measuring lipid layer thickness. *BMC Ophthalmol.* (2015) 15:53. doi: 10.1186/s12886-015-0036-9
124. Evaluation of incomplete blinking as a measurement of dry eye disease. *Ocul Surf.* (2019) 17:440–6. doi: 10.1016/j.jtos.2019.05.007
125. Wan T, Jin X, Lin L, Xu Y, Zhao Y. Incomplete blinking may attribute to the development of meibomian gland dysfunction. *Curr Eye Res.* (2016) 41:179–85. doi: 10.3109/02713683.2015.1007211
126. Markoulli M, Duong TB, Lin M, Papas E. Imaging the Tear Film: A Comparison Between the Subjective Keeler Tearscope-Plus^{TM} and the Objective Oculus® Keratograph 5M and LipiView® Interferometer. *Curr Eye Res.* (2018) 43:155–62. doi: 10.1080/02713683.2017.1393092
127. Lee JM, Jeon YJ, Kim KY, Hwang KY, Kwon YA, Koh K. Ocular surface analysis: A comparison between the LipiView® II and IDRA®. *Eur J Ophthalmol.* (2020) 2:1120672120969035.
128. Sun Xuguang. *Blepharitis and Meibomian Gland Dysfunction.* Beijing: People's Health Publishing House (2015). p. 2–10.
129. Zhang Mingchang, Liu Yang. Interpretation of dry eye examination in the 2017 consensus of dry eye experts of the International Association of tear film and ocular surface[J]. *Chin J Ophthalmol.* (2018) 54:87–9. doi: 10.3760/cma.j.issn.0412-4081.2018.02.003
130. Asia Dry Eye Society, ADES China branch, Cross strait Medical Exchange Association, Ophthalmology Committee, Ocular surface and lacrimopathy group, Ocular Surface and Dry Eye Group of Ophthalmologist Branch of Chinese Medical Doctor Association. Expert consensus on dry eye in China: Examination and diagnosis (2020). (2020) 56:741-7. doi: 10.3760/cma.j.cn112142-20200714-00477
131. Wang J, Li S, Yeh TN, Chakraborty R, Graham AD, Yu SX, et al. Quantifying meibomian gland morphology using artificial intelligence. *Optom Vis Sci.* (2021) 98:1094–103. doi: 10.1097/OPX.0000000000001767
132. Fromstein SR, Harthan JS, Patel J, Opitz DL. Demodex blepharitis: clinical perspectives. *Clin Optom.* (2018) 10:57–63. doi: 10.2147/OPTO.S142708
133. Amano S. Meibomian gland dysfunction: recent progress worldwide and in Japan. *Invest Ophthalmol Vis Sci.* (2018) 59:DES87-DES93. doi: 10.1167/iovs.17-23553
134. Fineide F, Arita R, Utheim TP. The role of meibography in ocular surface diagnostics: A review. *Ocul Surf.* (2021) 19:133–44. doi: 10.1016/j.jtos.2020.05.004
135. Efron N, Brennan NA, Morgan PB, Wilson T. Lid wiper epitheliopathy. *Prog Retin Eye Res.* (2016) 53:140–74. doi: 10.1016/j.preteyeres.2016.04.004
136. Shiraishi A, Yamanishi S, Yamamoto Y, Yamaguchi M, Ohashi Y. [Lid-wiper epitheliopathy in patients with dry eye symptoms]. *Nippon Ganka Gakkai Zasshi.* (2009) 113:596–600.
137. Korb DR, Herman JP, Blackie CA, Scaffidi RC, Greiner JV, Exford JM, et al. Prevalence of lid wiper epitheliopathy in subjects with dry eye signs and symptoms. *Cornea.* (2010) 29:377–83. doi: 10.1097/ICO.0b013e3181ba0cb2
138. Liang X, Li Y, Xiong K, Chen S, Li Z, Zhang Z, et al. Demodex infection changes ocular surface microbial communities, in which meibomian gland dysfunction may play a role. *Ophthalmol Ther.* (2021) 10:601–17. doi: 10.1007/s40123-021-00356-z
139. Huo Y, Mo Y, Wu Y, Fang F, Jin X. Therapeutic effect of intense pulsed light with optimal pulse technology on meibomian gland dysfunction with and without ocular Demodex infestation. *Ann Transl Med.* (2021) 9:238. doi: 10.21037/atm-20-1745
140. Kim J. The use of vital dyes in corneal disease. *Curr Opin Ophthalmol.* (2000) 11:241–7. doi: 10.1097/00055735-200008000-00005
141. Bron AJ, Evans VE, Smith JA. Grading of corneal and conjunctival staining in the context of other dry eye tests. *Cornea.* (2003) 22:640–50. doi: 10.1097/00003226-200310000-00008
142. Maurice DM. The use of fluorescein in ophthalmological research. *Invest Ophthalmol.* (1967) 6:464–77.
143. Roberts CW, Carniglia PE, Brazzo BG. Comparison of topical cyclosporine, punctal occlusion, and a combination for the treatment of dry eye. *Cornea.* (2007) 26:805–9. doi: 10.1097/ICO.0b013e318074e460

144. Korb DR, Herman JP, Finnemore VM, Exford JM, Blackie CA. An evaluation of the efficacy of fluorescein, rose bengal, lissamine green, and a new dye mixture for ocular surface staining. *Eye Contact Lens.* (2008) 34:61–4. doi: 10.1097/ICL.0b013e31811ead93
145. Feenstra RP, Tseng SC. Comparison of fluorescein and rose Bengal staining. *Ophthalmology.* (1992) 99:605–17. doi: 10.1016/S0161-6420(92)31947-5
146. Zeev MS, Miller DD, Latkany R. Diagnosis of dry eye disease and emerging technologies. *Clin Ophthalmol.* (2014) 8:581–90. doi: 10.2147/OPTH.S45444
147. Yoon KC, Im SK, Kim HG, You IC. Usefulness of double vital staining with 1% fluorescein and 1% lissamine green in patients with dry eye syndrome. *Cornea.* (2011) 30:972–6. doi: 10.1097/ICO.0b013e31820687dd
148. Begley C, Caffery B, Chalmers R, Situ P, Simpson T, Nelson JD. Review and analysis of grading scales for ocular surface staining. *Ocul Surf.* (2019) 17:208–20. doi: 10.1016/j.jtos.2019.01.004
149. Baudouin C, Barton K, Cucherat M, Traverso C. The measurement of bulbar hyperemia: challenges and pitfalls. *Eur J Ophthalmol.* (2015) 25:273–9. doi: 10.5301/ejo.5000626
150. Singh RB, Liu L, Anchouche S, Yung A, Mittal SK, Blanco T, et al. Ocular redness—I: etiology, pathogenesis, and assessment of conjunctival hyperemia. *Ocul Surf.* (2021) 21:134–44. doi: 10.1016/j.jtos.2021.05.003
151. Owen CG, Fitzke FW, Woodward EG. A new computer assisted objective method for quantifying vascular changes of the bulbar conjunctivae. *Ophthalmic Physiol Opt.* (1996) 16:43. doi: 10.1046/j.1475-1313.1996.96000373.x
152. Huntjens B, Basi M, Nagra M. Evaluating a new objective grading software for conjunctival hyperaemia. *Cont Lens Anterior Eye.* (2020) 43:137–43. doi: 10.1016/j.clae.2019.07.003
153. Schulze MM, Ng A, Yang M, Panjwani F, Srinivasan S, Jones LW, et al. Bulbar redness and dry eye disease: comparison of a validated subjective grading scale and an objective automated method. *Optom Vis Sci.* (2021) 98:113–20. doi: 10.1097/OPX.0000000000001638
154. Matsumoto Y, Ibrahim OMA. Application of *in vivo* confocal microscopy in dry eye disease. *Invest Ophthalmol Vis Sci.* (2018) 59:DES41–7. doi: 10.1167/iovs.17-23602
155. Benítez del Castillo JM, Wasfy MA, Fernandez C, Garcia-Sanchez J. An in vivo confocal masked study on corneal epithelium and subbasal nerves in patients with dry eye. *Invest Ophthalmol Vis Sci.* (2004) 45:3030–5. doi: 10.1167/iovs.04-0251
156. Benítez-Del-Castillo JM, Acosta MC, Wassfi MA, Díaz-Valle D, Gegúndez JA, Fernandez C, et al. Relation between corneal innervation with confocal microscopy and corneal sensitivity with noncontact esthesiometry in patients with dry eye. *Invest Ophthalmol Vis Sci.* (2007) 48:173–81. doi: 10.1167/iovs.06-0127
157. Villani E, Galimberti D, Viola F, Mapelli C, Ratiglia R. The cornea in Sjögren's syndrome: an in vivo confocal study. *Invest Ophthalmol Vis Sci.* (2007) 48:2017–22. doi: 10.1167/iovs.06-1129
158. Villani E, Galimberti D, Viola F, Mapelli C, Del Papa N, Ratiglia R. Corneal involvement in rheumatoid arthritis: an in vivo confocal study. *Invest Ophthalmol Vis Sci.* (2008) 49:560–4. doi: 10.1167/iovs.07-0893
159. Wakamatsu TH, Sato EA, Matsumoto Y, Ibrahim OM, Dogru M, Kaido M, et al. Conjunctival in vivo confocal scanning laser microscopy in patients with Sjögren syndrome. *Invest Ophthalmol Vis Sci.* (2010) 51:144–50. doi: 10.1167/iovs.08-2722
160. Matsumoto Y, Sato EA, Ibrahim OMA, Dogru M, Tsubota K. The application of in vivo laser confocal microscopy to the diagnosis and evaluation of meibomian gland dysfunction. *Mol Vis.* (2008) 14:1263–71.
161. Ibrahim OM, Matsumoto Y, Dogru M, Adan ES, Wakamatsu TH, Goto T, et al. The efficacy, sensitivity, and specificity of in vivo laser confocal microscopy in the diagnosis of meibomian gland dysfunction. *Ophthalmology.* (2010) 117:665–72. doi: 10.1016/j.ophtha.2009.12.029
162. Sato EA, Matsumoto Y, Dogru M, Kaido M, Wakamatsu T, Ibrahim OM, Obata H, Tsubota K. Lacrimal gland in Sjögren's syndrome. *Ophthalmology.* (2010) 117:1055.e3. doi: 10.1016/j.ophtha.2009.11.034
163. Villani E, Magnani F, Viola F, Santaniello A, Scorza R, Nucci P, et al. In vivo confocal evaluation of the ocular surface morpho-functional unit in dry eye. *Optom Vis Sci.* (2013) 90:576–86. doi: 10.1097/OPX.0b013e318294c184
164. Cox SM, Kheirkhah A, Aggarwal S, Abedi F, Cavalcanti BM, Cruzat A, et al. Alterations in corneal nerves in different subtypes of dry eye disease: An *in vivo* confocal microscopy study. *Ocul Surf.* (2021) 22:135–42. doi: 10.1016/j.jtos.2021.08.004
165. Ma B, Xie J, Yang T, Su P, Liu R, Sun T, Zhou Y, Wang H, Feng X, Ma S, Zhao Y, Qi H. Quantification of increased corneal subbasal nerve tortuosity in dry eye disease and its correlation with clinical parameters. *Transl Vis Sci Technol.* (2021) 10:26. doi: 10.1167/tvst.10.6.26
166. Ma J, Wei S, Jiang X, Chou Y, Wang Y, Hao R, et al. Evaluation of objective visual quality in dry eye disease and corneal nerve changes. *Int Ophthalmol.* (2020) 40:2995–3004.
167. Lin H, Li W, Dong N, Chen W, Liu J, Chen L, et al. Changes in corneal epithelial layer inflammatory cells in aqueous tear-deficient dry eye. *Invest Ophthalmol Vis Sci.* (2010) 51:122–8. doi: 10.1167/iovs.09-3629
168. Pan S, Chen Y, A. clinical study on the correlation between demodex infestation and ocular surface changes in patients with meibomian gland dysfunction. *Indian J Ophthalmol.* (2021) 69:2389–94. doi: 10.4103/ijo.IJO_3641_20
169. Binotti WW, Bayraktutar B, Ozmen MC, Cox SM, Hamrah P, A. Review of Imaging Biomarkers of the Ocular Surface. *Eye Contact Lens.* (2020) 46:S84–S105. doi: 10.1097/ICL.0000000000000684
170. Chinese Experts Consensus Members on Standardized Construction of Dry Eye Clinical CenDry Eye Rehabilitation Specialty,Visual Rehabilitation Committee of Chinese Rehabilitation Medicine Associat Jin Xiuming. Chinese experts consensus on standardized construction of dry eye clinical center. *Zhonghua Shiyan Yanke Zazhi.* (2021) 39:473–476. doi: 10.3760/cma.j.cn115989-20210223-00128
171. Song F, Hao S, Gu Y, Yao K, Fu Q. Research advances in pathogenic mechanisms underlying air pollution-induced ocular surface diseases. *Adv Ophthalmol Pract Res.* (2021) 1. doi: 10.1016/j.aopr.2021.100001

11

Orthokeratology Lens Wear for 2 Years in Children Did Not Alter Tear Film Lipid Thickness by Non-Invasive Interferometry

Haozhe Yu[1], *Yifei Yuan*[1], *Wenyu Wu*[1], *Weizhen Zeng*[1], *Louis Tong*[2,3,4], *Yu Zhang*[1*] and *Yun Feng*[1*]

[1] Department of Ophthalmology, Peking University Third Hospital, Beijing, China, [2] Singapore Eye Research Institute, Singapore, Singapore, [3] Department of Cornea and External Diseases, Singapore National Eye Centre, Singapore, Singapore, [4] Department of Ophthalmology, Duke-NUS Medical School, Singapore, Singapore

***Correspondence:**
Yu Zhang
zhangyured@sohu.com
Yun Feng
fengyun@bjmu.edu.cn

Purpose: Previous studies suggest that overnight orthokeratology (OOK) may be detrimental to tear function. We aimed to investigate the effect of OOK on lipid layer thickness (LLT), blink pattern, and meibomian gland and elucidate the relationship of these variables.

Methods: Thirty-seven participants who wore OOK lenses every night for at least 2 years and twenty-four healthy non-contact lens wearers (controls) were enrolled in this retrospective study. LipiView interferometry, blink pattern analysis, the ocular surface status, and morphology and function of the meibomian gland were determined.

Results : The OOK group and healthy controls had similar LLT, blink patterns, ocular surface status, and the function of the meibomian gland. OOK participants demonstrated higher meiboscore in the lower eyelids ($p < 0.05$) but not in the upper eyelids. Within the OOK group, LLT was significantly impacted by the partial blink rate ($p < 0.05$) and the total score of the upper meibomian gland ($p = 0.10$).

Conclusions: Wearing OOK for 2 or more years increased lower eyelid meibomian gland dropout but did not have a reduction of LLT.

Keywords: orthokeratology, lipid layer thickness, dry eye, LipiView, meibomian gland

INTRODUCTION

With the widespread availability of electronic devices, the prevalence of myopia in children is rising rapidly and is considered a major public health issue worldwide, especially in East Asia (1). It has been reported that 80% of high school graduates in China suffer from myopia, which greatly increases the incidence of blinding diseases like glaucoma and macula lutea, resulting in a disease burden of over $240 billion per year (2, 3). Several methods of preventing myopia have been proposed, of which Overnight Orthokeratology (OOK) has been proved to be one of the most effective and widely used options in recent years (4, 5). Through reshaping the corneal epithelial tissue to change refractive and present myopic defocus in the peripheral retina, OOK can effectively slow down the elongation of the axial length by +0.70 mm after a 2 year treatment (6, 7).

Several studies have reported on the potential impact of OOK on diseases of the ocular surface, including corneal staining and infectious keratitis (8). OOK wearers may suffer from contact lens-related dry eye, which manifests as increased tear evaporation rate, reduced tear film thickness, and increased frequency of incomplete blinks. Such dry eye problems are common reasons for the discontinuation of OOK-wear (9). It is generally accepted that these tear film complications might be attributed to meibomian gland dysfunction (MGD) instead of hypoxia given the high oxygen permeability design of the OOK (10, 11).

Despite several reports that explored the association between OOK and the structure and function of the meibomian gland in OOK-wears (12, 13), these relationships remain controversial because lipid layer analysis was rarely performed and the effect of long term OOK has not been sufficiently evaluated. Recently, LipiView interferometry, which can accurately determine tear lipid layer thickness and rate of incomplete blinks, has become available (14–16). This offers an opportunity to re-evaluate the relationship between OOK and MGD, along with other tear film parameters.

The main purpose of this study was to evaluate the changes in the meibomian gland, lipid layer, and incomplete blinking in OOK-wears based on LipiView to reveal the potential etiology of OOK-related dry eye.

METHODS

Design and Patients

This retrospective study was conducted at the Department of Ophthalmology, Peking University Third Hospital from January 2019 to September 2019. The inclusion criteria were as follows: (1) Age > 10 years; (2) myopia from −1.0D to −5.5 DS, and with-the-rule astigmatism of up to −1.75 DC or against-the-rule astigmatism of <-0.75 DC with keratometry from 41 to 46 D; (3) For the OOK group, patients should have been able to master the wearing of OOK lenses and had worn them for 2 years; and (4) for the control group, all patients wore no glasses or used mainly frames, rarely using contact lenses (<2 h/d and <2 d/1w). Consent of guardians was obtained for minors who met the aforementioned inclusion criteria. The exclusion criteria were patients who were previously diagnosed with dry eye disease (DED), had a daily screen time ≥ 2 h, had pathological changes of the lid margin or cornea, uvea, or retina, had other systemic diseases that may influence the ocular surface, and received other ocular treatment or surgeries.

The sample size was estimated through PASS software (NCSS, LLC., USA) with LLT as the primary outcome under the power of the test (1–β) = 0.8 and significance level (α) = 0.05. The difference in LLT between the OOK and control groups was set to be significant at 10 ± 15 mm according to previous research (16–18). The 1:1 equal sample size design was used in this study, and the sample size for each group was calculated to be 37. The study was approved by the Institutional Ethics Committee of Peking University Third Hospital (M2018171), and all procedures were conducted in accordance with the principles of the Declaration of Helsinki.

Ocular Examination

All subjects were asked to avoid using any eye cream and ocular medications for at least 24 h prior to the clinical measurements, and for the OOK group, contact lenses should be removed more than 4 h in advance. The ocular surface disease index (OSDI) was conducted to compare the DED-related symptoms between OOK and healthy control, and the total scores of 13, 23, and 33 represented the cut points of mild, moderate, and severe DED symptoms, respectively (19). The cornea staining and tear break-up time (TBUT) were conducted through a fluorescein strip (Meizilin Co., Ltd. China) to evaluate the ocular surface status and tear film stability. The score of cornea staining followed by the Oxford grading scheme and the TBUT < 10 s was considered consistent with the diagnosis of DED (20). For tear secretion evaluation, the Schirmer test sterile strips (Meizilin Co., Ltd. China) were inserted into the lower conjunctival sac, the wetting paper was measured after 5 min with the eye closed, and the wetting length > 10 mm were considered to be normal (21). The physiological function of the meibomian gland was assessed by observing the meibomian gland expressibility and its properties in the central five meibomian glands of the eyelids. Zero referred to all meibomian glands secreting normally or the meibum presenting as clear and transparent, while 3 stood for none of the meibomian gland secreting meibum or the meibum presenting toothpaste-like consistency (22). The total score of the meibomian gland was defined as the sum of meiboscore, meibomian gland expressibility, and its properties score.

LipiView Measurement

During the examination, the patients were asked to look at the front light-spot to ensure their pupils were directly in the center of the interferometer camera with natural blinking, and all the measurements were conducted by the same experienced examiner using LipiView Ocular Surface Interferometer (Johnson & Johnson, USA). The average lipid layer thickness (LLT), partial blinks and their rate (PBR, per 20s), and complete blinks of subjects were recorded, and the patients with an outcome conformance factor (CF) of <0.8 were asked to repeat the measurement. The morphology of the upper and lower eyelid meibomian gland in these subjects were observed using the photographic module of LipiView, and the extent of meibomian gland loss was scored as follows (meiboscore): 0 (no loss), 1 (loss area <33%), 2 (34%< loss area <66%), and 3 (loss area >67%) (23).

Statistical Method

Statistical analysis was performed by IBM SPSS Statistics 24.0 (IBM SPSS Inc., USA) and R software 4.0.4, and the measurement data subjected to normal distribution were presented as the mean ± SD (M ± SD) while the enumeration data were presented as the ratio (%). Their differences between the groups were compared through *t*-test (demographic data), linear mixed models (ophthalmic examination data), and Clustered Wilcoxon rank sum test (enumeration data), respectively (24, 25). The generalized estimating equation was used to assess the relationship among various factors and LLT (26). The significant level was set up as $\alpha = 0.05$.

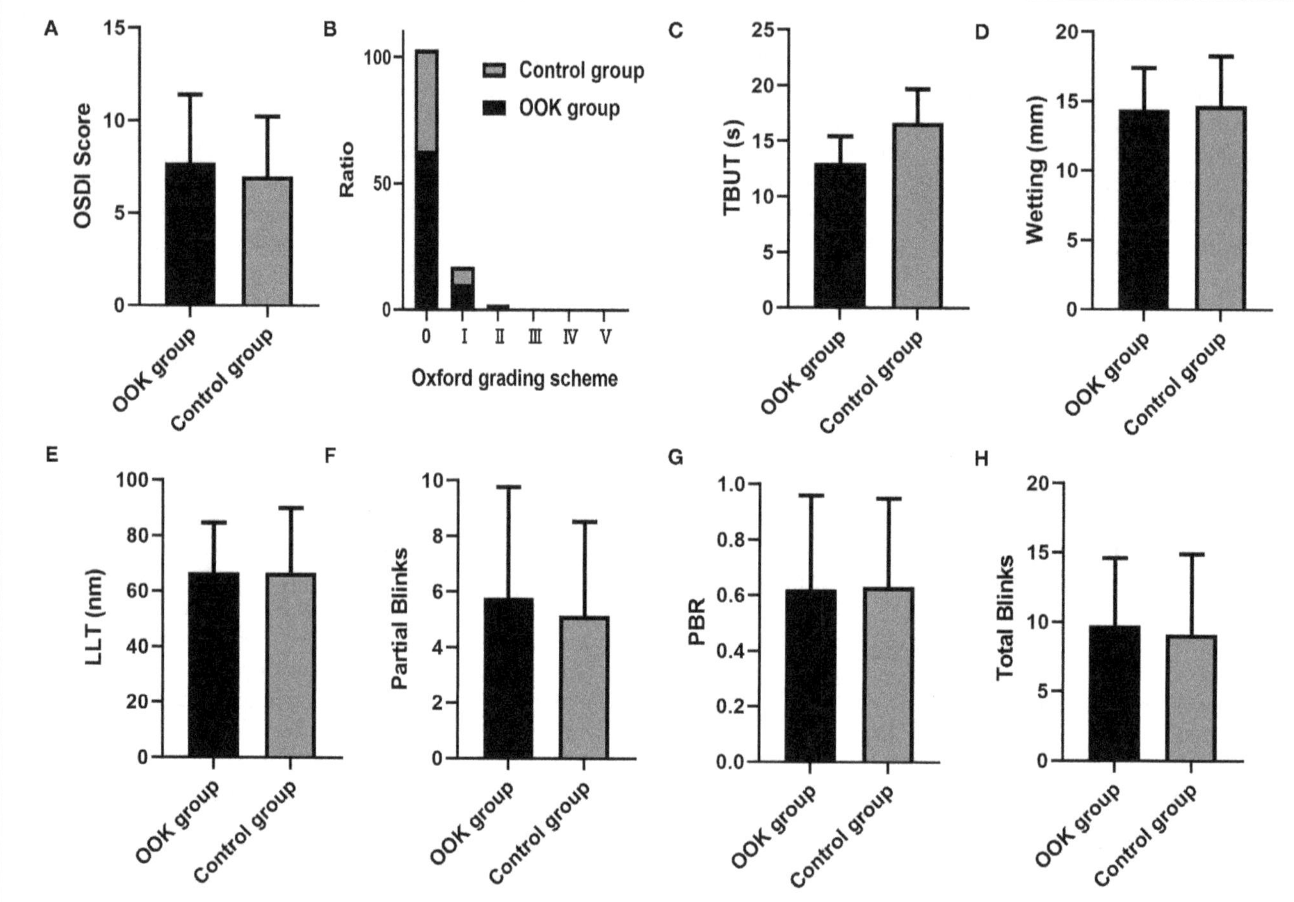

FIGURE 1 | Comparison of **(A)** ocular surface disease index (OSDI) score, **(B)** cornea staining score, **(C)** tear break-up time (TBUT), **(D)** tear secretion, **(E)** LLT, **(F)** partial blinks, **(G)** partial blinks and their rate (PBR), and **(H)** total blinks between orthokeratology (OOK) group and control group.

RESULTS

A total of sixty-one participants (122 eyes) were recruited into the study and completed the LipiView examination, which met sample size requirements. The OOK group consisted of thirty-seven cases (74 eyes) who had worn OOK lenses for 2 years with an average age year of 12.7 ± 1.9 and male/female = 20:17. Twenty-four cases (48 eyes) who were without a history of contact lens wearing and dry eye with an average age year of 12.9±7.7 and male/female = 13:11 were included in the control group. There was no statistical difference between each group in age ($p = 0.92$) and sex ($p = 0.99$). Additionally, the CF in both the OOK group (0.94 ± 0.06) and control group (0.93 ± 0.08) were higher than 0.8, indicating the high accuracy and reliability of the examination.

Intergroup Comparison of the Ocular Surface Examination

The results of the ocular surface examination and LipiView examination were summarized in **Figure 1**. There was no difference between OOK group and control group in OSDI (7.69 ± 3.71 vs. 6.98 ± 3.25, $p = 0.44$), cornea staining (score = 0: 85.1 vs. 83.4%, $p = 0.82$), TBUT (13.03 ± 2.40 vs. 13.67 ± 3.05, $p = 0.36$), Schirmer test (14.40 ± 3.02 vs. 14.71 ± 3.58, $p = 0.71$), LLT (66.53 ± 18.12 vs. 66.42 ± 23.52, $p = 0.77$), partial blinks (5.78 ± 3.98 vs. 5.14 ± 3.38, $p = 0.44$), PBR (0.62 ± 0.34 vs. 0.63 ± 0.32, $p = 0.91$), and total blinks (9.78 ± 4.83 vs. 9.14 ± 5.77, $p = 0.54$).

Comparison of Morphology and Function of Meibomian Gland

Figure 2 demonstrated the distribution of meibomian gland dropout in the OOK group and control group, and the meiboscore of each group was lower than 3. In the lower eyelids, the OOK group showed a higher proportion of light (51.35%) and medium (5.40%) loss of meibomain glands, while the meiboscore was limited to mild loss (1) without any case of moderate or severe loss in the control group (33.3%) ($p < 0.01$). There was no statistically significant difference in the upper meibomian gland dropout ($p = 0.25$), upper and lower score of meibum properties ($p = 0.71$, 0.83), and meibomian gland expressibility ($p = 0.79$, 0.13) in each group.

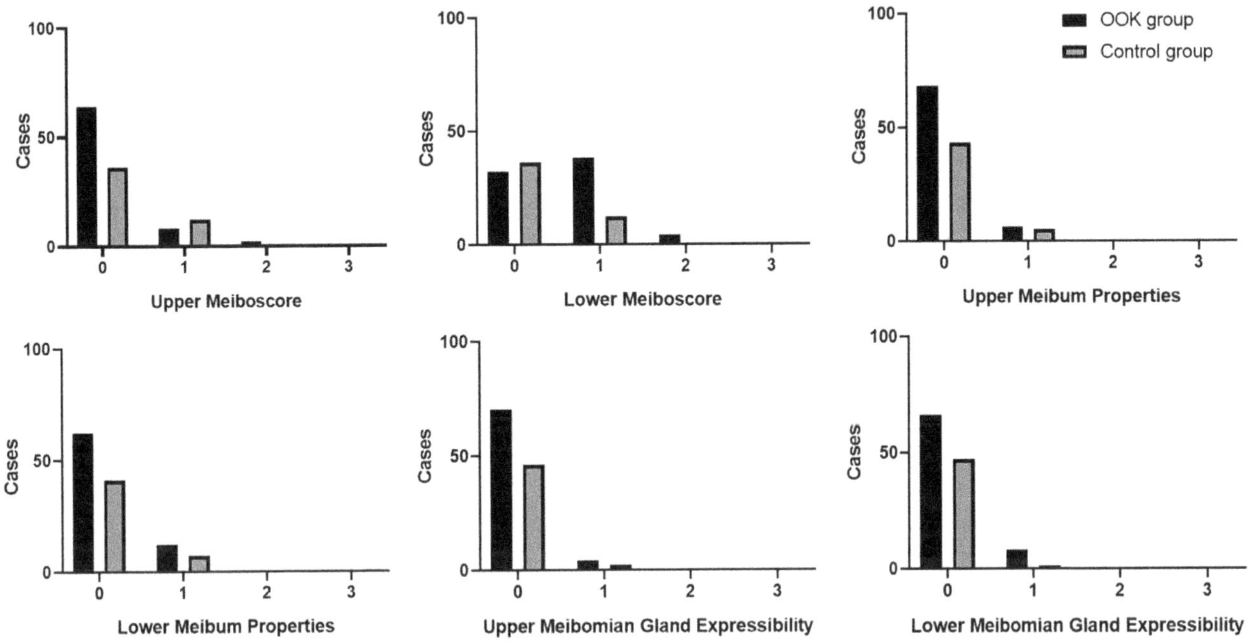

FIGURE 2 | Meiboscore, meibum properties, and meibomian gland expressibility of the upper and lower eyelid in the OOK group and control group.

TABLE 1 | Associations of lipid layer thickness (LLT) and other parameters in generalized estimating equations models.

Variable	OOK group		Control group	
	B	*P*	*B*	*P*
Age	−0.90	0.24	−0.56	0.45
Gender	0.91	0.83	0.11	0.74
Years of lens	3.88	0.94	–	–
Partial Blink	0.34	0.61	0.34	0.76
PBR	17.30	$P < 0.001$	3.24	0.76
Total blink	−0.50	0.13	0.91	0.08
Total score of upper meibomian gland*	−2.30	0.10	−11.37	$P < 0.05$
Total score of lower meibomian gland*	−1.43	0.25	−7.25	$P < 0.05$

*Compared with score = 0.

Correlation Between LLT and Other Factors

The generalized estimating equation model was established to evaluate the associations of LLT with demographic factors, blink-related parameters, and the total score of the meibomian gland (**Table 1**). The LLT was significantly affected by the total score of the meibomian gland as well as PBR in the control and OOK groups, respectively. In addition, it could be considered that the lower total score of the upper meibomian gland was related to higher LLT in the OOL group with a significance level of 0.10.

DISCUSSION

In this study, we found LLT to be unaffected by OOK-wear and lower eyelid meibomian gland atrophy to be increased.

The lipid layer located in the superficial layer of the tear film is mainly formed by meibomian lipids secreted from the upper and lower meibomian gland (27, 28). The lipid layer was associated with contact lens-related ocular dryness and discomfort because an abnormal lipid layer could result in a high tear evaporation rate, low tear breakup time, and high tear osmolarity value (29–31). The LLT measured by LipiView interferometry is considered an important indicator of tear lipid health and demonstrates a good correlation with meibomian gland function (32–34). In this study, we do not observe any effect of long-term wearing of OOK on the LLT and the ocular surface status which is consistent with previous reports of high comfort levels in OOK wearers (11, 35, 36).

Previous studies of OOK wearers have reported changes in meibomian gland morphology, tear cytokines, and ocular surface parameters (13, 35).

The meibomian gland plays a vital role in maintaining the stability of tear film, and an increased meiboscore is generally considered as the important risk factor for DED and contact lens-related discomfort (37, 38). Previous studies have examined the influence of OOK wearing on the morphology of the meibomian gland based on non-contact infrared meibography or Keratograph 5M and found that there is no significant difference in the meiboscore before and after wearing lenses (12, 39). The discrepancy might be attributed to the imaging quality of different instruments. Wong et al. (40) found that the LipiView was easier in evaluating the extent of the meibomian gland, owing to its high contrast and low reflectivity compared with Keratograph 5M. Alternatively, the duration of OOK lens wear may be shorter in previous studies and so, insufficient to cause meibomian gland dropout.

Mechanical trauma and inflammation are the main hypotheses in explaining the contact lens-related meibomian gland damage. Overnight lens wearing plus rapid-eye-movement might further prolong the eyelid/lens contact duration and increase friction between the lens and the meibomian gland (41). Pult et al. (42) and Eom et al. (43) found the destruction of the meibomian gland in MGD and DED patients to be more severe in the lower eyelid. The upper eyelid could be relaxed to a larger extent to compensate for the damage induced by OOK (43–45). It may be that the lower eyelid is more irregular (46), and so predisposed to greater meibomian gland dropout. Considering that the upper eyelid usually shows a larger area lens than the lower eyelid during sleep, its deformation might be less affected by wearing OOK lenses, which results in a more regular lid margin and lower meiboscore.

It is generally accepted that the duration of contact lens plays a more critical role on the meibomian gland, rather than lens material (47). If anything, however, OOK lens materials have higher oxygen permeability and induce less hypoxia and inflammation (48–50). In addition, the MGD was also considered to be posterior blepharitis involving various inflammatory processes. The major reason that there was no difference in physiological functions of the meibomian gland between OOK and healthy control might be attributed to such characteristics of OOK (51, 52).

Blink can maintain tear film stability of the ocular surface by promoting the reconstruction and development of the lipid layer (53, 54). can be covered by tears through complete blinking, preventing damage from DED. Therefore, partial blinking is deleterious (55). Several studies have reported increased partial blinks in contact lens wearers, which have also been reported in DED (56, 57). However, we did not show OOK affecting PBR, likely due to underpowering for this variable.

As seen in previous studies, there was an exact correlation of LLT with the total score of the meibomian gland in the healthy control from the regression analysis results, which could be attributed to how the meibomian gland secreted lipid layer and stabilized them (58). In the OOK group, the PBR demonstrated a significant positive effect on LLT. Nevertheless, the relationship between partial blink and LLT was still unclear because of its complex influencing factors from meibomian gland function, tear composition, and flow rate (27). Li et al. (59) reported that the LLT showed significant negative correlations with incomplete blinking rate, while Jie et al. (60) presented that there was not an association between them. In this study, a reason proposed was that the upper meibomian gland could produce a stable tear film alone after a partial blink and the lower meibomian gland did not contribute to it, while the LLT was essential for tear film stability (61, 62). Based on this, a partial blink was considered a compensatory response to an abnormal tear film (63). It can be speculated that the function of the upper and lower meibomian gland might be reconfigured after a long time of wearing OOK lenses, and the PBR became a protective factor of LLT and tear film in OOK wearers. Furthermore, the significance of the total score of the upper meibomian gland in regression analysis indicated that the LLT was more likely to be influenced by the upper eyelid than the lower, which further supported this hypothesis.

There are a few limitations to our study. This is single-center research, and the limited number of participants enrolled in this study might increase potential sampling bias. Moreover, there was a lack of longitudinal assessment about the effect of long-term wearing OOK on the ocular surface, LLT, blink-related parameters, and the meibomian gland. Future studies are needed to evaluate tear composition and distribution, and how these are influenced by LLT, PBR, and meibomian gland status.

ETHICS STATEMENT

The studies involving human participants were reviewed and approved by Peking University Third Hospital Medical Science Research Ethics Committee. Written informed consent to participate in this study was provided by the participants' legal guardian/next of kin.

AUTHOR CONTRIBUTIONS

YZ and YF designed the study. HY and YY wrote the initial draft. YY, WW, WZ, LT, and YF revised the manuscript. All authors made a substantial and intellectual contribution to the article and approved the submitted version.

REFERENCES

1. Cho P, Tan Q. Myopia and orthokeratology for myopia control. *Clin Exp Optometry.* (2019) 102:364–77. doi: 10.1111/cxo.12839
2. Jan C, Li L, Keay L, Stafford RS, Congdon N, Morgan I. Prevention of myopia, China. *Bull World Health Organ.* (2020) 98:435–7. doi: 10.2471/BLT.19.240903
3. Tang Y, Chen A, Zou M, Liu Z, Young CA, Zheng D, et al. Prevalence and time trends of refractive error in Chinese children: a systematic review and meta-analysis. *J Glob Health.* (2021) 11:1–11. doi: 10.7189/jogh.11.08006
4. Batres L, Bodas J, Carracedo G. Safety in corneal refractive therapy for myopia control. Oftalmologija. *Vostochnaja Evropa.* (2020) 10:440–50. doi: 10.34883/PI.2020.10.4.016

5. Wang S, Wang J, Wang N. Combined orthokeratology with atropine for children with myopia: a meta-analysis. *Ophthalmic Res.* (2021) 64:723–31. doi: 10.1159/000510779
6. Guan M, Zhao W, Geng Y, Zhang Y, Ma J, Chen Z, et al. Changes in axial length after orthokeratology lens treatment for myopia: a meta-analysis. *Int Ophthalmol.* (2020) 40:255–65. doi: 10.1007/s10792-019-01167-9
7. Nti AN, Berntsen DA. Optical changes and visual performance with orthokeratology. *Clin Exp Optometry.* (2020) 103:44–54. doi: 10.1111/cxo.12947
8. Kam KW, Yung W, Li GKH, Chen LJ, Young AL. Infectious keratitis and orthokeratology lens use: a systematic review. *Infection.* (2017) 45:727–35. doi: 10.1007/s15010-017-1023-2
9. Lim CHL, Stapleton F, Mehta JS. Review of Contact Lens–Related Complications. *Eye Contact Lens.* (2018) 44:S1–10. doi: 10.1097/ICL.0000000000000481
10. Li W, Sun X, Wang Z, Zhang Y. A survey of contact lens-related complications in a tertiary hospital in China. *Contact Lens and Anterior Eye.* (2018) 41:201–204. doi: 10.1016/j.clae.2017.10.007
11. Duong K, McGwin G Jr, Franklin QX, Cox J, Pucker AD. Treating uncomfortable contact lens wear with orthokeratology. *Eye Contact Lens.* (2021) 47:74–80. doi: 10.1097/ICL.0000000000000690
12. Na KS, Yoo YS, Hwang HS, Mok JW, Kim HS, Joo CK. The influence of overnight orthokeratology on ocular surface and meibomian glands in children and adolescents. *Eye Contact Lens.* (2016) 42:68–73. doi: 10.1097/ICL.0000000000000196
13. Yang L, Zhang L, Jian Hu R, Yu PP, Jin X. The influence of overnight orthokeratology on ocular surface and dry eye-related cytokines IL-17A, IL-6, and PGE2 in children. *Contact Lens Anterior Eye.* (2021) 44:81–8. doi: 10.1016/j.clae.2020.04.001
14. Park J, Kim J, Lee H, Park M, Baek S. Functional and structural evaluation of the meibomian gland using a LipiView interferometer in thyroid eye disease. *Can J Ophthalmol.* (2018) 53:373–9. doi: 10.1016/j.jcjo.2017.11.006
15. Lee JM, Jeon YJ, Kim KY, Hwang KY, Kwon YA, Koh K. Ocular surface analysis: a comparison between the LipiView® II and IDRA®. *Eur J Ophthalmol.* (2020) 31:2300–6. doi: 10.1177/1120672120969035
16. Zhang J, Wu Z, Sun L, Liu XH. Function and morphology of the meibomian glands using a lipiview interferometer in rotating shift medical staff. *J Ophthalmol.* (2020) 2020:3275143. doi: 10.1155/2020/3275143
17. Blackie CA, Solomon JD, Scaffidi RC, Greiner JV, Lemp MA, Korb DR. The relationship between dry eye symptoms and lipid layer thickness. *Cornea.* (2009) 28:789–94. doi: 10.1097/ICO.0b013e318191b870
18. Chou YB, Fan NW, Lin PY. Value of lipid layer thickness and blinking pattern in approaching patients with dry eye symptoms. *Can J Ophthalmol.* (2019) 54:735–40. doi: 10.1016/j.jcjo.2019.03.005
19. Lu F, Tao A, Hu Y, Tao W, Lu P. Evaluation of reliability and validity of three common dry eye questionnaires in Chinese. *J Ophthalmol.* (2018) 2018:2401213. doi: 10.1155/2018/2401213
20. Tiskaoglu NS, Yazic,i A, Karlidere T, Sari E, Oguz EY, Musaoglu M, et al. Dry eye disease in patients with newly diagnosed depressive disorder. *Curr Eye Res.* (2017) 42:672–76. doi: 10.1080/02713683.2016.1236966
21. Karakus S, Agrawal D, Hindman HB, Henrich C, Ramulu PY, Akpek EK. Effects of prolonged reading on dry eye. *Ophthalmology.* (2018) 125:1500–5. doi: 10.1016/j.ophtha.2018.03.039
22. Chatterjee S, Agrawal D, Sharma A. Meibomian gland dysfunction in a hospital-based population in central India. *Cornea.* (2020) 39:634–9. doi: 10.1097/ICO.0000000000002217
23. Arita R, Itoh K, Maeda S, Maeda K, Furuta A, Fukuoka S, et al. Proposed diagnostic criteria for obstructive meibomian gland dysfunction. *Ophthalmology.* (2009) 116:2058–63.e1. doi: 10.1016/j.ophtha.2009.04.037
24. Rosner B, Glynn RJ, Lee MLT. Incorporation of clustering effects for the wilcoxon rank sum test: a large-sample approach. *Biometrics.* (2003) 59:1089–98. doi: 10.1111/j.0006-341X.2003.00125.x
25. Herber R, Kaiser A, Grählert X, Range U, Raiskup F, Pillunat LE, et al. Statistical analysis of correlated measurement data in ophthalmology: tutorial for the application of the linear mixed model in SPSS and R using corneal biomechanical parameters. *Ophthalmologe.* (2020) 117:27–35. doi: 10.1007/s00347-019-0904-4
26. Ying GS, Maguire MG, Glynn R, Rosner B. Tutorial on biostatistics: linear regression analysis of continuous correlated eye data. *Ophthalmic Epidemiol.* (2017) 24:130–40. doi: 10.1080/09286586.2016.1259636
27. Georgiev GA, Eftimov P, Yokoi N. Structure-function relationship of tear film lipid layer: a contemporary perspective. *Exp Eye Res.* (2017) 163:17–28. doi: 10.1016/j.exer.2017.03.013
28. Cohen Y, Trokel S, Arieli Y, Epshtien S, Gefen R, Harris A. Mapping the lipid layer of the human tear film. *Cornea.* (2020) 39:132–5. doi: 10.1097/ICO.0000000000002101
29. Ewen King-Smith P, Hinel EA, Nichols JJ. Application of a novel interferometric method to investigate the relation between lipid layer thickness and tear film thinning. *Invest Ophthalmol Vis Sci.* (2010) 51:2418–23. doi: 10.1167/iovs.09-4387
30. Kojima T, Matsumoto Y, Ibrahim OMA, Wakamatsu TH, Uchino M, Fukagawa K, et al. Effect of controlled adverse chamber environment exposure on tear functions in silicon hydrogel and hydrogel soft contact lens wearers. *Invest Ophthalmol Vis Sci.* (2011) 52:8811–7. doi: 10.1167/iovs.10-6841
31. Siddireddy JS, Vijay AK, Tan J, Willcox M. The eyelids and tear film in contact lens discomfort. *Contact Lens Anterior Eye.* (2018) 41:144–53. doi: 10.1016/j.clae.2017.10.004
32. Sengor T, Kurna SA, Ozbay N, Ertek S, Aki S, Altun A. Contact lens-related dry eye and ocular surface changes with mapping technique in long-term soft silicone hydrogel contact lens wearers. *Euro J Ophthalmol.* (2012) 22(Suppl. 7):S17–23. doi: 10.5301/ejo.5000079
33. Finis D, Pischel N, Borrelli M, Schrader S, Geerling G. Factors influencing the measurement of tear film lipid layer thickness with interferometry. *Klin Monbl Augenheilkd.* (2014) 231:603–10. doi: 10.1055/s-0034-1368536
34. Li J, Ma J, Hu M, Yu J, Zhao Y. Assessment of tear film lipid layer thickness in patients with meibomian gland dysfunction at different ages. *BMC Ophthalmol.* (2020) 20:394. doi: 10.1186/s12886-020-01667-8
35. Carracedo G, Martin-Gil A, Fonseca B, Pintor J. Effect of overnight orthokeratology on conjunctival goblet cells. *Contact Lens Anterior Eye.* (2016) 39:266–9. doi: 10.1016/j.clae.2016.04.001
36. García-Porta N, Rico-Del-Viejo L, Martin-Gil A, Carracedo G, Pintor J, González-Méijome JM. Differences in dry eye questionnaire symptoms in two different modalities of contact lens wear: silicone-hydrogel in daily wear basis and overnight orthokeratology. *Biomed Res Int.* (2016) 2016:1242845. doi: 10.1155/2016/1242845
37. Arita R, Fukuoka S, Morishige N. Meibomian gland dysfunction and contact lens discomfort. *Eye Contact Lens.* (2017) 43:17–22. doi: 10.1097/ICL.0000000000000351
38. Kiyat P, Palamar M, Gerceker Turk B, Yagci A. Dry eye and quantitative and qualitative changes of meibomian glands in patients with pemphigus. *Cornea.* (2020) 39:1108–11. doi: 10.1097/ICO.0000000000002356
39. Wang X, Li J, Zhang R, Li N, Pang Y, Zhang Y, et al. The influence of overnight orthokeratology on ocular surface and meibomian gland dysfunction in teenagers with myopia. *J Ophthalmol.* (2019) 2019:5142628. doi: 10.1155/2019/5142628
40. Wong S, Srinivasan S, Murphy PJ, Jones L. Comparison of meibomian gland dropout using two infrared imaging devices. *Contact Lens Anterior Eye.* (2019) 42:311–7. doi: 10.1016/j.clae.2018.10.014
41. Vu CHV, Kawashima M, Yamada M, Suwaki K, Uchino M, Shigeyasu C, et al. Influence of meibomian gland dysfunction and friction-related disease on the severity of dry eye. *Ophthalmology.* (2018) 125:1181–8. doi: 10.1016/j.ophtha.2018.01.025
42. Pult H, Riede-Pult BH, Nichols JJ. Relation between upper and lower lids' meibomian gland morphology, tear film, dry eye. *Optometry Vis Sci.* (2012) 89:E310–5. doi: 10.1097/OPX.0b013e318244e487
43. Eom Y, Choi KE, Kang SY, Lee HK, Kim HM, Song JS. Comparison of meibomian gland loss and expressed meibum grade between the upper and lower eyelids in patients with obstructive meibomian gland dysfunction. *Cornea.* (2014) 33:448–52. doi: 10.1097/ICO.0000000000000092
44. Knop E, Knop N, Millar T, Obata H, Sullivan DA. The international workshop on meibomian gland dysfunction: report of the subcommittee on anatomy physiology, and pathophysiology of the meibomian gland. *Invest Ophthalmol Vis Sci.* (2011) 52:1938–78. doi: 10.1167/iovs.10-6997c
45. Yang B, Liu L, Cho P. Does long-term rigid contact lens wear lead to acquired blepharoptosis in Chinese eyes? *Eye Contact Lens.* (2020) 46:24–30. doi: 10.1097/ICL.0000000000000607

46. Ha M, Kim JS, Hong SY, Chang DJ, Whang WJ, Na KS, et al. Relationship between eyelid margin irregularity and meibomian gland dropout. *Ocul Surf.* (2021) 19:31–7. doi: 10.1016/j.jtos.2020.11.007
47. Gu T, Du B, Bi H, Zhou L, Liu G, Jin N, et al. Meibomian gland dropout, not distortion, can distinguish dry eyes from normal eyes in contact lens wearers. *Curr Eye Res.* (2020) 45:897–903. doi: 10.1080/02713683.2020.1731829
48. Efron N. Contact lens wear is intrinsically inflammatory. *Clin Exp Optometry.* (2017) 100:3–19. doi: 10.1111/cxo.12487
49. Morgan PB, Efron N, Woods CA, Santodomingo-Rubido J. International survey of orthokeratology contact lens fitting. *Contact Lens Anterior Eye.* (2019) 42:450–4. doi: 10.1016/j.clae.2018.11.005
50. Harbiyeli II, Bozkurt B, Erdem E, Ozcan HG, Cam B, Sertdemir Y, et al. Associations with meibomian gland loss in soft and rigid contact lens wearers. *Contact Lens Anterior Eye.* (2021) 7:101400. doi: 10.1016/j.clae.2020.12.005
51. Mizoguchi S, Iwanishi H, Arita R, Shirai K, Sumioka T, Kokado M, et al. Ocular surface inflammation impairs structure and function of meibomian gland. *Exp Eye Res.* (2017) 163:78–84. doi: 10.1016/j.exer.2017.06.011
52. Sabeti S, Kheirkhah A, Yin J, Dana R. Management of meibomian gland dysfunction: a review. *Surv Ophthalmol.* (2020) 65:205–17. doi: 10.1016/j.survophthal.2019.08.007
53. Bandlitz S, Purslow C, Murphy PJ, Pult H. Time course of changes in tear meniscus radius and blink rate after instillation of artificial tears. *Invest Ophthalmol Vis Sci.* (2014) 55:5842–7. doi: 10.1167/iovs.14-14844
54. Jeon YJ, Song MY, Kim KY, Hwang KY, Kwon YA, Koh K. Relationship between the partial blink rate and ocular surface parameters. *Int Ophthalmol.* (2021) 41:2601–8. doi: 10.1007/s10792-021-01819-9
55. King-Smith PE, Nichols JJ, Nichols KK, Fink BA, Braun RJ. Contributions of evaporation and other mechanisms to tear film thinning and break-up. *Optometry Vis Sci.* (2008) 85:623–30. doi: 10.1097/OPX.0b013e318181ae60
56. Martín-Montañez V, López-de la Rosa A, López-Miguel A, Pinto-Fraga J, González-Méijome JM, González-García MJ. End-of-day dryness, corneal sensitivity and blink rate in contact lens wearers. *Contact Lens Anterior Eye.* (2015) 38:148–51. doi: 10.1016/j.clae.2015.01.003
57. Guillon M, Theodoratos P, Patel K, Gupta R, Patel T. Pre-contact lens and pre-corneal tear film kinetics. *Contact Lens Anterior Eye.* (2019) 42:246–52. doi: 10.1016/j.clae.2019.02.001
58. Fukuoka S, Arita R. Tear film lipid layer increase after diquafosol instillation in dry eye patients with meibomian gland dysfunction: a randomized clinical study. *Sci Rep.* (2019) 9:9091. doi: 10.1038/s41598-019-45475-7
59. Li Y, Li S, Zhou J, Liu C, Xu M. Relationship between lipid layer thickness, incomplete blinking rate and tear film instability in patients with different myopia degrees after small-incision lenticule extraction. *PLoS ONE.* (2020) 15:e0230119. doi: 10.1371/journal.pone.0230119
60. Jie Y, Sella R, Feng J, Gomez ML, Afshari NA. Evaluation of incomplete blinking as a measurement of dry eye disease. *Ocul Surf.* (2019) 17:440–6. doi: 10.1016/j.jtos.2019.05.007
61. Harrison WW, Begley CG, Liu H, Chen M, Garcia M, Smith JA. Menisci and fullness of the blink in dry eye. *Optometry Vis Sci.* (2008) 85:706–14. doi: 10.1097/OPX.0b013e318181ae02
62. Yin Y, Gong L. Uneven meibomian gland dropout over the tarsal plate and its correlation with meibomian gland dysfunction. *Cornea.* (2015) 34:1200–5. doi: 10.1097/ICO.0000000000000533
63. Su Y, Liang Q, Su G, Wang N, Baudouin C, Labbé A. Spontaneous eye blink patterns in dry eye: clinical correlations. *Invest Ophthalmol Vis Sci.* (2018) 59:5149–56. doi: 10.1167/iovs.18-24690

12

Sleep Quality is Associated with Severe Meibomian Gland Disruption in Dry Eye

Yirui Zhu[1]*, Xiaodan Huang*[1]*, Lin Lin*[1]*, Mengshu Di*[1]*, Ruida Chen*[1,2]*, Fei Fang*[1,3] *and Xiuming Jin*[1*]

[1] *Eye Center, Affiliated Second Hospital, School of Medicine, Zhejiang University, Hangzhou, China,* [2] *Eye Department, Affiliated Dongyang Hospital, Wenzhou Medical University, Dongyang, China,* [3] *Department of ENT, Wuning County People's Hospital, Jiujiang, China*

Correspondence:
Xiuming Jin
lzyjxm@zju.edu.cn

Purpose: To investigate the association between sleep quality and meibomian gland dropout characteristics in dry eye patients.

Methods: This cross-sectional study involved 172 dry eye patients with no history of conditions or factors that could confound dry eye disease (DED) and/or meibomian gland dropout. Participants underwent a comprehensive anterior eye assessment. The validated Athens Insomnia Scale (AIS) and Pittsburgh Sleep Quality Index (PSQI) were used to assess sleep quality. The measured outcomes were dry eye symptoms via the Ocular Surface Disease Index (OSDI), tear breakup time (TBUT), corneal fluorescein staining, meibomian gland function, and extent of meibomian gland dropout.

Results: Of the dry eye participants, 34.9% had severe meibomian gland dropout (SMD) and 41.3% of the subjects had poor sleep quality. Patients with poor sleep quality had greater Meibomian gland dropout while the sleep AIS and PSQI scores were significantly correlated with Meibomian gland dropout ($r = 0.495$, $p < 0.001$; $r = 0.24$, $p = 0.002$; respectively). SMD patients had worse scores on all components of the PSQI (all $p < 0.001$, corrected for age and sex). Use of sleep medication, poor habitual sleep efficiency, and sleep disturbance were particularly prevalent in SMD patients as compared to Non-severe meibomian gland dropout (NSMD) patients. Multivariate logistic regression analysis revealed that sleep quality was eventually associated with female gender ($p = 0.042$), OSDI ($p = 0.004$), TBUT ($p = 0.036$), and Meibomian gland dropout score ($p < 0.001$).

Conclusion: It was found that greater meibomian gland dropout in poor sleep quality individuals is especially related to use of sleep medication, poor habitual sleep efficiency, and sleep disturbance. This finding suggests a need for long-term studies of anterior eye health in people with poor sleep quality.

Keywords: poor sleep quality, dry eye, MGD, meibomian gland dropout, Pittsburgh Sleep Quality Index (PSQI)

INTRODUCTION

Sleep dysfunction leads to disruption of physiological systems essential to maintaining good health. Sleep disturbances, such as difficulties with sleep onset (sleep latency), efficiency, or duration, are not only highly prevalent in over one-third of the general population, with 8–27% reporting experiencing chronic or severe sleep problems, but are also associated with increased risk for serious diseases and health conditions, dependence on medication, higher incidences of drugs or alcohol abuse, and greater utilization of medical services (1, 2).

Dry eye disease (DED) is a multifactorial disease of the tears and ocular surface that results in symptoms of discomfort, visual disturbance, and tear film instability (3). The chronic discomfort observed in DED directly decreases quality of life and interferes with the ability to carry out daily functions (4–6). Meibomian gland dysfunction (MGD) is a leading cause of evaporative DED. MGD is characterized by terminal duct obstruction and altered meibum secretion. These obstructions block the delivery of meibum into the lid margin and cause an increase in pressure within the gland. The increased pressure results in atrophic gland degeneration, meibomian gland dropout, and ultimately results in the disappearance of glandular tissue within the upper and lower tarsal plates (7). Abnormal meibum quality and quantity can lead to a decreased tear film lipid layer, tear hyperosmolarity, mechanical irritation through increased friction, and the onset of inflammatory cascades, all of which can lead to ocular surface damage (7–9). Meibomian gland dropout and altered quality of expressed meibum have been used to classify the severity of MGD (8).

DED is commonly observed in individuals with sleep disturbances and other related disorders. A large, community-based study conducted by our eye center showed a strong association between poor sleep quality and an increased severity of dry eye (10). Mengliang et al. (11) found that sleep quality plays an important role in the development of dry eye by influencing tear secretion and tear film stability by indirectly aggravating anxiety and depression. Furthermore, sleep deprivation in a mouse model study indicated that sleep deprivation induced dry eye by disrupting superficial corneal epithelial cells microvilli morphology, which is caused by sequential declines in the peroxisome proliferator-activated receptor alpha (PPARα), transient receptor potential vanilloid 6 (TRPV6) expression, and Ezrin phosphorylation status (12). Though these studies suggest that sleep deprivation may contribute to dry eye status, they have not identified differences in meibomian gland structure in subjects with and without sleep deprivation in dry eye patients. Additionally, few studies to date have further analyzed the relationship between meibomian glands architecture parameters and poor sleep quality.

This study had several objectives. First, the purpose of the present study was to compare meibomian gland dropout and meibum quality between dry eye patients with and without sleep deprivation. Second, we planned to determine the association between sleep quality and meibum grade scores. Finally, we sought to assess the strength of the association between sleep quality and meibomian gland dropout excluding other chronic conditions known to induce meibomian gland loss. Our findings explored increasing severity of meibomian gland dropout in dry eye patients with the likelihood of having poor sleep quality.

PATIENTS AND METHODS

Patients

This study was approved by the Institutional Review Board of the Affiliated Second Hospital of Zhejiang University. The research followed the tenets of the Declaration of Helsinki. In this cross-sectional study, patients with DED were recruited at the eye clinic of the Affiliated Second Hospital of Zhejiang University (Hangzhou, China) and underwent standardized assessments from June 1, 2020 to May 30, 2021 ($N = 172$). DED was diagnosed in accordance with the following characteristics: 1) dry eye symptoms; 2) positive corneal fluorescein staining; and 3) a Schirmer I test result <5 mm or a tear breakup time (TBUT) <5 s.

Patients were excluded from the study if they presented with conditions or factors that could confound DED and meibomian gland dropout including eyelid or ocular surface disorders, allergic conjunctivitis, glaucoma, macular degeneration, contact lens-wear, any active external ocular processes, eye tattoo history, or a history of ocular surgery. Subjects with systemic conditions knowingly associated with ocular surface disease were also excluded from the study. These included anxiety, depression, diabetes mellitus, autoimmune disease, thyroid disease, vitamin B12 deficiency, oral isotretinoin therapy, patients taking oral hormone level drugs, and patients diagnosed with obstructive sleep apnea.

Tear meniscus height (TMH) and meibography were performed by capturing infrared images with the noncontact meibography system Oculus Keratograph 5 M (Oculus, Wetzlar, Germany). The meibomian gland dropout was defined as the percentage of gland dropout in relation to the total tarsal area of the upper and lower eyelids. The patients were classified into two groups in accordance with the severity of meibomian gland dropout: (1) Non-severe meibomian gland dropout group (NSMD group; where the affected area was $<1/2$ of the total area occupied by meibomian glands); (2) severe meibomian gland dropout group (SMD group; where the affected area was $>2/3$ of the total area occupied by meibomian glands). The demographic characteristics of the patients in each group are shown in **Table 1**. For each individual, demographic information (age, sex, residence, level of education, working status, financial status) were collected.

Evaluation of Dry Eye Symptoms

Before any examination, all patients completed the Ocular Surface Disease Index (OSDI) questionnaire to assess the severity of ocular surface symptoms. The OSDI questionnaire consists of 12 questions regarding the presence and frequency of symptoms related to the ocular surface (13).

The OSDI total score (ranging from 0 to 100) can be calculated with a formula using the sum score of all completed questions. The final scale ranges from 0 to 12 (no disability), 13 to 22 (mild symptoms), 23 to 32 (moderate symptoms), and 33 to 100 (severe symptoms).

TABLE 1 | Demographic characteristics of study subjects: sleep characteristics and dry eye parameters.

Parameters	MG evaluation			Sleep evaluation		
	Group with NSMD	**Group with SMD**	***p*-value**	**Group with good sleep**	**Group with poor sleep**	***p*-value**
Number of subjects	112 (65.1%)	60 (34.9%)	–	101 (58.7%)	71 (41.3%)	–
Age, years	46.3 ± 11.1	51.0 ± 8.8	0.003*	46.2 ± 11.2	50.4 ± 9.1	0.003*
Gender			0.227			0.007*
Male	40 (35.7%)	16 (26.7%)	–	41 (40.6%)	15 (21.1%)	–
Female	72 (64.3%)	44 (73.3%)	–	60 (59.4%)	56 (78.9%)	–
Residence			0.506			0.13
Rural	67 (59.8%)	39 (65%)	–	67 (66.3%)	39 (54.9%)	–
Urban	45 (40.2%)	21 (35%)	–	34 (33.7%)	32 (45.1%)	–
Level of education			0.681			0.562
Illiteracy	9 (8.0%)	4 (6.7%)	–	8 (7.9%)	5 (7.1%)	–
Primary school	13 (11.6%)	11 (18.3%)	–	13 (12.8%)	11 (15.5%)	–
Middle school	38 (33.9%)	19 (31.7%)	–	30 (29.7%)	27 (38%)	–
College or more	52 (46.5%)	26 (43.3%)	–	50 (49.6%)	28 (39.4%)	–
Working status			0.961			0.233
Employed	78 (69.6%)	42 (70%)	–	74 (73.3%)	46 (64.8%)	–
Unemployed	34 (30.4%)	18 (30%)	–	27 (26.7%)	25 (35.2%)	–
Financial status			0.733			0.701
Low	21 (18.7%)	11 (18.3%)	–	17 (16.8%)	13 (18.3%)	–
Medium	63 (56.2%)	37 (61.7%)	–	57 (56.4%)	43 (60.6%)	–
High	28 (25.1%)	12 (20%)	–	27 (26.8%)	15 (21.1%)	–
OSDI	39.9 ± 22.3	53.2 ± 17.9	<0.001*	39.6 ± 21.4	51.7 ± 20.4	<0.001*
TBUT, s	5.2 ± 2.3	3.6 ± 1.8	<0.001*	5.1 ± 2.3	3.9 ± 2.1	<0.001*
Corneal staining	0.2 ± 0.5	0.4 ± 0.7	0.012*	0.3 ± 0.6	0.3 ± 0.7	0.738
TMH	0.17 ± 0.05	0.16 ± 0.05	0.343	0.17 ± 0.05	0.17 ± 0.07	0.351
MG quality	1.5 ± 0.9	2.2 ± 0.9	<0.001*	1.6 ± 0.9	1.9 ± 0.9	0.031*
MG expressibility	2.0 ± 0.8	2.9 ± 0.9	<0.001*	2.1 ± 0.9	2.6 ± 0.9	0.001*
MG dropout score	1.7 ± 1.8	9.9 ± 1.7	<0.001*	3.0 ± 3.6	6.9 ± 4.3	<0.001*
Sleep AIS score	3.5 ± 3.7	8.8 ± 4.9	<0.001*	2.0 ± 1.7	10.3 ± 3.6	<0.001*
Sleep PSQI score	3.7 ± 4.3	11.4 ± 6.9	<0.001*	2.0 ± 2.3	12.7 ± 5.3	<0.001*

**p-values < 0.05 were considered significant.*
NSMD, Non-severe meibomian gland dropout; SMD, severe meibomian gland dropout; MG, meibomian gland; TBUT, tear film break-up time; OSDI, ocular surface disease index; TMH, tear meniscus height.

Sleep Quality Assessment

The validated Athens Insomnia Scale (AIS) and Pittsburgh Sleep Quality Index (PSQI) were used to assess sleep quality. AIS is an eight-item self-assessment psychometric instrument designed for quantifying sleep difficulty. For each item, four answers are provided representing increasing difficulty with sleep. Among these options are no problem, minor problem, considerable problem, and serious problem or did not sleep at all. Answers are scored 0, 1, 2, and 3, respectively. The total score ranges from 0 to 24, with greater scores depicting poorer sleep quality. A total score of 6 or higher identifies 90% of the subjects suffering from nonorganic insomnia (14).

The PSQI is the most frequently used validated questionnaire for assessing sleep quality (15). This self-reported questionnaire of Chinese version assesses the average sleep quality over the patient's last month of sleep. It consists of 19 questions in seven domains: subjective sleep quality, sleep latency, sleep duration, habitual sleep efficiency, sleep disturbances, use of sleep medication, and daytime dysfunction. The scores in each of these seven domains, each on a 0–3 scale, are summed to generate a global score with a possible range of 0–21. A global score of >5 was used as the cut-off to distinguish good sleepers (≤5) from poor sleepers (>5) (15).

Evaluation of Dry Eye Signs

Dry eye tests were performed in both eyes in the following order: TBUT, corneal fluorescein staining, and MGD evaluation. As previously reported, corneal fluorescein staining was measured using commercially available sterile fluorescein paper strips (Jinming New Technological Development Co. Ltd., Tianjin, China) (16). The strip was moistened with 20 μL 0.9% sterile saline and gently pressed along the lower tarsal conjunctiva. The TBUT was then measured by counting the seconds after a blink before the tear film was broken. A median of three measurements per eye was taken. The TBUT ranged from 0 to 10. Corneal fluorescein staining score was assessed by grading

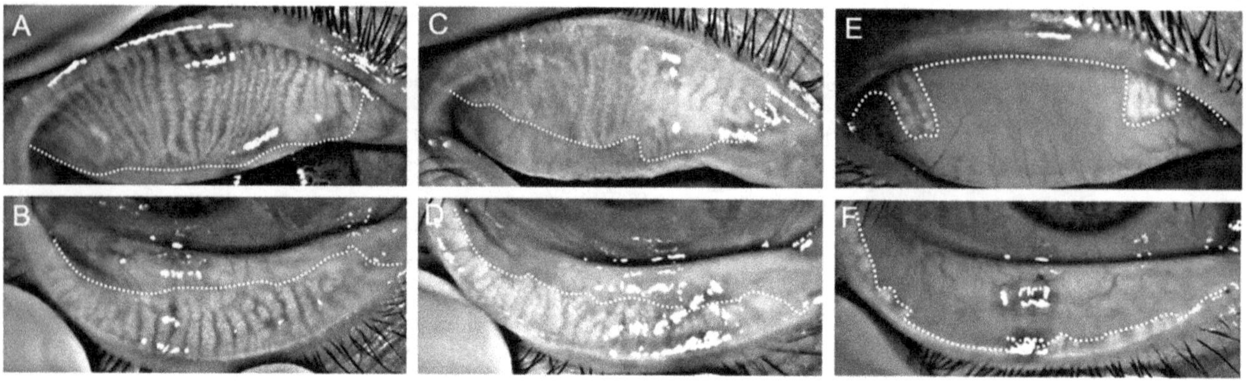

FIGURE 1 | Representative infrared meibography images from the superior **(A,C,E)** and inferior **(B,D,F)** eyelids of a control **(A–D)** and poor sleep **(E,F)** participant. Overall, the poor sleep quality participant demonstrates more extensive MG dropout than the control participant.

the upper, middle, and lower parts of the cornea on a nine-point scale: no staining = 0; <5 stained punctate dots = 1; 5 to 9 stained punctate dots = 2; and ≥ 10 stained punctate dots or filamentous staining = 3. Afterwards, the total score for corneal fluorescein staining was calculated as the summed score for all three parts of the cornea and ranged from 0 to 9 (17). Meibomian gland function was evaluated in accordance with the recommendations of the International Workshop on Meibomian Gland Dysfunction (18, 19). MGD was assessed by averaging the quality score (clear = 1; cloudy = 2; granular = 3; toothpaste = 4) and expressibility score of the meibum (minimal pressure = 0; light pressure = 1; moderate pressure = 2; heavy pressure = 3).

Evaluation of Meibomian Gland Morphology

As shown in **Figure 1**, partial or complete dropout of meibomian glands was scored using the following meiboscore grades: 0 = no loss; 1 = loss of an area of <1/3 of the total area; 2 = loss of an area between one-third and two-thirds of the total area; 3 = loss of an area of more than two-thirds of the total area. The meiboscores for the upper and lower eyelids were summed for each eye (20), and were evaluated by one examiner. Images were digitally analyzed using ImageJ software (National Institutes of Health). Photographs were analyzed in a random order by two double-blinded investigators to minimize observer bias.

Statistical Analysis

Data analysis was performed using SPSS statistical software (SPSS Inc., Chicago, IL, USA). Continuous variables were expressed as mean ± SD and categorical variables were expressed as absolute and relative (%) frequencies. The data of only the right eye from all subjects were used for analysis. The Mann-Whitney *U* test was used to compare the ocular surface changes. Categorical variables were compared with the χ^2 test. Correlations (Pearson and Spearman) were used to evaluate the strength of association between sleep and severity of meibomian gland dropout signs and symptoms. Logistic regression models were used to assess the relationship between poor sleep quality (PSQI score > 5 as the dependent variable) and meibomian gland dropout (meibomian gland dropout ≥2 as the independent variables). To investigate which components of sleep quality were most affected, we performed the same analysis for the seven components of the PSQI separately. The analysis was stratified by age in decades and sex. Multivariate logistic regression analysis was used to investigate the effects of various parameters on meibomian dropout. ORs and 95% CIs were presented. A *p*-value of <0.05 was considered statistically significant.

RESULTS

During the study period between June 1, 2020 and May 30, 2021, an initial dataset was collected on a total of 286 patients with dry eye that had an ocular surface evaluation and sleep quality assessment. After the filtering process, 172 patients were included.

Out of the 172 dry eye participants, 60 (34.9%) subjects had severe meibomian gland dropout and 71 (41.3%) subjects had poor sleep quality. The subjects in NSMD and SMD groups did not differ significantly in terms of gender ($p = 0.227$), residence ($p = 0.506$), level of education ($p = 0.681$), working status ($p = 0.961$), and gross income ($p = 0.733$). The mean age of SMD participants was 51.0 ± 8.8 years (range: 26–75) and 44 were women (73.3%). Patients with SMD were older ($p = 0.003$), experienced more dry eye symptoms ($p < 0.001$), had worse meibomian gland function ($p < 0.001$), and had poorer sleep quality ($p < 0.001$) as compared to patients without SMD (**Table 1**). Patients with poor sleep were generally older ($p = 0.003$), were more frequently women ($p = 0.007$), experienced more dry eye symptoms ($p < 0.001$), and had greater meibomian gland dropout ($p < 0.001$) as compared to patients without poor sleep (**Table 1**).

The mean sleep AIS score was significantly higher in subjects with SMD than in subjects with NSMD (8.8 ± 4.9 vs. 3.5 ± 3.7, $p < 0.001$). Similarly, patients with poor sleep quality had greater Meibomian gland dropout than patients without poor sleep (6.9 ± 4.3 vs. 3.0 ± 3.6, $p < 0.001$) and the sleep AIS score and PSQI score were significantly correlated to Meibomian gland dropout ($r = 0.495$, $p < 0.001$; $r = 0.24$, $p = 0.002$; respectively; **Table 2**).

TABLE 2 | Correlation between sleep quality and dry eye parameters.

Variables	OSDI	TBUT	Corneal staining	MG quality	MG expressibility	MG dropout
TBUT, s	$r = -0.284$					
	$p < 0.001^*$					
Corneal staining	$r = 0.245$	$r = -0.627$				
	$p = 0.001^*$	$p < 0.001^*$				
MG quality	$r = 0.062$	$r = -0.359$	$r = 0.246$			
	$p = 0.418$	$p < 0.001^*$	$p = 0.001^*$			
MG expressibility	$r = 0.254$	$r = -0.454$	$r = 0.343$	$r = 0.551$		
	$p = 0.001^*$	$p < 0.001^*$	$p < 0.001^*$	$p < 0.001^*$		
MG dropout	$r = 0.34$	$r = -0.691$	$r = 0.751$	$r = 0.303$	$r = 0.478$	
	$p < 0.001^*$	$p < 0.001^*$	$p < 0.001^*$	$p < 0.001^*$	$p < 0.001^*$	
Sleep AIS score	$r = 0.248$	$r = -0.434$	$r = 0.318$	$r = 0.2$	$r = 0.238$	$r = 0.495$
	$p = 0.001^*$	$p < 0.001^*$	$p < 0.001^*$	$p = 0.008^*$	$p = 0.002^*$	$p < 0.001^*$
Sleep PSQI score	$r = 0.292$	$r = -0.189$	$r = 0.079$	$r = 0.084$	$r = 0.17$	$r = 0.24$
	$p < 0.001^*$	$p = 0.013^*$	$p = 0.3$	$p = 0.271$	$p = 0.026^*$	$p = 0.002^*$

**p-values < 0.05 were considered significant.*
OSDI, ocular surface disease index; MG, meibomian gland; TBUT, tear film break-up time; PSQI, pittsburgh sleep quality index.

TABLE 3 | Association between sleep quality (all components of the PSQI) and MG dropout.

PSQI component	Without SMD	With SMD	*p* value	Corrected for age and sex only		Corrected for age, sex, education, residence, income, working status	
				OR (95% CI)	*p*-value	OR (95% CI)	*p*-value
Global score: Overall poor quality of sleep (PSQI > 5)	3.7 ± 4.3	11.4 ± 6.9	<0.001*	1.226 (1.145–1.312)	<0.001*	1.248 (1.158–1.346)	<0.001*
1. Subjective sleep quality (bad vs. good)	1.2 ± 1.1	2.3 ± 0.8	<0.001*	2.428 (1.696–3.476)	<0.001*	2.614 (1.773–3.853)	<0.001*
2. Suboptimal sleep latency (>2 vs. ≤2)	0.5 ± 0.8	1.4 ± 1.2	<0.001*	2.023 (1.439–2.843)	<0.001*	2.182 (1.521–3.132)	<0.001*
3. Suboptimal sleep duration (>6 h vs. ≤6 h)	0.6 ± 0.8	1.7 ± 1.2	<0.001*	2.902 (1.991–4.231)	<0.001*	3.205 (2.118–4.849)	<0.001*
4. Poor habitual sleep efficiency (<75% vs. ≥75%)	0.4 ± 0.6	1.6 ± 1.2	<0.001*	3.798 (2.464–5.857)	<0.001*	4.226 (2.631–6.787)	<0.001*
5. Sleep disturbance (>9 vs. ≤9)	0.5 ± 0.8	1.9 ± 1.1	<0.001*	3.439 (2.338–5.057)	<0.001*	4.495 (2.766–7.305)	<0.001*
6. Use of sleep medication (yes vs. no)	0.2 ± 0.4	1.1 ± 1.1	<0.001*	4.37 (2.532–7.541)	<0.001*	4.554 (2.581–8.037)	<0.001*
7. Daytime dysfunction (>2 vs. ≤2)	0.4 ± 0.7	1.4 ± 1.1	<0.001*	2.846 (1.911–4.24)	<0.001*	3.415 (2.152–5.421)	<0.001*

**p-values < 0.05 were considered significant.*
PSQI, pittsburgh sleep quality index; MG, meibomian gland; SMD, severe meibomian gland dropout; CI, confidence interval; OR, odds ratio.

Comparably, Meibomian gland dropout score was significantly associated with Meibomian gland quality ($r = 0.303$; $p < 0.001$), Meibomian gland expressibility ($r = 0.478$; $p < 0.001$), dry eye symptoms ($r = 0.34$; $p < 0.001$), TBUT ($r = -0.691$; $p < 0.001^*$), and corneal staining ($r = 0.751$; $p < 0.001$). Nevertheless, the sleep PSQI score was not significantly associated with corneal staining ($r = 0.079$; $p = 0.3$) or Meibomian gland quality ($r = 0.084$; $p = 0.271$).

Table 3 presents the relationship between sleep quality and Meibomian gland dropout. In SMD patients, poor sleep quality was much more prevalent than in NSMD groups (3.7 ± 4.3 vs. 11.4 ± 6.9; p <0.001; OR 1.21 [95% CI 1.13–1.29], corrected for age and sex only, $p < 0.001$; OR 1.21 [95% CI 1.13–1.30], corrected for age, sex, education, residence, income and working status, $p < 0.001$). **Table 3** further demonstrates the association between Meibomian gland dropout and different components of sleep quality. It reveals that SMD patients have worse scores than NSMD patients on all components of the PSQI (all $p <$ 0.001, corrected for age and sex). Use of sleep medication, poor habitual sleep efficiency, and sleep disturbance were particularly

TABLE 4 | Multivariate logistic regression analysis between sleep quality (PSQI score), demographics and dry eye parameters.

Parameters	OR	*p* value	95% CI	
			Lower	Upper
Age	0.001	$p = 0.991$	−0.118	0.119
Female gender	0.129	$p = 0.042^*$	0.068	3.519
Rural residence	0.044	$p = 0.496$	−1.118	2.296
Level of education	0.007	$p = 0.935$	−1.136	1.233
Gross income	0.032	$p = 0.684$	−1.256	1.909
Working status	0.122	$p = 0.154$	−0.658	4.120
OSDI	0.195	$p = 0.004^*$	0.018	0.098
TBUT, s	−0.145	$p = 0.036^*$	−0.790	−0.028
Corneal staining	−0.046	$p = 0.476$	−1.770	0.829
TMH	−0.037	$p = 0.572$	−18.437	10.213
MG quality	−0.014	$p = 0.857$	−1.140	0.950
MG expressibility	−0.047	$p = 0.580$	−1.424	0.800
MG dropout score	0.467	$p < 0.001^*$	0.481	0.928

**p-values < 0.05 were considered significant.*
PSQI, pittsburgh sleep quality index; MG, meibomian gland; TBUT, tear film break-up time; OSDI, ocular surface disease index; TMH, tear meniscus height; CI, confidence interval; OR, odds ratio.

prevalent in SMD patients as compared to NSMD patients. After correcting for age, sex, education, residence, income, and working status, SMD was still associated with lower sleep quality on all seven components. The multivariate logistic regression analysis included presence or absence of poor sleep as dependent parameters, with demographics and dry eye variables as independent parameters by dropping those parameters with a p value > 0.05. Sleep quality was eventually associated with female gender ($p = 0.042$) and poorer scoring on OSDI ($p = 0.004$), TBUT ($p = 0.036$), and Meibomian gland dropout scores ($p < 0.001$) (**Table 4**).

DISCUSSION

Although previous studies have conducted meibomian gland evaluation and quantification in individuals with poor sleep, during this study we undertook a novel and comprehensive approach in characterizing anterior ocular health and dry eye disease in people with and without poor sleep (11). In doing so, the major finding of this cross-sectional study revealed the presence of more extensive meibomian gland dropout in poor sleep quality individuals relative to that of the control participants.

It was determined that poor sleepers with worse outcomes in all components of the PSQI were more likely to have severe meibomian gland dropout. Moreover, patients with dry eye with poor sleep had shorter TBUT and higher meibum grade scores that were in accordance with previous studies that showed a positive association between dry eye and sleep quality (11). The result of severe meibomian gland dropout in participants with reduced quality of sleep may emphasize the clinical value of this association and help increase awareness of sleep disease as a serious disorder affecting multiple aspects of ocular surface health.

Meibomian glands provide key components to the tear film that help maintain a healthy ocular surface. When these glands are reduced, absent, or dysfunctional, the impact on the ocular surface can be immense (21). Clinical studies have reported that patients with obstructive MGD (defined as meibomian gland dropout, poor meibum expression, and lack of signs of inflammation) had increased tear evaporation rates compared with controls (22). If alterations in meibum lipid composition occur in MGD pathogenesis, meibum cannot function normally and can increase tear film evaporation, which results in evaporative dry eyes and corneal staining (23). Our study supports this understanding of pathogenesis based on the correlations between expressed meibum grade, TBUT, and corneal staining.

Meibomian gland dropout is typically caused by atrophic degeneration secondary to increased pressure within the gland because of orifice obstruction and meibomian gland duct obliteration in the late phase of the disease (8, 24). In a cross-sectional study, Bao et al., reported the possible mechanism of an immune-driven process underlying meibomian gland dropout in early HIV (25). Another prospective cross-sectional study found that meibomian gland dropout is related to indoor microbial concentration (26). As found in other studies, aging is also a known risk factor for MGD (27). With age, meibomian glands exhibit decreased meibocyte differentiation, decreased meibomian gland size, increased meibomian gland dropout, and increased inflammatory cell infiltration (28). Additionally, age is a significant factor when evaluating the clinical signs of dry eye and sleep quality (29, 30). Consistent with previous studies, we found that most older individuals showed more glandular loss and had poorer sleep. Therefore, we analyzed the relationship between meibomian gland dropout score and sleep quality after correcting for age.

Past studies investigating the association between poor sleep quality and dry eye have shown that the relationship is likely to be complex. Several studies have gone so far as to correlate DED not only with sleep quality, but sleep position (31, 32). Mengliang et al. reported that sleep quality plays an important role in the development of DED in influencing tear secretion and tear film stability by indirectly aggravating anxiety and depression, ultimately leading to higher self-reported symptom scores (11). Similarly, a large population-based study found that dry eye is associated with worse outcomes in all quantitative and qualitative aspects of sleep, and this relationship is present in all ages and sexes (33). An randomized control trial showed that the repeated use of warming eye masks had a positive effect on both tear function and mental health including depression and anxiety (34). An recent study suggested that the inability to close the eyelids during sleep was associated with worsened DED symptoms and poor sleep quality (35). The results might provide additional evidence for a clinical association between DED and sleep. This relationship between sleep quality and dry eye is partly explained by coexisting comorbidities such as autoimmune diseases, psychiatric disorders, endocrine disorders, and chronic pain syndromes. Therefore, patients were excluded from the study if they presented with conditions or factors that could confound DED and meibomian gland dropout. Within this current study, results showed noticeable changes in tear film break-up time and meibomian gland function in sleep deprivation subjects. In previous studies, sleep deprivation induced dry eye through the defective changes of superficial corneal epithelial cells in a mouse model (12). This study also revealed that meibomian gland morphology after sleep deprivation for 5–10 days was the same as that of normal mice. One possibility for explanation is that short-term sleep deprivation could not cause meibomian gland morphology change. Considering all of this, it is clear that all the mechanisms underlying the association between sleep quality and meibomian gland function are still not fully understood. Further studies in understanding the underlying biological mechanisms linked to sleep deprivation disorder are warranted.

In the present study it was demonstrated that SMD is clearly associated with various sleep parameters, particularly use of sleep medication, poor habitual sleep efficiency, and sleep disturbance. This highlights the impact of sleep quality on a patient's life, but also the need for holistic thinking when treating a patient with DED. It is important to address comorbid conditions such as systemic conditions, poor sleep, depression, and anxiety. As these conditions are thought to exacerbate one another and contribute to the overall burden of disease, treatment options should be considered.

Our study has several limitations. First, as this was a cross-sectional study, we were unable to infer causality on any of the reported associations. Longitudinal studies with a larger sample size are required to further clarify these relationships. Second, since some study participants could not answer the sleep quality questionnaire alone, these questions were asked by trained technicians for all subjects. Other limitations of this study also subject to recall bias of self-reported sleep parameters. Nevertheless, self-reported assessments of sleep have been shown to be valid measures compared with quantitative sleep assessments with actigraphy (36). Moreover, the effects of risk factors, such as menopause, body mass index, social status, and other possible confounding factors, should be considered to ensure a detailed understanding of the relationships among sleep status and SMD. In addition, we excluded individuals with a known diagnosis of autoimmune diseases, psychiatric disorders, endocrine disorders, and chronic pain syndromes, but did not conduct laboratory screening for this potential confounder in the present study.

In conclusion, poor sleep quality is significantly associated with severe meibomian gland dropout. These findings suggest that clinicians should be aware of this relationship and ask about dry eye symptoms and sleep quality, especially in highly symptomatic patients. Further prospective studies are needed to determine the directionality of this association and establish appropriate treatment strategies for patients with poor sleep quality and severe meibomian gland dropout.

ETHICS STATEMENT

The studies involving human participants were reviewed and approved by Institutional Review Board of the Affiliated Second Hospital of Zhejiang University. The patients/participants provided their written informed consent to participate in this study.

AUTHOR CONTRIBUTIONS

All authors listed have made a substantial, direct, and intellectual contribution to the work and approved it for publication.

ACKNOWLEDGMENTS

The authors acknowledge the financial support of the National Natural Science Foundation of China (Project numbers: 81870624 and 81700802), Key Research and Development Project of Zhejiang (Province Project number: 2020C03035), and Natural Science Foundation of Zhejiang Province (Q20H120063).

REFERENCES

1. Leger D, Poursain B. An international survey of insomnia: under-recognition and under-treatment of a polysymptomatic condition. *Curr Med Res Opin.* (2005) 21:1785–92. doi: 10.1185/030079905X65637
2. Foley D, Ancoli-Israel S, Britz P, Walsh J. Sleep disturbances and chronic disease in older adults: results of the 2003 National Sleep Foundation Sleep in America Survey. *J Psychosom Res.* (2004) 56:497–502. doi: 10.1016/j.jpsychores.2004.02.010
3. The definition and classification of dry eye disease: report of the Definition and Classification Subcommittee of the International Dry Eye WorkShop (2007). *Ocul Surf.* (2007) 5:75–92. doi: 10.1016/S1542-0124(12)70081-2
4. Li M, Gong L, Chapin WJ, Zhu M. Assessment of vision-related quality of life in dry eye patients. *Invest Ophthalmol Vis Sci.* (2012) 53:5722–7. doi: 10.1167/iovs.11-9094
5. Miljanovic B, Dana R, Sullivan DA, Schaumberg DA. Impact of dry eye syndrome on vision-related quality of life. *Am J Ophthalmol.* (2007) 143:409–15. doi: 10.1016/j.ajo.2006.11.060
6. Mertzanis P, Abetz L, Rajagopalan K, Espindle D, Chalmers R, Snyder C, et al. The relative burden of dry eye in patients' lives: comparisons to a U.S. normative sample. *Invest Ophthalmol Vis Sci.* (2005) 46:46–50. doi: 10.1167/iovs.03-0915
7. Gutgesell VJ, Stern GA, Hood CI. Histopathology of meibomian gland dysfunction. *Am J Ophthalmol.* (1982) 94:383–7. doi: 10.1016/0002-9394(82)90365-8
8. Nelson JD, Shimazaki J, Benitez-del-Castillo JM, Craig JP, McCulley JP, Den S, et al. The international workshop on meibomian gland dysfunction: report of the definition and classification subcommittee. *Invest Ophthalmol Vis Sci.* (2011) 52:1930–7. doi: 10.1167/iovs.10-6997b
9. Wu H, Wang Y, Dong N, Yang F, Lin Z, Shang X, et al. Meibomian gland dysfunction determines the severity of the dry eye conditions in visual display terminal workers. *PLoS One.* (2014) 9:e105575. doi: 10.1371/journal.pone.0105575
10. Yu X, Guo H, Liu X, Wang G, Min Y, Chen SS, et al. Dry eye and sleep quality: a large community-based study in Hangzhou. *Sleep.* (2019) 42:zsz160. doi: 10.1093/sleep/zsz160

11. Wu M, Liu X, Han J, Shao T, Wang Y. Association between sleep quality, mood status, and ocular surface characteristics in patients with dry eye disease. *Cornea.* (2019) 38:311–7. doi: 10.1097/ICO.0000000000001854
12. Tang L, Wang X, Wu J, Li SM, Zhang Z, Wu S, et al. Sleep deprivation induces dry eye through inhibition of PPARalpha expression in corneal epithelium. *Invest Ophthalmol Vis Sci.* (2018) 59:5494–508. doi: 10.1167/iovs.18-24504
13. Schiffman RM, Christianson MD, Jacobsen G, Hirsch JD, Reis BL. Reliability and validity of the ocular surface disease index. *Arch Ophthalmol.* (2000) 118:615–21. doi: 10.1001/archopht.118.5.615
14. Soldatos CR, Dikeos DG, Paparrigopoulos TJ. The diagnostic validity of the Athens insomnia scale. *J Psychosom Res.* (2003) 55:263–7. doi: 10.1016/S0022-3999(02)00604-9
15. Buysse DJ, Reynolds CF 3rd, Monk TH, Berman SR, Kupfer DJ. The Pittsburgh sleep quality index: a new instrument for psychiatric practice and research. *Psychiatry Res.* (1989) 28:193–213. doi: 10.1016/0165-1781(89)90047-4
16. Methodologies to diagnose and monitor dry eye disease: report of the Diagnostic Methodology Subcommittee of the International Dry Eye WorkShop. *Ocul Surf.* (2007) 5:108–52. doi: 10.1016/S1542-0124(12)70083-6
17. Toda I, Tsubota K. Practical double vital staining for ocular surface evaluation. *Cornea.* (1993) 12:366–7. doi: 10.1097/00003226-199307000-00015
18. Tomlinson A, Bron AJ, Korb DR, Amano S, Paugh JR, Pearce EI, et al. The international workshop on meibomian gland dysfunction: report of the diagnosis subcommittee. *Invest Ophthalmol Vis Sci.* (2011) 52:2006–49. doi: 10.1167/iovs.10-6997f
19. Geerling G, Tauber J, Baudouin C, Goto E, Matsumoto Y, O'Brien T, et al. The international workshop on meibomian gland dysfunction: report of the subcommittee on management and treatment of meibomian gland dysfunction. *Invest Ophthalmol Vis Sci.* (2011) 52:2050–64. doi: 10.1167/iovs.10-6997g
20. Arita R, Itoh K, Inoue K, Amano S. Noncontact infrared meibography to document age-related changes of the meibomian glands in a normal population. *Ophthalmology.* (2008) 115:911–5. doi: 10.1016/j.ophtha.2007.06.031
21. Ekin MA, Ugurlu SK, Imre SS, Kahraman HG. The role of meibomian gland dysfunction on the development of dry eye disease in patients with facial nerve palsy. *Arq Bras Oftalmol.* (2021). doi: 10.5935/0004-2749.20220021 [Epub ahead of print].
22. Goto E, Endo K, Suzuki A, Fujikura Y, Matsumoto Y, Tsubota K. Tear evaporation dynamics in normal subjects and subjects with obstructive meibomian gland dysfunction. *Invest Ophthalmol Vis Sci.* (2003) 44:533–9. doi: 10.1167/iovs.02-0170
23. Arciniega JC, Wojtowicz JC, Mohamed EM, McCulley JP. Changes in the evaporation rate of tear film after digital expression of meibomian glands in patients with and without dry eye. *Cornea.* (2011) 30:843–7. doi: 10.1097/ICO.0b013e31820cd291
24. Bron AJ, Tiffany JM. The contribution of meibomian disease to dry eye. *Ocul Surf.* (2004) 2:149–65. doi: 10.1016/S1542-0124(12)70150-7
25. Nguyen BN, Chung AW, Lopez E, Silvers J, Kent HE, Kent SJ, et al. Meibomian gland dropout is associated with immunodeficiency at HIV diagnosis: Implications for dry eye disease. *Ocul Surf.* (2020) 18:206–13. doi: 10.1016/j.jtos.2020.02.003
26. Rock S, Galor A, Kumar N. Indoor airborne microbial concentration and dry eye. *Am J Ophthalmol.* (2021) 223:193–204. doi: 10.1016/j.ajo.2020.10.003
27. Schaumberg DA, Nichols JJ, Papas EB, Tong L, Uchino M, Nichols KK. The international workshop on meibomian gland dysfunction: report of the subcommittee on the epidemiology of, and associated risk factors for, MGD. *Invest Ophthalmol Vis Sci.* (2011) 52:1994–2005. doi: 10.1167/iovs.10-6997e
28. Chhadva P, Goldhardt R, Galor A. Meibomian gland disease: the role of gland dysfunction in dry eye disease. *Ophthalmology.* (2017) 124:S20–6. doi: 10.1016/j.ophtha.2017.05.031
29. Stapleton F, Alves M, Bunya VY, Jalbert I, Lekhanont K, Malet F, et al. TFOS DEWS II epidemiology report. *Ocul Surf.* (2017) 15:334–65. doi: 10.1016/j.jtos.2017.05.003
30. Ohayon MM, Carskadon MA, Guilleminault C, Vitiello MV. Meta-analysis of quantitative sleep parameters from childhood to old age in healthy individuals: developing normative sleep values across the human lifespan. *Sleep.* (2004) 27:1255–73. doi: 10.1093/sleep/27.7.1255
31. Ayaki M, Kawashima M, Negishi K, Tsubota K. High prevalence of sleep and mood disorders in dry eye patients: survey of 1,000 eye clinic visitors. *Neuropsychiatr Dis Treat.* (2015) 11:889–94. doi: 10.2147/NDT.S81515
32. Alevi D, Perry HD, Wedel A, Rosenberg E, Alevi L, Donnenfeld ED. Effect of sleep position on the ocular surface. *Cornea.* (2017) 36:567–71. doi: 10.1097/ICO.0000000000001167
33. Magno MS, Utheim TP, Snieder H, Hammond CJ, Vehof J. The relationship between dry eye and sleep quality. *Ocul Surf.* (2021) 20:13–9. doi: 10.1016/j.jtos.2020.12.009
34. Uchino M, Kawashima M, Yamanishi R, Inoue S, Kawashima S, Tagami K, et al. The effects of a steam warming eye mask on the ocular surface and mental health. *Ocul Surf.* (2021) 21:129–33. doi: 10.1016/j.jtos.2021.05.007
35. Takahashi A, Negishi K, Ayaki M, Uchino M, Tsubota K. Nocturnal lagophthalmos and sleep quality in patients with dry eye disease. *Life.* (2020) 10:105. doi: 10.3390/life10070105
36. Lockley SW, Skene DJ, Arendt J. Comparison between subjective and actigraphic measurement of sleep and sleep rhythms. *J Sleep Res.* (1999) 8:175–83. doi: 10.1046/j.1365-2869.1999.00155.x

13

Long Non-coding RNAs Gabarapl2 and Chrnb2 Positively Regulate Inflammatory Signaling in a Mouse Model of Dry Eye

Yuhan Yang[1,2†], *Minjie Chen*[1†], *Zimeng Zhai*[1], *Yiqin Dai*[1], *Hao Gu*[2], *Xujiao Zhou*[1*] and *Jiaxu Hong*[1,2*]

[1] *Department of Ophthalmology, Eye and ENT Hospital, Fudan University, Shanghai, China,* [2] *Department of Ophthalmology, The Affiliated Hospital of Guizhou Medical University, Guiyang, China*

Correspondence:
Xujiao Zhou
xujiaozhou@126.com
Jiaxu Hong
Jiaxu.hong@fdeent.org

† *These authors have contributed equally to this work*

Purpose: To elucidate the expression profile and the potential role of long non-coding ribonucleic acids (RNAs) (lncRNAs) in a dry eye disease (DED) model.

Methods: A DED model was established in C57BL/6J mice with 0.2% benzalkonium chloride (BAC) twice a day for 14 days. The differentially expressed lncRNAs were detected by RNA-seq technology (Gene Expression Omnibus, GEO GSE186450) and the aberrantly expressed lncRNAs were further verified by RT-qPCR. Gene Ontology (GO) and Kyoto Encyclopedia of Genes and Genomes (KEGG) enrichment analyses were conducted to predicate the related candidate genes and potential pathological pathways. Cells from a human corneal epithelial cell line (HCECs) were cultured under hyperosmolarity. The regulation of inflammatory factors by silencing potential targeted lncRNAs was verified *in vitro* in HCECs.

Results: In our study, a significant increase in corneal fluorescence staining and a reduction in tear production were observed in DED mice at all follow-ups compared with the controls, and the differences were increasing over time. In total, 2,649 upregulated and 704 downregulated lncRNAs were identified in DED mice. We selected six aberrantly expressed and most abundant lncRNAs and performed RT-qPCR using the samples for RNA-seq. Chrnb2, Gabarapl2, and Usp31 were thereby confirmed as the most significantly altered lncRNAs. Pathway analysis revealed that the neuroactive ligand–receptor interaction signaling pathway was the most enriched, followed by the calcium signaling pathway and cytokine–cytokine receptor interaction. Following treatment of Gabarapl2 siRNA and Chrnb2 siRNA, tumor necrosis factor-α (TNF-α), interleukin (IL)-1β, and IL-6 were significantly downregulated in the HCECs.

Conclusion: Our study suggests that Chrnb2 and Gabarapl2 may be involved in the inflammation response by regulating TNF-α, IL-1β, and IL-6 in DED. These candidate lncRNAs may be both potential biomarkers and therapeutic targets for DED.

Keywords: long non-coding RNA (lncRNA), Gabarapl2 and Chrnb2, dry eye disease (DED), neuroactive ligand–receptor interaction signaling, inflammation

INTRODUCTION

Hundreds of millions of people throughout the world are affected by dry eye disease (DED), typically suffering symptoms such as blurred vision, ocular discomfort, and a stinging, burning, scratchy, or gritty sensation while reading, driving, or working with computers (1–5). Unsurprisingly (6), severe symptoms of DED are also associated with decreased work productivity and levels of activity (7). Dry eye is a multifactorial disease of the ocular surface characterized by a loss of homeostasis of the tear film and accompanied by ocular symptoms, in which tear film instability and hyperosmolarity, ocular surface inflammation and damage, and neurosensory abnormalities play etiological roles (5). Numerous cellular and molecular components have been found to contribute to immune-cell activation and associated inflammation in the pathogenesis of dry eye, including inflammatory cytokines, metalloproteinases, and chemokines and their receptors (8–11). Compared to inflammation, neuroinflammation is more persistent in DED environments (12). Nowadays, considerable attention is being paid to the role and mechanisms of ocular-surface nerve inflammation in DED pain sensitivity (13). Neuropathic pain is difficult to cure: all existing therapies, such as serotonin-noradrenaline reuptake inhibitors, anticonvulsants acting at calcium channels, and topical lidocaine and opioids, have only variable success in alleviating pain, while failing to tackle the underlying mechanisms (14, 15).

Long non-coding ribonucleic acids (RNAs) (lncRNAs), which consist of more than 200 nucleotides, are involved in protein translation and messenger RNA (mRNA) decay, which play important roles in regulating inflammatory pathways (16, 17). A growing number of studies has revealed that some lncRNAs participate in the pathogenesis of multiple diseases, including cancer, ocular alkali burns, and Sjögren's syndrome by regulating mRNA directly or indirectly (18–20). Long non-coding ribonucleic acids regulate gene expression through epigenetic regulation, transcriptional regulation, and post-transcriptional regulation, thus participating in various biological processes (BP) such as cell proliferation, differentiation, and apoptosis (21–26). In addition, the interaction of lncRNAs–microRNAs (miRs) participates in the progression of the inflammatory reaction. Myocardial infarction associated transcript 2 (Mirt2) blocks the NF-κB and JAK/STAT signaling pathways by facilitating miR-377 in response to IFN-γ-induced inflammatory insults in Sjögren's syndrome (27). Computational analyses have revealed that differentially expressed lncRNAs are involved in chemokine signaling pathways, the NF-κB signaling pathway, and the tumor necrosis factor (TNF) signaling pathway in labial salivary glands of Sjögren's syndrome patients. However, studies on lncRNAs in the cellular and molecular nerve inflammation pathogenesis of DED are still far from complete.

In the current study, we analyzed the expression profile of lncRNAs in a mouse model of DED using the whole-transcriptome sequencing technology. In our findings, Chrnb2 and Gabarapl2 were confirmed as the most significantly altered lncRNAs. Systemic bioinformatic analyses revealed that the neuroactive ligand–receptor interaction signaling pathway was the most enriched, followed by the calcium signaling pathway and cytokine–cytokine receptor interaction. *In vitro* human corneal epithelial cell line (HCEC) studies revealed that Gabarapl2 siRNA and Chrnb2 siRNA treatment could affect inflammatory factors. Chrnb2 and Gabarapl2 are the potential elements of lncRNAs involved in the pathogenesis of DED, implying a novel target for early therapy.

MATERIALS AND METHODS

DED Mouse Model

Sixty specific-pathogen-free (SPF) C57BL/6J mice (120 eyes), 6–8 weeks old, were randomized into two groups (control group $n = 25$, DED group $n = 35$). The mice were housed in an environmentally controlled room (25°C, with 60% humidity and 12 h/12 h light–dark cycle), with adequate rodent chow and water available. All experimental protocols conformed to the Association for Research in Vision and Ophthalmology statement on the use of animals. We performed surgery on the animals according to the guidelines of the Fudan University Ethics Committee (Ethical code: EENTIRB-2018-03-01). Both eyes in the DED group were administered with 5 μl of 0.2% benzalkonium chloride (BAC) twice a day for 14 days, while phosphate-buffered saline (PBS) was administered to the control group. Schirmer's I-test and the corneal fluorescein sodium staining score were recorded before and at days 7, 14, and 21 after treatment.

Detection of Basal Tear Secretion (Schirmer's I-Test)

Schirmer's I-test was performed with Zone-Quick Phenol-Red cotton thread. After general anesthesia with 1.25% avertin (0.2 ml/10 g) given intraperitoneally, 1 mm of the folded end of the phenol red cotton line was inserted into the lower lateral conjunctival fornix for 20 s. The color of phenol cotton changes from yellow to red with the secretion of tears. The wetted length (mm) of the strip indicated by red dye was read and recorded. The eyelids were closed after examination.

Corneal Fluorescein Sodium Staining Score

An experienced oculist took the measurement by a slit lamp with a cobalt blue light. After 90 s of staining with fluorescein sodium, the corneal epithelium was evaluated. We divided the cornea into four quadrants. Each quadrant was checked and the reading recorded. The sum of all quadrants is regarded as the final score. The scoring criteria were: 0 points for no staining; 1 point for fewer than 30 stained dots; 2 points for more than 30 non-diffuse stained dots; 3 points for severe diffuse staining but no plaque staining; and 4 points for a patchy stain.

RNA-Seq Database Construction Sequencing and Bioinformatics Analysis

Ribonucleic acid was extracted from the corneal tissue of DED mice, and the quality of RNA samples was strictly controlled. Agarose gel electrophoresis was used to analyze the RNA integrity and DNA contamination of the samples. Nanodrop was used to detect RNA concentration and purity. Agilent 2100 BioAnalyzer accurately detects RNA integrity. Ribosomal RNA was removed from total RNA, and then the RNA was broken into short fragments of 250–300 bp. The first complementary DNA (cDNA) strand was synthesized using the fragment RNA as the template and random oligonucleotide as the primer. The RNA strand was degraded by Rnase H. The second strand of cDNA was synthesized from deoxyribonucleotide triphosphates (dNTPs; dUTP, dATP, dGTP, and dCTP) under the DNA polymerase I system. The purified double-stranded cDNA was repaired at the end and "A" tail was added, before sequencing. AMPure XP Beads were used to screen 350–400 bp of cDNA. The second strand of cDNA containing U was degraded by USER enzyme, and PCR amplification was performed to obtain the library. The library was diluted to 1 ng/μl by Qubit. Then Agilent 2100 BioAnalyzer was used to detect the insert size of the library, the insert size being aproximately 250–300 bp. Illumina PE150 sequencing is performed after pooling according to effective concentration and data output requirements with paired-end 150 bp sequencing strategy. After quantitative analysis, the expression matrix of all samples was obtained, and then the significance analysis of expression difference at gene or transcript level was conducted to search for functional genes or transcripts related to the treatment group. EdgeR software was used to analyze the significance of expression differences. The significance level was determined by p-value or corrected p-value (padj).

Gene Ontology and Kyoto Encyclopedia of Genes and Genomes Pathway Analyses

In organisms, different genes coordinate their biological functions. Significant pathway enrichment can explore the most important biochemical metabolic pathways and signal transduction pathways involved in differentially expressed genes. ClusterProfiler software was used to select the widely used annotated gene databases Gene Ontology (GO) and Kyoto Encyclopedia of Genes and Genomes (KEGG) for pathway enrichment analysis of differential genes. Gene Ontology enrichment analysis was performed in molecular function (MF), cellular component (CC), and BP. Gene Ontology and KEGG enrichment analysis was performed for co-location and co-expression of differential lncRNAs, respectively, to predict the function of lncRNAs.

lncRNA–mRNA Co-expression Network

An lncRNA–mRNA expression correlation network was built based on the normalized signal intensity of differential expression in lncRNAs and mRNAs to explore the dysregulation of lncRNAs in DED mice. A co-expression network of control and DED mice was established. Differentially expressed lncRNAs and mRNAs that met the criteria were selected according to p-value < 0.05 and fold change >2 or <0.5. Correlations between lncRNA–lncRNA, lncRNA–mRNA, and mRNA mRNA pairs were assessed using Pearson's correlations.

Cell Cultures

The HCECs line was kindly provided by Dr. Weiyun Shi (Shandong Eye Hospital, Shandong Eye Institute, Shandong Academy of Medical Sciences, Jinan, China) (28–30). Human corneal epithelial cells were cultured in Dulbecco's Modified Eagle's Medium/Nutrient Mixture F12 Ham (DMEM/F12; Gibco, Carlsbad, CA, USA) containing 100 U/ml penicillin, 100 U/ml streptomycin (Gibco), and 10% heat-inactivated fetal bovine serum (FBS; Hyclone, Rockford, IL, USA). Cells were incubated in a humidified 37°C incubator containing 5% CO_2.

Small Interfering RNA Transfection

Chrnb2 and Gabarapl2 knockdown was achieved using small interfering RNA (siRNA). Small interfering RNA were designed and synthesized by RiboBio Technology (Guangzhou, China). Small interfering RNA was transfected using lipofectamine 3000 transfection reagent (Invitrogen, Cat. L3000015; Invitrogen, Waltham, MA, USA) according to the manufacturer's protocol. A total of 5×10^5 cells in 2 ml of medium were seeded in six-well plates. Forty-eight hours post-transfection, cells were harvested in TRIzol for RNA isolation.

RNA Extraction and RT-PCR Analysis

Total RNA from mice corneal tissue and HCECs were extracted using TRIzol reagent (Invitrogen) according to the manufacturer's instructions, and reverse transcriptions were synthesized using the PrimeScript RT reagent kit (Takara, Japan). RT-PCR analysis was performed using SYBR Premix Ex Taq (Takara) with an ABI Prism 7500 sequence detection system (Applied Biosystems, Waltham, MA, USA). The relative expression of interleukin (IL)-1β, IL-6, TNF-a, Chrnb2, and Gabarapl2 was normalized to the endogenous control GAPDH using the $2^{-\Delta\Delta Ct}$ method.

Statistical Analysis

Quantitative data were expressed as the mean ± standard error of the mean (SEM). Analysis of variance (ANOVA) was used to test for difference among four different follow-ups, and the Bonferroni test was used to identify which pairs were significantly different. The paired t-test or the matched-pairs signed-rank test was used to identify between-group differences. The statistical significance was assumed at $p < 0.05$.

RESULTS

DED in the Mouse Model

Seven days after the treatment with 0.2% BAC, obvious epithelial punctate defects were detected using a fluorescence sodium dye in DED mice compared with the control group (**Figures 1A–C**). We observed no difference in fluorescence score between the two groups by the slit-lamp examination before the treatment (d0) (**Figure 1C**). The fluorescein scores at day 7, day 14, and day 21 were significantly increasing over time in the cornea of the DED mice compared to control animals (5.98 ± 0.51 at day 7, 8.89 ± 0.67 at day 14, and 11.26 ± 0.74 at day 21; $p < 0.001$; **Figure 1E**). Tear production was similar before treatment between the two groups of animals (4.89 ± 0.81 mm/30 s). However, there was a rapid and significant reduction in tear production (2.23 ± 0.75, $p < 0.01$, **Figures 1D,F**) in the DED compared with the control animals.

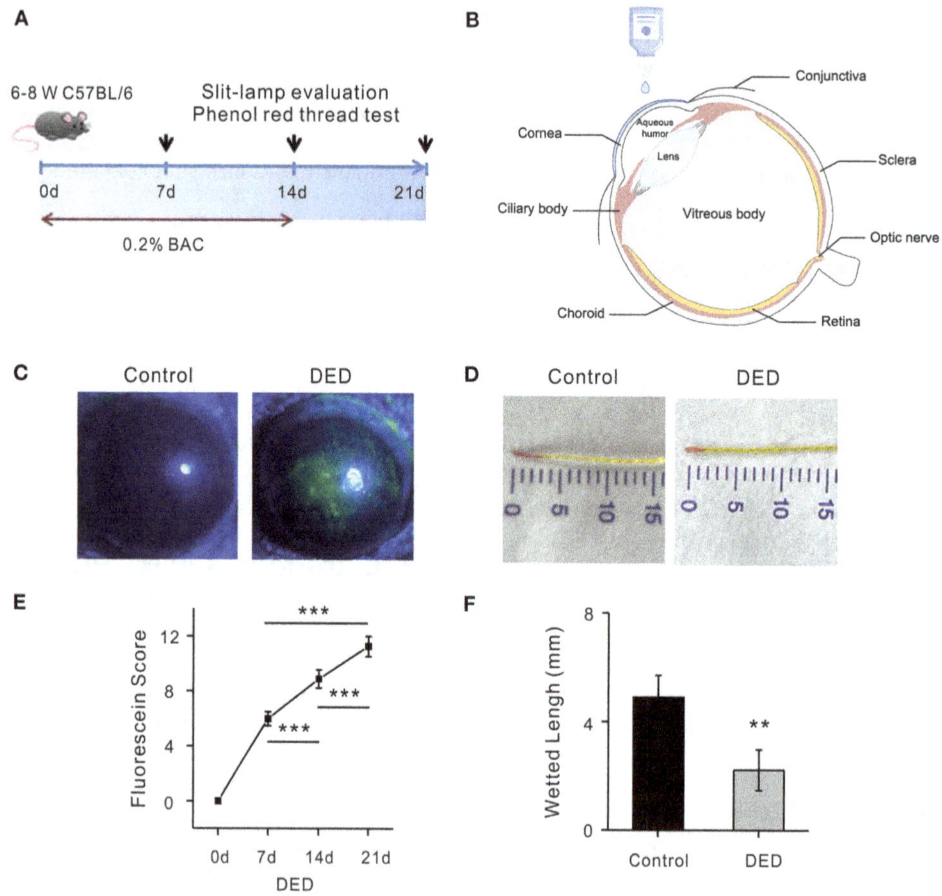

FIGURE 1 | Identification of DED in mouse model. **(A)** Administration of 0.2% BAC in both eyes for 14 days in DED group. Examinations were taken at day 0, day 7, day 14, and day 21. **(B)** Topical 5 μl of 0.2% BAC and PBS were applied twice a day. **(C)** Representative images of fluorescence sodium staining on day 14 in a DED cornea compared with images of the control cornea. **(D)** Representative images of tear production on day 14 after DED animal modeling. **(E)** The fluorescein scores at day 7, day 14, and day 21 were significantly increasing over time in the cornea of the DED mice (all $p < 0.001$). **(F)** Significant reduction of wetted length was observed in the DED group compared with the controls ($p < 0.01$). DED, dry eye disease; BAC, benzalkonium chloride; PBS, phosphate buffered saline.

Expression Profiling and Bioinformatic Functional Analysis of Differentially Expressed lncRNAs in the Mouse DED Model

RNA-seq was performed to identify lncRNAs involved in the cornea with the DED model. The lncRNAs were longer than 200 bp, with more than two exons (**Figures 2A,B**). The reproducibility between the biological and sequencing technical replicates was very high (Pearson correlation coefficients), at 0.931 (**Figure 2C**). The Venn diagram indicates the intersection of three computational approaches (CPC/CNCI/PFAM) for candidate lncRNA from putative protein-coding RNAs, and 4,071 aberrantly lncRNAs were predicted as potential lncRNAs using a Venn diagram (**Figure 2D**). The heatmap of hierarchical clustering revealed that the tissue-specific lncRNA expression patterns among samples were distinct (**Figure 3A**). Moreover, the Volcano plot revealed the 2,649 upregulated and 704 downregulated lncRNA expression profiles in each group (**Figure 3B**). Long non-coding ribonucleic acids regulates the expression of target genes (mRNAs) through co-location or co-expression. For the association analysis between lncRNA and mRNA, we performed cross set analysis on target genes with differentially expressed lncRNA and mRNA (**Figure 3C**). Next, the function of dysregulated lncRNAs and the potential target mRNAs were analyzed. Gene Ontology enrichment analyses were performed. If the Jensen–Shannon (JS) score >0.5, the significantly altered lncRNAs and mRNAs were selected. Subsequently, GO annotation was utilized to investigate the function of differentially expressed lncRNAs, yielding the number in GO terms. In BP, CC, and MF, the numbers of differentially expressed lncRNAs in sensory perception, metal ion homeostasis, extracellular matrix, and calcium ion binding were the highest (**Figure 3D**). **Table 1** shows the top six aberrantly expressed lncRNAs. **Table 2** indicates the primer sequences of the top six dysregulated known lncRNAs. In the mice corneal tissue, we evaluated the differences between groups with these six select genes by RT-qPCR (**Figures 3E,F**).

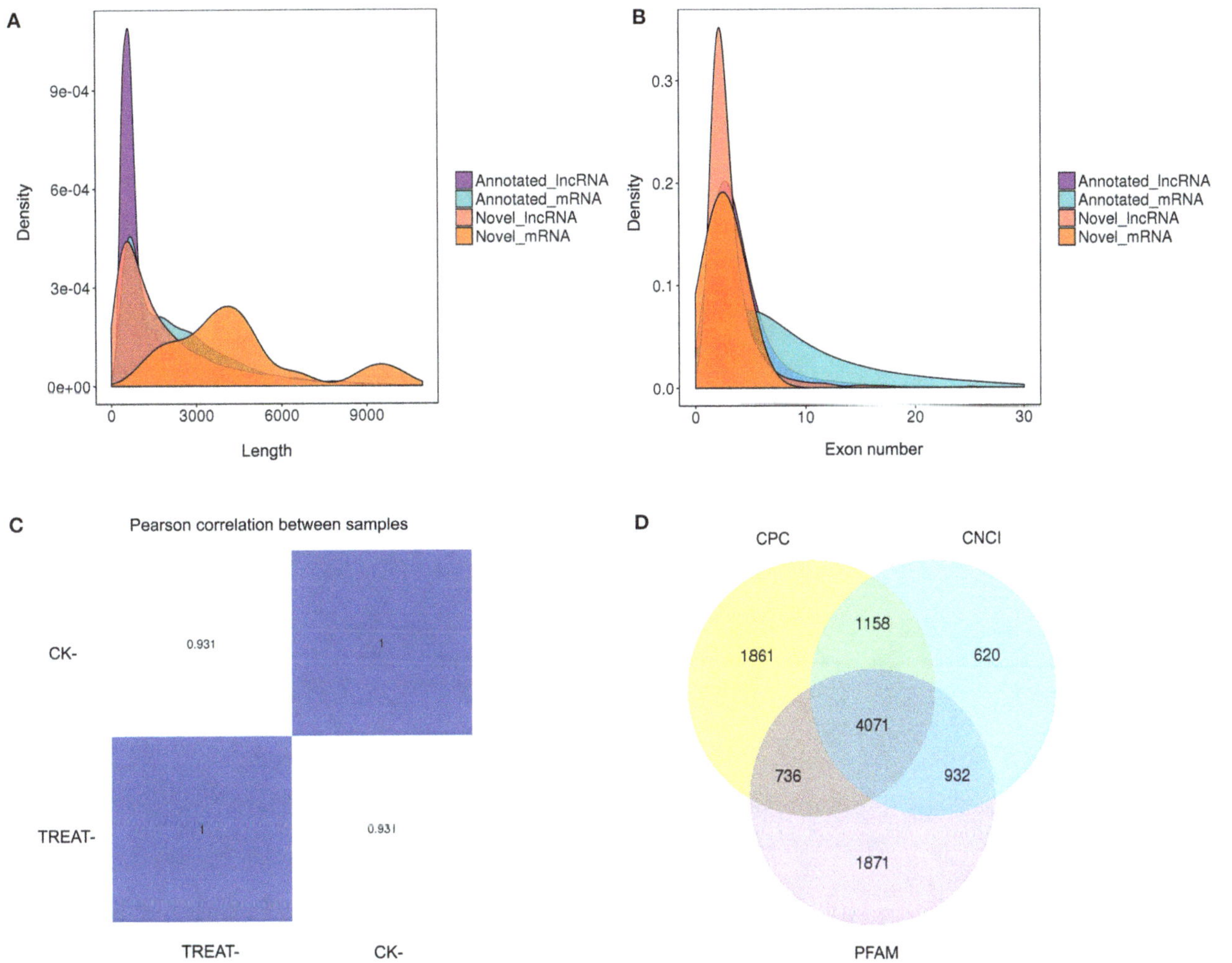

FIGURE 2 | Expression profiling of lncRNAs in the mouse DED model. **(A)** Histogram showing length distribution of novel lncRNA. **(B)** Histogram showing the number of lncRNA exons. **(C)** Heatmap of gene expression correlation; the numerical value refers to the correlation coefficient. **(D)** Venn diagram presenting overlapping potential lncRNAs of three computational approaches (CPC/CNCI/PFAM). DED, dry eye disease; lncRNAs, long non-coding RNAs.

The results showed that cholinergic receptor nicotinic beta 2 (Chrnb2) and autophagy target factor (gamma-aminobutyric acid (GABA) a receptor-associated protein-like 2, Gabarapl2) were significantly increased following DED compared with the control group ($p < 0.01$) (**Figure 3E**). Then, we verified the between-group differences with the top three downregulated lncRNAs, revealing significantly decreased expression levels of Usp31 ($p < 0.05$) (**Figure 3F**).

KEGG Pathway Analysis and Regulatory Mechanism of Differentially Expressed lncRNAs

Multiple active pathways were found in expressed lncRNAs by KEGG pathway analysis. Among them, the neuroactive ligand–receptor interaction signaling pathway was the most enriched, followed by cytokine–cytokine receptor interaction, the calcium signaling pathway, and the cell adhesion molecules (CAMs) signaling pathway (**Figures 4A–C**). Based on the above results, Chrnb2 and Gabarapl2 were the most significantly altered lncRNAs and may play a critical role in the molecular network of DED.

To establish the hyperosmolarity-induced HCECs dysfunction model, we exposed HCECs to sodium chloride (NaCl) at a concentration of 100 mM for 6 h. For further corroboration, we compared the expression levels of the two candidate lncRNAs in HCECs with or without NaCl treatment (the inflammation DED model *in vitro*). Consistent with the qRT-PCR results in the mice cornea *in vivo*, Chrnb2 and Gabarapl2 were remarkably elevated after NaCl treatment in HCECs (**Figures 5A,B**). To verify that candidate lncRNAs are involved in inflammatory insults, siRNA-mediated knockdown experiments on the two lncRNAs were performed *in vitro* in HCECs by transfection. The two candidate lncRNAs were designed to produce three siRNAs (Gabarapl2: si-Gabarapl2-1, si-Gabarapl2-2, si-Gabarapl2-3) and two siRNAs

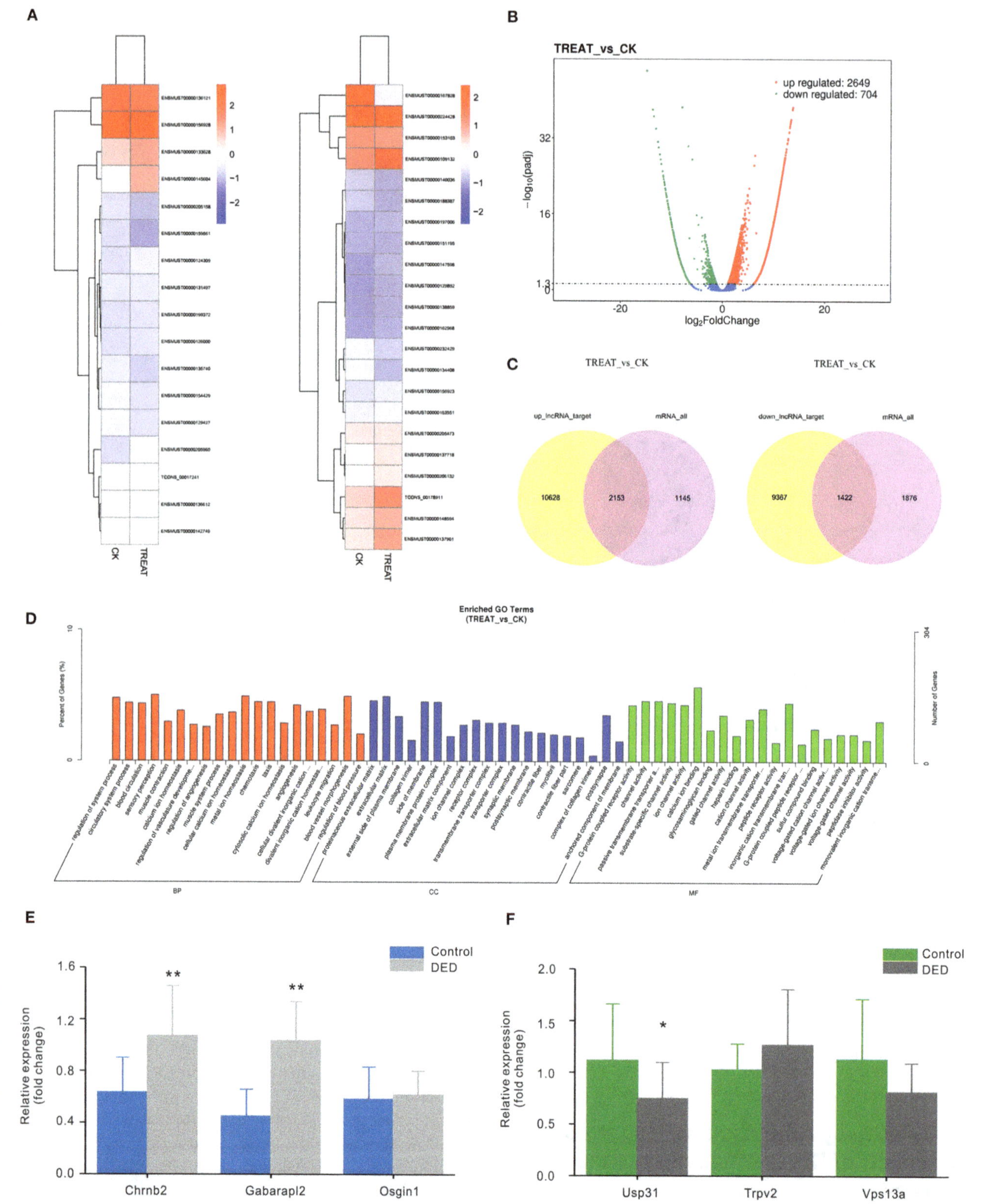

FIGURE 3 | Bioinformatic functional analysis of differentially expressed lncRNAs. **(A)** Heatmap of expression levels of tissue-specific lncRNAs. **(B)** Volcano plot of the different lncRNAs expression in each group. **(C)** Venn diagram showing co-location or co-expression of lncRNA-target genes (mRNAs). **(D)** The number of differentially expressed lncRNAs in BP, CC, and MF. **(E)** Expression levels of the top three upregulated lncRNAs in both groups via RT-qPCR. **(F)** Expression levels of the top three downregulated lncRNAs in both groups via RT-qPCR. CC, cellular component; MF, molecular function; BP, biological process. $^{*}p < 0.05$, $^{**}p < 0.01$. DED, dry eye disease.

TABLE 1 | The list of the top 6 dysregulated known lncRNAs.

Transcript ID	Gene name	Regulation	Log2 fold change	Locus	TREAT	CK	*p*-Value
ENSMUST00000199372	Chrnb2	Up	6.950176971	3:89752433–89763401	0.457683	0.002203	4.23E-21
ENSMUST00000133628	Gabarapl2	Up	2.105375715	8:111941068–111952742	3.161783	0.674989	1.15E-06
ENSMUST00000145604	Osgin1	Up	2.904841522	8:119437167–119446256	2.935011	0.360286	1.35E-10
ENSMUST00000205473	Usp31	Down	−1.895615293	7:121658782–121666815	0.403898	1.383633	1.72E-05
ENSMUST00000151195	Trpv2	Down	−10.13605601	11:62574486–62600299	0	0.093729	1.27E-17
ENSMUST00000224428	Vps13a	Down	−2.173306821	19:16734025–16780912	1.426892	5.919149	3.96E-07

TABLE 2 | Primers used in RT-PCR.

Transcript ID	Forward primer	Reverse primer
ENSMUST00 000199372	TGCTGACGGCATGTACGAAG	TGCTGGTCAAATGGGAAGTG
ENSMUST00 000133628	TCACTGTGGCTCAGTTCATG	TAGTTAGGCTGGACTGTGGG
ENSMUST00 000145604	CTCACATTAGACCCGTGCTTC	GACTGTCACTGTGGTCCCTCT
ENSMUST0 0000205473	GGAAGGAGACAGGCGTATGA	GGGACCAATGAGATGGCAAG
ENSMUST00 000151195	TGAGGCTTAGACAGCGTGAG	GGTAGTTCTTCATCCCAGAGG
ENSMUST00 000224428	GAGTGGTGGGCTTATGCTAT	TTCTTTGCCTCAACTTCTGC
GAPDH	GCACCACACCTTCTACAATG	GTGAGGGAGAGCATAGCC

(Chrnb2: si-Chrnb2-1, si-Chrnb2-2) according to primer sequence, respectively. The culture supernatant was collected for monitoring the inflammatory cytokines. As shown in **Figures 5C–H**, the expression levels of TNF-α, IL-1β, and IL-6 were significantly reduced in HCECs after transfection with si-Gabarapl2-2/si-Gabarapl2-3 (si-Gabarapl2-2: 0.98 ± 0.03 vs. 0.57 ± 0.11 in TNF-a, $n = 6$, $p < 0.001$; 0.98 ± 0.02 vs. 0.58 ± 0.10 in IL-1β, $n = 6$, $p < 0.001$; 0.99 ± 0.02 vs. 0.71 ± 0.13 in IL-6, $n = 6$, $p < 0.001$. si-Gabarapl2-3: 0.98 ± 0.03 vs. 0.54 ± 0.15 in TNF-a, $n = 6$, $p < 0.001$; 0.98 ± 0.02 vs. 0.49 ± 0.10 in IL-1β, $n = 6$, $p < 0.001$; 0.99 ± 0.02 vs. 0.65 ± 0.05 in IL-6, $n = 6$, $p < 0.001$), or si-Chrnb2-1 (si-Chrnb2-1: 0.99 ± 0.02 vs. 0.61 ± 0.21 in TNF-a, $n = 6$, $p < 0.01$; 0.98 ± 0.02 vs. 0.59 ± 0.16 in IL-1β, $n = 6$, $p < 0.001$; 0.99 ± 0.01 vs. 0.56 ± 0.24 in IL-6, $n = 6$, $p < 0.01$) in HCECs. The above results suggested that Gabarapl2 and Chrnb2 silence significantly repressed TNF-α, IL-1β, and IL-6.

DISCUSSION

Dysfunction of lncRNAs is highly associated with various human physiological processes, such as cell proliferation, development, metastasis, apoptosis, and immune response modulation (31–33). Additionally, the critical role of lncRNAs in the pathogenesis and regulation of ocular disorders such as glaucoma and cataract has been well-established (34, 35). In glaucoma, lncRNA-MALAT1 could inhibit retinal ganglion cell (RGC) apoptosis through activation of the PI3K/Akt signaling pathway (35). MIAT was found to act as a competing endogenous RNAs (ceRNA) and to form a feedback loop with Akt and miR-150-5p to inhibit TNF-α-induced proliferation and migration of human lens epithelial cells (HLECs) under oxidative stress (34). Subsequently, we explored the potential targeted lncRNA expression profile in a mouse model of DED. In the present study, we identified 3,353 significantly dysregulated lncRNAs in DED, further confirmed by PCR analysis. In total, 2,649 upregulated and 704 downregulated co-expressed lncRNAs were identified in the DED model. Notably, Chrnb2, Gabarapl2, and Usp31 were verified as the potential regulated lncRNAs compared with the control group. Knockdown of Chrnb2 or Gabarapl2 alleviated the pro-inflammatory signals in HCECs in the hypertonic state. All these results indicated that lncRNAs may participate in the mechanisms of DED.

Our correlation analysis between differentially expressed lncRNA and target gene mRNA showed that the Chrnb2 and the autophagy-related gene (GABA, a receptor-associated protein-like 2, Gabarapl2) were significantly up-regulated. Few studys have yet linked them to the eye diseases. Previous studies had found that Chrnb2 gene mutations induce autosomal dominant nocturnal frontal lobe epilepsy (36). Mice lacking expression of Chrnb2 display abnormal retinal waves and a dispersed projection of RGC axons to their dorsal lateral geniculate nuclei (dLGNs) (37). Gabarapl2 belongs to autophagy-related 8 (Atg8) gene family member. Autophagy-related 8 regulates GABA receptor-associated protein, GABARAP, GABARAP is one of the earliest and most important helper protein that mediates $GABA_A$ receptors transport from Golgi apparatus to the cell membrane (38, 39). In mammals, Atg8 has evolved into the LC3/Gabarap protein family, which consists of LC3A, LC3B, LC3C, Gabarap, Gabarapl1, and Gabarapl2 (40, 41). Sasau et al. revealed that Gabarap is involved in host immunization system, especially interferon-inducible GTPases (41).

Furthermore, we performed GO and KEGG enrichment analyses to explore signaling pathways and their relationship with biological systems, revealing that the neuroactive ligand–receptor interaction signaling pathway was the most significant pathway. This pathway was previously evidenced as functionally significant in neurotransmitter-mediated disorders such as alcohol dependence disorder (42), autism spectrum disorders (43), Parkinson's disease (44), and some types of lung cancer (45). Besides, the pathway was found to be enriched in proliferative diabetic retinopathy and age-related macular degeneration

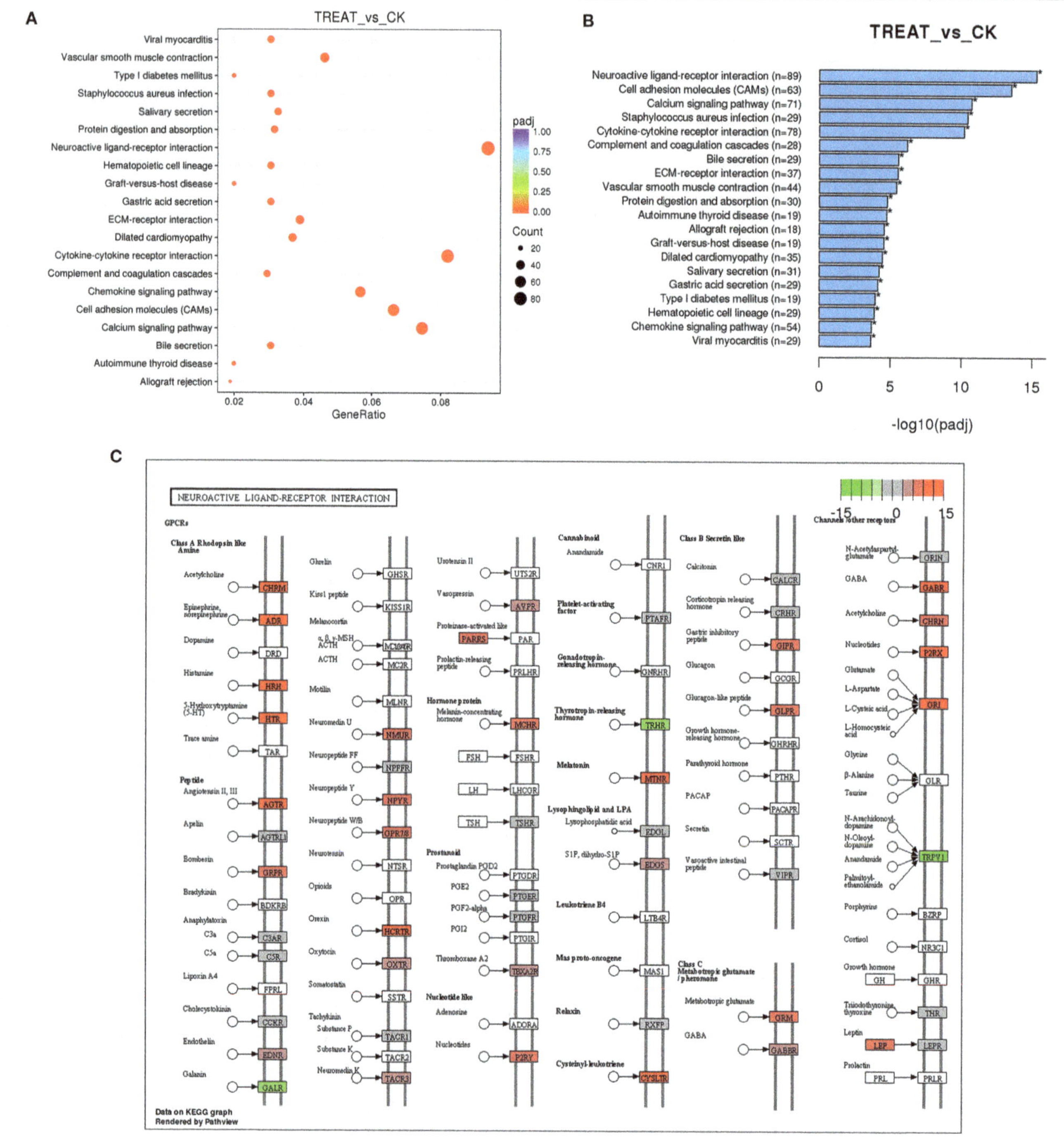

FIGURE 4 | Signaling pathway analysis of differentially expressed lncRNAs. **(A)** The KEGG pathway analysis demonstrates that the genes are enriched in multiple pathways. **(B)** Lists of the most affected pathways. **(C)** Neuroactive ligand–receptor interaction signaling pathway map. Red in **(C)** indicates upregulated genes; green in **(C)** indicates downregulated genes; lncRNAs, long non-coding RNAs; KEGG, Kyoto Encyclopedia of Genes and Genomes.

(46, 47). This pathway regulates multiple neuroreceptors and their associated distant signaling molecules, such as 5-hydroxytryptamine (5-HT, serotonin) and GABA. A previous study found DED patients have higher tear serotonin levels (48), whereas another study indicated that selective serotonin reuptake inhibitor (SSRI) promotes an inflammatory response on the ocular surface by increasing the tear serotonin levels (49). It may be concluded that the serotonin acted as a mediator during the etiology of DED. However, the upstream and downstream mechanisms of serotonin in DED have

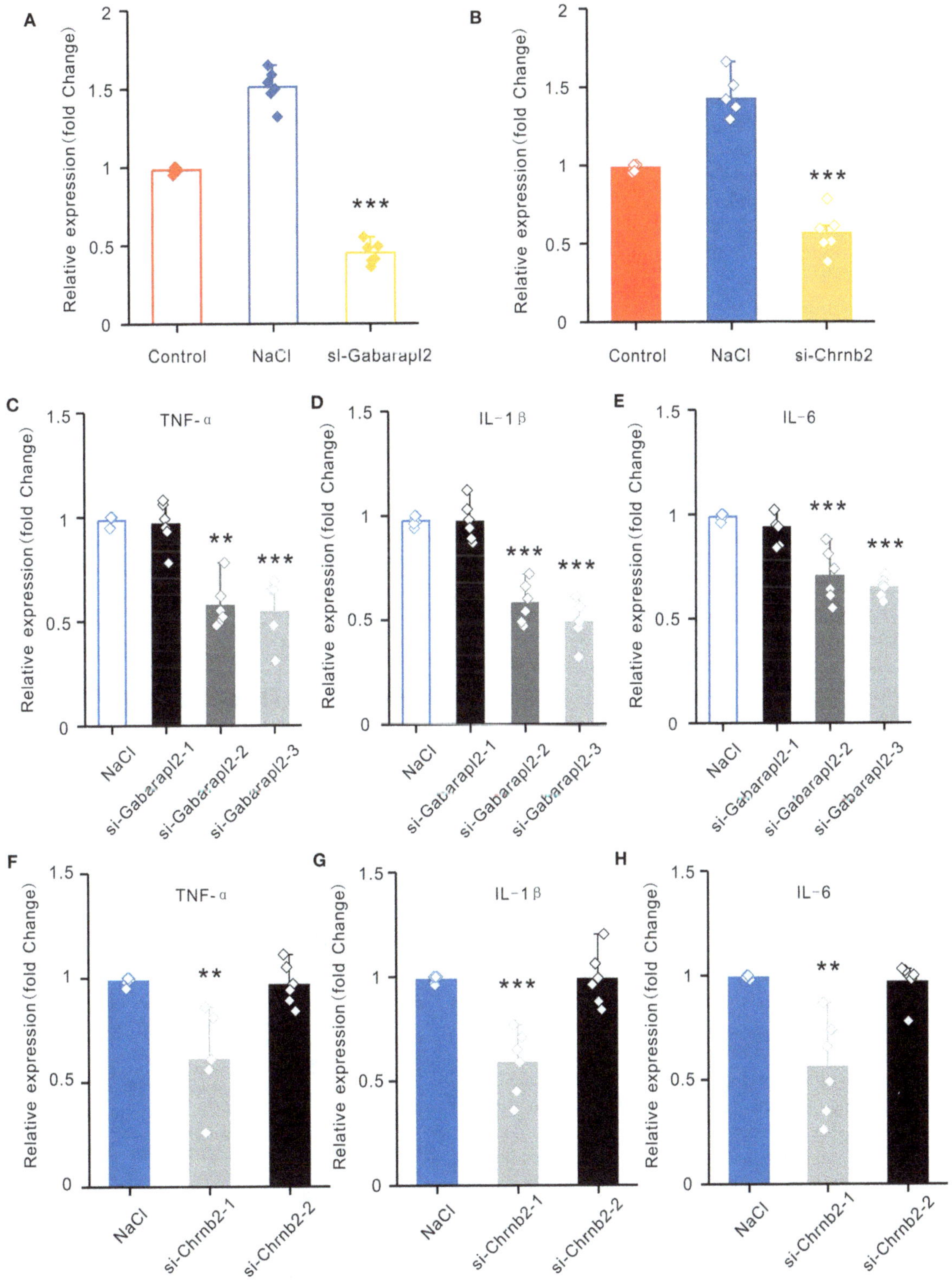

FIGURE 5 | Validation of lncRNAs Chrnb2 and Gabarapl2, regulating the inflammatory factor *in vitro*. **(A,B)** The expression levels of Chrnb2 and Gabarapl2 in HCECs after NaCl treatment. **(C–E)** After transfection with si-Gabarapl2, the mRNA levels of TNF-α, IL-1β, and IL-6 in HCECs following NaCl treatment. **(F–H)** After transfection with si-Chrnb2, the mRNA levels of TNF-α, IL-1β, and IL-6 in HCECs following NaCl treatment. $^{**}p < 0.01$, $^{***}p < 0.001$.

not been fully elucidated. Another parallel study on the mechanism of serotonin regulation of dry eye is ongoing. The enriched expression of GABA in the neuroactive ligand–receptor interaction signaling pathway hints toward further understanding. Researchers demonstrated that GABA- and 5-HT-immunoreactive neurons could constitute parallel inhibitory or excitatory pathways (50, 51). Further, GABA can regulate the release of serotonin and modulate serotonergic neurons in the nervous system (52, 53). Meanwhile, as the neurotransmitters, 5-HT and GABA usually participate in the physiological cycle together (54). According to the definition of DED by the Tear Film and Ocular Surface Society (TFOS) Dry Eye Workshop (DEW) II, the core mechanism of DED is tear hyperosmolarity, which is the hallmark of the disease (5). Tear hyperosmolarity, as well as inflammatory mediators, may induce DED symptoms and cause damage to the ocular surface, including epithelial cells, surface microvilli, and goblet cells (5, 11). Some lncRNAs can interact with RNA binding proteins (RBPs) and promote the release of corresponding cytokines (55–57), including IL-6, TNF-α, and IL-1β, which may play a significant role in the regulation of DED (58). Long-term and recurring nerve inflammations can also create a chain effect. The neuroactive ligand–receptor interaction signaling pathway may regulate the inflammatory process. 5-Hydroxytryptamine-related GABA regulatory enhances the phagocytic functions of monocytes/macrophages and induces them to produce pro-inflammatory cytokines, stimulating neutrophil chemotaxis (59). Thus, we speculated that tear hyperosmolarity could trigger 5-HT and GABA secretion, which stimulates production of pro-inflammatory cytokines, resulting in increased friction and also symptoms.

Meanwhile, the results showed that the cytokine–cytokine receptor interaction signaling and calcium signaling pathway were also enriched in the DED model. Nociceptors respond to cytokines and produce inflammatory mediators. Non-neuronal cells release pro-inflammatory mediators such as TNF and IL-1β, which live in close proximity to nociceptors following injury or insult, promoting pain transduction via the modulation of ion channels (transient receptor potential vanilloid 1, TRPV1) (12, 60–62). The expression levels of a lncRNA (uc.48+) were increased in the dorsal root ganglions (DRGs) of diabetic rats. Knockdown of uc.48+ alleviated TNF-α in DRGs of diabetic rats (63). A significant upregulation of genes associated with inflammatory and immune responses was found to be related to cytokine–cytokine receptor interactions in human corneal, conjunctival, and meibomian glands (64). Moreover, in a DED-related therapeutic study, diquafosol promoted corneal epithelial healing via intracellular calcium-mediated signaling (65). These findings indicate that both cytokine–cytokine receptor interaction signaling and calcium signaling pathways may participate in the inflammatory process of DED. Consistent with previous studies, our results also showed that the expression levels of Chrnb2 and Gabarapl2 were upregulated in HCECs after NaCl treatment, and mice corneas of DED and knockdown of Chrnb2 and Gabarapl2 could alleviate the expression of TNF-α, IL-1β, and IL-6 *in vitro* and *in vivo*. However, the exact molecular mechanism contributing to the etiology of DED is not fully defined, warranting further exploration.

In conclusion, our study first reported the lncRNA high-transcriptome sequencing analysis of DED. In view of our results, 3,353 dysregulated lncRNAs were explored. Among them, Chrnb2, Gabarapl2, and Usp31 were verified as potentially regulated lncRNAs. Further, we speculated that the neuroactive ligand–receptor interaction signaling pathway may be involved in the inflammatory process of DED via neurotransmitter secretion. TNF-α, IL-1β, and IL-6 were significantly reduced in HCECs after transfection with si-Chrnb2 or si-Gabarapl2. Thus, the current findings may lead to a greater depth of understanding of DED, providing potential regulatory mechanisms of lncRNAs in the DED and therapeutic targets based on the differentially expressed lncRNAs.

ETHICS STATEMENT

All experimental protocols conformed to the Association for Research in Vision and Ophthalmology statement on the use of animals. We performed surgery on the animals according to the guidelines of the Fudan University Ethics Committee (Ethical code: EENTIRB-2018-03-01).

AUTHOR CONTRIBUTIONS

YY and MC performed the *in vitro* experiments and analyzed the data. ZZ and YD performed the *in vivo* experiments. XZ and JH designed and supervised the project, and wrote the manuscript. All authors contributed to manuscript revision, read, and approved the submitted version.

REFERENCES

1. Miljanovic B, Dana R, Sullivan DA, Schaumberg DA. Impact of dry eye syndrome on vision-related quality of life. *Am J Ophthalmol.* (2007) 143:409–15. doi: 10.1016/j.ajo.2006.11.060
2. Jie Y, Xu L, Wu YY, Jonas JB. Prevalence of dry eye among adult Chinese in the Beijing Eye Study. *Eye (Lond).* (2009) 23:688–93. doi: 10.1038/sj.eye.6703101
3. Viso E, Rodriguez-Ares MT, Gude F. Prevalence of and associated factors for dry eye in a Spanish adult population (the Salnes Eye Study). *Ophthalmic Epidemiol.* (2009) 16:15–21. doi: 10.1080/09286580802228509
4. Farrand KF, Fridman M, Stillman IO, Schaumberg DA. Prevalence of diagnosed dry eye disease in the united states among adults aged 18 years and older. *Am J Ophthalmol.* (2017) 182:90–8. doi: 10.1016/j.ajo.2017.06.033
5. Stapleton F, Alves M, Bunya VY, Jalbert I, Lekhanont K, Malet F, et al. TFOS DEWS II epidemiology report. *Ocul Surf.* (2017) 15:334–65. doi: 10.1016/j.jtos.2017.05.003
6. Sayegh RR, Yu Y, Farrar JT, Kuklinski EJ, Shtein RM, Asbell PA, et al. Ocular discomfort and quality of life among patients in the dry eye assessment and management study. *Cornea.* (2021) 40:869–76. doi: 10.1097/ICO.0000000000002580
7. Greco G, Pistilli M, Asbell PA, Maguire MG, Dry Eye Assessment and Management Study Research Group. Association of severity of dry eye

disease with work productivity and activity impairment in the dry eye assessment and management study. *Ophthalmology.* (2021) 128:850–6. doi: 10.1016/j.ophtha.2020.10.015
8. Li DQ, Chen Z, Song XJ, Luo L, Pflugfelder SC. Stimulation of matrix metalloproteinases by hyperosmolarity via a JNK pathway in human corneal epithelial cells. *Invest Ophthalmol Vis Sci.* (2004) 45:4302–11. doi: 10.1167/iovs.04-0299
9. De Paiva CS, Corrales RM, Villarreal AL, Farley WJ, Li DQ, Stern ME, et al. Corticosteroid and doxycycline suppress MMP-9 and inflammatory cytokine expression, MAPK activation in the corneal epithelium in experimental dry eye. *Exp Eye Res.* (2006) 83:526–35. doi: 10.1016/j.exer.2006.02.004
10. Coursey TG, Bohat R, Barbosa FL, Pflugfelder SC, de Paiva CS. Desiccating stress-induced chemokine expression in the epithelium is dependent on upregulation of NKG2D/RAE-1 and release of IFN-gamma in experimental dry eye. *J Immunol.* (2014) 193:5264–72. doi: 10.4049/jimmunol.1400016
11. Clayton JA. Dry eye. *N Engl J Med.* (2018) 378:2212–23. doi: 10.1056/NEJMra1407936
12. Ji RR, Xu ZZ, Gao YJ. Emerging targets in neuroinflammation-driven chronic pain. *Nat Rev Drug Discov.* (2014) 13:533–48. doi: 10.1038/nrd4334
13. Hessen M, Akpek EK. Dry eye: an inflammatory ocular disease. *J Ophthalmic Vis Res.* (2014) 9:240–50.
14. Fornasari D. Pharmacotherapy for neuropathic pain: a review. *Pain Ther 6(Suppl 1).* (2017) 25–33. doi: 10.1007/s40122-017-0091-4
15. Li Z, Li X, Chen X, Li S, Ho IHT, Liu X, et al. Emerging roles of long non-coding RNAs in neuropathic pain. *Cell Prolif.* (2019) 52:e12528. doi: 10.1111/cpr.12528
16. Fitzgerald KA, Caffrey DR. Long noncoding RNAs in innate and adaptive immunity. *Curr Opin Immunol.* (2014) 26:140–6. doi: 10.1016/j.coi.2013.12.001
17. Bhat SA, Ahmad SM, Mumtaz PT, Malik AA, Dar MA, Urwat U, et al. Long non-coding RNAs: mechanism of action and functional utility. *Noncoding RNA Res.* (2016) 1:43–50. doi: 10.1016/j.ncrna.2016.11.002
18. Sharma U, Barwal TS, Malhotra A, Pant N, Vivek, Dey, D, et al. Long non-coding RNA TINCR as potential biomarker and therapeutic target for cancer. *Life Sci.* (2020) 257:118035. doi: 10.1016/j.lfs.2020.118035
19. Ye L, Shi H, Yu C, Fu J, Chen C, Wu S, et al. LncRNA Neat1 positively regulates MAPK signaling and is involved in the pathogenesis of Sjogren's syndrome. *Int Immunopharmacol.* (2020) 88:106992. doi: 10.1016/j.intimp.2020.106992
20. Jiang L, He W, Tang F, Tang N, Huang G, Huang W, et al. Epigenetic landscape analysis of the long non-coding RNA and messenger RNA in a mouse model of corneal alkali burns. *Invest Ophthalmol Vis Sci.* (2021) 62:28. doi: 10.1167/iovs.62.4.28
21. Wang Q, Gu L, Adey A, Radlwimmer B, Wang W, Hovestadt V, et al. Tagmentation-based whole-genome bisulfite sequencing. *Nat Protoc.* (2013) 8:2022–32. doi: 10.1038/nprot.2013.118
22. Gu L, Frommel SC, Oakes CC, Simon R, Grupp K, Gerig CY, et al. BAZ2A (TIP5) is involved in epigenetic alterations in prostate cancer and its overexpression predicts disease recurrence. *Nat Genet.* (2015) 47:22–30. doi: 10.1038/ng.3165
23. Bauer T, Trump S, Ishaque N, Thurmann L, Gu L, Bauer M, et al. Environment-induced epigenetic reprogramming in genomic regulatory elements in smoking mothers and their children. *Mol Syst Biol.* (2016) 12:861. doi: 10.15252/msb.20156520
24. Gu H, Guo Y, Gu L, Wei A, Xie S, Ye Z, et al. Deep learning for identifying corneal diseases from ocular surface slit-lamp photographs. *Sci Rep.* (2020) 10:17851. doi: 10.1038/s41598-020-75027-3
25. Gu L, Wang L, Chen H, Hong J, Shen Z, Dhall A, et al. CG14906 (mettl4) mediates m(6)A methylation of U2 snRNA in Drosophila. *Cell Discov.* (2020) 6:44. doi: 10.1038/s41421-020-0178-7
26. Blanco MA, Sykes DB, Gu L, Wu M, Petroni R, Karnik R, et al. Chromatin-state barriers enforce an irreversible mammalian cell fate decision. *Cell Rep.* (2021) 37:109967. doi: 10.1016/j.celrep.2021.109967
27. Xin M, Liang H, Wang H, Wen D, Wang L, Zhao L, et al. Mirt2 functions in synergy with miR-377 to participate in inflammatory pathophysiology of Sjogren's syndrome. *Artif Cells Nanomed Biotechnol.* (2019) 47:2473–80. doi: 10.1080/21691401.2019.1626413
28. Hong J, Shao T, Sun X, Li G, Xu J. Interferon-gamma up-regulates major-histocompatibility-complex class I-related chain A expression and enhances major-histocompatibility-complex class I-related chain A-mediated cytolysis of human corneal epithelium by natural killer cells *in vitro. J Interferon Cytokine Res.* (2012) 32:115–20. doi: 10.1089/jir.2011.0003
29. Wu D, Zhang J, Qian T, Dai Y, Mashaghi A, Xu J, et al. IFN-gamma regulates the expression of MICA in human corneal epithelium through miRNA4448 and NFkappaB. *Front Immunol.* (2018) 9:1530. doi: 10.3389/fimmu.2018.01530
30. Zhou X, Lv J, Li G, Qian T, Jiang H, Xu J, et al. Rescue the retina after the ischemic injury by polymer-mediated intracellular superoxide dismutase delivery. *Biomaterials.* (2021) 268:120600. doi: 10.1016/j.biomaterials.2020.120600
31. Atianand MK, Caffrey DR, Fitzgerald KA. Immunobiology of long noncoding RNAs. *Annu Rev Immunol.* (2017) 35:177–98. doi: 10.1146/annurev-immunol-041015-055459
32. Dykes IM, Emanueli C. Transcriptional and post-transcriptional gene regulation by long non-coding RNA. *Genomics Proteomics Bioinformatics.* (2017) 15:177–86. doi: 10.1016/j.gpb.2016.12.005
33. Fernandes JCR, Acuna SM, Aoki JI, Floeter-Winter LM, Muxel SM. Long non-coding RNAs in the regulation of gene expression: physiology and disease. *Noncoding RNA.* (2019) 5:17. doi: 10.3390/ncrna5010017
34. Shen Y, Dong LF, Zhou RM, Yao J, Song YC, Yang H, et al. Role of long non-coding RNA MIAT in proliferation, apoptosis and migration of lens epithelial cells: a clinical and *in vitro* study. *J Cell Mol Med.* (2016) 20:537–48. doi: 10.1111/jcmm.12755
35. Li HB, You QS, Xu LX, Sun LX, Abdul Majid AS, Xia XB, et al. Long non-coding RNA-MALAT1 mediates retinal ganglion cell apoptosis through the PI3K/Akt signaling pathway in rats with glaucoma. *Cell Physiol Biochem.* (2017) 43:2117–32. doi: 10.1159/000484231
36. Diaz-Otero F, Quesada M, Morales-Corraliza J, Martinez-Parra C, Gomez-Garre P, Serratosa JM. Autosomal dominant nocturnal frontal lobe epilepsy with a mutation in the CHRNB2 gene. *Epilepsia.* (2008) 49:516–20. doi: 10.1111/j.1528-1167.2007.01328.x
37. Rubin CM, van der List DA, Ballesteros JM, Goloshchapov AV, Chalupa LM, Chapman B. Mouse mutants for the nicotinic acetylcholine receptor ss2 subunit display changes in cell adhesion and neurodegeneration response genes. *PLoS ONE.* (2011) 6:e18626. doi: 10.1371/journal.pone.0018626
38. Wang H, Bedford FK, Brandon NJ, Moss SJ, Olsen RW. GABA(A)-receptor-associated protein links GABA(A) receptors and the cytoskeleton. *Nature.* (1999) 397:69–72. doi: 10.1038/16264
39. Karigo T, Kennedy A, Yang B, Liu M, Tai D, Wahle IA, et al. Distinct hypothalamic control of same- and opposite-sex mounting behaviour in mice. *Nature.* (2021) 589:258–63. doi: 10.1038/s41586-020-2995-0
40. Nath S, Dancourt J, Shteyn V, Puente G, Fong WM, Nag S, et al. Lipidation of the LC3/GABARAP family of autophagy proteins relies on a membrane-curvature-sensing domain in Atg3. *Nat Cell Biol.* (2014) 16:415–24. doi: 10.1038/ncb2940
41. Sasai M, Sakaguchi N, Ma JS, Nakamura S, Kawabata T, Bando H, et al. Essential role for GABARAP autophagy proteins in interferon-inducible GTPase-mediated host defense. *Nat Immunol.* (2017) 18:899–910. doi: 10.1038/ni.3767
42. Biernacka JM, Geske J, Jenkins GD, Colby C, Rider DN, Karpyak VM, et al. Genome-wide gene-set analysis for identification of pathways associated with alcohol dependence. *Int J Neuropsychopharmacol.* (2013) 16:271–8. doi: 10.1017/S1461145712000375
43. Wen Y, Alshikho MJ, Herbert MR. Pathway network analyses for autism reveal multisystem involvement, major overlaps with other diseases and convergence upon MAPK and calcium signaling. *PLoS ONE.* (2016) 11:e0153329. doi: 10.1371/journal.pone.0153329
44. Kong Y, Liang X, Liu L, Zhang D, Wan C, Gan Z, et al. High throughput sequencing identifies microRNAs mediating alpha-synuclein toxicity by targeting neuroactive-ligand receptor interaction pathway in early stage of Drosophila Parkinson's disease model. *PLoS ONE.* (2015) 10:e0137432. doi: 10.1371/journal.pone.0137432
45. Ji X, Bosse Y, Landi MT, Gui J, Xiao X, Qian D, et al. Identification of susceptibility pathways for the role of chromosome 15q251 in modifying lung cancer risk. *Nat Commun.* (2018) 9:3221. doi: 10.1038/s41467-018-05074-y
46. Dhirachaikulpanich D, Li X, Porter LF, Paraoan L. Integrated microarray and RNAseq Transcriptomic analysis of retinal pigment epithelium/choroid in age-related macular degeneration. *Front Cell Dev Biol.* (2020) 8:808. doi: 10.3389/fcell.2020.00808

47. Yao H, Xin D, Zhan Z, Li Z. Network pharmacology-based approach to comparatively predict the active ingredients and molecular targets of compound xueshuantong capsule and hexuemingmu tablet in the treatment of proliferative diabetic retinopathy. *Evid Based Complement Alternat Med.* (2021) 2021:6642600. doi: 10.1155/2021/6642600
48. Chhadva P, Lee T, Sarantopoulos CD, Hackam AS, McClellan AL, Felix ER, et al. Human Tear serotonin levels correlate with symptoms and signs of dry eye. *Ophthalmology.* (2015) 122:1675–80. doi: 10.1016/j.ophtha.2015.04.010
49. Zhang X, Yin Y, Yue L, Gong L. Selective serotonin reuptake inhibitors aggravate depression-associated dry eye via activating the NF-kappaB pathway. *Invest Ophthalmol Vis Sci.* (2019) 60:407–19. doi: 10.1167/iovs.18-25572
50. Giese M, Gestrich J, Massah A, Peterle J, Wei H, Stengl M. GABA- and serotonin-expressing neurons take part in inhibitory as well as excitatory input pathways to the circadian clock of the Madeira cockroach *Rhyparobia maderae. Eur J Neurosci.* (2018) 47:1067–80. doi: 10.1111/ejn.13863
51. Sahni S, Tickoo M, Gupta R, Vaswani M, Ambekar A, Grover T, et al. Association of serotonin and GABA pathway gene polymorphisms with alcohol dependence: a preliminary study. *Asian J Psychiatr.* (2019) 39:169–73. doi: 10.1016/j.ajp.2018.04.023
52. Tao R, Auerbach SB. Regulation of serotonin release by GABA and excitatory amino acids. *J Psychopharmacol.* (2000) 14:100–13. doi: 10.1177/026988110001400201
53. Hernandez-Vazquez F, Garduno J, Hernandez-Lopez S. GABAergic modulation of serotonergic neurons in the dorsal raphe nucleus. *Rev Neurosci.* (2019) 30:289–303. doi: 10.1515/revneuro-2018-0014
54. Jones BE. Arousal and sleep circuits. *Neuropsychopharmacology.* (2020) 45:6–20. doi: 10.1038/s41386-019-0444-2
55. Carpenter S, Aiello D, Atianand MK, Ricci EP, Gandhi P, Hall LL, et al. A long noncoding RNA mediates both activation and repression of immune response genes. *Science.* (2013) 341:789–92. doi: 10.1126/science.1240925
56. Rapicavoli NA, Qu K, Zhang J, Mikhail M, Laberge RM, Chang HY. A mammalian pseudogene lncRNA at the interface of inflammation and anti-inflammatory therapeutics. *Elife.* (2013) 2:e00762. doi: 10.7554/eLife.00762
57. Li Z, Chao TC, Chang KY, Lin N, Patil VS, Shimizu C, et al. The long noncoding RNA THRIL regulates TNFα expression through its interaction with hnRNPL. *Proc Natl Acad Sci USA.* (2014) 111:1002–7. doi: 10.1073/pnas.1313768111
58. Roda M, Corazza I, Bacchi Reggiani ML, Pellegrini M, Taroni L, Giannaccare G, et al. Dry eye disease and tear cytokine levels-a meta-analysis. *Int J Mol Sci.* (2020). 21:3111. doi: 10.3390/ijms21093111
59. Khan J, Ali G, Rashid U, Khan R, Jan MS, Ullah R, et al. Mechanistic evaluation of a novel cyclohexenone derivative's functionality against nociception and inflammation: an *in-vitro*, *in-vivo* and *in-silico* approach. *Eur J Pharmacol.* (2021) 902:174091. doi: 10.1016/j.ejphar.2021.174091
60. White FA, Sun J, Waters SM, Ma C, Ren D, Ripsch M, et al. Excitatory monocyte chemoattractant protein-1 signaling is up-regulated in sensory neurons after chronic compression of the dorsal root ganglion. *Proc Natl Acad Sci USA.* (2005) 102:14092–7. doi: 10.1073/pnas.0503496102
61. Zelenka M, Schafers M, Sommer C. Intraneural injection of interleukin-1beta and tumor necrosis factor-alpha into rat sciatic nerve at physiological doses induces signs of neuropathic pain. *Pain.* (2005) 116:257–63. doi: 10.1016/j.pain.2005.04.018
62. Basbaum AI, Bautista DM, Scherrer G, Julius D. Cellular and molecular mechanisms of pain. *Cell.* (2009) 139:267–84. doi: 10.1016/j.cell.2009.09.028
63. Wang S, Xu H, Zou L, Xie J, Wu H, Wu B, et al. LncRNA uc.48+ is involved in diabetic neuropathic pain mediated by the P2X3 receptor in the dorsal root ganglia. *Purinergic Signal.* (2016) 12:139–48. doi: 10.1007/s11302-015-9488-x
64. Chen D, Sahin A, Kam WR, Liu Y, Darabad RR, Sullivan DA. Influence of lipopolysaccharide on proinflammatory gene expression in human corneal, conjunctival and meibomian gland epithelial cells. *Ocul Surf.* (2018) 16:382–9. doi: 10.1016/j.jtos.2018.05.003
65. Byun YS, Yoo YS, Kwon JY, Joo JS, Lim SA, Whang WJ, et al. Diquafosol promotes corneal epithelial healing via intracellular calcium-mediated ERK activation. *Exp Eye Res.* (2016) 143:89–97. doi: 10.1016/j.exer.2015.10.013

14

Effect of Transcutaneous Upper Eyelid Blepharoplasty on Blink Parameters and Lipid Layer Thickness

Siyi Zhang[1,2], *Yan Yan*[1,2], *Yang Lu*[1,2], *Yixiong Zhou*[1,2*] *and Yao Fu*[1,2*]

[1] *Department of Ophthalmology, Shanghai Ninth People's Hospital, Shanghai JiaoTong University School of Medicine, Shanghai, China,* [2] *Shanghai Key Laboratory of Orbital Diseases and Ocular Oncology, Shanghai, China*

***Correspondence:**
Yixiong Zhou
35267130@qq.com
Yao Fu
drfuyao@126.com

Purpose: This study aimed to investigate the effect of transcutaneous upper eyelid blepharoplasty on lipid layer thickness (LLT) and blink parameters in young women during the early postoperative period.

Methods: This prospective study included 110 eyes of 55 young female patients (age range, 19–31 years) who underwent transcutaneous upper eyelid blepharoplasty. The LLT and blink parameters measured using a LipiView interferometer were recorded before the surgery and 1 week and 1 month after the surgery. Ocular Surface Disease Index (OSDI) score, noninvasive tear film breakup time (NITBUT), and palpebral fissure height (PFH) measurements were also performed at each time point.

Results: The number of blinks significantly decreased ($P < 0.001$), and the number of partial blinks and partial blink rate (PBR) significantly increased 1 week after the surgery ($P = 0.002$ and $P < 0.001$); they all returned to baseline in 1 month. The LLT and OSDI score increased significantly 1 week and 1 month after the surgery ($P < 0.001$ and $P < 0.001$). A significant increase in the NITBUT and a significant decrease in the PFH were observed 1 week after the surgery ($P < 0.001$ and $P < 0.001$), and the values returned to baseline 1 month after the surgery. No clinical correlation was found between blink parameters and ocular surface parameters.

Conclusions: Transcutaneous upper eyelid blepharoplasty led to a change in blink parameters and ocular surface parameters during the early postoperative period. However, this influence was temporary, and the transitory change in blink parameters had no effects on the ocular surface environment.

Keywords: upper blepharoplasty, blink, lipid layer thickness (LLT), dry eye, noninvasive tear film breakup time (NITBUT)

INTRODUCTION

Some Asians have a single upper eyelid or upper eyelid hypertrophy, which makes their eyes appear small and droopy, owing to the difference in fat distribution in the orbital septum and upper eyelid anatomical structures between Asians and the white race (1). Many Asians, especially young women, choose to undergo upper blepharoplasty to have a pair of attractive double eyelids. However, this surgical procedure is associated with many complications (2, 3), and dry eye disease

(DED) is one of the most common complications (4). A retrospective study of 892 patients indicated that dry eye symptoms following blepharoplasty were reported in 26.5% of patients (4). Yan et al. measured subjective and objective parameters of dry eye in patients who underwent upper blepharoplasty and found that upper eyelid blepharoplasty might temporarily affect tear film dynamics and aggravate dry eye symptoms in young women. However, these changes generally disappear 3 months after the surgery (5). Zloto et al. (6) also confirmed no significant differences between the postoperative and preoperative objective and subjective dry eye tests in patients with blepharoplasty 3 months after the surgery.

However, DED is a multifactorial ocular surface disease characterized by a loss of homeostasis of the tear film (7), and a stable preocular tear film is a hallmark of ocular health (8). The tear film consists of a mucin layer, an aqueous layer, and a lipid layer. The lipid layer is important in preventing the loss of aqueous layer through overspill and evaporation (8–11). Upper blepharoplasty involved surgical removal of the skin, orbicularis oculi muscle, and (or) orbital fat, and might lead to the formation of scar and injury to the innervation, resulting in incomplete blink and decreased blink rate (3, 12). The fullness of the blink affects the stability of the tear film and its distribution in the inter-blink period (13). Moreover, the mechanical action of the lid muscles during the blink contributes to the delivery of meibomian oil (9). Jie et al. (14) indicated that partial blink would contribute to meibomian gland obstruction and subsequent loss of tear film homeostasis. Therefore, an abnormal eyeblink pattern was considered as a part of DED pathogenesis. Previously, few studies focused on the specific influence of upper blepharoplasty on eyeblink and lipid layer (15). Whether the postoperative dry eye symptoms have a correlation with the change in blink parameters and lipid layer is unclear. Thus, the lipid layer thickness (LLT) and blink parameters before and after the surgery need to be evaluated, and the specific influence of transcutaneous upper blepharoplasty on the LLT and blink parameters needs to be confirmed.

Eyeblink is a fast eyelid movement that closes and opens the palpebral fissure (13, 16, 17); it is difficult to measure and analyze blink parameters. Recently, some new devices are being used to analyze eyeblink patterns. One of these is a LipiView interferometer (TearScience, NC, USA), which provides clinicians with the LLT of the tear film and partial blink rate (PBR) (14, 18, 19).

Therefore, this prospective study was designed to observe the effect of transcutaneous upper eyelid blepharoplasty on the LLT, blink parameters, and tear film stability, and also evaluate the relationship between blink parameters, LLT, and tear film stability using the LipiView interferometer.

METHODS

This single-institution prospective, observational clinical study was approved by the ethics committee of the Shanghai Ninth People's Hospital. The study began on January 1, 2019, and lasted for 10 months. It was conducted in accordance with the 1964 Helsinki declaration and its later amendments or comparable ethical standards. Prior written informed consent was obtained from all patients after receiving a detailed explanation of the study protocols and possible consequences associated with participation.

Participants

A total of 55 female patients (110 eyes) referred to the Department of Ophthalmology of Shanghai Ninth People's Hospital, who underwent upper eyelid blepharoplasty, were included in the study.

Patients with a history of ophthalmic surgeries (intraocular surgeries, eyelid surgeries, etc.); previous dry eye disease; systemic diseases as thyroid eye disease, disorders of the eyelids, and other ophthalmic diseases that required priority treatment; glaucoma; incomplete medical patient records, and age <18 years or >35 years were excluded from the study.

Surgical Procedures

The surgeries were performed by a single surgeon (Y.F.) using the same techniques. The incision line was marked about 6–10 mm above the upper lid. The orbicularis oculi muscle was removed inferior to the incision within 2–3 mm. Then, the septum was incised to expose and remove the fat tissue over the top of the tarsus. The incision was closed using a 6–0 silk suture through the skin and aponeurosis.

Clinical Evaluation

All patients were scheduled for examinations before the surgery and 1 week and 1 month after the surgery. At each scheduled time point, subjective symptoms were evaluated using the ocular surface disease index (OSDI) questionnaire, and then clinical examinations were performed in the following order: lipid layer thickness (LLT) measurement, blink parameter analysis, noninvasive tear breakup time (NITBUT), and palpebral fissure height (PFH). All the clinical examinations were performed by a single clinician (SZ) at the same room location at each visit.

The LLT and blink parameters were analyzed with the LipiView interferometer. The patients positioned their eyes in front of an illumination source and were asked to blink freely, and a 20-s video was captured and recorded. The interferometric color unit value reflected the local LLT with 1 color unit equivalent to 1 nm of lipid layer thickness. The number of blinks and partial blinks were recorded, and PBR was calculated as the rate between the two.

The NITBUT was recorded using the Keratograph 5M (Oculus, Optikgerate, Germany). The examination was carried out and repeated three times under the condition of natural eye opening, and the average value was recorded.

The PFH was measured using an imaging system designed based on a convolutional neural network. The images of the eyes were documented at each time point.

Statistical Analysis

Statistical analysis was performed with SPSS for Windows version 25.0 (SPSS Inc., IL, USA). Descriptive statistics were

TABLE 1 | Comparison of preoperative and postoperative ocular surface parameters (**$P < 0.001$).

Ocular surface parameters	Before the surgery	After the surgery		P value	
		1 week	1 month	1 week after the surgery vs. before the surgery	1 month after the surgery vs. before the surgery
OSDI	6.58 ± 0.36	8.89 ± 0.41	11.95 ± 0.55	<0.001**	<0.001**
LLT_{av}, nm	76.74 ± 2.51	89.44 ± 1.75	90.85 ± 1.72	<0.001**	<0.001**
$NITBUT_{av}$, s	8.91 ± 0.40	11.66 ± 0.36	8.72 ± 0.35	<0.001**	0.17
Number of blinks	7.40 ± 0.18	6.36 ± 0.17	7.43 ± 0.20	<0.001**	0.73
Number of partial blinks	4.22 ± 0.34	5.12 ± 0.24	4.29 ± 0.38	0.002**	0.57
PBR	0.58 ± 0.05	0.81 ± 0.03	0.58 ± 0.04	<0.001**	0.80
PFH, mm	9.45 ± 0.12	8.52 ± 0.13	9.31 ± 0.11	<0.001**	0.08

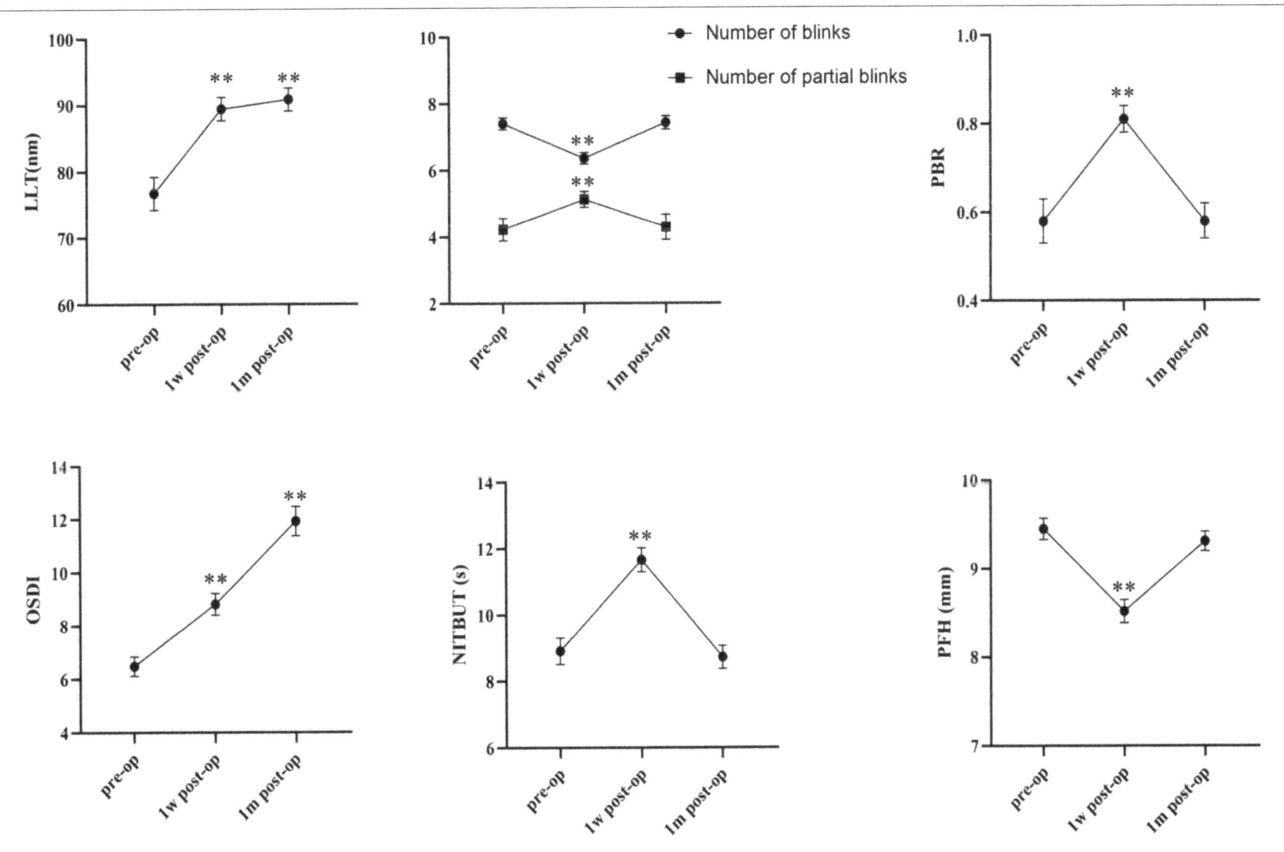

FIGURE 1 | Graph depicting mean and standard error (SE) for OSDI, LLT, NITBUT, PFH, number of blinks, number of partial blinks, and PBR before and after upper blepharoplasty (**$P < 0.001$) (pre-op, preoperative; post-op, postoperative; 1w, 1 week; 1m, 1 month).

expressed as mean ± standard error (SE). Data were examined for normality using the Shapiro–Wilk test. A generalized estimation equation (GEE) was used to compare the variables of interest among different visits. The working correlation for each GEE model was selected using the corrected quasi-likelihood under the independence model criterion. The Spearman correlation coefficient (r) was calculated to assess the relationship between blink parameters, LLT, NITBUT, and OSDI value. All tests were two-tailed, and a $P < 0.05$ was considered significant.

RESULTS

A total of 110 eyes of 55 female patients were identified. The mean age of the participants was 25.18 ± 2.99 (mean ± standard deviation) years (range, 19–31 years). The ocular findings based on routine ancillary tests performed in the cornea clinic are shown in **Table 1**.

A significant decrease was observed in number of blinks and PFH 1 week after the surgery; these values returned to baseline 1 month after the surgery (number of blinks: before the surgery, 7.40 ± 0.18; 1 week after the surgery, 6.36 ± 0.17, $P < 0.001$; 1 month after the surgery, 7.43 ± 0.20, $P = 0.73$; PFH: before the surgery, 9.45 ± 0.12; 1 week after the surgery, 8.52 ± 0.13, $P < 0.001$; 1 month after the surgery, 9.31 ± 0.11, $P = 0.08$). A significant increase in the number of partial blinks and PBR was observed 1 week after the surgery, and the values 1 month after the surgery had no significant differences compared with preoperative values (number of partial blinks: before the surgery, 4.22 ± 0.34; 1 week after the surgery, 5.12 ± 0.24, $P = 0.002$; 1 month after the surgery, 4.29 ± 0.38, $P = 0.57$; PBR: before the surgery, 0.58 ± 0.05; 1 week after the surgery, 0.81 ± 0.03, $P < 0.001$; 1 month after the surgery, 0.58 ± 0.04, $P = 0.80$). The OSDI value and LLT significantly increased 1 week after the surgery and increased further 1 month after the surgery (OSDI: before the surgery, 6.48 ± 0.36; 1 week after the surgery, 8.82 ± 0.41, $P < 0.001$; 1 month after the surgery, 11.93 ± 0.55, $P < 0.001$; LLT: before the surgery, 76.74 ± 2.51; 1 week after the surgery, 89.44 ± 1.75, $P < 0.001$; 1 month after the surgery, 90.85 ± 1.72, $P < 0.001$). The mean NITBUT increased significantly and returned to preoperative levels 1 week after the surgery (before the surgery, 8.91 ± 0.40; 1 week after the surgery, 11.66 ± 0.36, $P < 0.001$; 1 month after the surgery, 8.72 ± 0.35, $P = 0.17$; **Figure 1**).

The number of blinks had a statistically significant correlation with NITBUT and LLT ($r = -0.13$, $P = 0.02$; $r = -0.13$, $P = 0.02$). The PFH correlated significantly with the NITBUT ($r = -0.12$, $P = 0.03$); but the coefficients of correlation were less than 0.2 and had no clinical significance. No correlation was found between the other parameters (**Table 2**).

TABLE 2 | Correlation between blink parameters and ocular surface parameters (*$P < 0.05$).

		OSDI	NITBUT	LLT
Number of blinks	*r*	0.03	−0.13	−0.13
	P	0.59	0.02*	0.02*
Number of partial blinks	*r*	0.02	0.04	−0.02
	P	0.72	0.46	0.74
PBR	*r*	0.03	0.09	0.05
	P	0.64	0.11	0.40
PFH	*r*	−0.08	−0.12	−0.08
	P	0.13	0.03*	0.13

DISCUSSION

DED is caused by a variety of iatrogenic interventions, and one of the most emblematic situations is DED caused by surgical procedures (20). The increasing number of patients looking for cosmetic procedures has drawn more attention to DED caused or worsened by blepharoplasty (21). Studies indicated that the prevalence of DED after blepharoplasty ranged from 0 to 26.5% (3, 4, 22). Previous studies investigated the changes in tear film parameters after upper blepharoplasty (6, 23), but only a few of them paid attention to the changes in lipid layer and eyeblink parameters. Therefore, this study was performed to observe the specific influence of transcutaneous upper blepharoplasty on LLT, blink parameters, and tear film stability in young Asian women during the early postoperative period, using the LipiView interferometer and Keratograph 5M.

The results showed that blink patterns changed 1 week after the surgery and returned to baseline in 1 month. The number of blinks decreased while the number of partial blinks and PBR increased 1 week after the surgery. Eyeblink is a complex process influenced by many factors, such as ocular surface damage and exposure, corneal and lid margin sensitivity, muscular fatigue and tension, and so on (16). The active forces that produce the movement of the upper eyelid during a blink are generated only by the orbicularis oculi muscle and levator palpebral superior muscle. The transcutaneous upper blepharoplasty performed in the present study involved the removal of the orbicularis oculi muscle (2–3 mm) and periorbital fat. The surgical procedure caused tissue trauma, which led to inflammatory responses and postoperative periorbital swelling. During the early postoperative period, patients blinked less and incompletely due to the swelling and incision pain. However, this phenomenon was temporary. Patients were used to the condition, and the incision pain was greatly eased 1 month after the surgery. Hence, the blink patterns returned to baseline, indicating that the limited excision of the orbicularis oculi muscle did not affect blink patterns in young patients.

In this study, the postoperative LLT significantly increased compared with the preoperative value. The driving forces leading to meibum secretion onto the lid margin and tear film are responsible for the mechanical muscular action by muscle fibers of the pretarsal orbicularis muscle, located on the outside of the tarsus, and of the marginal muscle of Riolan, which encircles the terminal part of the meibomian gland (9). The transcutaneous blepharoplasty removed part of the orbicularis muscle, but did not involve the muscle of Riolan, thus retaining the maximum driving force on the meibomian glands. The meibum is secreted by the meibomian gland through the thickness of the lids due to pressure on the glands (10). The upper eyelid is thickened due to surgical damage, and the postoperative swollen eyelid contributes to the increased pressure on the meibomian glands. The PFH decreased during the early postoperative period, indicating a reduction in the ocular surface area. Therefore, the LLT increased 1 week and 1 month after the surgery due to increased meibum secretion and decreased ocular surface area.

Previous experiments have shown that tear film breakup occurs mainly as a result of evaporation from the tear film (8). The lipid layer is of great importance for the stabilization of the air/aqueous tear interface of the tear film (11). Thus, the NITBUT increased 1 week after the surgery and returned to baseline 1 month after the surgery, indicating that the effect of blepharoplasty on the tear film breakup time was temporary.

However, despite the increased LLT and NITBUT, the results showed that OSDI values increased 1 week and 1 month after the surgery, demonstrating the worsening of the subjective symptoms of the patients. Although the patients' objective signs improved, they still complained of suffering from more severe dry eye symptoms. The main complaints of the patient were the foreign body sensation and irritation. The decreased number of blinks and increased PBR would aggravate the foreign body sensation and irritation, and led to increase of OSDI values (16). And it was assumed that postoperative inflammation and incision pain might aggravate the subjective feeling.

In addition, no correlation was observed between blink parameters and ocular surface parameters. Previous studies showed that partial blink correlated with ocular surface parameters (14, 19). However, these studies were performed on middle-aged and elderly patients with DED, while the present study was conducted on normal young women. Young women had good muscle function with a small degree of partial blink. Therefore, the blink parameters had no correlation with ocular surface parameters. Moreover, the lack of correlation between LLT and other parameters was in accordance with previous findings, highlighting the difference between the thickness of the lipid layer and its quality.

This study was novel in focusing on the effect of transcutaneous upper blepharoplasty on LLT and blink parameters in young women, while previous studies were mostly carried out on elders and paid no attention to eyeblink parameters and LLT. However, the present study had certain limitations. In the present study, the blink parameters and NITBUT returned to baseline 1 month after the surgery, which was sufficient to observe the effect of upper blepharoplasty on blink parameters. However, the LLT did not return to baseline 1 month after the surgery, which might be related to eyelid edema. In the early stage, the eyelid edema had a dominant role. However, the effect of the removal of the orbicularis muscle on the LLT when edema was eliminated remains unknown. Long-term follow-up of postoperative patients is required to confirm the findings of this study.

ETHICS STATEMENT

The studies involving human participants were reviewed and approved by the Ethics Committee of the Shanghai Ninth People's Hospital. The patients/participants provided their written informed consent to participate in this study.

AUTHOR CONTRIBUTIONS

SZ: acquisition of data, drafting the article, final approval of the version to be published, and agreement to be accountable for all aspects of the work. YY: analysis and interpretation of data, drafting the article, final approval of the version to be published, and agreement to be accountable for all aspects of the work. YL: acquisition of data, revising it critically for important intellectual content, final approval of the version to be published, and agreement to be accountable for all aspects of the work. YZ: analysis and interpretation of data, revising it critically for important intellectual content, final approval of the version to be published, and agreement to be accountable for all aspects of the work. YF: substantial contributions to conception and design, revising it critically for important intellectual content, final approval of the version to be published, and agreement to be accountable for all aspects of the work. All authors contributed to the article and approved the submitted version.

REFERENCES

1. Jeong S, Lemke BN, Dortzbach RK, Park YG, Kang HK. The Asian upper eyelid: an anatomical study with comparison to the Caucasian eyelid. *Arch Ophthalmol.* (1999) 117:907–12. doi: 10.1001/archopht.117.7.907
2. Pacella SJ, Codner MA. Minor complications after blepharoplasty: dry eyes, chemosis, granulomas, ptosis, scleral show. *Plast Reconstr Surg.* (2010) 125:709–18. doi: 10.1097/PRS.0b013e3181c830c7
3. Leatherbarrow B, Saha K. Complications of blepharoplasty. *Facial Plast Surg.* (2013) 29:281–8. doi: 10.1055/s-0033-1349362
4. Prischmann J, Sufyan A, Ting JY, Ruffin C, Perkins SW. Dry eye symptoms and chemosis following blepharoplasty: a 10-year retrospective review of 892 cases in a single-surgeon series. *JAMA Facial Plast Surg.* (2013) 15:39–46. doi: 10.1001/2013.jamafacial.1
5. Yan Y, Zhou Y, Zhang S, Cui C, Song X, Zhu X, et al. Impact of full-incision double-eyelid blepharoplasty on tear film dynamics and dry eye symptoms in young asian females. *Aesthetic Plast Surg.* (2020) 44:2109–116. doi: 10.1007/s00266-020-01874-0
6. Zloto O, Matani A, Prat D, Leshno A, Ben Simon G. The effect of a ptosis procedure compared to an upper blepharoplasty on dry eye syndrome. *Am J Ophthalmol.* (2020) 212:1–6. doi: 10.1016/j.ajo.2019.11.021
7. Craig JP, Nichols KK, Akpek EK, Caffery B, Dua HS, Joo CK, et al. TFOS DEWS II definition and classification report. *Ocular Surf.* (2017) 15:276–83. doi: 10.1016/j.jtos.2017.05.008
8. Willcox MDP, Argueso P, Georgiev GA, Holopainen JM, Laurie GW, Millar TJ, et al. TFOS DEWS II tear film report. *Ocul Surf.* (2017) 15:366–403. doi: 10.1016/j.jtos.2017.03.006
9. Knop E, Knop N, Millar T, Obata H, Sullivan DA. The international workshop on meibomian gland dysfunction: report of the subcommittee on anatomy, physiology, and pathophysiology of the meibomian gland. *Invest Ophthalmol Vis Sci.* (2011) 52:1938–78. doi: 10.1167/iovs.10-6997c
10. Foulks GN, Bron AJ. Meibomian gland dysfunction: a clinical scheme for description, diagnosis, classification, and grading. *Ocular Surf.* (2003) 1:107–26. doi: 10.1016/S1542-0124(12)70139-8
11. Georgiev GA, Eftimov P, Yokoi N. Structure-function relationship of tear film lipid layer: a contemporary perspective. *Exp Eye Res.* (2017) 163:17–28. doi: 10.1016/j.exer.2017.03.013
12. Hamawy AH, Farkas JP, Fagien S, Rohrich RJ. Preventing and managing dry eyes after periorbital surgery: a retrospective review. *Plast Reconstr Surg.* (2009) 123:353–9. doi: 10.1097/PRS.0b013e31819346ea
13. Braun RJ, King-Smith PE, Begley CG, Li L, Gewecke NR. Dynamics and function of the tear film in relation to the blink cycle. *Prog Retin Eye Res.* (2015) 45:132–64. doi: 10.1016/j.preteyeres.2014.11.001
14. Jie Y, Sella R, Feng J, Gomez ML, Afshari NA. Evaluation of incomplete blinking as a measurement of dry eye disease. *Ocul Surf.* (2019) 17:440–46. doi: 10.1016/j.jtos.2019.05.007
15. Abell KM, Cowen DE, Baker RS, Porter JD. Eyelid kinematics following blepharoplasty. *Ophthalmic Plast Reconstr Surg.* (1999) 15:236–42. doi: 10.1097/00002341-199907000-00003

16. Rodriguez JD, Lane KJ, Ousler GW III, Angjeli E, Smith LM, Abelson MB. Blink: characteristics, controls, and relation to dry eyes. *Curr Eye Res.* (2018) 43:52–66. doi: 10.1080/02713683.2017.1381270
17. Cruz AAV, Garcia DM, Pinto CT, Cechetti SP. Spontaneous Eyeblink activity. *Ocular Surf.* (2011) 9:29–41. doi: 10.1016/S1542-0124(11)70007-6
18. Jung JW, Park SY, Kim JS, Kim EK, Seo KY, Kim TI. Analysis of factors associated with the tear film lipid layer thickness in normal eyes and patients with dry eye syndrome. *Invest Ophthalmol Vis Sci.* (2016) 57:4076–83. doi: 10.1167/iovs.16-19251
19. Su Y, Liang Q, Su G, Wang N, Baudouin C, Labbe A. Spontaneous eye blink patterns in dry eye: clinical correlations. *Invest Ophthalmol Vis Sci.* (2018) 59:5149–56. doi: 10.1167/iovs.18-24690
20. Gomes JAP, Azar DT, Baudouin C, Efron N, Hirayama M, Horwath-Winter J, et al. TFOS DEWS II iatrogenic report. *Ocul Surf.* (2017) 15:511–38. doi: 10.1016/j.jtos.2017.05.004
21. Zhang SY, Yan Y, Fu Y. Cosmetic blepharoplasty and dry eye disease: a review of the incidence, clinical manifestations, mechanisms and prevention. *Int J Ophthalmol.* (2020) 13:488–92. doi: 10.18240/ijo.2020.03.18
22. Terella AM, Wang TD, Kim MM. Complications in periorbital surgery. *Facial Plast Surg.* (2013) 29:64–70. doi: 10.1055/s-0033-1333838
23. Soares A, Faria-Correia F, Franqueira N, Ribeiro S. Effect of superior blepharoplasty on tear film: objective evaluation with the Keratograph 5M - a pilot study. *Arq Bras Oftalmol.* (2018) 81:471–74. doi: 10.5935/0004-2749.20180094

15

Incidence and Risk Factors of Dry Eye in Children and Adolescents With Diabetes Mellitus: A 3-Year Follow-Up Study

Zhangling Chen [1,2], Ying Xiao [3], Yu Qian [4], Qiurong Lin [4], Zhaoyu Xiang [4], Lipu Cui [4], Jiaqi Sun [4], Sicong Li [4], Xinran Qin [4], Chenhao Yang [3] and Haidong Zou [1,4,5,6,7,8]**

[1] Department of Ophthalmology, Shanghai General Hospital of Nanjing Medical University, Shanghai, China, [2] Department of Ophthalmology, Shanghai Songjiang District Central Hospital, Shanghai, China, [3] Department of Ophthalmology, Children's Hospital of Fudan University, Shanghai, China, [4] Department of Ophthalmology, Shanghai General Hospital, Shanghai Jiao Tong University School of Medicine, Shanghai, China, [5] Shanghai Key Laboratory of Fundus Diseases, Shanghai, China, [6] Shanghai Eye Diseases Prevention & Treatment Center, Shanghai Eye Hospital, Shanghai, China, [7] National Clinical Research Center for Eye Diseases, Shanghai, China, [8] Shanghai Engineering Center for Precise Diagnosis and Treatment of Eye Diseases, Shanghai, China

***Correspondence:**
Haidong Zou
zouhaidong@sjtu.edu.cn
Chenhao Yang
ychben@hotmail.com

Purpose: To investigate the incidence and risk factors of dry eye in children with diabetes mellitus (DM) over a period of 3 years.

Methods: Children and adolescents with DM (age: 3–14 years) from the Shanghai Children and Adolescent Diabetes Eye (SCADE) study cohort who did not have dry eye in January 2018 were followed-up for 3 years and re-examined in January 2021, and the incidence rate and risk factors for dry eye were calculated.

Results: Forty children and adolescents with DM came for follow-up in 2021. Nine of them were diagnosed with dry eye, resulting in a 3-year incidence rate of 22.5% and an annual mean incidence rate of 7.5% for dry eye. Univariate regression analysis confirmed that decreased corneal sensation (OR [Odds Ratio] = 25.60; 95%CI [Confidence Interval] = 1.31~501.69; $P = 0.03$) was the risk factor for dry eye incidence. Long course of DM (OR = 1.80; 95%CI = 0.96~3.38; $P = 0.07$), eye pain (OR = 12.27; 95%CI = 0.65~231.48; $P = 0.09$), and dry eye in parents (OR = 15.99; 95%CI = 0.76~337.75; $P = 0.08$) may interfere with the incidence of dry eye in them.

Conclusions: The incidence of dry eye in children and adolescents with DM is high.

Keywords: children and adolescents, diabetes, dry eye, morbidity, risk factors

INTRODUCTION

The prevalence of diabetes mellitus (DM) is increasing every year globally. The International Diabetes Federation revealed that in 2011, the number of DM patients worldwide was 370 million, and the number may reach ~550 million by 2030, of which 80% will be from developing countries (1). In 2017, the numbers of children and adolescents (age: <20 years) with type 1 DM in the world and China were 1,106,500 and 47,000, respectively (2). The risk of chronic eye disease always increases with the progression of DM, for example, dry eye, which is a multifactorial disease of the tear and eyeball surface, causing ocular discomfort, visual impairment, tear osmotic pressure increase, and ocular surface inflammation (3). Risk factors for dry eye in the adults include reduced lacrimal gland secretion, changes in tear composition, instable tear film, decreased density of the corneal and conjunctival nerves, reduced number of conjunctival goblet cells, and meibomian gland dysfunction (4–6). The worldwide prevalence of dry eye is ~7–33% (7). Manaviat et al. (8) found that dry eye symptoms happened in 54.3% of the adult patients with type 2 DM, much higher than that of the normal individuals.

Previous epidemiology studies of dry eye in children with DM only reported the prevalence (9, 10), and found the relationship between dry eye and fasting blood glucose, HbA1c values (11), and ocular surface impairment; (9, 12, 13) however, no study has investigated the incidence of dry eye in children with DM or without. In 2018, our team established the Shanghai Children and Adolescent Diabetes Eye Study (SCADE Study) cohort, then we found that the prevalence of dry eye was much higher in children with DM (28.95%) than in normal children (5.00%) in 2018 (10). Since then, we followed these children annually. In the present study, the incidence rate and risk factors of dry eye in them over a 3-year period time are reported.

METHODS

Research Objective

The participants in the SCADE study cohort without dry eye in January 2018 came for follow up in January 2021 were enrolled in the present study. Inclusion criteria were set as follows: (1) providing written informed consent; (2) aged 6–17 years in 2021; (3) diagnosed with type 1 DM; and (4) fulfill the questionnaire and underwent all eye examinations. Exclusion criteria were set as follows: (1) other ocular and systemic diseases that affect tear secretion and quality, such as eyelid diseases (trichiasis, eyelid eversion, ptosis, and eyelid incompleteness) and conjunctival diseases (acute and chronic infectious conjunctivitis, allergic conjunctivitis, and conjunctival calculus); (2) a history of eye trauma within 6 months; (3) a history of eye surgery within 6 months; (4) severe eye complications caused by DM; (6) receiving eye treatment with eye drops; and (7) with systemic diseases such as systemic lupus erythematosus, Sjogren's syndrome, and Grave's disease. This study was conducted in accordance with the ethical standards of the Helsinki Declaration, and all participants (or their guardians) provided informed consent. This study was approved by the Institutional Review Committee and the Ethics Committee of Shanghai General Hospital, Shanghai Jiao Tong University School of Medicine (approval number: 2018KY209).

Questionnaires and Examination Items

We used two questionnaires: the Ocular Surface Disease Index (OSDI) and Dry Eye Questionnaire (DEQ), including questions on name, sex, date of birth, height, weight, cell phone number, address, date of examination, presence of diabetes, diabetes type, presence of diabetes complications, history of eye disease (trichiasis and allergic conjunctivitis), ocular trauma, ocular surgery, or medication, presence of eye discomfort (foreign body sensation, fatigue, pain force fluctuations, and frequent blinking), use of contact lens, reading and writing posture, presence of sleep disorders, mental status, dietary preferences, use of air conditioner, passive smoking, daily time spent on electronic screens, refractive errors, and dry eye in parents.

The following examinations were conducted: (1) The best-corrected visual acuity was measured using the LogMAR visual acuity chart (Wenzhou Xingkang, Zhejiang, China), which meets international standards. Cyclopentolate hydrochloride eye drops (Alcon, Belgium) were used for dilation. Refraction was measured using a computerized automatic optometry device (KR-8900, Topcon, Japan), and the final refraction was measured using a comprehensive optometry device (CV-5000, Topcon). (2) A slit-lamp biomicroscope (SL130, Zeiss, Germany) was used to examine the eyelid, conjunctiva, cornea, anterior chamber, iris, pupil, lens, tear film rupture time, and corneal fluorescein staining. (3) Qualitative examination of corneal sensation was performed using a long and thin cotton thread that was twisted out from the tip of a disinfected cotton swab by bending the tip on a cotton stick at 45°. The cornea of the eye under examination was approached from the side with the tip of the cotton thread and gently touched. Patients with normal corneal sensation had immediate blink reflex or perception. (4) The Schirmer I test was performed to assess tear secretion without superficial anesthesia. (5) Biometric examination (IOL Master 700, Zeiss, Germany) was performed to determine the ocular axis, radius of corneal curvature, anterior chamber depth, lens thickness, central corneal thickness, and corneal diameter. (6) A non-contact tonometer (NT-510, NIDEK, Japan) was used to measure the intraocular pressure (IOP) in both eyes. (7) Corneal endothelium counter (TOPCON, SP-2000P) was used to record the number of corneal endothelia in both eyes.

Dry Eye Diagnosis Index

Tear secretion test (Schirmer *I*-test): The tip of the Schirmer paper (Jingming, Tianjin, China) (5 × 35 mm) was folded into the conjunctival sac, the eyes closed normally, and the length of the tear soaked paper was measured after 5 min.

Break-up Time (BUT) measurement: The saline moistened fluorescein paper (Jingming, Tianjin) was lightly touched to the conjunctiva of the patients; consequently, patients blinked three to four times, spreading the fluorescein evenly on the cornea. The time from the last blink of the eye to the appearance of the first black spot on the corneal surface was the tear film rupture time, which was measured three times to obtain the average value.

Cornea fluorescein staining (CFS): The cornea was observed after uniform staining with fluorescein. No corneal staining was recorded as negative, whereas presence of corneal staining was considered positive.

Diagnostic Criteria

According to the 2020 Chinese expert consensus on examination and diagnosis of dry eye (14), diagnosis of dry eye can be made based on the following criteria: (1) the patient complaining of one of the subjective symptoms such as eye dryness, foreign body sensation, burning sensation, fatigue, discomfort, redness, and fluctuation of vision and having an OSDI of ≥13 points and a BUT of ≤5 s or a Schirmer *I*-test value of ≤5 mm/5 min. (2) Patients with dry eye-related symptoms, an OSDI score of ≥13 points, a BUT of >5 s and ≤10 s or a Schirmer I test value of >5 mm/5 min and ≤10 mm/5 min, and positive staining with fluorescein sodium. Any eye meeting one of the aforementioned criteria was diagnosed as dry eye.

Quality Control

All children were examined at the Shanghai Eye Disease Prevention & Treatment Center. All eye examinations were performed by the same trained ophthalmologist to ensure consistency in the results.

Statistical Analysis

IBM SPSS Statistics 22.0 statistical software was used for analysis. The measurement data were tested for K-S normality and the measurement data with normal distribution were presented as mean ± standard deviation and an independent sample *t-test* was performed for between group comparisons. The measurement data with non-normal distribution are presented as median (25%, 75%) and a non-parametric independent sample *U*-test was performed for between group comparisons. Enumerative data were compared between the groups using the Pearson

TABLE 1 | Characteristics and eye examination results of 40 children with DM.

Characteristics	Subjects with dry eye	Subjects without dry eye	Statistics#	P
Total number	9	31		
Gender/male (cases)	2	16	$x^2 = 1.39$	0.24
Age (years)	12.60 ± 2.69	12.56 ± 3.28	$t = 0.03$	0.97
The course of DM (years)	8.04 (6.25, 9.88)	4.76 (3.81, 7.28)	$U = 219.5$	0.01
BMI* (kg/m²)	19.26 ± 2.32	20.23 ± 2.81	$t = 0.94$	0.35
OSDI (scores)	17.00 (16.50, 19.50)	10.00 (8.00, 12.00)	$U = 278$	<0.01
HbA1c (mg/ml)	7.33 ± 1.26	8.22 ± 1.65	$t = 1.00$	0.33
Better-seeing eye BUT (s)	5.00 (4.50, 7.50)	10.00 (9.00, 12.00)	$U = 15$	<0.01
Better-seeing eye Schirmer *I*-test (mm/5 min)	8.00 (4.50, 15.00)	18.00 (15.00, 25.00)	$U = 42$	<0.01
Corneal hypoparesis (cases)	8	6	$x^2 = 11.93$	<0.01
Corneal fluorescein staining/positive (cases)	5	1	$x^2 = 11.16$	<0.01

BMI, Body mass index.
#t is an independent sample t-test, U is a non-parametric independent sample U-test, and x^2 is a chi-square test.

TABLE 2 | The questionnaire information of 40 children with DM.

Items	Subjects with dry eye	Subjects without dry eye	Statistics (X^2)*	P
History of eye surgery/yes (cases)	0	0	–	–
History of eye trauma/yes (cases)	0	0	–	–
History of ocular medication/yes (cases)	2	3	1	0.32
Eating habits/meat (cases)	8	15	3.17	0.08
Allergic conjunctivitis/yes (cases)	2	3	0.13	0.72
Trichiasis/yes (cases)	0	0	–	–
Eye pain/yes (cases)	6	5	6.58	0.01*
Foreign body sensation in the eyes/yes (cases)	4	3	3.68	0.55
Vision fluctuation/yes (cases)	3	12	0.07	0.77
Refractive errors/yes (cases)	5	20	0.24	0.63
Use of contact lenses/yes (cases)	0	1	–	1
Reading and writing posture/right (cases)	5	10	1.62	0.2
Sleep disorders/yes (cases)	1	5	0.12	0.71
Using air conditioning/yes (cases)	8	24	0.57	0.45
Passive smoking/yes (cases)	0	2	–	1
Use electronic screen/mild (cases)	7	19	0.13	0.72
Eye strain/yes (cases)	7	20	0.56	0.46
Mental pressure/yes (cases)	3	13	0.22	0.64
Like blinking eyes/yes (cases)	3	7	0.43	0.51
Dry eye in parents/yes (cases)	7	10	4.2	0.04*

**x^2 is a chi-square test.*

χ^2-test, continuity corrected χ^2-test, or Fisher's exact test. First, univariate analysis was performed to analyze the eye examination results and questionnaire survey results, independent variables with a $P < 0.05$ in univariate analysis were used to perform binary logistic regression analysis. The incidence of dry eye was considered the dependent variable. A $P < 0.05$ was considered statistically significant.

RESULTS

A total of 123 children and adolescent patients with DM are enrolled in the SCADE study. Because of the COVID-19 pandemic, only 40 of them (32.5%) were enrolled in the present study. The eye examination results of them are presented in **Table 1**. Among them, 55% (22/40) were girls and 45% (18/40) were boys. In 2018, none of the patients were diagnosed with dry eyer, and nine of them were diagnosed with dry eye by 2021, with both eyes meeting the criteria for dry eye. Among them, 77.8% (7/9) were girls, and 22.2% (2/9) were boys. The 3-year of rate of dry eye in children with DM was then calculated as 22.5% (9/40), with an average annual incidence rate of 7.5%.

The results of univariate analysis for the incidence of dry eye in children with DM are presented in **Tables 2, 3**. Statistically significant differences were observed in the course of diabetes mellitus, corneal sensation (sensitive/less sensitive), eye pain (with/without), and dry eye in parents (with/without) in children with DM ($P < 0.05$). Further logistic regression analysis confirmed that the risk factor of the incidence of dry eye in children with DM was reduced corneal sensation ($P < 0.05$), as shown in **Table 4**.

DISCUSSION

An increase in the number of children and adolescents with DM poses a serious economic burden on society; hence, measures to control the risk factors and reduce the morbidity rate of dry eye in them should be taken. According to previous study (13), when blood glucose keeps stable, the ocular surface impairment of patients may still aggravate in children with type 1 DM. The strict study design and uniform definitions and standards in our 3-year prospective study reveal the incidence and risk factors of dry eye in pediatric diabetes.

Previous studies have reported that the factors related to the prevalence of dry eye in adult patients with DM were age, sex, course of disease, corneal perception, fasting blood glucose (FBG), and glycosylated hemoglobin levels (HBA1c) (10, 15, 16). It is believed that the prevalence of dry eye in patients with DM increases with the increase of age, and the prevalence of dry eye in adult patients with DM is as high as 54.3% (8). Female patients with DM are more likely to suffer from dry eye (15). The prevalence of dry eye was higher in patients with high FBG and HBA1c (16).

The risk factors of high incidence of dry eye in children with DM is not the same as previous results in adults with DM. Previous cross-sectional study (10) showed that the corneal sensation was lower in children diagnosed with dry eye than those without. In the present prospective study, reduced corneal

TABLE 3 | Better-seeing Eye examination results of 40 children with DM.

Items	Subjects with dry eye	Subjects without dry eye	Statistics	P
The number of children with DM	9	31		
Equivalent spherical lens degree (D)*	−1.40 ± 1.96	−2.72 ± 2.75	$t = 1.33$	0.19
Corneal endothelial cell count (/mm^2)	3188.00 ± 426.69	3058.80 ± 378.66	$t = 0.82$	0.43
Ocular axial length (mm)	23.90 ± 0.81	24.57 ± 1.34	$t = -1.42$	0.16
Horizontal corneal radius of curvature, R1 (mm)	7.93 ± 0.27	7.95 ± 0.28	$t = -0.2$	0.85
Vertical corneal radius of curvature, R2 (mm)	7.64 ± 0.25	7.70 ± 0.30	$t = -0.59$	0.56
Corneal horizontal diameter (mm)	12.24 ± 0.41	12.13 ± 0.34	$t = 0.76$	0.46
Central corneal thickness (nm)	539.22 ± 33.16	552.55 ± 29.69	$t = -1.16$	0.25
Anterior chamber depth (mm)	3.65 ± 0.27	3.65 ± 0.26	$t = 0$	1
Lens thickness (mm)	3.52 ± 0.15	3.46 ± 0.24	$t = 0.76$	0.45

Equivalent spherical refraction = sphere + 1/2 cylinder.

TABLE 4 | Results of multivariate logistic regression analysis for dry eye in children with DM.

	β	S.E.	Wald	P	OR	95% CI
Corneal sensation (decrease)	3.24	1.52	4.56	0.03	25.6	1.31–501.69
The course of DM (years)	0.59	0.32	3.3	0.07	1.8	0.96–3.38
Eye pain (yes)	2.51	1.5	2.8	0.09	12.27	0.65–231.48
Dry eye in parents (yes)	2.77	1.56	3.17	0.08	15.99	0.76–337.75
Constant	−9.71	3.49	7.74	0.01	0	

sensation is confirmed as the only statistically significant risk factor of dry eye. A clinical study conducted by Alise et al. showed that the degree of reduced corneal sensitivity in adult patients with DM was positively correlated with the severity of dry eye (17). The possible mechanisms involved may be that high-level glycosylated end metabolites may cause metabolic damage to the peripheral corneal nerve (18) and thus, reduce the corneal perceptual sensitivity and tear secretion in patients with DM (19–21). Additionally, corneal perception is positively correlated with blink reflex (22, 23) and the decrease in blink reflex can accelerate tear evaporation and lead to an increase in tear osmotic pressure.

Other factors may affect the incidence of dry eye (P close to 0.05) are the following: firstly, the course of DM: previous studies in adult populations have found that the longer the course of DM, the more severe damage of accessory lacrimal gland cells and the less the basic secretion of tears, and therefore, the increased prevalence of dry eye (24–26). Akinci et al. (9) believed that the duration of disease in patients with type 1 DM was the only factor related to tear secretion and tear film stability. Secondly, eye pain: Xiang et al. (27) believed that corneal neuralgia was a pre-clinical manifestation of dry eye. We believe that the cornea tissue damage may release inflammatory factors, stimulate corneal pain receptors, cause eye pain, and aggravate dry eye. Thirdly, family history: after further inquiry, we confirmed that none of the parents of the children with dry eye were DM patients or with other systemic diseases related to dry eye. Therefore, we speculated that this was related to the living environment, living habits, dietary structure, and micro-ecological structure of the children; however, further study is required to confirm these speculations.

Since all the subjects in this study were children aged 6–17 years, the age distribution difference and sample size were both small, and therefore, the age factor had no significant influence on the incidence of dry eye in children and adolescents with DM. In this study, all young patients wore insulin pumps, and then fasting and postprandial blood glucose were well-controlled. These may be the reason for no correlation between blood glucose and HbA1c levels and the incidence of dry eye in children with DM.

The shortcomings of this study are the following: no gold standard for the diagnosis of dry eye in children is currently available and therefore, we used the standard diagnosis criteria of dry eye in the adult population with diabetes mellitus. The participants of the SCADE cohort were students who had a tight course schedule, and furthermore, affected by the COVID-19 pandemic, many parents of the children included in the 2018 SCADE study withdrew from this investigation, resulting in a small sample size of the present study.

In conclusion, the incidence of dry eye in children with DM is high. Children with reduced corneal sensation, long course of diabetes, dry eye in parents, or eye pain should be examined for dry eye for early diagnosis and treatment to improve prognosis and the quality of life. Society, especially parents of these children, should be made aware of this through publicity and education. Simultaneously, it is necessary to establish a screening mode and better file management system, formulate prevention and treatment norms, and strengthen the scientific management of dry eye in children with DM.

ETHICS STATEMENT

The studies involving human participants were reviewed and approved by the Institutional Review Committee and the Ethics Committee of the First People's Hospital Affiliated to Shanghai Jiao Tong University (approval number: 2018KY209). Written informed consent to participate in this study was provided by the participants' legal guardian/next of kin.

AUTHOR CONTRIBUTIONS

ZC: substantial contributions to the conception or design of the work or the acquisition, analysis, or interpretation of data for the work. HZ: drafting the work or revising it critically for important intellectual content, final approval of the version to be published, and agreement to be accountable for all aspects of the work in ensuring that questions related to the accuracy or integrity of any part of the work are appropriately investigated and resolved. YX, YQ, QL, ZX, LC, JS, SL, XQ, and CY: participate in survey and data collection. All authors contributed to the article and approved the submitted version.

REFERENCES

1. American Diabetes Association. Standards of medical care in diabetes-2013. *Diabetes Care.* (2013) 36:S11–66. doi: 10.2337/dc13-S011
2. Cho NH, Shaw JE, Karuranga S, Huang Y, Rocha Fernandes JD, da Ohlrogge AW, et al. IDF Diabetes Atlas: global estimates of diabetes prevalence for 2017 and projections for 2045. *Diabetes Res Clin Pract.* (2018) 138:271–81. doi: 10.1016/j.diabres.2018.02.023
3. Zhao KX, Yang PZ, Fan XQ, Sun XH, Liu YZ, Zhao GQ, et al. *Ophthalmology.* 9th Ed. Beijing: People's Medical Publishing House (2018). p. 82–4.
4. Gao CL, Lu FQ. Epidemiological characteristics of dry eye in ophthalmology department. *J Shanxi Med Univ.* (2011) 42:667–9. doi: 10.3969/J.ISSN.1007-6611.2011.08.016
5. Meng LH. Preliminary investigation on the prevalence of dry eye in ophthalmology clinic and health guidance. *Int J Ophthalmol.* (2011) 11:2005–6. doi: 10.3969/j.issn.1672-5123.2011.11.045
6. Qiao YB, Yi H, Nie X. Epidemiological investigation of dry eye disease in 620 cases of ophthalmic clinic. *Chongqing Med J.* (2013) 42:1623–5. doi: 10.3969/j.issn.1671-8348.2013.14.021
7. Gayton JL. Etiology,prevalence,and treatment of dry eye disease. *Clin Ophthalmol.* (2009) 3:405–12. doi: 10.2147/OPTH.S5555
8. Manaviat MR, Rashidi M, Afkhami-Ardekani M, Shoja MR. Prevalence of dry eye syndrome and diabetic retinopathy in type 2 diabetic patients. *BMC Ophthalmol.* (2008) 8:284–91. doi: 10.1186/1471-2415-8-10
9. Akinci A, Cetinkaya E, Aycan Z. Dry eye syndrome in diabetic children. *Eur J Ophthalmol.* (2007) 17:873–8. doi: 10.1177/112067210701700601

10. Wang S, Jia Y, Li T, Wang A, Gao L, Yang CH, et al. Dry eye disease is more prevalent in children with diabetes than in those without diabetes. *Curr Eye Res.* (2019) 44:1299–305. doi: 10.1080/02713683.2019.1641827
11. Akil H, Buluş AD, Andiran N, Alp MN. Ocular manifestations of Type 1 diabetes mellitus in pediatric population. *Indian J Ophthalmol.* (2016) 64:654–8. doi: 10.4103/0301-4738.194336
12. Gunay M, Celik G, Yildiz E, Bardak H, Koc N, Kirmizibekmez H, et al. Ocular surface characteristics in diabetic children. *Curr Eye Res.* (2016) 41:1526–31. doi: 10.3109/02713683.2015.1136421
13. Inanc M, Kiziltoprak H, Hekimoglu R, Tekin K, Ozalkak S, Koc M, et al. Alterations of tear film and ocular surface in children with type 1 diabetes mellitus. *Ocul Immunol Inflamm.* (2020) 28:362–9. doi: 10.1080/09273948.2019.1571212
14. Liu ZG, Sun XG, Zhang MC, Xu JJ, Hong J, Deng YP, et al. Asia dry eye association, professional committee of ophthalmology of cross-strait medical and health exchange association, Chinese branch, ophthalmology and dryness group, ophthalmology and dryness group, ophthalmology branch of Chinese medical doctor association (in Chinese with english abstract). *J Ophthalmol* (2020) 56:741–7. doi: 10.3760/cma.j.cn112142-20200714-00477
15. Kaiserman I, Kaiserman N, Nakar S, Vinker S. Dry eye in diabetic patients. *Am J Ophthalmol.* (2005) 139:498–503. doi: 10.1016/j.ajo.2004.10.022
16. Ozdemir M, Buyukbese MA, Cetinkaya A, Ozdemir G. Risk factors for ocular surface disorders in patients with diabetes mellitus. *Diabetes Res Clin Pract.* (2003) 59:195–9. doi: 10.1016/S0168-8227(02)00244-9
17. Alise K, Maryam F, Shazli A, Andrew M, Handrean S, Rayaz AM. Keratocyte density is reduced and related to corneal nerve damage in diabetic neuropathy. *Invest Ophthalmol Vis Sci.* (2018) 59:3584–90. doi: 10.1167/iovs.18-23889
18. Mansoor H, Tan HC, Lin MT, Mehta JS, Liu YC. Diabetic corneal neuropathy. *AJ Clin Med.* (2020) 9:3956. doi: 10.3390/jcm9123956
19. Bourcier T, Acosta MC, Borderie V, Borras F, Gallar J, Bury T, et al. Decreased corneal sensitivity in patients with dry eye. *Invest Ophthalmol Vis Sci.* (2005) 46:2341–5. doi: 10.1167/iovs.04-1426
20. Achtsidis V, Eleftheriadou I, Kozanidou E. Dry eye syndrome in subjects with diabetes and association with neuropathy. *Diabetes Care.* (2014) 37:e210–1. doi: 10.2337/dc14-0860
21. Nepp J, Abela C, Polzer I, Derbolav A, Wedrich A. Is there a correlation between the severity of diabetic retinopathy and keratoconjunctivitis sicca? *Cornea.* (2000) 19:487–91. doi: 10.1097/00003226-200007000-00017
22. De Cillà S, Ranno S, Carini E, Fogagnolo P, Ceresara G, Orzalesi N, et al. Corneal subbasal nerves changes in patients with diabetic retinopathy: an in vivo confocal study. *Invest Ophthalmol Vis Sci.* (2009) 50:5155–8. doi: 10.1167/iovs.09-3384
23. Baek J, Doh SH, Chung SK. Assessment of the tear meniscus using optical coherence tomography in patients with type 2 diabetes mellitus. *Cornea.* (2015) 34:1534–40. doi: 10.1097/ICO.0000000000000651
24. Derakhshan A, Abrishami M, Khajedaluee M, Omidtabrizi A, Moghaddam SG. Comparison between tear film osmolar cocentration and other tear film function parameters in patients with diabetes mellitus. *Korean J Ophthalmol.* (2019) 33:326–32. doi: 10.3341/kjo.2013.0146
25. Lane JD, Krumholz DM, Sack RA, Morris C. Tear glucose dynamics in diabetes mellitus. *Curr Eye Res.* (2006) 31:895–901. doi: 10.1080/02713680600976552
26. Erdur SK, Aydin R, Ozsutcu M, Olmuscelik O, Eliacik M, Demirci G, et al. The relationship between metabolic syndrome, its components, and dry eye: a cross-sectional study. *Curr Eye Res.* (2017) 42:1115–7. doi: 10.1080/02713683.2017.1280511
27. Lin X, Liu ZL, Wu JL, Liu ZG. A review of sensory neuropathic pain in the dry eye. *Chin J Ophthalmol.* (2018) 54:144–7. doi: 10.3760/cma.j.issn.0412-4081.2018.02.016

16

Changes of Dry Eye Related Markers and Tear Inflammatory Cytokines After Upper Blepharoplasty

Songjiao Zhao [1], Nan Song [2†] and Lan Gong [1,3*†]*

[1] Department of Ophthalmology, Eye, Ear, Nose and Throat Hospital of Fudan University, Shanghai, China, [2] Department of Facial Plastic and Reconstructive Surgery, Eye, Ear, Nose and Throat Hospital of Fudan University, Shanghai, China, [3] Myopia Key Laboratory of Ministry of Health, Eye, Ear, Nose and Throat Hospital of Fudan University, Shanghai, China

***Correspondence:**
Nan Song
greenkingsn@163.com
Lan Gong
13501798683@139.com

† These authors have contributed equally to this work and share last authorship

Objectives: To investigate the changes of dry eye-related clinical manifestations, ocular surface parameters, and tear inflammatory cytokines after upper blepharoplasty.

Methods: Forty eyes of 20 who underwent upper blepharoplasty were divided into either the group with or the group without preexisting dry eye before upper blepharoplasty. Ocular Surface Disease Index (OSDI), Schirmer I test, tear meniscus height, lipid layer thickness, non-invasive tear break-up time (NIKBUT), fluorescein tear film break-up time (FBUT), corneal fluorescein staining, meibum expression, lid margin changes, and tear inflammatory cytokines were assessed preoperatively and at 1, 3, and 6 months postoperatively. Correlations between inflammatory cytokines and dry eye-related parameters were determined.

Results: The OSDI scores increased significantly at 1 month ($p = 0.040$) and subsequently decreased to the preoperative levels at 6 months postoperatively in subjects with dry eye. First (f)-NIKBUT and FBUT were significantly shortened at 1, 3, and 6 months postoperatively in subjects with dry eye (f-NIKBUT: $p < 0.001$, $p = 0.010$, $p = 0.042$; FBUT: $p = 0.002$, $p = 0.005$, $p = 0.037$, respectively), but were only shortened at 1 month ($p = 0.028$, $p = 0.005$) and returned to baseline levels at 6 months postoperatively in subjects without preexisting dry eye. A significant increasing trend of interleukin (IL)-6 was found in both dry eye and subjects without preexisting dry eye ($p = 0.016$, $p = 0.008$), while IL-8 and tumor necrosis factor alpha (TNF-α) were only found to be increased in subjects with dry eye postoperatively ($p = 0.031$, $p = 0.031$). The levels of IL-8 and TNF-α were positively correlated with OSDI scores ($p = 0.046$, $p = 0.043$, respectively) and negatively correlated with f-NIKBUT and FBUT ($p = 0.026$, $p = 0.006$, respectively).

Conclusions: Upper blepharoplasty might increase the release of tear inflammatory cytokines and tear film instability that contribute to the development of postoperative dry eye in the early postoperative poriod and the changes most relieved in 6 months. Preexisting dry eye is a higher risk factor for worse and persistent ocular surface damage after upper blepharoplasty.

Keywords: dry eye, ocular surface, tear inflammatory cytokines, postoperative, upper blepharoplasty

INTRODUCTION

Upper blepharoplasty is one of the most popular esthetic surgeries in Asia to create an upper eyelid crease and improve appearance and functional visual field (1). This procedure generally involves the removal of redundant upper eyelid skin, orbital fat, and/or the orbicularis oculi muscle to achieve periorbital rejuvenation (2). Changes in upper eyelid anatomy and movement dynamics may be attributed to the development of dry eye disease after upper blepharoplasty, with a reported incidence of 0–12.9% (3–5). Dry eye is a multifactorial disease of the ocular surface in which tear film instability and hyperosmolarity, ocular surface inflammation and damage, and neurosensory abnormalities play etiological roles (6). Typical symptoms of postoperative dry eye are similar to those of common dry eye, including dryness, redness, burning, foreign body sensation, and occasional blurred vision (7). Although dry eye is considered a relatively rare, mild, and transient complication of upper blepharoplasty, the severity of dry eye symptoms could affect psychosomatic symptoms and quality of life (8, 9). In addition, few cases can develop into chronic, persistent dry eye syndrome, which severely affects the physical and mental health of patients (3). To prevent and manage dry eye after upper blepharoplasty, investigating the potential pathogenesis *via* preoperative and postoperative evaluation of the ocular surface is pivotal.

Postoperative dry eye triggered by upper blepharoplasty is generally considered to be related to the decline of tear film stability. Several potential mechanisms contributing to this phenomenon have been proposed: the uneven distribution of tear film caused by the change in interaction between the eyelid and ocular surface (10); decreased lipid secretion and increased tear evaporation induced by the reduced blink rate and incomplete blinking; and postoperative lagophthalmos (3, 11–13). However, a recent study showed that palpebral aperture or blink dynamics changes are not the main cause of dry eye following upper blepharoplasty (14). We wondered whether there are other factors associated with the development of this complication. The updated definition of dry eye specifies the critical role of ocular surface inflammation in the course of the disease (6). Several studies identified an inflammatory cascade that may occur following ocular and intraocular surgeries, such as LASIK and cataract surgery, which lead to direct damage of the ocular surface (15, 16). Another recent study showed that frontalis suspension surgery resulted in the elevation of inflammatory cytokine levels on the ocular surface in the early period postoperative (17). Existing research on dry eye after upper blepharoplasty focused on tear film stability and tear fluid dynamics. However, changes in ocular surface inflammation after upper blepharoplasty have not been reported.

In this study, we evaluated the changes in dry eye-related markers and tear inflammatory cytokines in patients who underwent upper blepharoplasty. Furthermore, the correlations between inflammatory cytokines and dry eye-related markers were determined. We aimed to characterize the effects of upper blepharoplasty on the ocular surface microenvironment and investigate the potentially novel pathogenesis of postoperative dry eye following upper blepharoplasty.

Abbreviations: OSDI, Ocular Surface Disease Index; TMH, tear meniscus height; NIKBUT, non-invasive tear break-up time; f-NIKBUT, first non-invasive tear break-up time; av-NIKBUT, average non-invasive tear break-up time; FBUT, fluorescein tear film break-up time; FL, fluorescein staining; IFN-γ, interferon-gamma; IL, interleukin; LLT, lipid layer thickness; TNF-α, tumor necrosis factor alpha.

MATERIALS AND METHODS

Patient Characteristics

Twenty patients (19 women, 1 man; age range, 21–35 years) who underwent bilateral upper blepharoplasty at the Eye, Ear, Nose, and Throat Hospital of Fudan University from August 2020 to January 2021 were recruited for this prospective study. The study was conducted in accordance with the World Medical Association Declaration of Helsinki. The study was approved by the ethics committee of the Eye, Ear, Nose, and Throat Hospital of Fudan University (number 2019093-1), and written informed consent was obtained from all patients who participated.

All surgical candidates underwent a thorough ocular surface assessment by an ophthalmologist before surgery and at 1, 3, and 6 months after surgery. The candidates were divided into two groups according to whether they had preexisting dry eye disease. The diagnostic criteria for dry eye disease included the presence of at least one of the following symptoms, dryness, burning sensation, grittiness, photophobia, pain, and tickle, and one of the following signs: Schirmer I test $\leq$ 5 mm/5 min; tear film break-up time $<$ 5 s; positive fluorescein staining with either 5 mm/5 min $<$ Schirmer I test $\leq$10 mm/5 min or 5 s $\leq$ tear film break-up time $<$ 10 s. Eighteen eyes of nine enrolled subjects met the criteria for dry eye and were classified as the dry eye group. The remaining 22 eyes of 11 patients were in the group without preexisting dry eye. The exclusion criteria included a history of eyelid surgery, a history of ocular surgery within 6 months, neuromuscular abnormalities, a history of wearing contact lenses, ocular/eyelid diseases such as acute inflammation or infection, glaucoma, lagophthalmos; systemic diseases that would probably affect the ocular surface, such as Sjögren's syndrome; and inability to follow or cooperate during the examinations.

Surgical Techniques

All subjects underwent cosmetic, bilateral upper blepharoplasty by the same senior oculoplastic surgeon (Nan Song) under topical anesthesia with 2% lidocaine. In brief, the operation process involves the following steps: excision of excess upper eyelid skin and a strip of preseptal orbicularis oculi muscle, removal of excess fat, and exposure of septoaponeurosis junctional thickening, which is stitched with the lower edge orbicularis oculi muscle using 6-0 non-absorbable suture, and the eyelid is closed with 7-0 absorbable suture. No anti-inflammatory eye drops were used after surgery.

Ocular Surface Evaluation

All subjects underwent a thorough ocular examination with the help of an ophthalmologist in the following conditions: the interval between the tests was >15 min; the examination room was quiet, with a constant temperature of 25°C and 50%

humidity; and none of the patients used any eye drops on the day of the examination.

Ocular Surface Disease Index

Dry eye symptoms were assessed using the OSDI questionnaire. Twelve questions were included to quantify the discomfort in a 1-week period, covering three subscales: ocular symptoms, vision-related function, and environmental stimulant. The OSDI score ranges from 0 to 100, and a higher OSDI score indicates greater disability.

Non-invasive Tear Break-Up Time and Tear Meniscus Height

NIKBUT and TMH were measured using an OCULUS Keratograph 5M (Wetzlar, Germany) equipped with modified TF-scan software. All subjects were requested to blink twice and then keep their eyes open as much time as possible until the next blink. The outputs included the first non-invasive tear break-up time (f-NIKBUT) and the average non-invasive tear break-up time (av-NIKBUT). The tear meniscus height was measured three times, as previously reported (18) using infrared images taken at the central point of the lower lid margin. The procedure was repeated three times for each eye in a dark room.

Lipid Layer Thickness

Lipid layer thickness was measured non-invasively by tear interferometry using a LipiView instrument (TearScience, Morrisville, NC, United States). All subjects were instructed to blink naturally to record a 15 s video of the tear film interference pattern and analyze the thickness of the lipid layer. The procedure was repeated three times for each eye.

Fluorescein Tear Film Break-Up Time

After instilling fluorescein into the lower fornix using fluorescein strips (Jingming, Tianjing, China), the subjects were asked to blink naturally several times and then keep their eyes open for as long as possible until the next blink. The time between the last blink and the occurrence of the first dry spot on the cornea was observed under cobalt blue light and recorded as FBUT. The procedure was repeated three times for each eye.

Corneal Fluorescein Staining

After measuring the FBUT, corneal FL was performed. To quantify punctate staining, the corneal surface was divided into five areas, as proposed by the US National Eye Institute (19). The grade of punctate staining in each area was recorded as 0–3, 0, no staining; 1, < 15 dots; 2, 16 −20 dots; 3, > 30 dots, strip/bulk staining, or corneal filaments. The total FL scores ranged from 0 to 15.

Schirmer I Test

The Schirmer test without anesthesia (Schirmer I test) was used to assess basic tears. A 40 mm Schirmer paper strip (Jingming, Tianjing, China) was placed into the temporal one-third portion of the lower conjunctival fornix. The subjects were asked to close their eyes gently and sit quietly for 5 min. The length of the wetting part from the folded notch was recorded.

TABLE 1 | Demographic data and clinical characteristics of normal and dry eye.

	Normal (*n* = 22)	Dry eye (*n* = 18)	*P*-value
Age	25.64 ± 1.44	28.11 ± 1.31	0.229
Sex	10F/1M	9F	
OSDI score	2.66 ± 1.49	12.51 ± 2.25	**0.001**
Schirmer I test (mm/5 min)	18.09 ± 1.19	7.17 ± 0.87	**<0.001**
TMH(mm)	0.32 ± 0.02	0.21 ± 0.01	**<0.001**
FBUT(s)	9.18 ± 0.32	5.78 ± 0.53	**<0.001**
f-NIKBUT(s)	11.85 ± 0.77	8.07 ± 0.77	**0.001**
Av-NIKBUT(s)	16.46 ± 0.87	9.69 ± 0.93	**<0.001**
FL score	0.14 ± 0.07	0.39 ± 0.14	0.110
Meibomian gland evaluation			
Meibum expression	0.36 ± 0.49	0.83 ± 0.62	**0.011**
Lid margin changes	0.83 ± 0.79	1.54 ± 1.01	**0.044**
LLT (nm)	71.17 ± 3.68	61.72 ± 3.65	0.082
Blink frequency (blink/min)	18.08 ± 1.04	17.00 ± 0.98	0.481
Incomplete blink rate (%)	39.55 ± 8.18	44.44 ± 9.26	0.694

TMH, Tear meniscus height; FBUT, Fluorescein break-up time; f-NIKBUT, first-non-invasive keratograph tear film break-up time; Av-NIKBUT, average-non-invasive keratograph tear film break-up time; FL score, Fluorescein staining score; LLT, Lipid layer thickness. The bold values means significant results.

Meibomian Gland Evaluation

Evaluation of meibomian gland function was performed under slit lamp using a grading method using meibum expression and lid margin changes (20). The upper eyelid was digitally pressed and the meibum expression was graded based on the expressibility and meibum quality as 0–2: 0, clear and normal volume; 1, opaque with hyperviscosity and/or reduced; and 2, not expressed. Lid margin changes were graded based on the irregularity of the lid margin, telangiectasia, plugging of meibomian orifices, and replacement of the mucocutaneous junction, ranging from 0 to 4 (20).

Tear Inflammation Cytokines

Tear Sample Collection

Disposable 2.2 μL tear collectors (Seinda, Guangdong, China) were used to obtain tear fluid at the lateral canthus before surgery and at 1, 3, and 6 months postoperatively. A total sample of 15 μL without being diluted was collected without anesthesia or irritation of the cornea, conjunctiva, or lid margin. Tear samples were transferred into 0.5 mL microtubes (Axygen, Union City, United States), immediately placed on ice, and then stored at −80°C for further experiments.

Assays for Tear Inflammation Cytokines

Luminex liquid suspension chip detection was performed using Wayen Biotechnologies (Shanghai, China). MILLIPLEX MAP High Sensitivity T Cell Magnetic Bead Panel (Merck EMD Millipore, Billerica, MA, United States) for interleukin (IL)-1β, IL-6, IL-8, tumor necrosis factor alpha (TNF-α), and interferon-gamma (IFN-γ) was used according to the manufacturer's instructions. Briefly, tear samples were incubated in microbead-embedded 96-well plates overnight at 4°C and subsequently incubated with detection antibody for 1 h at room temperature. Next, streptavidin-phycoerythrin was added into each well of the plate and incubated for 30 min at room temperature, and the values were read using a Luminex 200 system (Luminex Corporation, Austin, TX, United States).

Statistical Analyses

Data analyses were performed using SPSS 24.0 (IBM Corp., Armonk, NY, United States). The tabulated results are expressed as the mean ± standard deviation. The generalized estimating equation (21) was used to adjust the correlation between the right and left eyes and to compare the preoperative examination values between the group without and the group with dry eye (**Table 1**). The differences between preoperative and postoperative OSDI scores, TMH, NIKBUT, FBUT, FL score, Schirmer I test, and tear inflammatory cytokines were compared using Wilcoxon signed-rank test (**Figures 1, 2**). The correlations between measurements were performed using the Spearman rank correlation test (**Figure 3**). Statistical significance was set at $p < 0.05$.

RESULTS

Demographic and Preoperative Dry Eye-Related Markers

Forty eyes of 20 subjects underwent bilateral upper blepharoplasty. Twenty-two eyes of 11 subjects without preexisting dry eye with a mean age of 26.00 ± 4.47 years (10 females, 1 male) were included and compared with 18 eyes of nine subjects who had dry eye (mean age: 27.67 ± 4.58 years; 9 females; $p = 0.423$). All the subjects were satisfied with the operation results, and no other complications such as wound infection or lagophthalmos occurred within 6 months postoperatively.

By comparing the preoperative dry eye-related markers, subjects with dry eye showed more severe clinical manifestations than subjects without dry eye. The OSDI score in subjects with dry eye disease was significantly higher than that in subjects without dry eye ($p = 0.001$). The values of the Schirmer I test, TMH, FBUT, f-NIKBUT, and av-NIKBUT in subjects with dry eye were significantly lower than those in subjects without dry eye ($p < 0.001, p < 0.001, p < 0.001, p = 0.001, p < 0.001$). The grades of meibum expression and lid margin changes were significantly higher in subjects with dry eye than in eyes without dry eye ($p = 0.028, p = 0.006$). The FL score, LLT, and blink dynamics showed no significant differences between subjects with and without dry eye. The demographic data and preoperative ocular surface parameters are listed in **Table 1**.

The Effect of Upper Blepharoplasty on Dry Eye-Related Markers

To evaluate the effect of upper blepharoplasty on the ocular surface, the preoperative parameters were compared to those at 1, 3, and 6 months postoperatively in subjects with dry eye and subjects without dry eye, respectively.

Ocular Surface Disease Index

The OSDI scores significantly increased at 1 month ($p = 0.040$) and subsequently decreased to the preoperative levels at 6 months postoperatively in subjects with dry eye. No significant change was observed in the OSDI scores in subjects without dry eye from the preoperative value. Subjects with dry eye had higher OSDI scores at any follow-up time than subjects without dry eye ($p < 0.001$) (**Figure 1A**).

Tear Production

Tear production was assessed using the Schirmer I test and the TMH. Compared with the preoperative measurements, no significant difference was found in the Schirmer I test or TMH at any follow-up time in both subjects with and without dry eye. Subjects with dry eye showed less tear production at any follow-up time than subjects without dry eye ($p < 0.001$) (**Figures 1B,C**).

Tear Film Stability

Tear film stability was evaluated by NIKBUT, FBUT, and LLT. The values of f-NIKBUT and FBUT in subjects with dry eye were significantly reduced at 1, 3, and 6 months postoperatively compared with the preoperative measurements (f-NIKBUT: $p < 0.001$, $p = 0.010$, $p = 0.042$, respectively; FBUT: $p = 0.002$, $p = 0.005$, $p = 0.037$, respectively) (**Figures 1D,E**). In contrast to subjects with dry eye, f-NIKBUT and FBUT were significantly shortened at 1 month postoperatively ($p = 0.028, p = 0.005$) and returned to baseline levels at 6 months postoperatively in subjects without dry eye. No significant difference was observed in av-NIKBUT at any follow-up time in either subjects with or without dry eye compared to preoperative measurements (**Figure 1F**). A shorter tear film break-up time was demonstrated in subjects with dry eye than in subjects without dry eye at any postoperative follow-up time ($p < 0.001$). The lipid layer plays a critical role in preventing excessive evaporation and stabilizing the tear film surface. Subjects with dry eye had a thinner lipid layer than eyes without dry eye at 3 and 6 months postoperatively ($p = 0.042$, $p = 0.003$). However, the LLT values did not significantly change with time in both subjects with and without dry eye (**Figure 1G**).

Corneal Epithelium Injury

Corneal epithelium injury was quantified using the FL score. The FL scores showed no significant change at any follow-up time after surgery in both subjects with and without dry eye (**Figure 1H**).

Meibomian Gland Function

The meibomian gland function was evaluated using meibum expression and lid margin changes. In comparison with the preoperative parameters, meibum expression scores were significantly higher in subjects without dry eye at 1 and 3 months postoperatively ($p = 0.012, p = 0.016$), but remained unchanged in subjects with dry eye (**Figure 1I**). No remarkable change was found in the lid margin after surgery in both subjects with and without dry eye (**Figure 1J**).

Blink Dynamics

Blink dynamics were assessed using blink frequency and incomplete blink rate. No significant changing trend was found in the blink frequency or incomplete blink rate following upper blepharoplasty (**Figures 1K,L**).

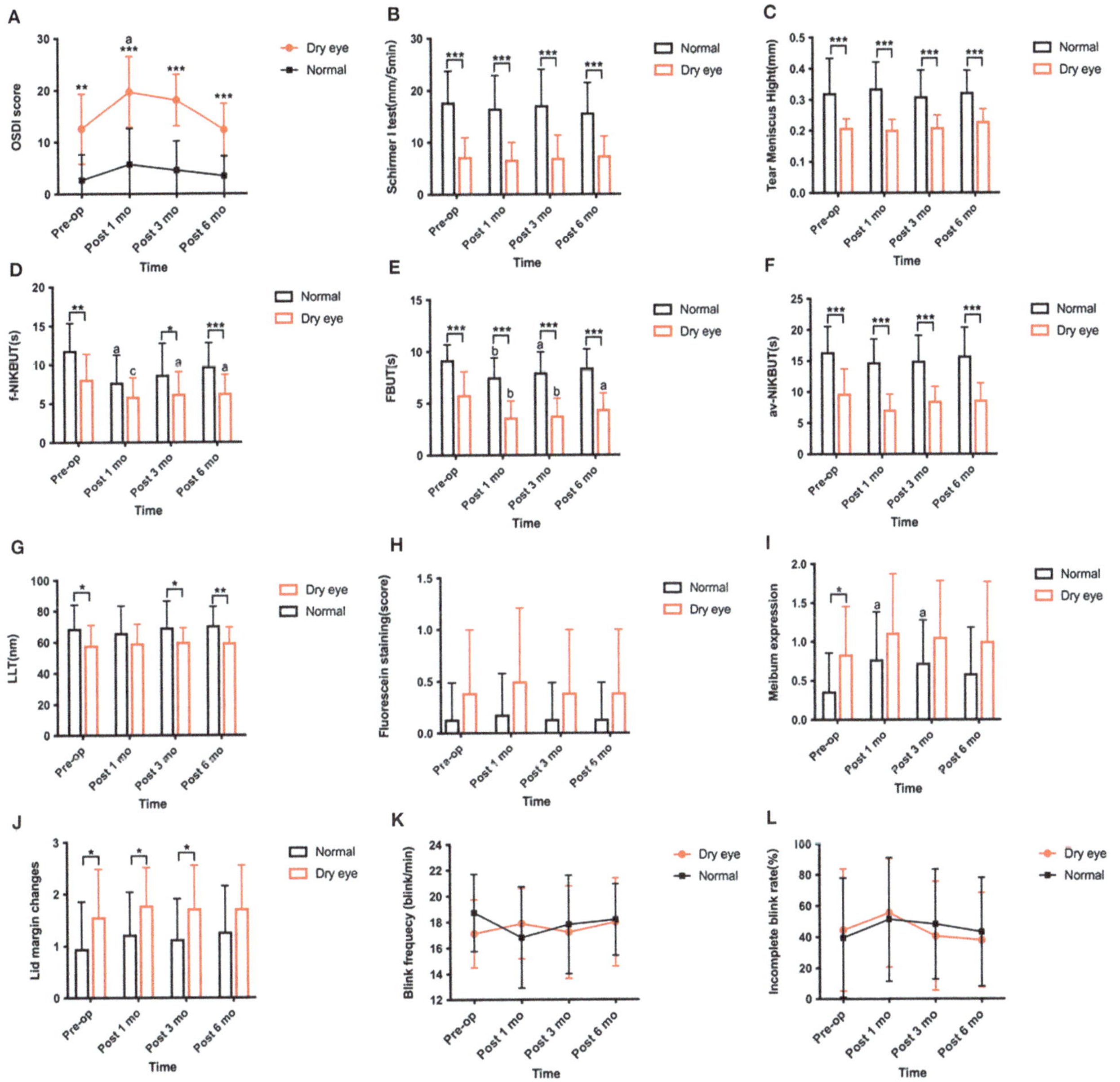

FIGURE 1 | Changes in dry eye related parameters preoperatively, 1, 3, and 6 months postoperatively from preoperative value. **(A)** Change in the Ocular Surface Disease Index (OSDI) score. The OSDI score is significantly increased in subjects with dry eye at 1 month postoperatively ($p = 0.040$) and subsequently decreased to preoperative level at 6 months postoperatively. No significant change shows in subjects without dry eye from preoperative value. Subjects with dry eye have higher OSDI scores at any follow up time than normal ($p < 0.001$). **(B,C)** Changes in Schirmer I test and tear meniscus height (TMH). No significant difference is found in Schirmer I test or TMH at any follow up time in both subject with and without dry eye. Subjects with dry eye show a less tear production at any follow up time than normal ($p < 0.001$). **(D)** Changes in first non-invasive tear break-up time (f-NIKBUT) from preoperative value. f-NIKBUT in dry eye subjects is significantly shortened at 1, 3, and 6 months postoperatively ($p < 0.001$, $p = 0.010$, $p = 0.042$). In subjects without dry eye, the f-NIKBUT is significantly shortened at 1 month postoperatively ($p = 0.028$) and returns to baseline levels at 6 months postoperatively. Subjects with dry eye shows a decreased f-NIKBUT than normal at 3 and 6 months postoperatively ($p = 0.037$, $p < 0.001$). **(E)** Changes in fluorescein tear film break-up time (FBUT) from preoperative value. FBUT in subjects with dry eye is significantly shortened at 1, 3, and 6 months postoperatively compared with the preoperative measurements ($p = 0.002$, $p = 0.005$, $p = 0.037$). FBUT is significantly shortened at 1 month postoperatively ($p = 0.005$) and returns to baseline levels at 6 months postoperatively in subjects without dry eye. **(F–H)** Changes in average non-invasive tear break-up time (av-NIKBUT), lipid layer thickness (LLT) and corneal fluorescein staining from preoperative values. No significant changes are found in av-NIKBUT, LLT and fluorescein staining scores at any follow up time postoperatively. **(I,J)** Changes in meibum expression and lid margin changes. Meibum expression scores are significantly higher in normal subjects at 1 and 3 months postoperatively ($p = 0.012$, $p = 0.016$), while no significant change is found in subjects with dry eye. Lid margin changes show no significant change at any follow up time in subjects with and without dry eye. **(K,L)** Changes in blink frequency and incomplete blink rate. No significant changes are shown in blink frequency and incomplete blink rate at any follow up time in subjects with and without dry eye ($^{*}p < 0.05$, $^{**}p < 0.01$, $^{***}p < 0.001$). a, b, c: significant differences between preoperative and postoperative values. $^{a}p < 0.05$, $^{b}p < 0.01$, $^{c}p < 0.001$.

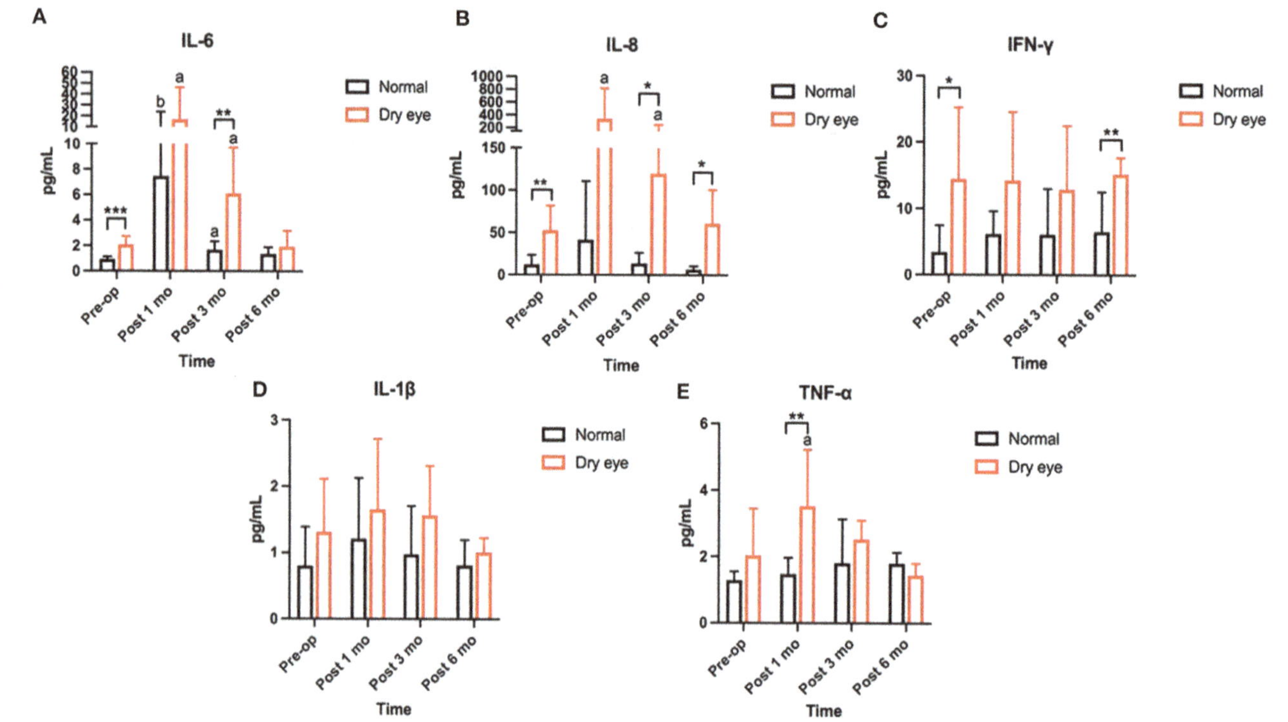

FIGURE 2 | Changes in concentration of tear inflammatory cytokines from the preoperative value. **(A,B)** The baseline levels of IL-6, IL-8, and IFN-γ are significantly higher in subjects with dry eye than in subjects without dry eye ($p < 0.001$, $p = 0.003$). Increasing trends of IL-6 and IL-8 are found at 1 ($p = 0.016$, $p = 0.031$) and 3 months ($p = 0.016$, $p = 0.047$) postoperatively in subjects with dry eye. At 6 months postoperatively, the levels of IL-6 and IL-8 are gently declined but still higher than the baseline levels ($p = 0.004$, $p = 0.047$). In subjects without dry eye, only IL-6 has significantly increased at 1 and 3 months postoperatively ($p = 0.008$, $p = 0.016$). **(C)** The concentration of interferon-gamma (IFN-γ) is significantly higher in dry eye subjects than in normal subjects preoperatively and 6 months postoperatively ($p = 0.019$, $p = 0.003$). No significant change is found in IFN-γ from preoperative levels in subjects with and without dry eye. **(D)** The concentration of interleukin (IL)-1β shows no significant changes at preoperative and any follow up time in subjects with and without dry eye. **(E)** The concentration of tumor necrosis factor alpha (TNF-α) is significantly increased at 1 month ($p = 0.031$) and returns to the baseline level at 3 months in subjects with dry eye. No significant change is found in subjects without dry eye (*significant difference between subjects with and without dry eye. $^{*}p < 0.05$, $^{**}p < 0.01$, $^{***}p < 0.001$; a, b: significant differences between preoperative and postoperative values. $^{a}p < 0.05$, $^{b}p < 0.01$).

The Effect of Upper Blepharoplasty on Tear Inflammatory Cytokines

Five inflammatory cytokines IL-1β, TNF-α, IL-6, IL-8, and IFN-γ, were examined and compared between subjects with and without dry eye. The baseline levels of IL-6, IL-8, and IFN-γ were significantly higher in subjects with dry eye than in subjects without dry eye ($p < 0.001, p = 0.003, p = 0.019$) (**Figures 2A–C**). No significant differences in the preoperative levels of IL-1β and TNF-α were found between the subjects with and without dry eye (**Figures 2D,E**). Increasing trends of IL-6 and IL-8 were found at 1 ($p = 0.016$, $p = 0.031$) and 3 months ($p = 0.016$, $p = 0.047$) postoperatively in subjects with dry eye (**Figures 2A,B**). The level of TNF-α significantly increased at 1 month ($p = 0.031$) and returned to the baseline level at 3 months postoperatively in subjects with dry eye (**Figure 2E**); at 6 months postoperatively, the levels of IL-6 and IL-8 declined slightly but were still higher than the baseline levels ($p = 0.004, p = 0.047$) (**Figures 2A,B**). In subjects without dry eye, only IL-6 significantly increased at 1 and 3 months postoperatively ($p = 0.008, p = 0.016$) (**Figure 2A**). The expression of IL-6, IL-8, and TNF-α returned to baseline levels at 6 months postoperatively (**Figures 2A,B,E**). No significant fluctuations were found in IL-1β and IFN-γ at the any of the following time (**Figures 2C,D**).

The Correlations Between Tear Inflammatory Cytokines and Dry Eye Related Markers

The significantly affected dry eye-related markers were correlated with significant changes in IL-6, IL-8, IFN-γ, and TNF-α levels. The concentration of IL-8 were positively correlated with the OSDI score and meibum expression score ($r = 0.259$, $p = 0.046$; $r = 0.407$, $p = 0.001$ respectively), and negatively correlated with f-NIKBUT ($r = -0.288$, $p = 0.026$) (**Figure 3A**). The level of TNF-α was positively correlated with the OSDI score ($r = 0.385$, $r = 0.043$), while it was negatively correlated with FBUT ($r = -0.509$, $p = 0.006$) (**Figure 3B**). However, the levels of IL-6 and IFN-γ were not significantly correlated with any of the dry eye-related markers (**Figures 3C,D**).

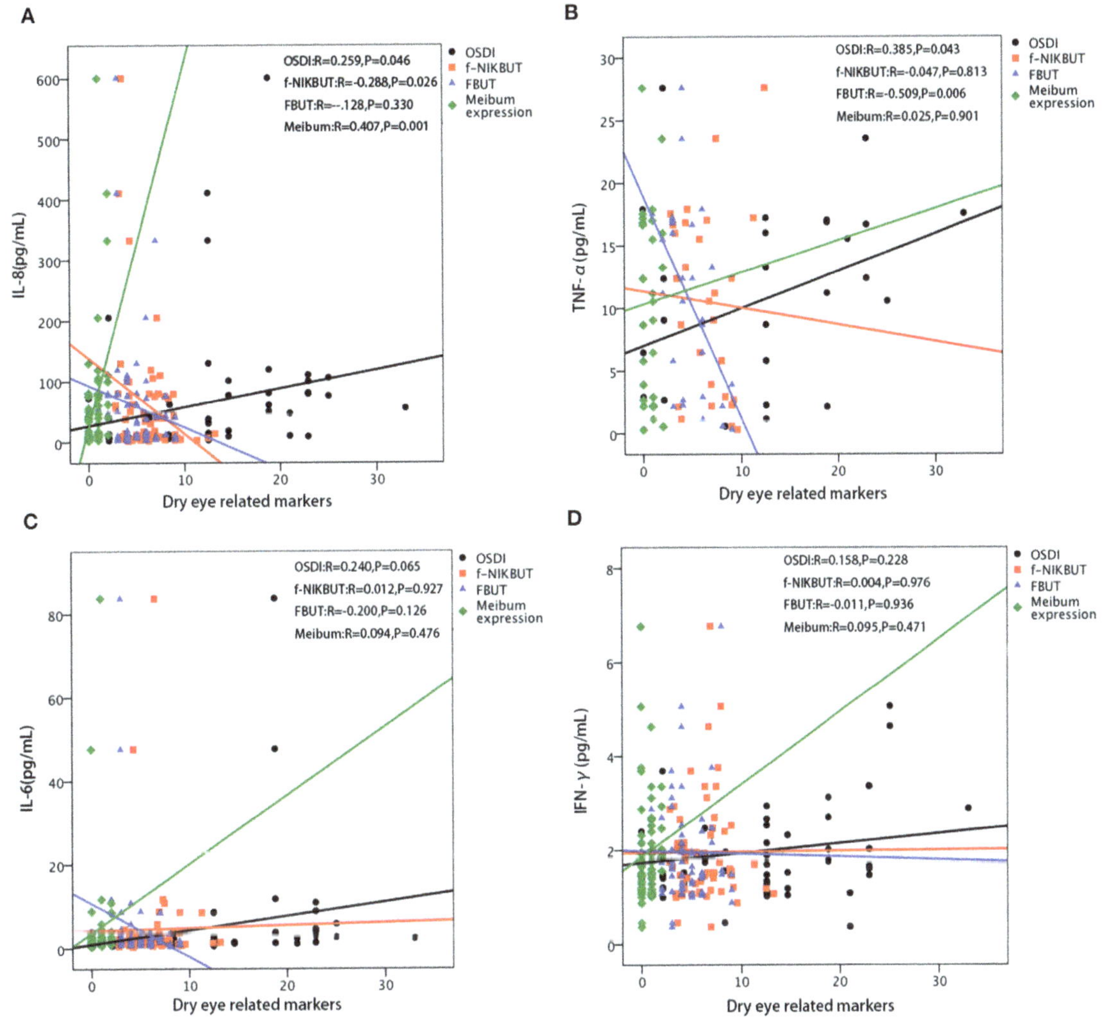

FIGURE 3 | Correlations between each inflammatory cytokines and dry eye related parameters. **(A)** The level of interleukin (IL)-8 is positively correlated with the Ocular Surface Disease Index (OSDI) score ($r = 0.259$, $p = 0.046$) and meibum expression score ($r = 0.407$, $p = 0.001$), while negatively correlated with first non-invasive tear break-up time (f-NIKBUT) ($r = -0.228$, $p = 0.026$). No significant correlation is found between IL-8 and fluorescein tear film break-up time (FBUT). **(B)** The level of tumor necrosis factor alpha (TNF-α) is positively correlated with the OSDI score ($r = 0.385$, $p = 0.043$), while negatively correlated with FBUT ($r = -0.509$, $p = 0.006$). No significant correlations are found between TNF-α and f-NIKBUT, and meibum expression score. **(C)** The level of IL-6 is not significantly correlated with the OSDI score, f-NIKBUT, FBUT, and meibum expression score. **(D)** The level of interferon-gamma (IFN-γ) is not significantly correlated with OSDI, f-NIKBUT, FBUT and meibum expression score.

DISCUSSION

Damage to ocular surface homeostasis following upper blepharoplasty contributes to the development of non-infective postoperative complications, such as dry eye. The emergence of dry eye or worsening of preexisting dry eye may occur in patients with upper blepharoplasty (5). Although usually mild and self-limited, a small fraction of postoperative dry eye might have a course longer than 1 month, even 3 months, according to previous studies (3–5, 22).

In this study, we demonstrated that aggravating symptoms and worse tear film stability induced by upper blepharoplasty were more dramatic and persisted for more than 6 months in patients with preexisting dry eye, whereas those changes were always mild and resolved within 3 months in patients without dry eye. This was consistent with the report of Prischmann et al. (3) that people with preexisting dry eye history were at a higher risk for generating dry eye following cosmetic blepharoplasty. Similar results were reported by Park et al. (23) in cataract surgery in which patient with preexisting dry eye had a higher OSDI score and a lower tear break-up time than those without dry eye after surgery. An explanation for this phenomenon is that the lowered sensory nerve thresholds of the ocular surface generally exist in people with preexisting dry eye, rendering them more susceptible to surgical irritation (24). It is noteworthy that a vicious circle exists in corneal sensation and tear film instability that might aggravate each other to promote the development of dry eye (24, 25).

In addition to unstable tear film, dry eye was characterized by ocular surface inflammation. Proinflammatory cytokines IL-1, IL-6, IL-8, and HLA-DR activators TNF-α and IFN-γ were shown to be strongly correlated with dry eye markers, leading to ocular surface damage and goblet cell reduction (26). Surgical procedures might induce the release of ocular inflammatory cytokines, promoting the development of postoperative dry eye. Li et al. (17) demonstrated that IL-1β, IL-6, IL-8, TNF-α, and IL-17A in conjunctival epithelial cells increased dramatically during the early postoperative period of frontalis suspension surgery. Park et al. (23) showed significant elevations of IL-1β, IL-6, IL-8, macrophage chemoattractant protein-1, TNF-α, and IFN-γ in lacrimal tears after cataract surgery. Zhang et al. (15) compared the levels of NGF, TGF-β1, IL-1α, and TNF-α in tears after femtosecond lenticule extraction and LASIK, and found increasing trends in both surgeries. In our study, similar increasing trends were found in the levels of IL-6, IL-8, and TNF-α following upper blepharoplasty. Positive correlations were found in our study between symptoms and inflammatory cytokines (IL-8 and TNF-α), which agreed with the correlations reported by Li et al. (17) and Zhang et al. (15). TNF-α is secreted by macrophages, binding to TNF receptor1 (TNFR1), and TNF receptor2 (TNFR2) to trigger several inflammatory signaling pathways such as NF-κB signals (27). IL-8 is an important member of IL family, showing strong attractive chemotactic effects to T cells and neutrophil cells (28). Amplification of whether TNF-α or IL-8 might lead to the damage of lacrimal gland and meibomian gland. Iatrogenic injury of the eyelid skin and orbicularis oculi muscle in upper blepharoplasty is likely to induce lymphocyte accumulation and the release of inflammatory cytokines, activating the inflammation cascade. Each of these inflammatory cytokines potentially contributes to the activation of sensory nerve terminals by directly inducing ongoing nerve activity or reducing sensory nerve thresholds (24). Therefore, the increased irritation following upper blepharoplasty is partially attributed to an increased inflammation level, except for tear film instability.

Lam et al. (29) showed that meibomian gland dysfunction is associated with increased levels of IL-6, IL-8, TNF-α, and IFN-γ. In this study, we found that the levels of IL-8 and TNF-α were negatively correlated with tear film break-up time, and IL-8 was negatively correlated with meibum quality and expressibility, which is in accordance with the results of Park et al. (23) reported after cataract surgery. These results verified that worse meibomian gland function was associated with a higher level of inflammation (29). Upper blepharoplasty-induced inflammation may lead to meibomian gland obstruction and abnormal meibum release. Moreover, persistent chemosis due to postoperative inflammation might destroy the goblet cells and lead to an unstable tear film (3, 4).

It is generally considered that cosmetic blepharoplasty, especially trimming the orbicularis oculi muscle, might change the dynamics of eyelid closure, tear pumping, and tear distribution, causing a decreased blink rate and tear production, and increased tear evaporation (5, 13, 30). Kim et al. (31) found a significant increase in the Schirmer test at 1 month postoperatively, while Watanabe et al. (32) showed a decrease in tear volume after cosmetic blepharoplasty. However, no significant changes in tear production, including the Schirmer I test and TMH, were observed in our study. In addition, we found that eyelid dynamics represented by blink frequency and an incomplete blink rate were not significantly changed by eyelid surgery, which is consistent with the study performed by Mak et al. (14). They proposed that blink dynamics did not change after upper blepharoplasty and were unlikely to be the cause of dry eye following this surgery (14). Although mechanical alteration of the corneoscleral and conjunctival interface in eyelid surgery was considered sufficient to aggravate or unmask a subclinical condition, our study found that excision of a small portion of the preseptal orbicularis oculi muscle did not obviously affect the lacrimal pump function and blink patterns.

There are several limitations of this study including the relatively small number of subjects and inadequate analysis of inflammatory cytokines. In addition, no evaluation was conducted on the effects of perioperative agents, such as anti-inflammatory agents. Postoperative management is challenging and should be discussed preoperatively. Thus, further studies should be conducted with a longer follow-up period, a larger number of subjects with and without anti-inflammatory agents and more comprehensive examination and analysis of inflammatory cytokines to illustrate the definite role of inflammation in the postoperative dry eye, and to investigate the appropriate management of patients undergoing cosmetic blepharoplasty.

To the best of our knowledge, this study is the first to identify that ocular surface inflammation induced by upper blepharoplasty plays a critical role in the development of postoperative dry eye, and is closely related to irritation symptoms, tear film instability, and meibomian gland dysfunction. Furthermore, preexisting dry eye is considered a higher risk factor to generate worse and persistent ocular surface damage. It is necessary for surgeons to complete a preoperative assessment, recognize preoperative dry eye, and address rational drug use such as artificial tears and topical anti-inflammatory agents during the perioperative period. It is beneficial for patients undergoing upper blepharoplasty to reduce postoperative dry eye and improve patient satisfaction and quality of life. Moreover, to improve the preoperative assessment, elevated inflammatory cytokines might be a more sensitive marker for the development of dry eye than traditional parameters, especially in those with separated symptoms and signs.

ETHICS STATEMENT

The studies involving human participants were reviewed and approved by Ethics Committee of the Eye, Ear, Nose and Throat Hospital of Fudan University (2019093-1). The patients/participants provided their written informed consent to participate in this study.

AUTHOR CONTRIBUTIONS

LG, NS, and SZ: conception, design, writing, review, and revision of the manuscript. LG and SZ: development of methodology. NS: surgical operation. SZ: acquisition of data (patients follow up and examination) and analysis and interpretation of data. All authors contributed to the article and approved the submitted version.

ACKNOWLEDGMENTS

We would like to thank Editage (www.editage.com) for English language editing.

REFERENCES

1. Castro E, Foster JA. Upper lid blepharoplasty. *Facial Plastic Surg.* (1999) 15:173–81. doi: 10.1055/s-2008-1064317
2. Chen WP. Visual, physiological, and aesthetic factors and pitfalls in asian blepharoplasty. *Aesthetic Surg J.* (2016) 36:275–83. doi: 10.1093/asj/sjv186
3. Prischmann J, Sufyan A, Ting JY, Ruffin C, Perkins SW. Dry eye symptoms and chemosis following blepharoplasty: a 10-year retrospective review of 892 cases in a single-surgeon series. *JAMA Facial Plastic Surg.* (2013) 15:39–46. doi: 10.1001/2013.jamafacial.1
4. Hamawy AH, Farkas JP, Fagien S, Rohrich RJ. Preventing and managing dry eyes after periorbital surgery: a retrospective review. *Plastic Reconstructive Surg.* (2009) 123:353–9. doi: 10.1097/PRS.0b013e31819346ea
5. Saadat D, Dresner SC. Safety of blepharoplasty in patients with preoperative dry eyes. *Arch Facial Plastic Surg.* (2004) 6:101–4. doi: 10.1001/archfaci.6.2.101
6. Craig JP, Nichols KK, Akpek EK, Caffery B, Dua HS, Joo CK, et al. TFOS DEWS II definition and classification report. *Ocular Surface.* (2017) 15:276–83. doi: 10.1016/j.jtos.2017.05.008
7. Wolffsohn JS, Arita R, Chalmers R, Djalilian A, Dogru M, Dumbleton K, et al. TFOS DEWS II diagnostic methodology report. *Ocular Surface.* (2017) 15:539–74. doi: 10.1016/j.jtos.2017.05.001
8. Asiedu K, Dzasimatu SK, Kyei S. Impact of dry eye on psychosomatic symptoms and quality of life in a healthy youthful clinical sample. *Eye Contact Lens.* (2018) 44(Suppl. 2):S404–9. doi: 10.1097/ICL.0000000000000550
9. Gomes JAP, Azar DT, Baudouin C, Efron N, Hirayama M, Horwath-Winter J, et al. TFOS DEWS II iatrogenic report. *Ocular Surface.* (2017) 15:511–38. doi: 10.1016/j.jtos.2017.05.004
10. Bron AJ, de Paiva CS, Chauhan SK, Bonini S, Gabison EE, Jain S, et al. TFOS DEWS II pathophysiology report. *Ocular Surface.* (2017) 15:438–510. doi: 10.1016/j.jtos.2017.05.011
11. Jie Y, Sella R, Feng J, Gomez ML, Afshari NA. Evaluation of incomplete blinking as a measurement of dry eye disease. *Ocular Surface.* (2019) 17:440–6. doi: 10.1016/j.jtos.2019.05.007
12. Pacella SJ, Codner MA. Minor complications after blepharoplasty: dry eyes, chemosis, granulomas, ptosis, and scleral show. *Plastic Reconstructive Surg.* (2010) 125:709–18. doi: 10.1097/PRS.0b013e3181c830c7
13. Zhang SY, Yan Y, Fu Y. Cosmetic blepharoplasty and dry eye disease: a review of the incidence, clinical manifestations, mechanisms and prevention. *Int J Ophthalmol.* (2020) 13:488–92. doi: 10.18240/ijo.2020.03.18
14. Mak FHW, Ting M, Edmunds MR, Harker A, Edirisinghe M, Duggineni S, et al. Videographic analysis of blink dynamics following upper eyelid blepharoplasty and its association with dry eye. *Plastic Reconstructive Surg Global Open.* (2020) 8:e2991. doi: 10.1097/GOX.0000000000002991
15. Zhang C, Ding H, He H, Jin H, Liu LP, Yang XW, et al. Comparison of early changes in ocular surface markers and tear inflammatory mediators after femtosecond lenticule extraction and FS-LASIK. *Int J Ophthalmol.* (2021) 14:283–91. doi: 10.18240/ijo.2021.02.16
16. Kato K, Miyake K, Hirano K, Kondo M. Management of postoperative inflammation and dry eye after cataract surgery. *Cornea.* (2019) 38(Suppl. 1):S25–33. doi: 10.1097/ICO.0000000000002125
17. Li K, Zhang XC, Cai XX, Quan YD, Lu R. The inflammation influence on corneal surface after frontalis suspension surgery. *Int J Ophthalmol.* (2018) 11:1489–95. doi: 10.18240/ijo.2018.09.10
18. Wei A, Le Q, Hong J, Wang W, Wang F, Xu J. Assessment of lower tear meniscus. *Optometry Vision Sci.* (2016) 93:1420–5. doi: 10.1097/OPX.0000000000000986
19. Lemp MA. Report of the National Eye Institute/Industry workshop on clinical trials in dry eyes. *CLAO J.* (1995) 21:221–32.
20. Den S, Shimizu K, Ikeda T, Tsubota K, Shimmura S, Shimazaki J. Association between meibomian gland changes and aging, sex, or tear function. *Cornea.* (2006) 25:651–5. doi: 10.1097/01.ico.0000227889.11500.6f
21. Liang KY, Zeger SL. Regression analysis for correlated data. *Annu Rev Public Health.* (1993) 14:43–68. doi: 10.1146/annurev.pu.14.050193.000355
22. Shao C, Fu Y, Lu L, Chen J, Shen Q, Zhu H, et al. Dynamic changes of tear fluid after cosmetic transcutaneous lower blepharoplasty measured by optical coherence tomography. *Am J Ophthalmol.* (2014) 158:55–63.e1. doi: 10.1016/j.ajo.2014.03.016
23. Park Y, Hwang HB, Kim HS. Observation of influence of cataract surgery on the ocular surface. *PLoS ONE.* (2016) 11:e0152460. doi: 10.1371/journal.pone.0152460
24. Belmonte C, Nichols JJ, Cox SM, Brock JA, Begley CG, Bereiter DA, et al. TFOS DEWS II pain and sensation report. *Ocular Surface.* (2017) 15:404–37. doi: 10.1016/j.jtos.2017.05.002
25. Willcox MD, Argüeso P, Georgiev GA, Holopainen JM, Laurie GW, Millar TJ, et al. TFOS DEWS II tear film report. *Ocular Surface.* (2017) 15:366–403. doi: 10.1016/j.jtos.2017.03.006
26. Yamaguchi T. Inflammatory response in dry eye. *Investigative Ophthalmol Visual Sci.* (2018) 59:Des192–9. doi: 10.1167/iovs.17-23651
27. Oliver Metzig M, Fuchs D, Tagscherer KE, Gröne HJ, Schirmacher P, Roth W. Inhibition of caspases primes colon cancer cells for 5-fluorouracil-induced TNF-α-dependent necroptosis driven by RIP1 kinase and NF-κB. *Oncogene.* (2016) 35:3399–409. doi: 10.1038/onc.2015.398
28. Xia L, Zhang S, Zhou J, Li Y. A crucial role for B and T lymphocyte attenuator in preventing the development of CD4+ T cell-mediated herpetic stromal keratitis. *Mol Vision.* (2010) 16:2071–83. doi: 10.1186/1471-2415-10-26
29. Lam H, Bleiden L, de Paiva CS, Farley W, Stern ME, Pflugfelder SC. Tear cytokine profiles in dysfunctional tear syndrome. *Am J Ophthalmol.* (2009) 147:198–205. e1. doi: 10.1016/j.ajo.2008.08.032
30. Yang P, Ko AC, Kikkawa DO, Korn BS. Upper eyelid blepharoplasty: evaluation, treatment, and complication minimization. *Semin Plastic Surg.* (2017) 31:51–7. doi: 10.1055/s-0037-1598628
31. Kim HH, De Paiva CS, Yen MT. Effects of upper eyelid blepharoplasty on ocular surface sensation and tear production. *Can J Ophthalmol J.* (2007) 42:739–42. doi: 10.3129/i07-141
32. Watanabe A, Selva D, Kakizaki H, Oka Y, Yokoi N, Wakimasu K, et al. Long-term tear volume changes after blepharoptosis surgery and blepharoplasty. *Investigative Ophthalmol Visual Sci.* (2014) 56:54–8. doi: 10.1167/iovs.14-15632

17

Meibomian Gland Morphology Changes After Cataract Surgery: A Contra-Lateral Eye Study

Pingjun Chang [1,2,3], Shuyi Qian [1,2,3], Zhizi Xu [4], Feng Huang [1,2,3], Yinying Zhao [1,2,3], Zhangliang Li [1,2,3] and Yun-e Zhao [1,2,3]*

[1] Eye Hospital and School of Ophthalmology and Optometry, Wenzhou Medical University, Wenzhou, China, [2] National Clinical Research Center for Ocular Diseases, Wenzhou, China, [3] Eye Hospital of Wenzhou Medical University, Hangzhou Branch, Hangzhou, China, [4] Hangzhou Xiaoshan Liuliqiao Hospital, Hangzhou, China

***Correspondence:**
Yun-e Zhao
zyehzeye@126.com

Purpose: To evaluate the morphology changes of meibomian glands (MGs) after cataract surgery.

Setting: Hangzhou Branch of the Eye Hospital of Wenzhou Medical University, Zhejiang, China.

Methods: In this contra-lateral eye study, 40 patients received unilateral cataract surgery for age-related cataract. All the patients underwent the evaluation of non-invasive break-up time (NIBUT) and lower tear meniscus height (TMH) before the surgery and 6 months post-operatively. The MGs were evaluated via ImageJ and Meibomian Gland Bio-image Analyzer. MG dropout, length, width, area, gland diameter deformation index (DI), and gland signal index (SI) were recorded.

Results: MG length, width, area, DI, and SI were significantly decreased after cataract surgery in the study group (operated eyes, $P < 0.001$, $P = 0.003$, $P < 0.001$, $P = 0.001$, and $P < 0.001$, respectively) and showed no significant changes in the control group (non-operated eyes) (all $P > 0.05$). MG loss increased more in the study group ($P = 0.030$), and the changes in TMH and NIBUT were not significantly different between the two eyes (both $P > 0.05$).

Conclusion: Cataract surgery aggravated meibomian gland morphology, such as MG loss, MG length, width, area, and SI, and produced no change in NIBUT and TMH at 6 months post-operatively.

Keywords: meibomian gland morphology, meibomian gland dysfunction, dry eye disease, meibomian gland atrophy, cataract surgery, self-contrast study, automated algorithm

INTRODUCTION

Phacoemulsification with intraocular lens implantation is a standard procedure for the treatment of cataract. However, the post-operative visual acuities were improved, but a number of patients often complained about dry eye symptoms. Meibomian gland dysfunction (MGD) is the main cause of evaporative dry-eye disease, which leads to tear lipid deficiency and tear film instability (1, 2). The previous studies reported that cataract surgery is associated with high incidence of MGD (3, 4).

Several studies have investigated MGD after cataract surgery; however, few have evaluated specific morphological changes (4–7). Han et al. (4) reported that cataract surgery aggravated MG function but had no effect on the MG structure. MG morphology was evaluated by the grade of MG loss, and no quantitative parameters for each gland were assessed in their study. Nevertheless, a number of studies have demonstrated the relationship between MG morphology changes and MGD (5, 8). By analyzing the morphological changes using optical coherence tomography meibography (OCT-M), Liang et al. (8) revealed that MG length and width were decreased in the patients with MGD. The morphological changes of the meibomian gland (MG), such as shortening, dilation, distortion, and atrophy are sensitive and early indicators of MGD (9, 10).

In recent years, infrared non-contact meibography, confocal microscopy, and optical coherence tomography meibography are introduced to precisely visualize the MG structure. Keratograph 5M (K5M, Oculus, Wetzlar, Germany) is the most widely used infrared non-contact meibography for clinical MG morphology image acquisition (11).

Other factors, such as aging, sex, environmental factors, poor sleep quality, and sleeping position are associated with MGD (12–15), thus it is necessary to include the unoperated contralateral eye as the control when assessing the influence of cataract surgery. The previous studies did not involve the contralateral eyes as a control group to exclude confounding factors.

To our knowledge, this is the first contra-lateral study to evaluate the MGD and morphological changes in the patients who underwent cataract surgery. We analyzed multiple parameters offered by a new automated algorithm (16) to estimate the function and morphology of the MGs. Additionally, we explored the association between the MG structure and clinical tests in these patients.

PATIENTS AND METHODS

Patients

This study enrolled patients who underwent unilateral cataract phacoemulsification with intraocular lens implantation at the Hangzhou Branch of the Eye Hospital of Wenzhou Medical University from May 2017 to October 2019. The operated eyes were enrolled as the study group and the contra-lateral eyes as the control group. All the procedures followed the tenets of the Declaration of Helsinki. The ethics approval was obtained from

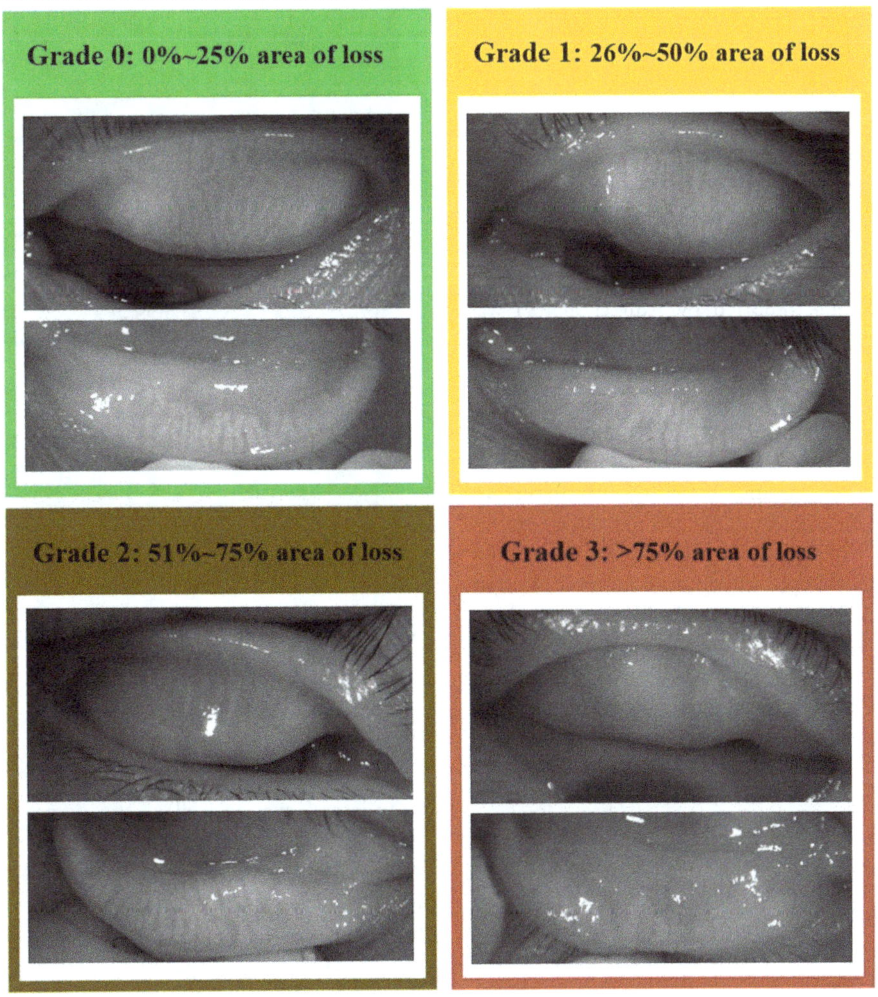

FIGURE 1 | The meibograde grading system reported by Adil et al. was referred to do subjective grading of meibomian gland (MG) loss.

the Ethics Committee of the Eye Hospital, Wenzhou Medical University, Wenzhou, China (ID: 2020-058-K-52).

The patients who had a similar degree of MG atrophy in both the eyes with grade 1 or 2 MG loss (defined as the proportion of the area of meibomian gland in its relation to the total area of the tarsus) were included (**Figure 1**). The patients who had previous ocular diseases, history of ocular surgery or contact lens wear, and who used topical or systemic medications that may affect the ocular surface were excluded.

Cataract Surgery

All surgeries were performed by a single surgeon (Zhao YE). The conjunctival sac was irrigated with 5% Povidone-iodine. Topical anesthesia was administered with 0.5% proparacaine hydrochloride eye drops. After capsulorhexis and phacoemulsification through a 2.2 mm incision, a 1-piece intraocular lens was placed in the capsular bag. At the end of surgery, the corneal incision was sealed with stromal hydration.

Post-operatively, all the patients were prescribed 0.5% topical levofloxacin (Cravit; Santen Pharmaceutical, Osaka, Japan) four times daily for 2 weeks and tobramycin-dexamethasone eye drops (Tobradex®, Alcon Couvreur NV, Puurs, Belgium) four times daily for the first week and tapered for the following 3 weeks.

Parameter Collections

Meibography was performed using a Non-contact Meibography System (Kerotography 5M, Oculus, Wetzlar, Germany) within 5 days before the operation and at ~6 months after the operation.

The MG loss area was calculated using ImageJ software (National Institute of Health; http://imagej.nih.gov/ij, **Figure 2**). Meibograde grading scheme reported by Adil et al. (9) was referred to evaluate the MG loss: grade 0, 0–25% area of loss; grade 1, 26–50% area of loss; grade 2, 51–75% area of loss; and grade 3, >75% area of loss (**Figure 1**).

MG parameters, such as length, width, area, gland diameter deformation index (DI), and gland signal index (SI) were analyzed using Meibomian Gland Bio-image Analyzer V3 software (16) (**Figure 3**) on the basis of the meibography images acquired by Kerotography 5M (K5M). This new automated algorithm developed by Xiao et al. offered multiple parameters for objective evaluation of MG morphology. The algorithm consists of three main steps: (I) region of interest (ROI) acquisition; (II) segmentation and identification of MGs within the ROI; and (III) quantitative parameter analysis. The five central MGs of upper lid were adopted to measure the length, width, area, DI, and SI changes of the MGs.

Additionally, the tear meniscus height (TMH) and the average non-invasive break-up time (NIBUT) was measured by K5M. The measurements were performed three times, and the average of the three attempts was used for analyses.

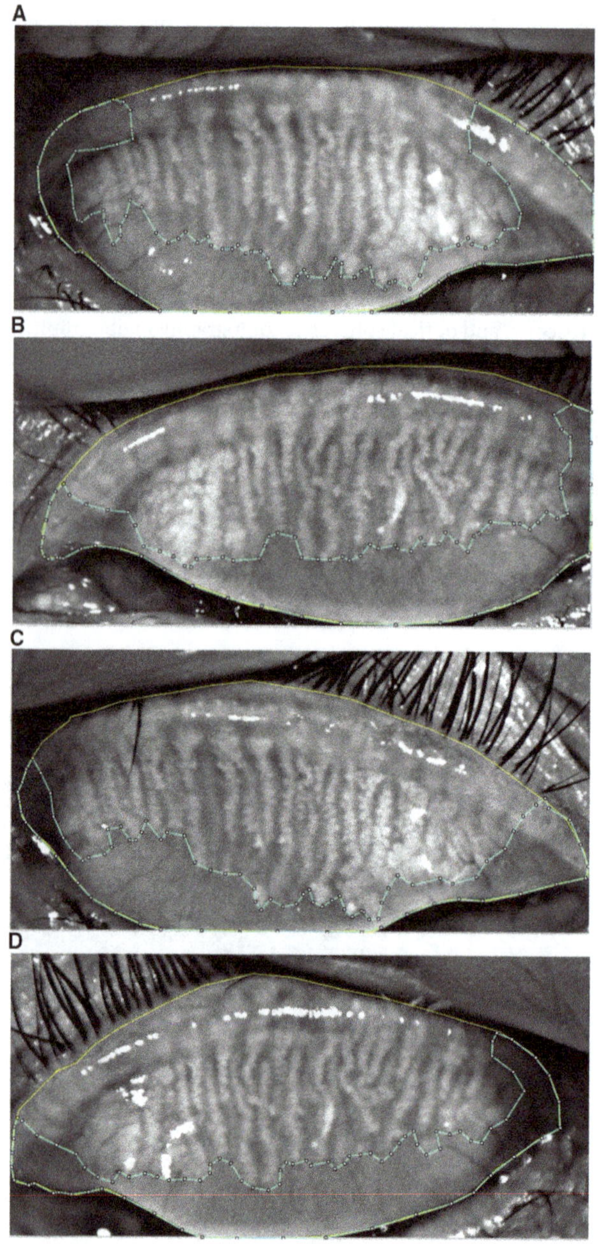

FIGURE 2 | The upper eyelid (yellow) and the edge of MG loss (blue) was drawn in the MG morphology images acquired from K5M. MG loss was calculated by the ImageJ software in the study group at baseline **(A)**, the control group at baseline **(B)**, the post-operative study group **(C)**, and the post-operative control group **(D)**.

Statistical Analysis

The normal distribution of the data was verified using the Shapiro–Wilk test. The differences between the operated eye and contralateral eye, as well as the differences between the pre-operative and post-operative parameters, were assessed using the paired-samples *t*-test or Wilcoxon signed-rank test according to the data normality. Spearman's rank correlation coefficient was used to assess the correlations between the changes in TMH, NIBUT, and MG morphology in each group. The statistical analyses were performed using SPSS for Windows version 26.0 (IBM Corp., NY, USA). The criterion for statistical significance was $P < 0.05$.

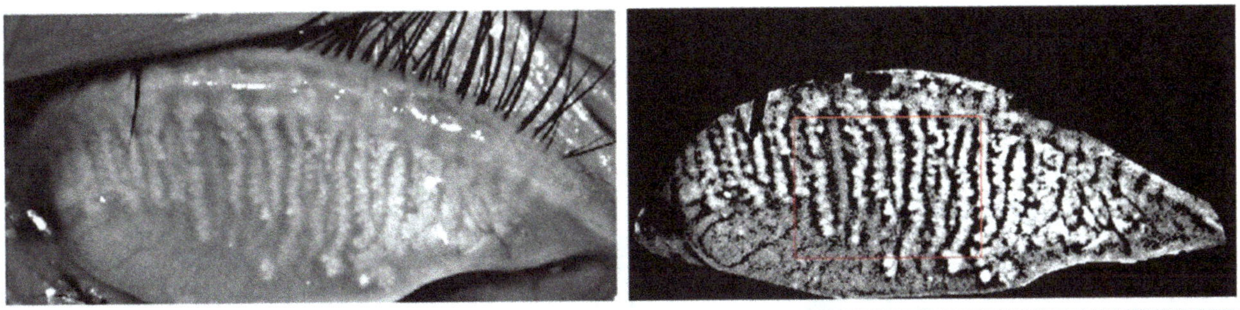

Number	Width (mm)	Length (mm)	Area (mm²)	DI	SI
2	0.36	4.79	1.50	5.58	7.74
3	0.41	3.21	1.12	8.90	8.09
4	0.40	3.38	1.28	4.72	8.68
5	0.45	5.09	2.05	6.46	9.84
6	0.34	5.18	1.64	6.51	6.98
Mean	0.39	4.33	1.52	6.43	8.27

FIGURE 3 | Meibomian Gland Bio-image Analyzer V3 software dealt with images from K5M and dampened the random noises and highlighted the visibility of glands. The width, length, area, DI, and SI of central five MGs were obtained after choosing the central part of the image and marked the MGs.

TABLE 1 | The changes in parameters before and at 6 months after cataract surgery in both groups.

	Baseline			6 months			P_{study}	$P_{control}$	P_{Δ}
	Study group	Control group	P_{base}	Study group	Control group	$P_{6\ mon}$			
MG loss (%)	35.05 ± 12.56	36.29 ± 12.78	0.278	37.84 ± 12.43	37.82 ± 12.56	0.984	0.004	0.015	0.030
MG length (mm)	4.15 ± 1.09	3.72 ± 0.89	0.017	3.64 ± 0.85	3.76 ± 0.92	0.466	<0.001	0.698	0.001
MG width (mm)	0.48 ± 0.14	0.49 ± 0.11	0.706	0.43 ± 0.09	0.50 ± 0.16	0.001	0.003	0.694	0.007
MG area (mm²)	1.67 ± 0.65	1.53 ± 0.47	0.204	1.36 ± 0.53	1.59 ± 0.64	0.035	<0.001	0.506	0.002
DI	8.60 ± 4.36	9.40 ± 3.54	0.242	6.89 ± 2.94	9.97 ± 5.32	<0.001	0.001	0.717	0.004
SI	5.36 ± 1.48	5.56 ± 1.44	0.351	4.60 ± 1.28	5.53 ± 1.14	<0.001	<0.001	0.846	<0.001
TMH (mm)	0.25 ± 0.13	0.23 ± 0.11	0.209	0.26 ± 0.14	0.26 ± 0.13	0.518	0.460	0.032	0.685
NIBUT(s)	6.76 ± 4.35	6.57 ± 3.64	0.658	6.51 ± 4.09	6.28 ± 4.10	0.360	0.555	0.492	0.736

The paired-samples t-test was applied for normal distribution, and the Wilcoxon matched-pair signed rank test was applied for abnormal distribution. P_{base}: The study group vs. the control group at baseline; P_{6mon}: The study group vs. the control group at 6 months post-operatively; P_{study}: The parameters at baseline vs. at 6 months post-operatively in the study group; $P_{control}$: The parameters at baseline vs. at 6 months post-operatively in the control group; P_{Δ}: Change of the parameters in the study group vs. that in the control group.
MG, Meibomian gland; DI, gland diameter deformation index; SI, gland signal index; TMH, tear meniscus height; NIBUT, non-invasive break-up time.

RESULTS

Demographics

A total of 80 eyes of 40 patients (25 men and 15 women) were included in this study. The mean age of the patients was 71.20 ± 9.73 years (range 38 to 87 years). The mean MG loss was 35.05 ± 12.56% in the study group (meibograde 1: 28 eyes; meibograde 2: 12 eyes) and 36.29 ± 12.78% in the control group (meibograde 1: 30 eyes; and meibograde 2: 10 eyes), respectively (P = 0.278, **Table 1**). At baseline, no significant differences were found between the two groups in TMH, NIBUT, and MG parameters except for MG length (the study group: 4.15 ± 1.09 versus the control group: 3.72 ± 0.89, $P = 0.017$, **Table 1**).

Changes in the Parameters After Cataract Surgery

As shown in **Table 1**, MG loss worsened in both the study group and the control group ($P = 0.004$ and $P = 0.015$, respectively). Despite similar MG loss were observed between baseline and post-operative in the two groups (both $P > 0.05$), we found that the change in MG loss was more severe in the study group ($P = 0.03$). Significant changes were observed after cataract surgery between the two groups in MG width, MG area, DI, and SI ($P = 0.001$, $P = 0.035$, $P < 0.001$, and $P < 0.001$, respectively). MG length, MG width, MG area, DI, and SI were significantly decreased after surgery in the study group ($P < 0.001$, $P =$

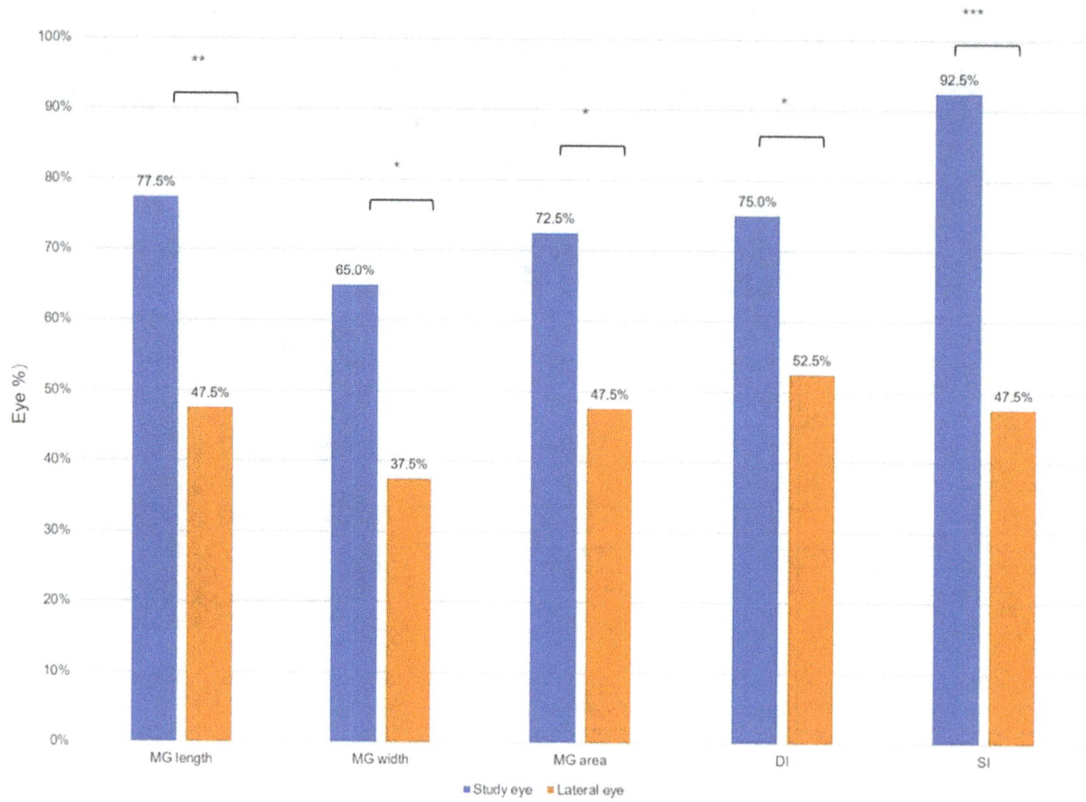

FIGURE 4 | The proportion of eyes whose ocular surface parameters value were decreased after the cataract surgery. Wilcoxon signed-rank test: *$P < 0.05$, **$P < 0.01$, and ***$P < 0.001$.

0.003, $P < 0.001$, $P = 0.001$, and $P < 0.001$, respectively) and showed no significant changes in the control group (all $P > 0.05$). The decrease in MG length, MG width, MG area, DI, and SI in the study group were significantly larger than those in the control group ($P = 0.001$, $P = 0.007$, $P = 0.002$, $P = 0.004$, and $P < 0.001$, respectively). However, no significant difference was found when comparing NIBUT, TMH, and the changes of these two parameters between the two groups at baseline and 6 months post-operatively. Moreover, NIBUT and TMH were not significantly changed in either group except that the control group displayed increased post-operative TMH values ($P = 0.032$)

As shown in **Figure 4**, the proportion of eyes whose parameter values decreased after cataract surgery. More eyes in the study group displayed decrease of MG width (65.0 vs. 37.5%, $P = 0.012$), MG length (77.5 vs. 47.5%, $P = 0.003$), MG area (72.5 vs. 47.5%, $P = 0.033$), DI (75.0 vs. 52.5%, $P = 0.029$), and SI (92.50 vs. 47.5%, $P < 0.001$) than those in the control group.

Correlations Between NIBUT, TMH, and MG Morphology

Spearman's rank correlation coefficient was used to assess the correlations. **Table 2** showed there was a positive correlation between NIBUT and MG length ($r = 0.186$, $P = 0.025$), MG area ($r = 0.188$, $P = 0.023$), and MG loss ($r = 0.185$, $P = 0.025$), whereas a negative correlation between NIBUT and SI ($r = -0.229$, $P = 0.005$) (**Figure 5**). Additionally, a significant correlation was found between MG loss and TMH ($r = 0.221$, $P = 0.005$).

TABLE 2 | Correlation coefficients of clinical tests and meibomian gland (MG) morphology.

	TMH (mm)		NIBUT(s)	
	r	*P*	*r*	*P*
MG length (mm)	−0.016	0.844	0.186	0.025
MG width (mm)	0.002	0.980	0.033	0.695
MG area (mm^2)	−0.015	0.846	0.188	0.023
DI	−0.152	0.055	−0.016	0.849
SI	−0.097	0.221	−0.229	0.005
MG loss(%)	0.221	0.005	0.185	0.025

TMH, tear meniscus height; NIBUT, non-invasive break-up time; MG, Meibomian gland; DI, gland diameter deformation index; SI, gland signal index.

DISCUSSION

MGD is one of the most common ocular surface diseases, which aggravates dry eye symptoms and leads to dissatisfaction

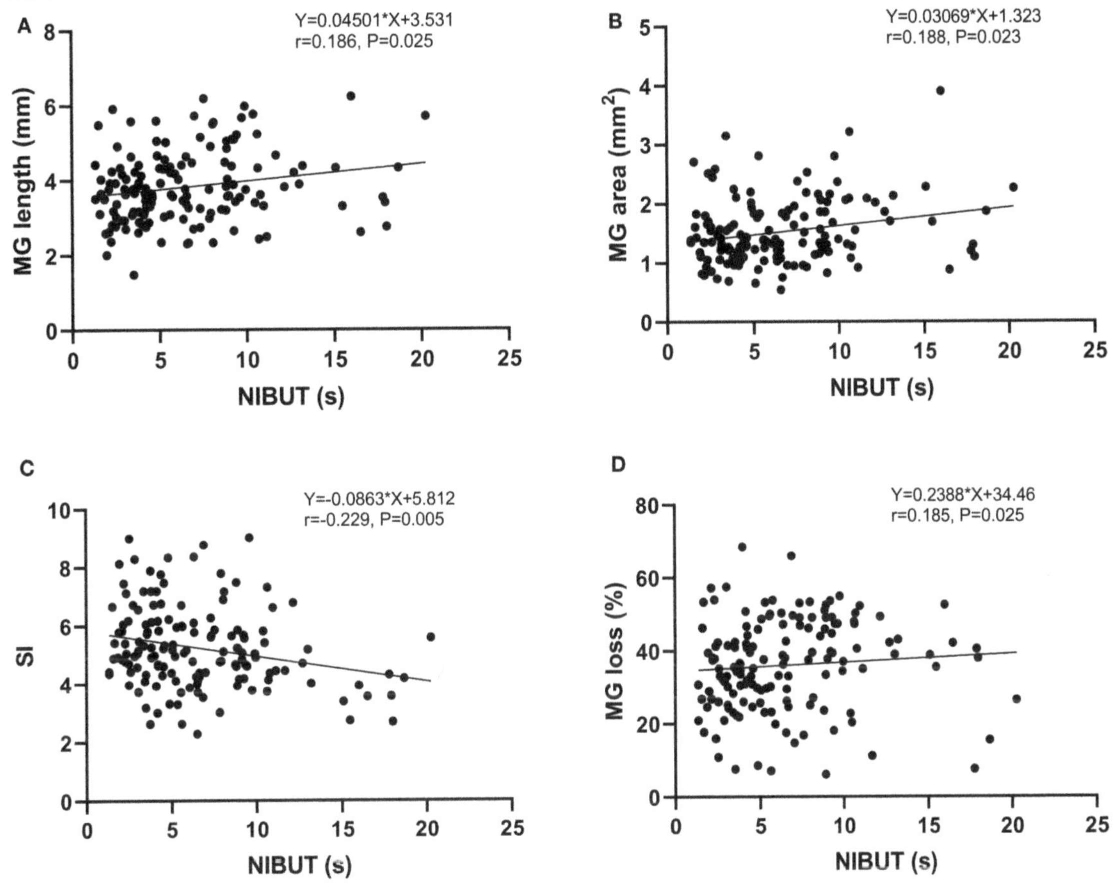

FIGURE 5 | Analysis of the Spearman's rank correlation between the NIBUT and MG length **(A)**, MG area **(B)**, SI **(C)**, and MG loss **(D)**.

in people who undergo cataract surgery. We performed the clinical tests and meibography based on the K5M to observe the functional and morphological changes in the MG after cataract surgery. To obtain more reliable and repeatable results, a fully automated algorithm was used for the objective evaluation of meibography, and a contra-lateral comparison was designed to exclude other factors.

A previous prospective observational study reported that cataract surgery aggravated MG function without changing the structure (4). They analyzed the MG loss at 1 and 3 months after cataract surgery. However, we found MG loss aggravation at 6 months after cataract surgery. Different follow-up time, the sample size and analysis approach might be the probable cause of different outcomes. After discovering more MG loss post-operatively, we evaluated the details of MG structure for further analysis and observed meibomian glands deterioration 6 months post-operatively. Using the automated algorithm reported by Xiao P. et al. (16), it is possible to analyze and compare the details of MG structure, such as length, width, area, DI, and SI.

In the present study, after analyzing the central five glands in the upper lid, we observed significant decreases in MG length, width, area, DI, and SI in the study group. The parameters, such as length, width, and area described the general morphology of MG, the decrease of which further proved deterioration of MG loss assessed by ImageJ software. Gland irregularity was first defined as the differential area compared with a "standard gland" through an automated morphological method in a previous study (17). They verified that gland irregularity was a good parameter for predicting gland function. In this study, we used DI to quantify the uneven width of the MG and found decreased values in the operated eyes. The probable explanation was that the measuring range got smaller due to the decrease of MG area. SI quantified the gland signal level according to the secretion, consistency, and color of meibum inside meibomian glands, which can potentially be used to evaluate meibum secretion activity (16). The decrease in SI in the study group indicated less meibum secretion of MG after cataract surgery.

No significant difference was found between the two groups in MG loss at baseline or 6 months post-operatively. Interestingly, the contra-lateral group also showed MG loss aggravation 6 months post-operatively, slightly less than the study group ($P = 0.015$ vs. $P = 0.004$). The possible reason is that lack of eyelid cleaning in both eyes in the early post-operative stage may result in eyelid margin deterioration, and then result in meibomian glands loss. When comparing MG morphology, there was no difference in MG width, area, DI, and SI values at baseline, but the post-operative values showed significantly lower in the study group. MG length showed no difference between the two groups post-operatively, it may be due to the higher pre-operative MG length value in the study group. Furthermore, all the morphological parameters changed more in the study group than in the control group.

As previously reported, MGD is associated with higher MG loss (9). We investigated TMH and NI-BUT as the functional parameters in the present study and revealed no significant changes in long-term post-operative NIBUT and TMH compared with the pre-operative levels or the contralateral eyes. We found no significant difference when comparing the NIBUT and TMH between the two groups at baseline and 6 months post-operatively. Although TMH increased in the control group post-operatively, TMH changes were not significantly different between the two groups. No significant NIBUT changes were found in either group after cataract surgery. Being consistent to our results, a study by Choi et al. (5) reported no significant difference at 1 and 3 months after surgery in TBUT when compared with the baseline data. A recent study by Lin et al. (18) showed that there was no difference in TMH between the patients with MGD and normal controls. However, some studies reported that TBUT and TMH decreased 3 months post-operatively (4, 7, 19). Based on the observation of 192 eyes of 96 patients, Cetinkaya et al. (20) noted that phacoemulsification surgery may aggravate dry eye test values in the patients with chronic dry eye in the short term (1st day, 1st week, and 1st month post-operatively), and these values will return to the pre-operative levels in the long term (3rd month, 6th month, 1st year, and 2nd year post-operatively). The possible reason of the controversial viewpoints was that most of the studies followed up in the early post-operative periods of cataract surgery, for example, 1 or 3 months post-operatively, while we included the 6-month data after the surgery. We speculate that the NIBUT value gradually compensated and returned to the baseline level, thus at 6 months post-operatively, it displayed slightly shorter than that at baseline without statistically significance.

The MG morphology parameters showed some weak correlations with the clinical tests. There was a positive correlation between TMH and MG loss ($r = 0.221$, $p = 0.005$). Furthermore, there was a positive correlation between NIBUT and MG length ($r = 0.186$, $p = 0.025$), MG area ($r = 0.188$, $p = 0.023$) and MG loss ($r = 0.185$, $p = 0.025$), whereas a negative correlation between NIBUT and SI ($r = -0.229$, $p = 0.005$). Several researchers reported significant strong correlation coefficients (21–23). Hence, TMH and NIBUT could partly represent the function of mebomian glands, especially NIBUT. Theoretically, MG loss indicating MGD that is negatively correlated with NIBUT. It is controversial with our results, although it was weakly correlated. The reason might be as follows: clinically, MG loss does not necessarily mean the MGD if there are no dry eye symptoms. Furthermore, NIBUT may gradually return to the baseline level in the long term after surgery while the changes of MG were irreversible.

The present study reported that MG morphology was aggravated even at 6 months post-operatively, and revealed the morphological changes more specifically, filling the lack of long-term investigation. However, this study has several limitations. First, this study only included 6-month post-operative examinations, so it was unable to determine the changing process after cataract surgery. Second, the lid margin, meibum expressibility were not investigated in this study. Third, we did not perform the Ocular Surface Disease Index (OSDI) Questionnaire, refraction or visual acuity tests in these patients, these parameters and their correlations with MG morphology aggravation need further study in the future. What's more, although we evaluated gland morphology in detail, this study only enrolled central five glands in the upper lid, unable to conclude the morphological changes in all glands. Hence, it is necessary to conduct a study that includes more parameters and glands in the lower lid at several time points.

In conclusion, our study revealed that cataract surgery was associated with MG loss aggravation, and MG morphology deterioration, such as a decrease in length, width, area, and gland signal index. Post-operative NIBUT and TMH did not significantly change in the long term. Therefore, it is important for the clinicians to monitor the MG morphological parameters before and after cataract surgery.

ETHICS STATEMENT

The studies involving human participants were reviewed and approved by the Ethics Committee of the Eye Hospital, Wenzhou Medical University (ID: 2020-058-K-52). The patients/participants provided their written informed consent to participate in this study.

AUTHOR CONTRIBUTIONS

PC and Y-eZ: study concept and design. SQ, ZX, and FH: data collection. PC, SQ, and YZ: analysis and interpretation of data. SQ and ZX: writing the manuscript. PC: critical revision of the manuscript. ZL: statistical expertise. Y-eZ: administrative, technical, or material support and supervision. All authors contributed to the article and approved the submitted version.

REFERENCES

1. McCulley JP, Shine WE. Meibomian gland function and the tear lipid layer. *Ocul Surf.* (2003) 1:97–106. doi: 10.1016/S1542-0124(12)70138-6
2. Baudouin C, Messmer EM, Aragona P, Geerling G, Akova YA, Benitez-del-Castillo J, et al. Revisiting the vicious circle of dry eye disease: a focus on the pathophysiology of meibomian gland dysfunction. Br J Ophthalmol. (2016) 100:300–6. doi: 10.1136/bjophthalmol-2015-307415
3. Cochener B, Cassan A, Omiel L. Prevalence of meibomian gland dysfunction at the time of cataract surgery. *J Cataract Refract Surg.* (2018) 44:144–8. doi: 10.1016/j.jcrs.2017.10.050
4. Han KE, Yoon SC, Ahn JM, Nam SM, Stulting RD, Kim EK, et al. Evaluation of dry eye and meibomian gland dysfunction after cataract surgery. *Am J Ophthalmol.* (2014) 157:1144–50.e1. doi: 10.1016/j.ajo.2014.02.036

5. Choi YJ, Park SY, Jun I, Choi M, Seo KY, Kim EK, et al. Perioperative ocular parameters associated with persistent dry eye symptoms after cataract surgery. *Cornea.* (2018) 37:734–9. doi: 10.1097/ICO.0000000000001572
6. Jung JW, Han SJ, Nam SM, Kim TI, Kim EK, Seo KY. Meibomian gland dysfunction and tear cytokines after cataract surgery according to pre-operative meibomian gland status. *Clin Exp Ophthalmol.* (2016) 44:555–62. doi: 10.1111/ceo.12744
7. Kim JS, Lee H, Choi S, Kim EK, Seo KY, Kim TI. Assessment of the tear film lipid layer thickness after cataract surgery. *Semin Ophthalmol.* (2018) 33:231–6. doi: 10.1080/08820538.2016.1208764
8. Liang Q, Pan Z, Zhou M, Zhang Y, Wang N, Li B, et al. Evaluation of optical coherence tomography meibography in patients with obstructive meibomian gland dysfunction. *Cornea.* (2015) 34:1193–9. doi: 10.1097/ICO.0000000000000563
9. Adil MY, Xiao J, Olafsson J, Chen X, Lagali NS, Raeder S, et al. meibomian gland morphology is a sensitive early indicator of meibomian gland dysfunction. *Am J Ophthalmol.* (2019) 200:16–25. doi: 10.1016/j.ajo.2018.12.006
10. Arita R, Fukuoka S, Morishige N. New insights into the morphology and function of meibomian glands. *Exp Eye Res.* (2017) 163:64–71. doi: 10.1016/j.exer.2017.06.010
11. Yoo YS, Na KS, Kim DY, Yang SW, Joo CK. Morphological evaluation for diagnosis of dry eye related to meibomian gland dysfunction. *Exp Eye Res.* (2017) 163:72–7. doi: 10.1016/j.exer.2017.07.005
12. Chlasta-Twardzik E, Gorecka-Niton A, Nowinska A, Wylegala E. The influence of work environment factors on the ocularsurface in a one-year follow-up prospective clinical study. *Diagnostics.* (2021) 11:392. doi: 10.3390/diagnostics11030392
13. Hashemi H, Asharlous A, Aghamirsalim M, Yekta A, Pourmatin R, Sajjadi M, et al. Meibomian gland dysfunction in geriatric population: tehran geriatric eye study. *Int Ophthalmol.* (2021) 41:2539–46. doi: 10.1007/s10792-021-01812-2
14. Alevi D, Perry HD, Wedel A, Rosenberg E, Alevi L, Donnenfeld ED. Effect of sleep position on the ocular surface. *Cornea.* (2017) 36:567–71. doi: 10.1097/ICO.0000000000001167
15. Hanyuda A, Sawada N, Uchino M, Kawashima M, Yuki K, Tsubota K, et al. Relationship between unhealthy sleep status and dry eye symptoms in a Japanese population. the JPHC NEXT study. *Ocul Surf.* (2021) 21:306–12. doi: 10.1016/j.jtos.2021.04.001
16. Xiao P, Luo Z, Deng Y, Wang G, Yuan J. An automated and multiparametric algorithm for objective analysis of meibography images. *Quant Imaging Med Surg.* (2021) 11:1586–99. doi: 10.21037/qims-20-611
17. Llorens-Quintana C, Rico-Del-Viejo L, Syga P, Madrid-Costa D, Iskander DR. meibomian gland morphology: the influence of structural variations on gland function and ocular surface parameters. *Cornea.* (2019) 38:1506–12. doi: 10.1097/ICO.0000000000002141
18. Lin X, Fu Y, Li L, Chen C, Chen X, Mao Y, et al. A novel quantitative index of meibomian gland dysfunction, the meibomian gland tortuosity. *Transl Vis Sci Technol.* (2020) 9:34. doi: 10.1167/tvst.9.9.34
19. Song P, Sun Z, Ren S, Yang K, Deng G, Zeng Q, et al. Preoperative management of MGD alleviates the aggravation of MGD and dry eye induced by cataract surgery: a prospective, randomized clinical trial. *Biomed Res Int.* (2019) 2019:2737968. doi: 10.1155/2019/2737968
20. Cetinkaya S, Mestan E, Acir NO, Cetinkaya YF, Dadaci Z, Yener HI. The course of dry eye after phacoemulsification surgery. *BMC Ophthalmol.* (2015) 15:68. doi: 10.1186/s12886-015-0058-3
21. Pult H, Riede-Pult BH. Non-contact meibography: keep it simple but effective. *Cont Lens Anterior Eye.* (2012) 35:77–80. doi: 10.1016/j.clae.2011.08.003
22. Pult H, Riede-Pult BH, Nichols JJ. Relation between upper and lower lids' meibomian gland morphology, tear film, and dry eye. *Optom Vis Sci.* (2012) 89:E310–5. doi: 10.1097/OPX.0b013e318244e487
23. Osae EA, Ablorddepey RK, Horstmann J, Kumah DB, Steven P. Assessment of meibomian glands using a custom-made meibographer in dry eye patients in Ghana. *BMC Ophthalmol.* (2018) 18:201. doi: 10.1186/s12886-018-0869-0

18

Improved Dry Eye Symptoms and Signs of Patients With Meibomian Gland Dysfunction by a Dietary Supplement

Kangcheng Liu [1†], Yau Kei Chan [2†], Xia Peng [1], Ruolan Yuan [1], Min Liao [1], Jingwen Liang [1], Xiangbo Tang [1], Yi Xu [1], Yingjun Cai [1], Qiangxiang Li [3] and Hua Wang [1]*

[1] Eye Center of Xiangya Hospital, Hunan Key Laboratory of Ophthalmology, Central South University, Changsha, China, [2] Department of Ophthalmology, Li Ka Shing Faculty of Medicine, The University of Hong Kong, Hong Kong, China, [3] Ningxia Geriatric Disease Clinical Research Center, People's Hospital of Ningxia Hui Autonomous Region, Yinchuan, China

***Correspondence:**
Hua Wang
wanghua1026@csu.edu.cn

† These authors share first authorship

Purpose: To explore the therapeutic effect of a dietary supplement on dry eye with meibomian gland dysfunction (MGD).

Methods: Sixty patients with MGD-related dry eye were included in this prospective and randomized, placebo-controlled study. All the subjects were treated with eye hot compress, artificial tears, and antibiotic ointment. After that, the patients received dietary supplementary or placebo daily for 12 weeks. The dry eye signs, function of MG, and visual quality of the patients were assessed at 4, 8, and 12 weeks after the treatment.

Results: Twelve weeks after the treatment, patients who received dietary supplement had a significantly better improvement of dry eye symptoms, in terms of ocular surface diseases index and tear breaking-up time (TBUT), than those who received placebo ($P < 0.05$). The functions of MG, in terms of meibum quality and MG exclusion and MG obstruction scores, were significantly improved in both dietary supplement and placebo groups ($P < 0.05$). Patients who received dietary supplement had a significantly better improvement in the MG structure, in terms of acinar diameter and acinar density, than those who received placebo ($P < 0.05$). The number of inflammatory cells near MG was significantly lower in the dietary supplement group when compared with the placebo group ($P < 0.05$). The objective visual quality was significantly improved in the dietary supplement group, but not in the placebo group ($P < 0.05$).

Conclusion: The dietary supplement can effectively improve the symptoms and signs of MGD-related dry eye, reduce the inflammatory reaction of MG, restore the gland structure, and indirectly improve the visual quality.

Keywords: dietary supplements, meibomian gland dysfunction (MGD), dry eye, Retaron®, symptoms and signs

INTRODUCTION

Meibomian gland dysfunction (MGD) is a chronic, diffuse meibomian gland lesion. The main features of MGD are the obstruction of the terminal duct of the meibomian glands and the abnormal quality or quantity of the meibum secretion (1). This disease causes tear film abnormalities with inflammatory reactions, resulting in eye irritation. The cornea gets damage and visual function is affected in severe MGD (1). When MGD occurs, the change of meibum, the main component of the lipid layer of the tear film, affects the steady state of the tear film and results in evaporative dry eye. Since the publication of the Tear Film and Ocular Surface Society Dry Eye Workshop (TFOS DEWS) report, numerous studies have conducted to investigate the correlation between MGD and dry eye (2). MGD is believed to be the most common cause of dry eye (3, 4). Epidemiological surveys of MGD patients from different ages, genders, and races showed that the prevalence of MGD over 40 years is from 38 to 68% (5–7). Other epidemiological surveys based on different ethnic groups have found that around 53.6–89.7% of patients in the dry eye population are with MGD (8, 9). Therefore, the functional improvement of MG becomes the major strategy to treat MGD-related dry eye patients (10).

The current treatment of MGD-related dry eye includes physical and oral drug therapies, such as eye drops, hot eye compresses, and MG massage (11). However, these treatments also have own limitations. Hot eye compresses need to maintain a constant temperature to liquefy the secretions that block MG, which is troublesome in real practice (12, 13). Similarly, although MG massage has a better theoretical therapeutic effect, it is easy to cause damage to the MG or cornea, and more severely secondary infection. Moreover, patient compliance is poor (14). At present, systemic oral bioactives, such as various vitamins and antibiotics, are needed for patients with severe MGD or MGD with seborrheic dermatitis, rosacea, and other skin lesions (15). As patients require a long-term use of antibiotics, they may suffer from the emergence of drug-resistant bacteria, bacterial imbalance and double infections, and other serious side effects (15). Meanwhile, among the commercially available drugs that treat dry eye diseases, most of them have poor acceptance from the stakeholders. Therefore, it is of great importance to find a bioactive that can safely and effectively treat MGD-related dry eye.

Dietary supplements have been widely used as an adjunct therapy for patients with various diseases (16). Many clinical studies have shown that dietary supplements can safely and effectively be used as adjuvant therapy (17). The American epidemiological survey shows that as many as 53% of the U.S. population have routine intake of dietary supplements, showing a very high population acceptance to the dietary supplements (18). The identification of dietary supplements that can treat MGD-related dry eye safely and effectively will have important clinical value and significance. Retaron® is a new dietary supplement formulation on the market that has recently obtained the national safety standard identification in China. Its main ingredients include omega-3 free fatty acids, lutein, aronia extract, vitamin C, and vitamin E. It has potent antioxidant and anti-inflammatory effects, which play an important role in promoting retinal development and improving visual function (19). In this study, we investigated the effect of the dietary supplement as an adjunct treatment of MGD-related dry eye. Our hypothesis was that the use of dietary supplement can improve dry eye symptoms and signs, reduce the inflammatory reaction of MG, and restore the gland structure in patients with MGD.

TABLE 1 | Formula of dietary supplement Retaron® in the study.

Formula	Retaron®
β-Carotene	–
Lutein	10 mg
Zeaxanthin	2 mg
Vitamin C	100 mg
Vitamin E	20 mg
Zinc	10 mg
Copper	–
Selenium	25 μg
Taurine	50 mg
Aronia extract	50 mg
Omega-3 free fatty acids, 250 mg DHA/30 mg EPA	500 mg

MATERIALS AND METHODS

Study Population

Between September 2018 and May 2019, 60 patients with binocular MGD-related dry eye were recruited from the ocular surface specialist outpatient clinic at Xiangya Hospital Ophthalmology Center. The diagnostic criteria of MGD and dry eye are based on Chinese Expert Consensus on the Diagnosis and Treatment of MGD (2017) (20) and TFOS DEWS II (2017) (21).

The inclusion criteria include (1) the age of patients in between 18 and 80 years and (2) the best-corrected visual acuity in both eyes that is higher than 0.1. The exclusion criteria include (1) systemic diseases such as systemic lupus erythematosus, rheumatism, and diabetes; (2) history of eye surgery and trauma; (3) other eye diseases; (4) systemic and ocular medications; (5) pregnant or lactating women; (6) patients who are allergic to the ingredients of the dietary supplement formulation or the drugs involved in this study; and (7) people who cannot take care of themselves and cooperate with treatment and follow-up.

Informed Consent

All patients have agreed and signed the consent form to be included in the study. This study followed the Declaration of Helsinki, conformed to the principles of medical ethics, and was approved by the Ethics Committee of Xiangya Hospital of Central South University (Document number: 201912528).

Study Design

The MGD-related dry eye patients included in this study were randomly divided into two groups, the experimental dietary supplement group (60 eyes of 30 cases) and placebo control group (60 eyes of 30 cases). Both the groups were respectively treated with oral dietary supplementary formulation Retaron® (**Table 1**) and placebo capsule daily for 12 weeks. The eyelid margins of all patients were applied with tobramycin and dexamethasone ophthalmic ointment (once per night) for the first 2 weeks, followed by levofloxacin ophthalmic gel (once per night) for the next 10 weeks. Eye hot compress (once per night) and eye drops of 0.1% sodium hyaluronate (four times a day) were applied in adjunct with the dietary supplement for 12 weeks.

Clinical Examinations

All subjects were followed up for 12 weeks with a 4-week interval. To avoid systematic errors, all the inspections and operations described below were completed by the same experienced ophthalmologist or technician. All subjects underwent routine examinations, such as vision, optometry, intraocular pressure, and fundus, at each follow-up.

Dry eye symptoms and signs were evaluated by Ocular Surface Disease Index (OSDI) Questionnaire Scale, (20) tear breaking-up time (TBUT), and corneal fluorescein (FL) staining. TBUT is an index used to evaluate the stability of the tear film. For each patient at each time point, TBUT was obtained by averaging the values from three measurements. TBUT value > 10 s is regarded as normal. Corneal FL staining helped us to examine the severity of corneal epithelial damage and was quantitatively evaluated using the 4-quadrant 12-point method as previously described (22).

The MG obstruction (23) of each eyelid was evaluated using a slit lamp microscope and anterior segment camera system with the following self-defined scoring system (24): 0 point, unobstructed opening; 1 point, MG with <1/3 obstruction; 2 points, between 1/3 and 2/3 obstruction; and 3 points, over 2/3 obstruction.

All the five MGs in the upper eyelid of each subject were squeezed, and the function of MG was assessed by the following MG discharge capacity score (20): 0 point, all five glands have discharge; 1 point: three or four glands have discharge; 2 points, only one or two glands have discharge; and 3 points, no gland with discharge. The meibum was evaluated according to the viscosity and turbidity of meibum using the meibum quality score: (20) 0 point, clear, transparent liquid; 1 point, turbid liquid; 2 points, turbid granular discharge; and 3 points, thick discharge like toothpaste.

The acinar morphology and inflammation of MG were examined using *in vivo* confocal microscopy (IVCM) (Heidelberg, Germany) and evaluated by (1) the diameter of MG opening, (2) acinar diameter, (3) acinar density, and (4) local inflammatory cell count (25, 26). For each parameter, ten photographs were randomly evaluated, and the average value of the ten measurements of the four previously mentioned parameters was recorded.

The visual quality of the patients was objectively assessed using the Optical Quality Analysis System (Visiometrics, Spain). Several visual quality assessment parameters were assessed, including modulation transfer function cutoff frequency (MTF_{cutoff}), Strehl ratio (SR), and objective scatter index (OSI). MTF_{cutoff} reflects the resolution of the optical system, and its value is directly proportional to the visual quality. The value below 30 c/deg is considered as abnormal visual quality. SR is the ratio of the light intensity at the Gaussian image point of the actual refractive medium to the light intensity at the Gaussian phase point of the normal refractive medium. The higher the SR value, the closer it is to an aberration-free optical system. Below 0.15, the visual quality is considered abnormal. OSI reflects the degree of turbidity of the refractive medium. Values higher than 2.0 are regarded as abnormal, and higher values represent more turbid refractive media.

Statistical Analysis

Statistical analysis was performed using SPASS 19.00 (IBM Corp, Armonk, NY, United States). The Kolmogorov–Smirnov test was used to test the normality of the data. Normally distributed data were expressed as mean ± SD, and non-normally distributed data were expressed as median and interquartile range. If the data conformed to be normally distributed, the comparisons between groups at each time point were tested by repeated-measures ANOVA (multiple time points) and independent-sample *t*-test (two time points). If the data did not meet the "spherical symmetry" assumption, the Greenhouse–Geisser estimate was used for correction. The LSD *t*-test (multiple time points) and paired *t*-test (two time points) were used for group comparison at each time point. If the data did not conform to be normally distributed, the Mann–Whitney *U*-test and the Kruskal-Wallis test were used for pairwise comparisons between groups at each time point. The test level was $\alpha = 0.05$, and $P < 0.05$ was considered statistically significant.

RESULTS

Clinical Outcomes

A total of 60 subjects (120 eyes) were included in this study, namely, 30 subjects (60 eyes) in the dietary supplement group and 30 subjects (60 eyes) in the control group. Before the treatment, there were no significant differences in age, best-corrected visual acuity, or intraocular pressure between the two groups ($P > 0.05$ for all indices) (**Table 2**).

Dry Eye Symptoms and Signs

Before the treatment, there was no significant difference between the two groups in terms of the symptoms and signs of dry eye as quantified by OSDI and FL scores and TBUT ($P > 0.05$ for all indices). Twelve weeks after the treatment, punctate staining of corneal epithelium disappeared in both groups (**Figure 1D**), and both the OSDI and FL scores of the two groups of subjects were significantly lower than the baseline values ($P < 0.001$) (**Figures 1A,C**). However, TBUT score of the two groups was significantly higher than the baseline values ($P < 0.001$) (**Figure 1B**). Moreover, the dietary supplement group showed better outcomes, with lower OSDI and FL scores, and a higher TBUT, when compared with the control group ($P < 0.05$ for all indices) (**Figure 1**).

TABLE 2 | Comparison of the demography of the two groups of patients.

	Range	Dietary supplement group	Control group	P
Sex (Male/female)	/	10/14	13/17	N/A
Age (years)	18–80	44.23 ± 14.03	46.83 ± 12.03	0.444
BCVA[U]	0.1–1.5	1.2 (1.0, 1.2)	1.2 (1.0, 1.2)	0.954
IOP (mmHg)	10–21	17.10 ± 2.07	16.03 ± 2.31	0.065

[U]*Data are tested by Mann–Whitney U-test.*
BCVA, best-corrected visual acuity; IOP, intraocular pressure.

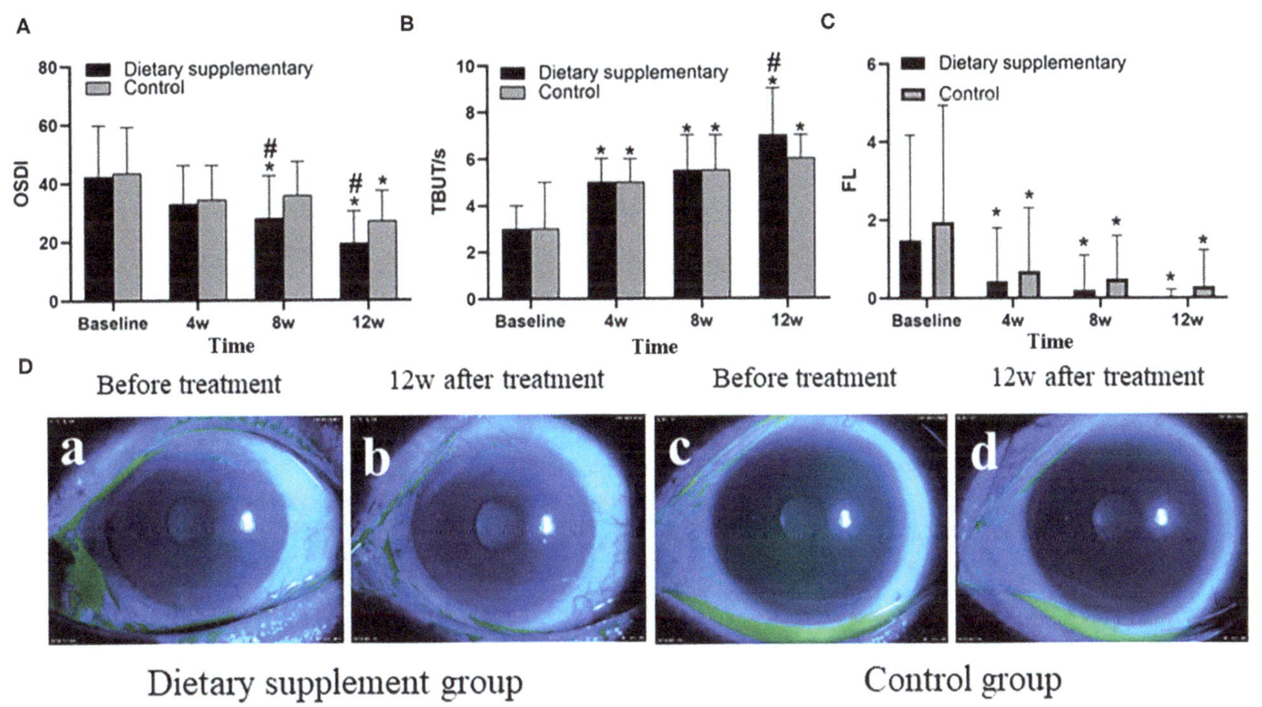

FIGURE 1 | The **(A)** OSDI, **(B)** TBUT, and **(C)** FL of the two groups. **(D)** Anterior segment images of corneal FL staining between the two groups before and after the treatment. *$P < 0.05$ vs. before the treatment; #$P < 0.05$ vs. control group.

The Function of MG and MG Obstruction

Before the treatment, the upper eyelid margin congestion and MG obstruction were significant in both groups, and the meibum was viscous and turbid and difficult to be excreted when the MG was compressed (**Figure 2D**-a,c). There was no difference between the two groups in MG obstruction, MG discharge function, and meibum quality ($P > 0.05$ for all indices). After 12 weeks of treatment, the upper eyelid margin congestion was reduced in both groups, and MG obstruction was significantly improved. The meibum was also clear and easy to be excreted when the MG was compressed (**Figure 2D**-b,d). The MG exclusion score, meibum quality score, and the obstruction score of the two groups were significantly improved after the treatment at 8 and 12 weeks ($P \leq 0.001$ for all time points). However, there is no significant difference between the two groups at the same time point ($P > 0.05$ for all indices) (**Figures 2A–C**).

Morphological Structure of MG and Local Inflammatory Response

Before the treatment, there was no significant difference between the two groups in inflammatory cell number (**Figures 3A,E**-a,c), MG opening diameter (**Figures 3B,E**-i,k), acinar density (**Figures 3C,E**-e,g), and acinar diameter (**Figures 3D,E**-e,g) ($P > 0.05$ for all indices). Twelve weeks after the treatment, the number of inflammatory cells (**Figures 3A,E**-b), acinar density (**Figures 3C,E**-f), and acinar diameter (**Figures 3D,E**-f) in the dietary supplement group were significantly improved ($P \leq 0.001$ for all indices) and were significantly better than in the control group ($P \leq 0.001$ for all indices) (**Figures 3A,C–E**-d,h). The diameter of MG in both groups was not significantly improved when compared with the baseline level ($P > 0.05$ for two groups) (**Figures 3B,E**-j,l).

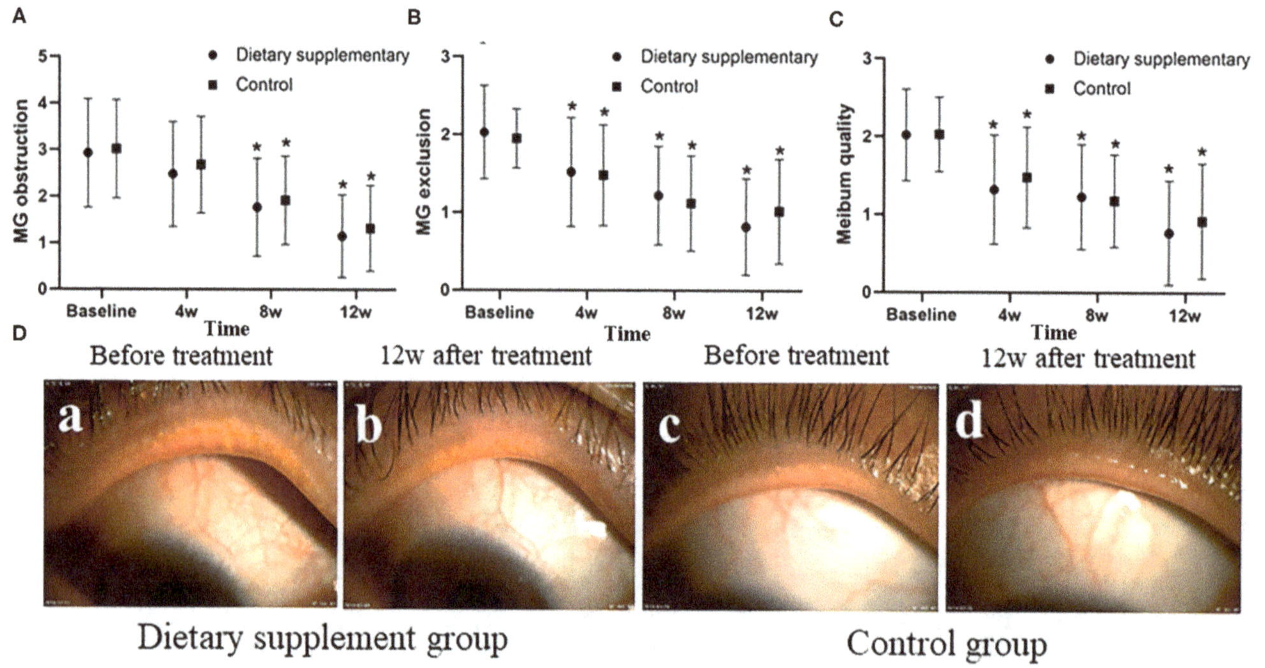

FIGURE 2 | The function of MG and MG obstruction between two groups. **(A)** The MG obstruction score, **(B)** the MG exclusion, and **(C)** the meibum quality score. **(D)** Anterior segment images of palpebral margin between the two groups before and after the treatment. *$P < 0.05$ vs. before the treatment.

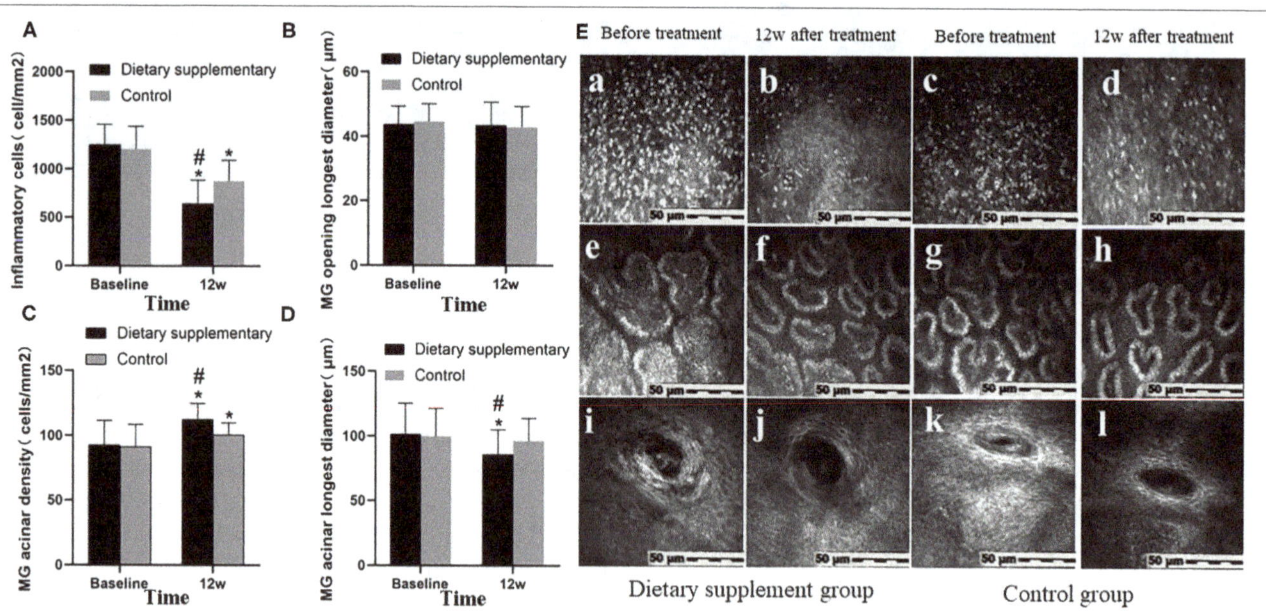

FIGURE 3 | The IVCM between two groups. **(A)** Inflammatory cell number. **(B)** The longest diameter of MG opening. **(C)** MG acinar density. **(D)** MG acinar longest diameter. **(E)** IVCM images of MG before and after treatment in both groups. (a–d) Inflammatory cells. (e–h) Acinar morphology and density. (i–l) The shape of MG opening. *$P < 0.05$ vs. before treatment; #$P < 0.05$ vs. control group.

Objective Visual Quality

Before the treatment, there was no significant difference in the three visual quality parameters, namely, $P_{MTFcutof}$, P_{SR}, and P_{OSI}, between the two groups ($P > 0.05$ for all indices). Twelve weeks after the treatment, the MTF_{cutoff} and SR of the dietary supplement group were significantly improved ($P < 0.001$ for MTF_{cutoff} and SR). In contrast, the improvement of the control group, when compared with the baseline, was not significant (P

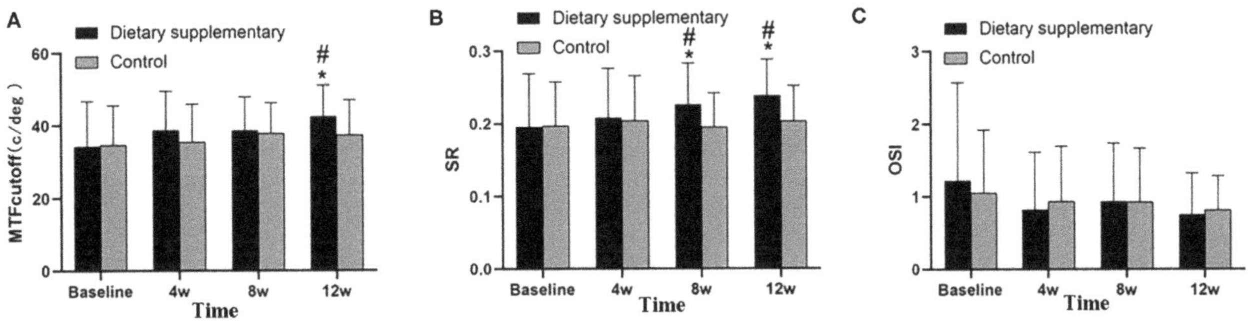

FIGURE 4 | Objective visual quality between two groups. **(A)** MTF_{cutoff}, **(B)** SR, and **(C)** OSI. *P < 0.05 vs. before treatment; #P < 0.05 vs. control group.

> 0.05 for MTF_{cutoff} and SR). Moreover, the difference between the two groups was significant ($P_{MTFcutoff} = 0.003$, $P_{SR} < 0.001$) (**Figures 4A,B**). However, there was no significant difference in OSI between two groups ($P_{OSI} > 0.05$ for two groups) (**Figure 4C**).

Adverse Reactions

During the follow-up, no obvious local or systemic adverse reactions were observed in all subjects.

DISCUSSION

The MG is a special exocrine gland. The meibum secreted by the acinar epithelium forms a lipid layer on the tear film surface to make the tear film stable. When the MG is blocked or atrophic, this causes pathological changes in both the quality and quantity of the meibomian ester and its excretion, and finally leads to MGD. At the same time, MGD is often accompanied by local inflammatory reaction, which will eventually lead to lipid deficiency-type dry eye. Current studies have confirmed that MGD is one of the most important causes of dry eye (4).

Dietary supplements have been widely used for long time in all age groups worldwide, especially in developed countries, where dietary supplement use is as high as 11.7–66% (27). It plays an important role in balancing the nutrition of the normal population and the auxiliary treatment of the sick population, and it has been proved safe and effective. In our study, dietary supplement was used as an adjunct therapy to treat and to explore the safety and efficacy on MGD-related dry eye. Our results indicated that the adjunct therapy using dietary supplement can improve the ocular symptoms and signs, MG structure, local inflammatory response, and objective visual quality of MGD-related dry eye patients, but no significant advantage in the improvement of the properties and excretion capacity of meibum.

Meibomian gland produces and secretes meibomian ester in a constant manner, which makes it a high oxygen consumption tissue. Long-term and excessive oxidative reaction is an important reason for the dysfunction of MG. Oxidative stress is often accompanied by local inflammation of the MG. The clinical manifestations are mucous and muddy meibum, abnormal increase or decrease in secretion, gland obstruction and pathological dilatation, ester embolization obstruction at the opening, congestion and edema at the edge of eyelid, and neovascularization, which may lead to lipid deficiency-type dry eye (28). Our study showed that the symptoms and signs of the dry eye, MG structure, local inflammatory response, and objective visual quality were all significantly improved after the treatment. The possible mechanism is that the active ingredients in the dietary supplement formulation, which have strong antioxidant and anti-inflammatory effects, promote the repair of acinar epithelial and peripheral nerve damage. Ares 2 formula contains vitamin C, vitamin E, beta carotene, zinc, and copper, which are similar to the dietary supplement we used in this study. Eskina et al. observed the improvement of visual quality by using the drug complex responding to the Ares 2 formula (29). Told et al. confirmed that dietary supplement Retaron® can play an antioxidant role in the human body, thus affecting the retinal dynamic function (30). However, their study did not assess the therapeutic effect of the dietary supplement on the ocular surface microenvironment.

Among the components in the dietary supplement we tested in this study, the high concentration of polyphenol compounds and cyanidin-3-O-glucoside chloride in aronia extracts can quickly and effectively remove oxygen free radicals and play a strong antioxidant effect (31). In addition, aronia extract contains active components such as nitric oxide synthase-2 and cyclooxygenase-2, which can effectively inhibit inflammatory and oxidative reactions (32). Cavet et al. also confirmed that polyphenols have anti-inflammatory and antioxidant effects on human corneal epithelial cells, which can be used to treat eye inflammation caused by diseases and have a potential value in the treatment of dry eyes (33).

Omega-3 free fatty acids can optimize the transformation of meibum from saturated fatty acids to unsaturated fatty acids under pathological conditions (4), so it may effectively promote the generation and excretion of meibomian esters, improve the obstruction of glandular ducts, and reduce the local inflammatory reaction, thus restoring the structure of MG. By improving the properties of eyelid esters and reducing the inflammation at the edge of the eyelid, the stability of the lipid layer of the tear film should be gradually restored, and therefore, the symptoms and signs of dry eyes could be indirectly improved and eventually improve the visual quality. Macsai evaluated the ocular symptoms of MGD patients and found that the use of omega-3 fatty acids improved the scores of OSDI, TBUT, and meibomian, which was similar to the results of our study (34). Meanwhile, Deinema et al. also confirmed that omega-3 fatty acids can reduce tear osmolality and improve tear film stability in patients with dry eye, thus improving the symptoms of dry eye (35). However, our results showed that there were no obvious advantages in the improvement of meibomian ester and MG excretion after dietary supplement was added, which might be related to the short-term treatment and observation period, and small sample size in this study. We will increase the sample size and extend the study period in the future, which may lead to more representative and conclusive results.

In summary, for the treatment of MGD-related dry eye that is based on conventional treatment strategies, the addition of dietary supplement can further improve the symptoms and signs of dry eye, reduce the inflammatory response of MG, restore the glandular structure, and improve the visual quality, without any systemic or local adverse reactions. However, there were no significant advantages in the improvement of meibomian ester and MG excretion. Dietary supplement is expected to be a safe and effective systemic drug in the treatment of MGD-related dry eye.

ETHICS STATEMENT

This study followed the Declaration of Helsinki, conformed to the principles of medical ethics, and was approved by the Ethics Committee of Xiangya Hospital of Central South University (Document Number: 201912528). The patients/participants provided their written informed consent to participate in this study.

AUTHOR CONTRIBUTIONS

KL and YC: data acquisition and/or research execution, data analysis and/or interpretation, and manuscript preparation. XP and ML: data acquisition and/or research execution, data analysis and/or interpretation. RY: data analysis and/or interpretation, manuscript preparation. JL, XT, and YX: data acquisition and/or research execution. YC and QL: data analysis and/or interpretation. HW: research design, data acquisition and/or research execution, data analysis and/or interpretation, and manuscript preparation. All authors contributed to the article and approved the submitted version.

REFERENCES

1. Vu CHV, Kawashima M, Yamada M, Suwaki K, Uchino M, Shigeyasu C, et al. Influence of meibomian gland dysfunction and friction-related disease on the severity of dry eye. *Ophthalmology.* (2018) 125:1181–8. doi: 10.1016/j.ophtha.2018.01.025
2. The International Dry Eye WorkShop. Design and conduct of clinical trials: report of the clinical trials subcommittee of the international dry eye workshop (2007). *Ocular Surface.* (2007) 5:153–62. doi: 10.1016/S1542-0124(12)70084-8
3. Galor A, Feuer W, Lee DJ, Florez H, Venincasa VD, Perez VL. Ocular surface parameters in older male veterans. *Invest Ophthalmol Vis Sci.* (2013) 54:1426–33. doi: 10.1167/iovs.12-10819
4. Jones L, Downie LE, Korb D, Benitez-Del-Castillo JM, Dana R, Deng SX, et al. TFOS DEWS II management and therapy report. *Ocul Surf.* (2017) 15:575–628. doi: 10.1016/j.jtos.2017.05.006
5. Jie Y, Xu L, Wu YY, Jonas JB. Prevalence of dry eye among adult Chinese in the Beijing eye study. *Eye.* (2009) 23:688–93. doi: 10.1038/sj.eye.6703101
6. Viso E, Rodriguez-Ares MT, Gude F. Prevalence of and associated factors for dry eye in a Spanish adult population (the Salnes Eye Study). *Ophthalmic Epidemiol.* (2009) 16:15–21. doi: 10.1080/09286580802228509
7. Han SB, Hyon JY, Woo SJ, Lee JJ, Kim TH, Kim KW. Prevalence of dry eye disease in an elderly Korean population. *Arch Ophthalmol.* (2011) 29:633–8. doi: 10.1001/archophthalmol.2011.78
8. Stapleton F, Alves M, Bunya VY, Jalbert I, Lekhanont K, Malet F, et al. TFOS DEWS II epidemiology report. *Ocul Surf.* (2017) 5:334–65. doi: 10.1016/j.jtos.2017.05.003
9. Viso E, Gude F, Rodríguez-Ares MT. The association of meibomian gland dysfunction and other common ocular diseases with dry eye: a population-based study in Spain. *Cornea.* (2011) 30:1–6. doi: 10.1097/ICO.0b013e3181da5778
10. Mendoza R L. Clinical trials with multiple endpoints can establish a correlation, but not (yet) causality, between dietary supplementation with omega-3 fatty acids and keratoconjunctivitis sicca. *J Med Econ.* (2018) 21:733–44. doi: 10.1080/13696998.2018.1478838
11. Lee L, Garrett Q, Flanagan JL, Vaddavalli PK, Papas EB. Treatment practices and outcomes of meibomian gland dysfunction at a tertiary center in Southern India. *Eye Contact Lens.* (2018) 44:S138–S43. doi: 10.1097/ICL.0000000000000356
12. Alghamdi YA, Camp A, Feuer W, Karp CL, Wellik S, Galor A. Compliance and subjective patient responses to eyelid hygiene. *Eye Contact Lens.* (2017) 43:213–7. doi: 10.1097/ICL.0000000000000258
13. Giannaccare G, Taroni L, Senni C, Scorcia V. Intense pulsed light therapy in the treatment of meibomian gland dysfunction: current perspectives. *Clin Optometry.* (2019) 11:113–26. doi: 10.2147/OPTO.S217639
14. Wang DH, Liu XQ, Hao XJ, Zhang YJ, Zhu HY, Dong ZG. Effect of the meibomian gland squeezer for treatment of meibomian gland dysfunction. *Cornea.* (2018) 37:1270–8. doi: 10.1097/ICO.0000000000001682
15. Voils SA, Evans ME, Lane MT, Schosser RH, Rapp RP. Use of macrolides and tetracyclines for chronic inflammatory diseases. *Ann Pharmacother.* (2005) 39:86–94. doi: 10.1345/aph.1E282
16. Alsharairi NA. The effects of dietary supplements on asthma and lung cancer risk in smokers and non-smokers: a review of the literature. *Nutrients.* (2019) 11:725. doi: 10.3390/nu11040725
17. Saccà SC, Cutolo CA, Ferrari D, Corazza P, Traverso CE. The eye, oxidative damage and polyunsaturated fatty acids. *Nutrients.* (2018) 10:668. doi: 10.3390/nu10060668
18. Avigan MI, Mozersky RP, Seeff LB. Scientific and regulatory perspectives in herbal and dietary supplement associated hepatotoxicity in the United States. *Int J Mol Sci.* (2016) 17:331. doi: 10.3390/ijms17030331
19. Shaik-Dasthagirisaheb YB, Varvara G, Murmura G, Saggini A, Caraffa A, Antinolfi P, et al. Role of vitamins D, E and C in immunity and inflammation. *J Biol Regulat Homeost Agents.* (2013) 27:291–5. doi: 10.1016/B978-0-12-386960-9.00025-3
20. China Dry Eye Society. Chinese expert consensus on the diagnosis and treatment of MGD Chinese *J Ophthalmol.* (2017) 53:657–61. doi: 10.3760/cma.j.issn.0412-4081.2017.09.005

21. Craig JP, Nichols KK, Akpek EK, Caffery B, Dua HS, Joo CK, et al. TFOS DEWS II definition and classification report. *Ocular Surface.* (2017) 15:276–83. doi: 10.1016/j.jtos.2017.05.008
22. Wang S, Zhao H, Huang C, Li Z, Li W, Zhang X, et al. Impact of chronic smoking on meibomian gland dysfunction. *PLoS ONE.* (2016) 11:e0168763. doi: 10.1371/journal.pone.0168763
23. Korb DR, Henriquez AS. Meibomian gland dysfunction and contact lens intolerance. *J Am Optom Assoc.* (1980) 51:243–51.
24. Agnifili L, Mastropasqua R, Fasanella V, Brescia L, Scatena B, Oddone F, et al. Meibomian gland features and conjunctival goblet cell density in glaucomatous patients controlled with prostaglandin/timolol fixed combinations: a case control, cross-sectional study. *J Glaucoma.* (2018) 27:364–70. doi: 10.1097/IJG.0000000000000899
25. Zhao H, Chen JY, Wang YQ, Lin ZR, Wang S. *In vivo* confocal microscopy evaluation of meibomian gland dysfunction in dry eye patients with different symptoms. *Chin Med J.* (2016) 129:2617–22. doi: 10.4103/0366-6999.192782
26. Chen T, Li Q, Tang X, Liao M, Wang H. *In vivo* confocal microscopy of cornea in patients with Terrien's marginal corneal degeneration. *J Ophthalmol.* (2019) 2019:3161843. doi: 10.1155/2019/3161843
27. Gahche JJ, Bailey RL, Potischman N, Ershow AG, Herrick KA, Ahluwalia N, et al. Federal monitoring of dietary supplement use in the resident, civilian, noninstitutionalized US population, national health and nutrition examination survey. *J Nutr.* (2018) 148:1436s—44s. doi: 10.1093/jn/nxy093
28. Bron AJ, de Paiva CS, Chauhan SK, Bonini S, Gabison EE, Jain S, et al. TFOS DEWS II pathophysiology report. *Ocul Surf.* (2017) 15:438–510. doi: 10.1016/j.jtos.2017.05.011
29. Eskina EN, Belogurova AV, Gvetadze AA, Smorchkova AS. Practical application of ophthalmic nutraceuticals in patients with dry form of age-related macular degeneration. *Vestn Oftalmol.* (2020) 36:86–92. doi: 10.17116/oftalma202013604186
30. Told R, Schmidl D, Palkovits S, Boltz A, Gouya G, Wolzt M, et al. Antioxidative capacity of a dietary supplement on retinal hemodynamic function in a human lipopolysaccharide (LPS) model. *Invest Ophthalmol Vis Sci.* (2014) 56:403–11. doi: 10.1167/iovs.14-15581
31. Sidor A, Gramza-Michałowska A. Black Chokeberry *Aronia melanocarpa* L.-A qualitative composition, phenolic profile and antioxidant potential. *Molecules.* (2019) 24:3710. doi: 10.3390/molecules24203710
32. Ohgami K, Ilieva I, Shiratori K, Koyama Y, Jin XH, Yoshida K, et al. Anti-inflammatory effects of aronia extract on rat endotoxin-induced uveitis. *Invest Ophthalmol Vis Sci.* (2005) 46:275–81. doi: 10.1167/iovs.04-0715
33. Cavet ME, Harrington KL, Vollmer TR, Ward KW, Zhang JZ. Anti-inflammatory and anti-oxidative effects of the green tea polyphenol epigallocatechin gallate in human corneal epithelial cells. *Mol Vis1.* (2011) 7:533–42. doi: 10.1515/BC.2002.010
34. Macsai MS. The role of omega-3 dietary supplementation in blepharitis and meibomian gland dysfunction (an AOS thesis). *Trans Am Ophthalmol Soc.* (2008) 106:336–56.
35. Deinema LA, Vingrys AJ, Wong CY, Jackson DC, Chinnery HR, Downie LE. A randomized, double-masked, placebo-controlled clinical trial of two forms of omega-3 supplements for treating dry eye disease. *Ophthalmology.* (2017) 124:43–52. doi: 10.1016/j.ophtha.2016.09.023

19

Treatment of Dry Eye With Intracanalicular Injection of Hydroxybutyl Chitosan

Tong Lin[1,2,3†], *Wushuang Wang*[1,2,3†], *Yang Lu*[1,2,3] *and Lan Gong*[1,2,3*]

[1] Department of Ophthalmology, Eye, Ear, Nose, and Throat Hospital of Fudan University, Shanghai, China, [2] NHC Key Laboratory of Myopia (Fudan University), Laboratory of Myopia, Chinese Academy of Medical Sciences, Shanghai, China, [3] Shanghai Key Laboratory of Visual Impairment and Restoration, Fudan University, Shanghai, China

***Correspondence:**
Lan Gong
13501798683@139.com

† These authors have contributed equally to this work

Background: Punctal/intracanalicular plugs on the market nowadays are all designed before clinical use in treating dry eye disease (DED). To provide an individualized lacrimal drainage system occlusion method and reduce the complications, we developed a "liquid plug" strategy by intracanalicular injection of hydroxybutyl chitosan (HBC) solution, a thermosensitive, phase-changing biomaterial. This study evaluated the efficacy and safety of the HBC plug in treating dry eye disease by comparing it with the VisiPlug absorbable intracanalicular plug.

Methods: A monocenter, randomized, controlled clinical trial was performed. Fifty patients with DED were randomized 1:1 to undergo either the HBC injection treatment or the VisiPlug treatment. Ocular Surface Disease Index (OSDI) questionnaire, tear break-up time (TBUT), corneal fluorescence staining (CFS), tear meniscus height (TMH), and phenol red thread test were evaluated at Day 0 (baseline, before treatment) and Weeks 1, 4, and 12.

Results: The two groups had a balanced baseline of age, gender, and DED-related characteristics. Both occlusion methods could relieve the symptoms and signs of DED. Significant improvement was found in OSDI, phenol red thread test, and tear meniscus height ($P < 0.05$ compared to baseline) but not in corneal fluorescence staining and tear break-up time ($P > 0.05$). There is no statistically significant difference between HBC injection and VisiPlug at Weeks 1 and 4 ($P > 0.05$). However, at week 12, the HBC injection was not as effective as the VisiPlug in maintaining phenol red thread test (HBC: 5.35 ± 3.22 mm, VisiPlug: 8.59 ± 4.35 mm, $P = 0.009$) and tear meniscus height (HBC: $206.9 \pm 47.95\,\mu m$, VisiPlug: $242.59 \pm 60.30\,\mu m$, $P = 0.041$). The numbers of ocular adverse events were relatively low in both groups.

Conclusions: The HBC injection showed similar efficacy and safety compared to VisiPlug. The intracanalicular injection of HBC solution proves to be a promising, individualizing method to treat DED.

Clinical Trial Registration: This study is registered with the Chinese Clinical Trial Registry (https://www.chictr.org.cn/enindex.aspx), Identifier: ChiCTR1800016603.

Keywords: dry eye disease, hydroxybutyl chitosan, intracanalicular occlusion, ocular surface, treatment

INTRODUCTION

Dry eye disease (DED) is a multifactorial disease of the ocular surface characterized by a loss of homeostasis of the tear film and accompanied by ocular symptoms, in which tear film instability and hyperosmolarity, ocular surface inflammation and damage, and neurosensory abnormalities play etiological roles (1). DED can greatly affect people's life and worse symptoms of DED are associated with decreased work productivity levels (2). About 21% of the adults in China are suffering from DED, which causes a great burden to society (3). Management and therapy of DED include treatments for tear insufficiency, tear conservation approaches, treatments for lid abnormalities, anti-inflammation therapy, and others (4). A sequence of treatments is often recommended according to the stage of the disease. In moderate or severe DED cases where tear replacement approaches alone are not enough, lacrimal drainage system occlusion is regarded as a simple and effective tear conservation method (5).

Lacrimal drainage system occlusion is commonly undertaken using punctal/intracanalicular plugs, including absorbable and non-absorbable plugs. Though featuring numerous materials (6–9), plugs available on the market currently are all shaped into a certain design before clinical use and are difficult to apply to individual treatment. Notably, the most common complication of punctal occlusion, spontaneous plug extrusion, is often caused by undersized plugs, which could lead to decreased efficacy and economic losses to DED patients (10). Thus, an individualized design of plug is necessary for better efficacy as well as fewer complications.

Recently, we have designed a novel type of "liquid plugs" using hydroxybutyl chitosan (HBC), a thermosensitive and dissolving material with good biocompatibility (11). When injected into the canaliculus, the HBC solution instantly formed a hydrogel plug at the body temperature and turned into an absorbable intracanalicular HBC plug. With the thermosensitive phase-changing feature, the HBC plug can fit all kinds of canaliculi. In our previous study, it was effective for treating the rabbit DED model (12). By comparing to the VisiPlug absorbable intracanalicular plug, this clinical study was undertaken to confirm the efficacy and safety of HBC plug and also to explore the difference between the HBC plug and other traditional absorbable punctal plug in treating DED.

METHODS

Study Design

A monocenter, randomized, controlled clinical trial was performed to evaluate the difference of safety and efficacy between the intracanalicular injection of HBC solution (Qisheng Biologic Agent Limited Company in Shanghai, China) and the absorbable intracanalicular plug, VisiPlug (Lacrimedics, Inc., United States), in DED patients. The study was performed in the Eye & ENT Hospital of Fudan University, was registered in the Chinese Clinical Trial Registry (Identifier: ChiCTR1800016603), was conducted in compliance with the Declaration of Helsinki, and was approved by the ethical committee of Eye & ENT Hospital of Fudan University. Written informed consent was obtained from all participants.

The clinical trial consisted of the intracanalicular occlusion treatment as well as a 12-week visit after the treatment (**Figure 1**). After informed consent was obtained, DED patients who met all criteria began the study and were randomized into either HBC plug treatment group or VisiPlug treatment group in a 1:1 ratio. In the HBC group, the HBC solution was injected into the puncta of the upper and lower canaliculi in both eyes, respectively. In the VisiPlug group, the plugs were placed into the puncta of the upper and lower canaliculi in both eyes. Patients could maintain the artificial tears therapy as before. Patients attended a total of 5 study visits: visit 0, day−14, screening; visit 1, day 0, randomization and treatment (baseline); visit 2, week 1; visit 3, week 4; visit 4, week 12; study exit.

Patients

A total of 50 DED patients between 18 and 75 years of age were enrolled in the clinical trial after screening. The inclusion criteria were as follows: diagnosed with dry eye according to the criteria of the International Dry Eye Workshop (13), visual acuity > 0.1, and not using any topical eye drugs except artificial tears. The exclusion criteria were as follows: inflammation or infection of lacrimal drainage system, obstruction or stenosis of nasolacrimal duct, conjunctival relaxation, being allergic to the ingredients of hydroxybutyl chitosan such as marine food (since HBC is a derivative of chitin, a high molecular compound purified from shrimp shell), abnormal lid anatomy, active inflammation or infection of cornea and conjunctiva, ocular surgery or trauma within 6 months, having undergone permanent punctal occlusion or absorbable punctal occlusion within 6 months, history of myopia laser surgery, use of contact lens within 1 month, glaucoma, autoimmune diseases, and severe cardiovascular, hepatic, renal or hematopoietic diseases.

HBC Injection Protocol

The hydroxybutyl chitosan solution is preserved in sterile tubes at 4–8°C. Before injection, drop topical anesthetics to the conjunctival sac to release the unpleasant feeling during the operation. Syringe the upper and lower lacrimal passages in

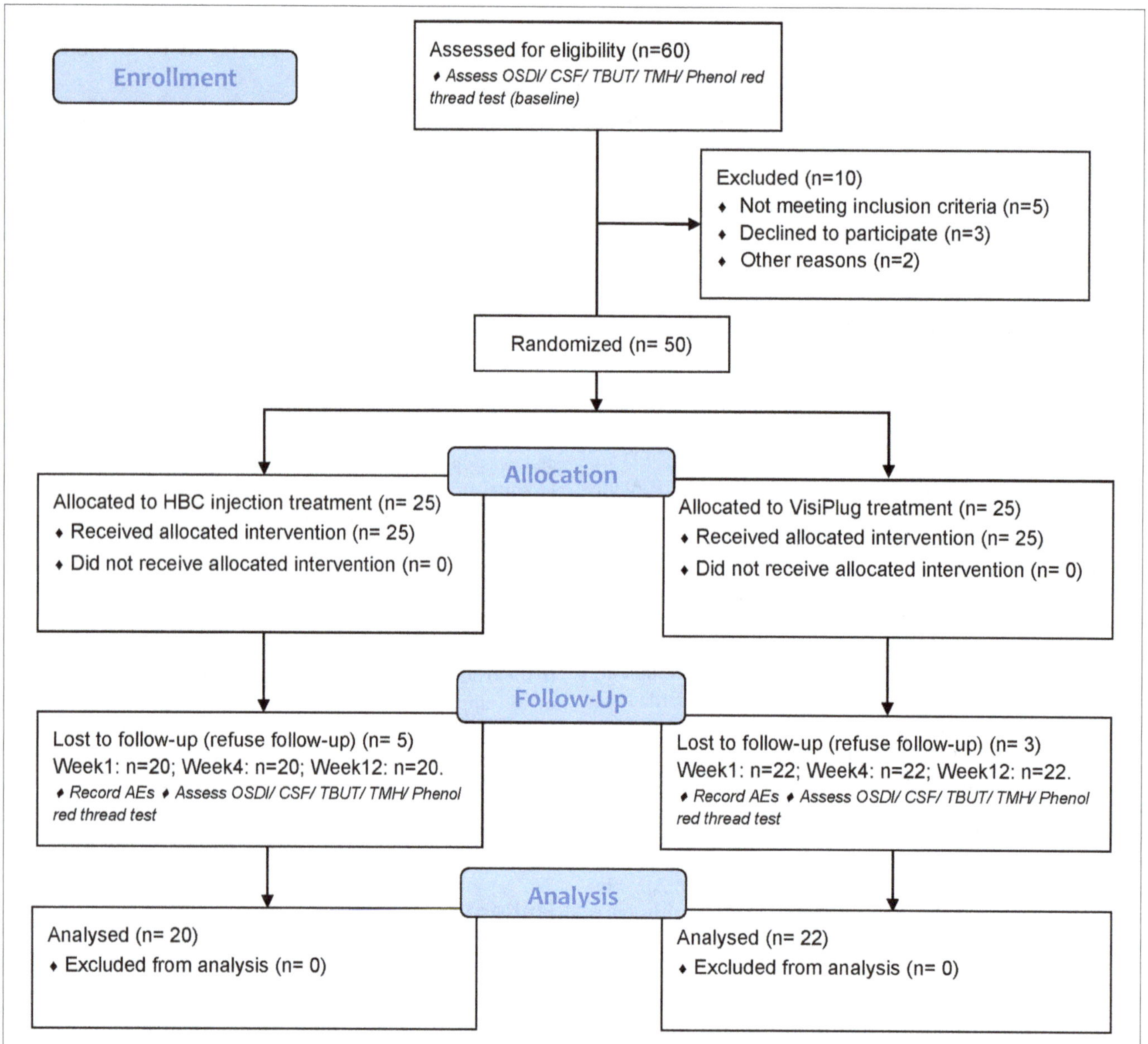

FIGURE 1 | CONSORT flow diagram of the study.

both eyes with saline before injection to ensure the passages are unobstructed. Attach a rinse needle to the tubes containing HBC solution and insert the needle 2–3 mm into the punctum. Inject the HBC solution into the puncta of the upper and lower canaliculi in both eyes until overflow. At the same time, press the dacryocyst sac to avoid downflow of the HBC solution. After injection, press the dacryocyst sac for another 1 min and give antibiotic eye drops to prevent infection. The treatments for all participants were conducted by the same operator.

Outcome Measures

Outcome measures include safety and changes related to efficacy. All the patients underwent an Ocular Surface Disease Index (OSDI) questionnaire, tear break-up time (TBUT), corneal fluorescence staining (CFS), OCT imaging for tear meniscus height (TMH), and phenol red thread test at Day 0 (baseline) and Weeks 1, 4, and 12. Ocular adverse events (AEs) related to the treatment are recorded.

Dry Eye Questionnaire

Ocular Surface Disease Index was used to assess the subjective symptoms at each visit. The questionnaire consisted of the bothersome symptoms, visual function, and environmental triggers subscales. The subjective symptoms were scored on a 5-point scale, with a score of 0 indicating least severe, and a score of 4 indicating most severe. A derived index score of ≤ 100 was calculated for each evaluation based on the total number of questions answered (14).

Tear Break-Up Time

TBUT was used to assess the tear film stability. A fluorescein-impregnated strip (Jingming, Tianjin, China) was wetted with saline solution before use. Placed the wetted strip in the lower conjunctival sac and the patient was asked to blink several times. TBUT was defined as the time between the last complete blink and the first black spot appearing in the stained tear film on the cornea. It was measured three times to get the mean TBUT.

Corneal Fluorescence Staining

According to the NEI criteria, CFS characteristics in five corneal zones were scored on a 4-point scale as follows: 0 = no staining, 1 ≤ 5 staining points, 2 ≥ 5 staining points but <10 staining points, and 3 ≥ 10 staining points or the appearance of corneal filaments (15).

Phenol Red Thread Test

Tear secretion was measured by the phenol red thread test without topical anesthesia. The phenol red thread (Jingming, Tianjin, China) was placed approximately 1/3 of the distance from the lateral canthus of the lower eyelid. The length of the wetted thread was measured as the lacrimal secretion 15 s after placement.

Tear Meniscus Height

The lower TMH was measured using an anterior segment OCT system (RTVue-100, Optovue Inc., Freemont, CA, United States) (16). The single-line scanning mode by the anterior segment-wide angle lens was selected (scanning line length, 3 mm; scanning direction, 90°–270°). Patients were instructed to stabilize their heads by an adjustable chin rest and then look straight ahead at an external light-emitting diode target in front of the eye examined. The patients were told to blink normally to evenly distribute the tear film and minimize ocular surface dehydration. Immediately after the patient blinked, scanning started at the 6 o'clock position of the cornea. The participants were asked to hold their blink during the scan. Three consecutive scans were performed during each examination, with a scanning interval of 3–5 s. The TMH was determined from the OCT images with the RTVue-100 image analysis software, which was defined as the straight-line distance between the upper extreme and the lower extreme of the tear boundary line.

Statistical Analysis

Statistical data were analyzed using SPSS 19.0 (SPSS, Chicago, IL, United States). Results were expressed as means ± SD. Differences were considered to be significant at a level of $P < 0.05$, using t-tests or Chi-square tests for inter-group comparisons and repeated measures analysis of variance or non-parametric tests for intra-group comparisons.

RESULTS

Fifty patients were enrolled in the trial and were randomized into two groups: the HBC group (intracanalicular HBC injection) and the VisiPlug group; 25 patients in each group, respectively. Eight patients dropped out after treatment since they refused follow-up. Twenty patients of the HBC group and 22 patients of the VisiPlug group (total 42 patients) completed the clinical trial (**Table 1**).

TABLE 1 | Characteristics of the study population and the baseline.

	HBC group	VisiPlug group	*P*-value
Patients enrolled, *n*	25	25	
Patients completing the study, *n* (%)	20 (80%)	22 (88%)	
Gender, *n* (%)			0.108
Male	4 (20%)	10 (45.5%)	
Female	16 (80%)	12 (54.5%)	
Mean age (years)	44.60 ± 14.82	44.86 ± 13.47	0.952
OSDI	51.21 ± 26.75	40.81 ± 20.59	0.163
Phenol red thread test	3.75 ± 2.17	4.45 ± 2.24	0.308
TBUT	6.47 ± 3.08	6.08 ± 2.61	0.658
Tear meniscus height	184.40 ± 48.83	200.18 ± 41.30	0.263
CFS	0.75	0	0.069

OSDI, Ocular Surface Disease Index; TBUT, tear break-up time; CFS, corneal fluorescein staining.

The distribution of age, gender, and baseline DED indexes (OSDI, TBUT, CFS, TMH, and phenol red thread test) between the two treatment groups were all well balanced (**Table 1**). No significant differences were found. The mean age of all the 42 patients was 44.7 ± 13.8 years. Among them, 28 (66.7%) were women.

Efficacy

The assessment of efficacy puts emphasis on both the efficacy of intracanalicular HBC injection and the difference between the HBC group and the VisiPlug group in treating DED.

The subjective symptoms of DED were relieved in both groups (**Figure 2**). One week after treatment, the OSDI score was 22.15 ± 19.18 in the HBC group and 19.02 ± 9.72 in the VisiPlug group, which significantly decreased compared to the baseline of each group (HBC: 51.21 ± 26.75; VisiPlug: 40.81 ± 20.59; both $P < 0.001$), indicating an onset effect of as early as 1 week. At Weeks 4 and 12, the OSDI score basically maintained in the VisiPlug group (week 4: 19.19 ± 11.71; week 12: 18.65 ± 12.35; $P < 0.05$ compared to baseline). While in the HBC group, the OSDI score slightly increased at week 12 (week 4: 18.55 ± 22.83; week 12: 25.78 ± 21.43; $P < 0.05$ compared to baseline). No statistical difference of the OSDI score was found between the HBC group and the VisiPlug group at any time ($P > 0.05$). So, it is believed that the HBC injection and the VisiPlug could improve the symptom of DED equally.

Improvements were also observed in the phenol red thread test after treatment (**Figure 3**). Generally, phenol red thread test increased greatly at week 1 (HBC: 10.95 ± 5.89 mm, VisiPlug: 10.18 ± 5.72mm) from the baseline (HBC: 3.75 ± 2.17 mm, VisiPlug: 4.45 ± 2.24 mm), and then began to decrease at week 4 (HBC: 7.40 ± 4.93 mm, VisiPlug: 9.36 ± 6.43 mm) and week 12 (HBC: 5.35 ± 3.22 mm, VisiPlug: 8.59 ± 4.35 mm). Notably,

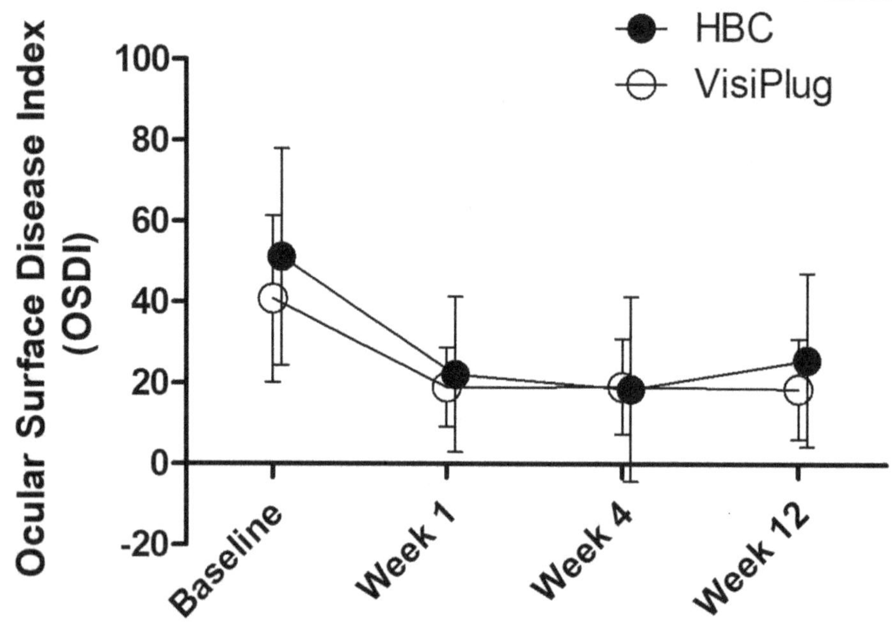

FIGURE 2 | Mean changes of Ocular Surface Disease Index (OSDI) after the treatment in the HBC group and the VisiPlug group. Both groups showed decreased OSDI score compared to baseline ($P < 0.05$) at Weeks 1, 4, and 12. No difference was found between the groups ($P > 0.05$).

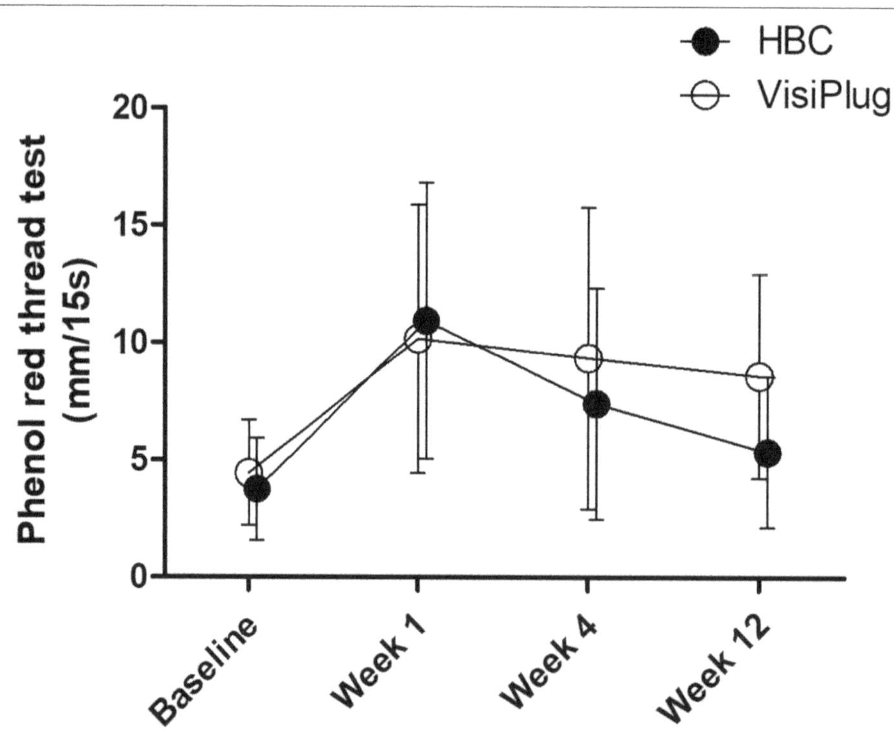

FIGURE 3 | Mean changes of phenol red thread test after the treatment in the HBC group and the VisiPlug group. Both groups showed improvement in phenol red thread test compared to baseline ($P < 0.05$) at Weeks 1, 4, and 12. VisiPlug was better than HBC at Week 12 ($P = 0.009$).

there is a significant difference between the two groups at week 12 ($P = 0.009$). The results showed that both groups were effective in improving tear secretion. However, 12 weeks after treatment, the HBC group was not as effective as the VisiPlug group. We suppose that it is caused by the difference in the degradation speed of different absorbable materials.

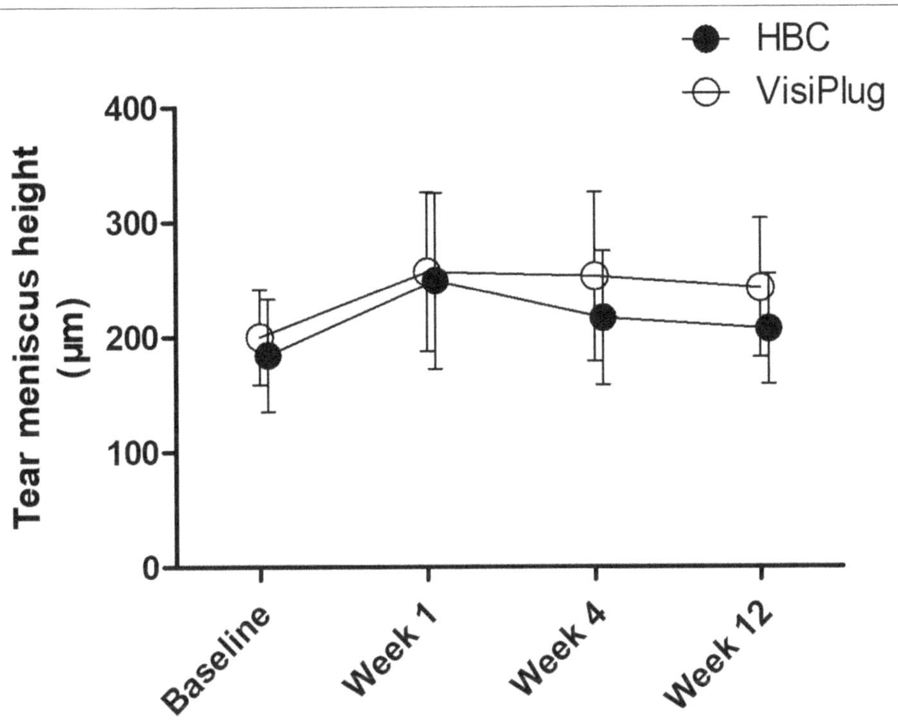

FIGURE 4 | Mean changes of tear meniscus height (TMH) after the treatment in the HBC group and the VisiPlug group. Both groups showed improvement in TMH compared to baseline ($P < 0.05$) at Weeks 1, 4, and 12. VisiPlug was better than HBC at Week 12 ($P = 0.041$).

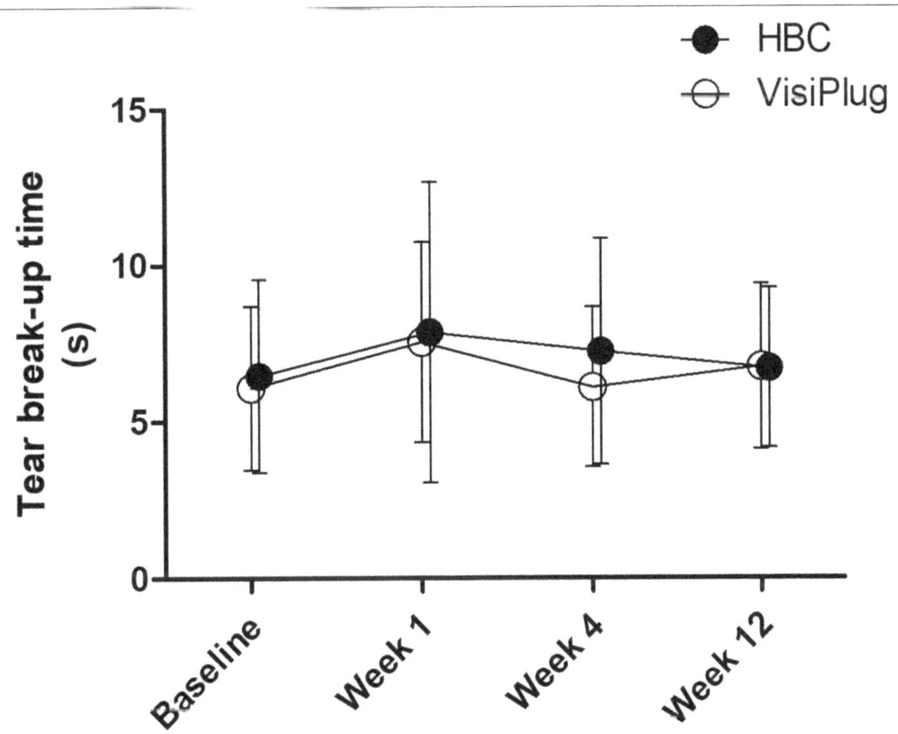

FIGURE 5 | Mean changes of tear break-up time (TBUT) after the treatment in the HBC group and the VisiPlug group. Both groups had little influence on TBUT compared to baseline ($P > 0.05$)

Both treatment groups showed an improvement in TMH (**Figure 4**). After treatment, patients in the VisiPlug group had a higher TMH (Week 1: 256.77 ± 69.05 μm; Week 4: 252.68 ± 73.4 μm; Week 12: 242.59 ± 60.30 μm) compared to the baseline (200.18 ± 41.30 μm, all $P < 0.05$). Likewise, TMH in the HBC group increased after HBC injection (Week 1: 249.05 ± 76.54 μm; Week 4: 216.60 ± 58.24 μm; Week 12: 206.9 ± 47.95 μm) compared to the baseline (184.40 ± 48.83 μm, all $P < 0.05$). Similarly, TMH also reflects the tear secretion, so that the VisiPlug treatment was better than the HBC injection in improving TMH at Week 12 ($P = 0.041$).

Both groups seemed to have little effect on TBUT (**Figure 5**). Although some improvement was found at Week 1 (HBC: 7.87 ± 4.81 s; VisiPlug: 7.55 ± 3.21 s) compared to the baseline (HBC: 6.47 ± 3.08 s; VisiPlug: 6.08 ± 2.61 s), there was no statistical difference (HBC: $P = 0.127$; VisiPlug: $P = 0.060$). TBUTs at Weeks 4 and 12 also had no difference with baseline in both groups.

No significant change in CSF was observed in both the inter-group comparisons or the intra-group comparisons, either. It is probably caused by the fact that all the patients enrolled showed little or no CFS score even before the treatment (HBC 0.75; VisiPlug 0).

Safety

During the clinical trial, no serious AE was reported in the HBC group or the VisiPlug group. The AEs include epiphora, increased secretion, conjunctival congestion, foreign body sensation, eye itching, and blurred vision. All of them were of mild intensity, which relieved automatically without any treatment. They are specifically listed in **Table 2**.

DISCUSSION

A highly comfortable and individualized design of intracanalicular plugs is hard to achieve if they have already been shaped into a certain size before use. Liquid materials can just fit the canaliculus of every person without spatial restriction and are hopeful to occlude canaliculi if they can form a gel after injection *in vivo*. An innovative thermosensitive phase-changing biomaterial, hydroxybutyl chitosan (HBC), makes the idea possible. Research studies showed that HBC can change from a liquid phase to a hydrogel solid phase in a short time. At body temperature (37°C), the phase-changing process will finish in 50 s (11). When it becomes a hydrogel plug, HBC can act as a water barrier (17). These two features make HBC an ideal material for "liquid plug."

In a previous study, we proposed the feasibility of applying HBC to intracanalicular occlusion and explored its efficacy in a pilot study of eight DED patients (12). To further confirm its efficacy, we enlarged the population to 42 patients and compared the HBC injection to a plug we commonly use nowadays, VisiPlug. In this study, the HBC injection showed similar efficacy as VisiPlug. The HBC injection could improve the symptoms and signs of DED just as the traditional absorbable plugs did during the visit time from Weeks 1 to 12. However, we found that the HBC injection was not as effective as VisiPlug in improving TMH and phenol red thread test at Week 12, which means the therapeutic effect of improving tear secretion may decrease faster in HBC injection as the time goes. Since the duration of the therapeutic effect is related to the degradation speed of the absorbable materials (18), we believe that the phenomenon is due to a faster degradation speed of HBC injection than VisiPlug. As the material degrades, more volume of tears pass through the lacrimal drainage system. Based on the clinical data, we suppose the effect of HBC will last for at least 4 weeks. To maintain the efficacy, DED patients may need a relatively frequent HBC injection therapy.

Both the HBC injection and the VisiPlug are methods that treat DED through lacrimal drainage occlusion. So, HBC injection had similar AEs as traditional absorbable intracanalicular plugs (19–21) in this study, including epiphora, increased secretion, conjunctival congestion, foreign body sensation, eye itching, and blurred vision. Besides these, there was no other special peculiar adverse event or complication after HBC injection in this study. We also did not find any difference in the rate or severity of AEs between them, except for the foreign body sensation (HBC: 0%; VisiPlug: 9%). We know that after injection, HBC will turn into a gel-like plug of which the size is just the same as the canaliculi of the patient, so fewer foreign body sensation events may owe to the special characteristics of HBC. The "liquid plug" design will bring more comfort to DED patients after occlusion therapy. In the previous study, we have already confirmed the biosafety of HBC to the ocular surface and an acceptable, transient inflammation reaction to the canalicular (12). We believe the safety of HBC injection is convincing.

The most important advantage of HBC injection occlusion over other traditional plugs is its individualized and flexible feature. Operators do not need to consider the problems of size or accidents such as spontaneous plug extrusion. Another potential advantage we believe is that HBC injection is less likely to cause infection: HBC can exhibit antibacterial activities just like chitosan (22). Furthermore, the phase transformation will lead to a retraction in volume, which can avoid complete obstruction of canaliculi (23). A more extensive application is needed to support this opinion.

One limitation of our findings is that we lack an appropriate method to monitor the HBC plug after injection. MR is used

TABLE 2 | Adverse events observed after occlusion treatments.

	HBC group ($n = 20$)	VisiPlug group ($n = 22$)
Epiphora	3 (15%)	5 (22.7%)
Increased secretion	2 (10%)	3 (13.6%)
Conjunctival congestion	1 (5%)	1 (4.5%)
Foreign body sensation	0 (0%)	2 (9.0%)
Eye itching	1 (5%)	1 (4.5%)
Vision blurred	1 (5%)	0 (0%)

AE, adverse event.
AE is defined as an ocular adverse event occurring after the occlusion treatment.

previously to image the plug (12) (water in the gel can be imaged in the T2 sequence) but may be not suitable for long-term observation since the water content decreases as time goes on. Future explorations should emphasize these problems.

CONCLUSIONS

The intracanalicular HBC injection was able to relieve both symptoms and signs of dry eye disease with great safety. No significant difference was found between the HBC injection and VisiPlug either in the efficacy of symptom improvement or in the safety. Taking advantage of the thermosensitive and dissolving properties of HBC, the *in situ* injection of HBC solution into the lacrimal drainage system proves to be a promising, individualized occlusion method to treat dry eye disease.

ETHICS STATEMENT

The studies involving human participants were reviewed and approved by the Ethical Committee of Eye & ENT Hospital of Fudan University. The patients/participants provided their written informed consent to participate in this study.

AUTHOR CONTRIBUTIONS

TL and LG designed the study. TL, YL, and LG performed recruitment, treatment, and follow-up for dry eye patients. TL and WW analyzed the data. TL, WW, and LG wrote and revised the manuscript. All authors approved the final manuscript.

ACKNOWLEDGMENTS

The authors acknowledge financial support from Shanghai Sailing Program, the National Natural Science Foundation of China and Shanghai Rising Stars of Medical Talents Youth Development Program. The authors also acknowledge the synthesis and supply of HBC solution from Qisheng Biologic Agent Limited Company in Shanghai.

REFERENCES

1. Craig JP, Nichols KK, Akpek EK, Barbara Caffery OD, Dua HS, Joo CK, et al. TFOS DEWS II definition and classification report. *Ocul Surf.* (2017) 15:276–83. doi: 10.1016/j.jtos.2017.05.008
2. Greco G, Pistilli M, Asbell PA, Maguire MG. Dry Eye assessment and management study research group. association of severity of dry eye disease with work productivity and activity impairment in the dry eye assessment and management study. *Ophthalmology.* (2021) 128:850–6. doi: 10.1016/j.ophtha.2020.10.015
3. Jie Y, Xu L, Wu YY, Jonas JB. Prevalence of dry eye among adult Chinese in the beijing eye study. *Eye.* (2009) 23:688–93. doi: 10.1038/sj.eye.6703101
4. Jones L, Downie LE, Korb D. Benitez-del-Castillo JM, Dana R, Deng SX, et al. TFOS DEWS II management and therapy report. *Ocul Surf.* (2017) 15:575–628. doi: 10.1016/j.jtos.2017.05.006
5. Marcet MM, Shtein RM, Bradley EA, Deng SX, Meyer DR, Bilyk JR, et al. Safety and efficacy of lacrimal drainage system plugs for dry eye syndrome: a report by the american academy of ophthalmology. *Ophthalmology.* (2015) 122:1681–7. doi: 10.1016/j.ophtha.2015.04.034
6. Miyata K, Otani S, Miyai T, Nejima R, Amano S. Atelocollagen punctal occlusion in dry eye patients. *Cornea.* (2006) 25:47–50. doi: 10.1097/01.ico.0000164783.10667.a4
7. Chen F, Shen M, Chen W, Wang J, Li M, Yuan Y, et al. Tear meniscus volume in dry eye after punctal occlusion. *Invest Ophthalmol Vis Sci.* (2010) 51:1965–9. doi: 10.1167/iovs.09-4349
8. Egrilmez S, Aslan F, Karabulut G, Kabasakal Y, Yagci A. Clinical efficacy of the SmartPlug^{TM} in the treatment of primary Sjogren's syndrome with keratoconjunctivitis sicca: one-year follow-up study. *Rheumatol Int.* (2011) 31:1567–70. doi: 10.1007/s00296-010-1527-x
9. Mazow ML, McCall T, Prager TC. Lodged intracanalicular plugs as a cause of lacrimal obstruction. *Ophthalmic Plast Reconstr Surg.* (2007) 23:138–142. doi: 10.1097/IOP.0b013e318031d62a
10. Nishii M, Yokoi N, Komuro A, Sugita J, Nakamura Y, Kojima K. et al. Comparison of extrusion rate for two different design of punctal plugs. *Nihon Ganku Gakkai Zasshi.* (2003) 107:322–5.
11. Wei CZ, Hou CL, Gu QS, Jiang LX, Zhu B, Sheng AL, et al. thermosensitive chitosan-based hydrogel barrier for post-operative adhesions' prevention. *Biomaterials.* (2009) 30:5534–40. doi: 10.1016/j.biomaterials.2009.05.084
12. Lin T, Lu Y, Zhang X, Gong L, Wei C. Treatment of dry eye by intracanalicular injection of a thermosensitive chitosan-based hydrogel: evaluation of biosafety and availability. *Biomater Sci.* (2018) 6:3160–9. doi: 10.1039/C8BM01047A
13. Wolffsohn JS, Arita R, Chalmers R, Djalilian A, Dogru M, Dumbleton K, et al. TFOS DEWS II diagnostic methodology report. *Ocul Surf.* (2017) 15:539–74. doi: 10.1016/j.jtos.2017.05.001
14. Schiffman RM, Christianson MD, Jacobsen G, Hirsch JD, Reis BL. Reliability and validity of the ocular surface disease index. *Arch Ophthalmol.* (2000) 118:615–21. doi: 10.1001/archopht.118.5.615
15. Lemp MA. Report of the National Eye Institute/Industry workshop on clinical trials in dry eyes. *CLAO J.* (1995) 21:221–32.
16. Lin T, Gong L, Liu X, Ma X. Fourier-domain optical coherence tomography for monitoring the lower tear meniscus in dry eye after acupuncture treatment. *Evid Based Complement Alternat Med.* (2015) 2015:492150. doi: 10.1155/2015/492150
17. Zhang E, Guo Q, Ji F, Tian X, Cui J, Song Y, et al. Thermoresponsive polysaccharide-based composite hydrogel with antibacterial and healing-promoting activities for preventing recurrent adhesion after adhesiolysis. *Acta Biomater.* (2018) 74:439–53. doi: 10.1016/j.actbio.2018.05.037
18. Hadassah J, Bhuvaneshwari N, Singh D, Sehgal PK. Preparation and clinical evaluation of succinylated collagen punctal plugs in dry eye syndrome: a pilot study. *Ophthalmic Res.* (2010) 43:185–92. doi: 10.1159/000272022
19. Kim BM, Osmanovic SS, Edward DP. Pyogenic granulomas after silicone punctal plugs: a clinical and histopathologic study. *Am J Ophthalmol.* (2005) 139:678–84. doi: 10.1016/j.ajo.2004.11.059
20. Rumelt S, Remulla H, Rubin PA. Silicone punctal plug migration resulting in dacryocystitis and canaliculitis. *Cornea.* (1997) 16:377–9. doi: 10.1097/00003226-199705000-00022
21. Balaram M, Schaumberg DA, Dana MR. Efficacy and tolerability outcomes after punctal occlusion with silicone plugs in dry eye syndrome. *Am J Ophthalmol.* (2001) 131:30–6. doi: 10.1016/S0002-9394(00)00620-6
22. Felt O, Carrel A, Baehni P, Buri P, Gurny R. Chitosan as tear substitute. a wetting agent endowed with antimicrobial efficacy. *J Ocul Pharmacol Ther.* (2000) 16:261–70. doi: 10.1089/jop.2000.16.261
23. Jehangir N, Bever G, Mahmood SM, Moshirfar M. Comprehensive review of the literature on existing punctal plugs for the management of dry eye disease. *J Ophthalmol.* (2016) 2016:9312340. doi: 10.1155/2016/9312340

20

Estimated Annual Economic Burden of Dry Eye Disease Based on a Multi-Center Analysis in China

*Wanju Yang[1], Yanzhu Luo[1,2,3], Shangcao Wu[1], Xiaoxia Niu[4], Yanshuang Yan[5], Chen Qiao[1,3], Wei Ming[1,3], Ying Zhang[1], Haoyu Wang[1,3], Dan Chen[1,3], Mengying Qi[1,3], Lan Ke[1,3], Ying Wang[1,3], Liping Li[1,3], Shaowei Li[6] and Qingyan Zeng[1,2,3,6,7]**

[1] Aier Eye Hospital of Wuhan University, Wuhan, China, [2] Aier School of Ophthalmology, Central South University, Changsha, China, [3] Department of Cornea and Ocular Surface Diseases, Wuhan Aier Hankou Eye Hospital, Wuhan, China, [4] Department of Cornea and Ocular Surface Diseases, Harbin Aier Eye Hospital, Harbin, China, [5] Department of Cornea and Ocular Surface Diseases, Guangzhou Aier Eye Hospital, Guangzhou, China, [6] Aier Cornea Institute, Beijing, China, [7] Aier School of Ophthalmology and Optometry, Hubei University of Science and Technology, Xianning, China

***Correspondence:**
Qingyan Zeng
zengqingyan1972@163.com

Purpose: To conduct a multi-center analysis and assess the economic burden due to dry eye disease (DED) in China.

Design: A retrospective and cross-sectional study.

Methods: Patients ($n = 598$) with diagnosed DED were recruited from 3 eye centers (in central, southeast, and northeast China) from 1 January 2018 to 31 December 2018. Data were collected regarding the examination, pharmacological therapy, and non-pharmacological therapy fees. Sub-group analyses were stratified by eye center, DED severity, types of DED, number of visits to physicians, and residential area. A logistic regression analysis was conducted to investigate the variables influencing total costs.

Results: The per capita costs devoted to DED at the 3 centers were 422.6, 391.3, and 265.4 USD, respectively. The costs of non-pharmacological therapy accounted the largest part in three centers (75.6, 76.4, 76.5%, respectively). Patients with severe DED sustained the largest economic burden. Patients with mixed type of DED spent the most comparing to patients with either evaporative or aqueous-deficient types of DED. Patients spent more during the first visit compared with subsequent visits. Patients living in urban areas spent significantly more than did those living in rural areas ($P = 0.001$). The logistics regression analysis showed that total costs were significantly influenced by DED severity, number of visits to physicians, and area of residence (beta = 2.83, 0.83, 1.48; $P < 0.0001$).

Conclusions: DED is a chronic ocular disease that timely non-cost counseling, early diagnosis, and efficacious treatment can reduce its economic burden on patients and the society.

Keywords: dry eye disease, burden of disease, costs, multi-center analysis, China

INTRODUCTION

Dry eye disease (DED) is a chronic and progressive multifactorial disorder of the ocular surface characterized by unstable tear film; or imbalanced microenvironment caused by abnormal tear quality, quantity, and dynamics. It can be accompanied by inflammatory reactions of the ocular surface, tissue damage, and neurological abnormalities, which result in a variety of symptoms of ocular discomfort, visual dysfunction, or both (1). Among people seeking eye care in the United States, DED has become the fifth most prevalent ocular condition in women and ninth most prevalent in men (2).

The prevalence of DED ranges from 5.28 to 33.7% worldwide (3–5). The Dry Eye Workshop (DEWS) committee reported that the prevalence of DED in Southeast Asia is as high as 20.0 to 52.4% (6). In New Zealand, signs of clinical dry eye were present in almost half of a cohort of 45-year-olds (7). In China, a meta-analysis revealed that DED diagnosed by symptoms alone affected 31.40%, or corresponding to 394.13 million affected individuals in the country (4).

DED can be caused by a variety of reasons, including aging, female population (6, 8), environmental factors (e.g., extreme temperature and reduced humidity) (9), and daily-life behaviors [smoking (10), digital screen exposure (11, 12), reduced caffeine consumption, and contact lenses (13)]. Surgical and para-surgical causes such as refractive (14, 15) and cataract surgeries (16, 17) can promote DED, as well as certain medications (18, 19) such as beta-blockers, antihistamines, oral contraceptives, and anti-glaucoma eye drops. A history of thyroid disease, and poorer self-rated health (16), have also been associated with DED.

Many therapies have been demonstrated to improve the signs and symptoms of DED (20). However, global studies suggest that long-term treatment of DED imposes a substantial economic burden on patients and society. In the United States in 2008, the overall burden of DED for the healthcare system was 3.84 billion United States dollars (USD), the cost of managing DED per patient was 11,302 USD, and the overall societal cost was 55.4 billion USD. The costs categories included ocular lubricant treatment, cyclosporine, punctal plugs, physician visits, and nutritional supplements (21). A retrospective study conducted in Germany showed that total costs were ~117 million euro for a DED cohort of 35,026 patients. The costs were analyzed based on the healthcare resource used by the DED patients, including visits to the general practitioner or ophthalmologist, pharmacological treatment, and ocular procedures (uncommon) (22). A systemic literature review evaluated and compared the burden of DED across France, Germany, Italy, Spain, United Kingdom, United States, and Japan (23). Clegg et al. (24) reported that the direct economic burden of managing DED in European countries in 2003 ranged from 270 USD to 1,100 USD per patient and the costs mainly included diagnostic test, specialists visits, prescribed drugs, and surgery. While DED costs vary among countries, the economic burden of DED across regions is comparable. Yet, there is limited data regarding the annual economic burden of DED in Asia, especially China. Besides, seldom research reported the costs of non-pharmacological therapies.

This study aims to conduct a multi-center comprehensive estimation of the costs associated with DED for the year 2018 in China and provides insight into the burden of DED on patients and society.

Abbreviations: ANOVA, analysis of variance; DED, dry eye disease; DEWS, The Dry Eye Workshop; GDP, gross domestic product; SSDE, Sjögren's syndrome dry eye; TFOS, Tear Film and Ocular Surface Society; USD, United States dollars.

MATERIALS AND METHODS

Data Source

The study was approved by the ethics committees of 3 eye centers, Wuhan Aier Hankou Eye Hospital (Center-1, central China), Guangzhou Aier Eye Hospital (Center-2, southeast China), and Ha'erbin Eye Hospital (Center-3, northeast China), respectively. The study was conducted in accordance with the tenets of the Declaration of Helsinki, and the enrolled patients provided signed informed consent.

The participants were recruited from outpatients visiting the above 3 eye centers, from 1 January 2018 to 31 December 2018. The inclusion criteria were: (1) subjects aged ≥18 years, (2) had received a diagnosis of DED without other ocular diseases (such as cataract or glaucoma), and (3) were managed and followed-up in the study centers without any interventions from other hospitals or pharmacies. Individuals with any of the following were excluded: (1) eye surgeries in the past 6 months, (2) infectious corneal diseases during follow-up visits, or (3) ended follow-up during the study year.

DED diagnosis and severity criteria were that of the dry eye consensus of the Chinese Medical Association in 2013, and defined as mild, moderate, or severe (**Table 1**). Classification of DED was consistent with the TFOS (Tear Film and Ocular Surface Society) DEWS II Definition and Classification Report.

Data Collection

The outpatient medical record systems of the 3 hospitals were searched for the cost information of the enrolled patients during the 1-year follow-up. The costs included 3 categories of fees: examinations, pharmacological therapy, and non-pharmacological therapy.

The examination fees included the costs of the general ophthalmological examinations (i.e., intraocular pressure and slit lamp inspection with fluorescein staining) and examinations related to DED (i.e., quantitative and qualitative evaluations of the tear film, and the morphology and function of the meibomian glands). The pharmacological therapy fees consisted of the cost of eye drops to treat DED during the year. Non-pharmacological therapy costs included costs of ophthalmic physiotherapy (i.e., meibomian gland massage, palpebral margin cleaning, eyelid nebulization therapy, and intense pulsed light) and costs of purchased products for treatment (i.e., lacrimal punctual plugs, moisture chamber glasses, corneal bandage lenses, and warm compress eye masks).

TABLE 1 | Diagnosis and severity criteria of DED.

Symptoms		Mild subjective symptoms with negative corneal fluorescein staining
Signs		• Meeting one of the following objective signs: • Tear break-up time ≤5 s, or Schirmer's *I*-test ≤5 mm/5 min; • Tear break-up time >5 s up to 10 s, or Schirmer's *I*-test* between nil up to 5 mm/5 min, with positive corneal and conjunctival fluorescein staining
Severity	Mild	Mild subjective symptoms with negative corneal fluorescein staining
	Moderate	Moderate and severe subjective symptoms with positive corneal fluorescein staining; corneal staining disappeared after treatment
	Severe	Moderate and severe subjective symptoms with positive corneal fluorescein staining; staining did not completely disappear after treatment

**Schirmer's I-test is without topical anesthesia.*

Statistical Analysis

All the data were analyzed using SPSS 22.0 (SPSS IBM, New York, NY, USA) software. A $P < 0.05$ was considered statistically significant. Demographic comparisons among the 3 centers (from the central, southeast, and northeast districts) were performed *via* chi-squared test for dichotomous variables, analysis of variance (ANOVA) for continuous variables, and non-parametric tests for non-normally distributed data.

The subjects were categorized, both overall (the 3 centers) and for each center individually, to determine the respective median values of the total costs.

Comparisons were made of the per capita cost related to DED with the gross domestic product (GDP), and with the income of the city where the medical center is located. Economic burden is shown as USD ($), according to the 2018 currency exchange rate (6.61 Chinese Yuan/USD; National Bureau of Statistics of China, https://data.stats.gov.cn/easyquery.htm?cn=C01&zb=A060J&sj=2018).

In the univariate analyses, cost comparisons between subgroups stratified by different variables were conducted by Mann-Whitney Test (2 categories) or Kruskal-Wallis *H*-Test (multiple categories). The variables included the following: DED severity (mild, moderate, severe); types of DED (evaporative, aqueous-deficient, and mixed DED); number of visits to physicians (first visit, subsequent visit); residential area (urban, rural).

Logistic regression models were used to estimate cost differences between the groups that were lower or higher than the median value. Variables related to DED severity, number of visits to physicians, and residential area were included in the models.

RESULTS

Demographics

The study population comprised 598 patients overall, with 199, 199, and 200 patients in Center-1, Center-2, and Center-3, respectively (**Table 2**). The 3 centers differed significantly by age, gender ratio, and number of visits to physicians ($P \leq 0.0001$, 0.018, <0.0001). There were 132 mild, 53 moderate, and 14 severe cases of DED in Center-1; 148 mild, 51 moderate, and no severe cases in Center-2; and 142 mild, 40 moderate, and 18 severe cases in Center-3. Regarding to the type of DED, there were 49 evaporative dry eye, 9 aqueous-deficient dry eye, and 141 mixed dry eye subjects in Center-1; 199 mixed dry eye subjects in Center-2; and 37 evaporative dry eye, 96 aqueous-deficient dry eye, and 67 mixed dry eye subjects in Center-3. The number of visits were 1 to 5, 1 to 4, and 4 at Center-1, Center-2, and Center-3.

Per Capita Annual Costs Analysis

The per capita total costs related to DED at Center-1, Center-2, and Center-3 were $422.6, $391.3, and $265.4 ($P = 0.043$), respectively (**Table 3**). The percentages in per capita residual income were 3.16, 2.31, 2.44%; and GDP (year 2018) were 1.66, 1.05, and 2.65%.

The examination fees differed significantly among the centers ($P < 0.0001$), as well as the pharmacological therapy fees ($P < 0.0001$), but the non-pharmacological fees were comparable ($P = 0.098$). The costs of non-pharmacological therapy accounted the largest part in three centers (75.6, 76.4, 76.5, respectively).

Sub-Group Analysis

The annual (2018) per capita costs related to DED among the subgroups was reported (**Table 4**). Compared with patients with mild or moderate DED, those with severe DED incurred the highest examination, pharmacological therapy, and non-pharmacological therapy fees. Compared with patients with evaporative or aqueous-deficient DED, those with mixed DED incurred the highest examination, non-pharmacological therapy, and total fees. There was no significant difference on the pharmacological therapy fee among three types of DED. Patients spent significantly more at the first visit on the examination fee, pharmacological therapy fee, non-pharmacological therapy fee, and the total fee (P =0.010, 0.049, <0.0001, <0.0001). Patients living in urban areas spent more than those living in rural areas on the examination fee, pharmacological therapy fee, non-pharmacological therapy fee, and the total fee (P <0.0001, <0.0001, <0.0001, <0.0001).

Logistics Regression Analysis

The logistics regression analysis showed that, for the centers overall, DED severity, number of visits to physicians, and residential area had a significant influence on total costs (beta = 2.83, 0.83, 1.48, respectively, $P < 0.0001$). The significant variable that influenced total costs at Center-1 was disease severity only (beta = 1.37, $P < 0.0001$); at Center-2, the influential variables were disease severity (beta = 2.84, $P < 0.0001$) and number of visits to physicians (beta = 1.51, $P = 0.003$); at Center-3, disease

TABLE 2 | Demographic characteristics of patients at 3 eye centers[a].

	Center-1	Center-2	Center-3	P
Subjects	199	199	200	–
Age, y	48.01 ± 13.71	42.22 ± 16.19*	47.57 ± 14.11#	<0.0001[b]
Gender, female/male	140/59	113*/86*	130/70	0.018[c]
Numbers of follow-ups (median, range)	2, 1–15	2, 1–31	4, 4–12*#	<0.0001[d]
Number of visits to physicians (first/subsequent visit)	147/52	137/62	179*/21*	<0.0001[c]
DED severity (mild/moderate/severe)	132/53/14	148/51/0*	142/40/18	<0.0001[c]
Type of DED (evaporative/aqueous-deficient/mixed)	49/9/141	199*/0*/0*	37/96*#/67*#	<0.0001[c]
Residential area (rural/urban)	64/135	37*/162*	68/132	0.001[c]

[a]Data is reported as n, unless indicated otherwise; [b]ANOVA; [c]chi-squared test; [d]Kruskal-Wallis H.
*Compare with Center-1, $P < 0.05$; #Compare with Center-2, $P < 0.05$; Bonferroni test was performed.
Center-1, Wuhan Aier Hankou Eye Hospital, Wuhan, central China; Center-2, Guangzhou Aier Eye Hospital, Guangzhou, southeast China; Center-3, Ha'erbin Aier Eye Hospital, Ha'erbin, northeast China.

TABLE 3 | Percentages of annual per capita DED costs in residual income and GDP (year 2018)[a].

Annual per capita DED costs	Center-1	Center-2	Center-3	P[b]
Examination fee	$53.0 ± 35.5 (12.5%)	$36.9 ± 30.1 (9.4%)*	$29.3 ± 24.5 (11.0%)*#	**<0.0001**
Pharmacological therapy fee	$50.1 ± 51.0 (11.9%)	$55.5± 55.1 (14.2%)*	$33.1 ± 21.6 (12.5%)#	**<0.0001**
Non-pharmacological therapy fee	$319.5 ± 302.6 (75.6%)	$298.9 ± 382.9 (76.4%)	$203.1 ± 129.5 (76.5%)	0.098
Total fee	$422.6 ± 324.8	$391.3 ± 422.6	$265.4 ± 145.0*	**0.014**
Per capita residual income in each area[c]	$13,362.6 (3.2%)	$16,919.7 (2.3%)	$10,857.9 (2.4%)	–
Per capita GDP[d]	$25,417.1 (1.7%)	$37,278.6 (1.1%)	$10,017.2 (2.7%)	–

*Compare with Center-1, $P < 0.05$; #Compare with Center-2, $P < 0.05$; Bonferroni test was performed.
[a]Reported as US dollars ($), the 2018 currency exchange rate 6.61 Chinese Yuan/USD; [b]Kruskal-Wallis H-test; [c]total fees related to residual income in each area; [d]total fees related to per capita GDP. The bold values means there was significant difference.

severity (beta = 2.84, $P < 0.0001$) and residential area (beta = 1.65, $P = 0.004$) were of greatest importance.

DISCUSSION

To the best of our knowledge, this is the first multi-center analysis of the annual economic burden imposed by DED in China. The global economic burden due to DED, to the patient and society, is not trivial. In the last decade, various methods have been used to analyze the economic burden on patients with DED worldwide (**Table 5**) (21, 22, 25, 27–30), but little is known about the situation in China (31).

In the current study, data were collected from 3 eye centers, in central, southeast, and northeast China, respectively. The annual total costs (per capita) associated with DED ranged from $264.5 to $422.6, which appeared lower than the studies discussed above. However, the economic and medical status in different regions is an important factor that affects economic burden. We found that the per capita costs of DED accounted for 2.31–3.16% of per capita residual income, and 1.05–2.65% of per capita GDP, in the different districts. When taking into account the prevalence of DED in China (affecting 394.13 million individuals) (4), the overall burden of DED for the healthcare system translates to $104.2 billion to $166.6 billion per year, which was much higher than the estimated annual economic burden in the US society overall [$55.4 billion (21)]. Therefore, the economic burden of DED on the Chinese people is such that more reasonable policymaking is needed regarding state-set medication prices and medical care reimbursement.

There were significant differences in the annual per capital DED costs, examination fee, and pharmacological therapy fee among three centers. The non-pharmacological therapy fee was still higher in Center-1 than other two centers, although the difference was not significant. One of the reasons is that the DED specialized outpatient clinic was set in Center-1 in 2014 and patients in Wuhan city were more willing to accept complicated examinations and non-pharmacological therapies. Costs in Center-3 located in Ha'erbin were all much lower than Center-1 and Center-2 as the city was less developed and the overall outpatient costs were much lower.

As far as we know, this study is the first multi-center analysis to report non-pharmacological costs, that is, those associated with ophthalmic physiotherapy conducted in clinics and those treatment products purchased. The non-pharmacological costs accounted for the largest share of the total costs in all three centers to ($319.5, $298.9, $203.1, 75.6, 76.4, 76.5%, respectively).

TABLE 4 | Summary of the annual (2018) per capita costs related to DED among the subgroups (USD).

	Examination fee	Pharmacological therapy fee	Non-pharmacological therapy fee	Total fee
DED severity				
Mild	$35.6 ± 31.3 (13.8%)	$36.9 ± 32.6 (14.3%)	$186.3 ± 191.8 (72.0%)	$258.4 ± 214.7
Moderate	$49.0 ± 31.0 (8.3%)*	$67.2 ± 65.6 (11.3%)*	$476.7 ± 398.7 (80.4%)*	$592.2 ± 429.6*
Severe	$51.9 ± 32.5 (8.1%)*	$74.2 ± 49.8 (11.6%)*	$513.1 ± 300.8 (80.3%)*	$639.1 ± 291.6*
P^a	<0.0001	<0.0001	<0.0001	<0.0001
Types of DED				
Evaporative	$35.9 ± 31.2 (9.7%)	$49.3 ± 54.0 (13.3%)	$286.4 ± 354.1 (77.1%)	$371.6 ± 391.7
Aqueous-Deficient	$32.1 ± 25.8 (14.9%)	$41.5± 39.9 (19.3%)	$141.6 ± 77.8 (65.8%)^	$215.2 ± 116.9
Mixed	$48.7 ± 33.6 (11.7%)^#	$44.4 ± 35.8 (10.7%)	$323.0 ± 254.5 (77.6%)^#	$416.1 ± 272.1^#
P^a	<0.0001	0.800	<0.0001	<0.0001
Number of visits to physicians				
First visit	$40.8 ± 30.1 (10.7%)	$47.6 ± 46.4 (12.4%)	$294.3 ± 305.0 (76.9%)	$382.7 ± 338.9
Subsequent visit	$36.0 ± 37.3 (12.8%)	$41.4 ± 44.5 (14.8%)	$203.1 ± 247.3 (72.4%)	$280.6 ±259.9
P^b	0.010	0.049	<0.0001	<0.0001
Residential area				
Rural area	$33.5 ± 30.9 (12.7%)	$38.3 ± 41.7 (14.5%)	$192.5 ± 201.7 (72.8%)	$264.3 ± 227.8
Urban area	$42.2 ± 32.0 (10.6%)	$49.3 ± 47.3 (12.4%)	$305.7 ± 319.3 (77.0%)	$397.2 ± 349.7
P^b	<0.0001	<0.0001	<0.0001	<0.0001

*[a]Kruskal-Wallis H-test; [b]Mann-Whitney Test; *Compare with Mild, $P < 0.05$ and Bonferroni was performed; ^Compare with Evaporative, $P < 0.05$, #Compare with Aqueous-deficient, $P < 0.05$, and Bonferroni test was performed.*

Examples of ophthalmic physiotherapy conducted in clinics are meibomian gland expression (MGX), palpebral margin cleaning, eyelid nebulization therapy, and intense pulsed light (IPL) treatment. Treatment products purchased by patients include lacrimal punctual plugs, moisture chamber glasses, corneal bandage lens, and warm compress eye masks. Among them, MGX and IPL were most widely used according to our preliminary single center analysis (32). As meibomian gland disease related DED becomes more common, technologies for efficacious management are important (33) and IPL was found safe for DED therapy (34). However, they are currently quite costly, and more advances in methods and strategies for DED management that may reduce costs are warranted.

From the logistic regression analysis of the current study, it was found that the total costs of the patient were significantly influenced by DED severity. Compared with patients with mild or moderate DED, those with severe DED incurred the highest medical expense. Although DED is not curable, timely and efficient treatment can relieve the symptoms. However, one study found that patients tended to discontinue follow-ups as DED prolonged after diagnosis (35). Thus, timely and comprehensive education on patient is essential to prevent their discouragement on following treatment. Besides, early intervention is important to prevent DED progression, which can potentially improve quality of life and work productivity, reducing the indirect costs of DED in more severe stages.

Patients with mixed type of DED spent the most and then followed patients with evaporative and aqueous-deficient DED. The possible reason was that the symptoms of patients with aqueous-deficient DED could be alleviated by pharmacological therapies which were much inexpensive. While patients with mixed or evaporative DED were more likely to be treated with non-pharmacological therapies or combining multiple kinds of therapied which could result in more costs.

In addition to DED severity and type, we also found that number of visits to physicians influenced the costs. Although much less subjects had follow-up visits, the costs of subsequent visits were comparable to the costs of subjects' first visit, especially the examinations and pharmacological therapy fee. As DED is not curable and in need of long-term treatment to alleviate symptoms, further research is essential to investigate on cheaper examination technologies and more efficient therapies so that patients could spend less on follow-up visits during their lifetime. Besides, in China, some costs on DED non-pharmacological therapy were not covered by patients' insurance. Thus, the support from the government and insurance companies is also important to reduce the burden on patients.

Compared with patients living in rural areas, those living in urban areas spent more on DED examinations and treatment. It is reasonable that patients with these later characteristics may be more annoyed by DED and more willing to seek medical treatment. In addition, such patients are more likely to experience longer exposures to electronic devices, which is a risk factor of DED onset and deterioration. Therefore, for these subjects, more detailed non-cost counseling is necessary to prevent disease progression.

Our study has several strengths. It gains credibility by being multicenter, with 3 eye centers in central, southeast, and northeast China. This aspect makes it more representative and comprehensive. Another strength is that the cost data was collected not from self-questionnaires, but from the outpatient medical record systems of the hospitals, which is more objective. Finally, subgroup and logistic regression analyses were conducted to investigate the significance of the variables that influence

TABLE 5 | Studies on the economic burden of DED published between 2010 and 2020.

	Year, location	Methods	Study population	Cost analysis
North America				
Yu et al. (21)	2008, USA	Survey, cross-sectional study, decision analytic model	2171 DED Pts	• Direct PCC: $783 • Indirect PCC: $11,302
Galor et al. (25)	2001–2006, USA	Survey, retrospective study	147 DED Pts	• DED medication PCC: • 2001–2002, $55/y • 2003–2004, $137/y • 2005–2006, $299/y • Yearly overall, $217.3 ± 23.4
Europe				
Tachkov et al. (26)	2016–2017, Sofia	Prospective, observational, decision troo analysis	64 eyes with POAG & DED	Median costs of DED treatment €179.9 ± 9.4
Darbà et al. (27)	1997–2015, Spain	Multi-centers, insurance claims analysis, retrospective study	36,081 DED Pts	• Total costs: increased from €4.9 to €30.3 M during the study period • Mean annual cost per Pt: €7,379 increase
Siffel et al. (22)	2008–2015, Germany	Insurance claims analysis, retrospective study	85,560 DED Pts with at least one confirmed diagnosis	• Total PCC: €3,809 ± 8,195 • Outpatient visits PCC: €932 ± 1,229 • Acute day ward visits PCC: €50 ± 328 • Pharmacological treatments PCC: €816 ± 3,415
Asia				
Mizuno et al. (28)	2005–2008, Japan	Multi-center, survey, cross-sectional study	118 DED Pts	• Annual PCC: $530 • Clinical PCC: $165 • Pharmacological PCC: $323 • Punctual plug PCC: $42
Nagata et al. (29)	2014–2015, Japan	Survey, cross-sectional study	266 subjects with eye condition including DED	Annual PCC of eye conditions including DED: $253.3
Waduthantri et al. (30)	2008–2009, Singapore	Pharmacy & clinic inventory database analysis, retrospective	54,052 DED Pts	• 2008, $22.11 • 2009, $23.59
Yao and Le (31)	2016, SE China	Survey, cross-sectional study	34 SSDE & 30 non-SSDE subjects	• Annual Medication costs: SSDE ¥7,637.2 ± 6,079.0, non-SSDE ¥1,179.1 ± 990.4 • Annual out-of-pocket money: SSDE ¥2,627.8 ± 1,857.0, non-SSDE ¥481.9 ± 393.3 • Annual indirect expense: SSDE ¥828.0 ± 1,866.0, non-SSDE ¥487.2 ± 1,404.0 • Expense on auxiliary therapy: SSDE ¥2,757.1 ± 2,496.0
Present study, 2021	2018, C, SE, NE China	Multi-centers, outpatient medical record system analysis, retrospective study	598 DED Pts	• Total PCC: $422.6, $391.3, and $265.4 in 3 centers • Sub-groups: • Severity: mild cf. moderate cf. severe = mild $258.4 ± 214.7; moderate $592.2 ± 429.6; severe $639.1 ± 291.6 • Types: evaporative cf. aqueous-deficient cf. mixed= evaporative $371.6 ± 391.7; moderate $215.2 ± 116.9; severe $4,616.1 ± 272.1 • Visit: first $382.7 ± 338.9; subsequent $280.6 ± 259.9 • Residence: rural $264.3 ± 227.8; urban $397.2 ± 349.7

C, central; NE, northeast; PCC, per capita cost; Pt, patient; SE, southeast.

the costs associated with DED. However, there are also some limitations. One limitation is that only the direct medical costs related to DED were collected or calculated. The effect of indirect costs, such as low employment, absence from work, and impaired productivity, will be investigated in the future. Another factor of note is that the actual economic burden of DED could have been underestimated, as we only collected data for 1 year. Future study using decision tree or Markov model is needed. Besides, the sample size was relatively small and we only included centers in China which may influence the generalizability of our study outside China.

CONCLUSIONS

Patients due to DED sustain a heavy economic burden for the healthcare system in China, which translates to $104.2–$166.6

billion per year when taking into account the prevalence of DED in China (affecting 394.13 million individuals). DED is a chronic ocular disease that costs more on patients in more severe disease stage. Thus, timely non-cost counseling, early diagnosis, and efficacious treatment are essential to retard the disease progression and potentially reduce the economic burden.

ETHICS STATEMENT

The studies involving human participants were reviewed and approved by Ethics Committees of Wuhan Aier Hankou Eye Hospital (Center-1), Guangzhou Aier Eye Hospital (Center-2), and Ha'erbin Eye Hospital (Center-3). The patients/participants provided their written informed consent to participate in this study.

AUTHOR CONTRIBUTIONS

WY, YL, SL, and QZ conceived and designed research. YL, XN, YY, CQ, WM, YZ, HW, DC, MQ, LK, YW, and LL collected data and conducted research. WY and SW analyzed and interpreted data. WY and QZ wrote the initial paper. SL and QZ revised the paper. QZ had primary responsibility for final content. All authors read and approved the final manuscript.

REFERENCES

1. Craig JP, Nichols KK, Akpek EK, Caffery B, Dua HS, Joo CK, et al. TFOS DEWS II definition and classification report. *Ocul Surf.* (2017) 15:276–83. doi: 10.1016/j.jtos.2017.05.008
2. Bradley JL, Özer Stillman I, Pivneva I, Guerin A, Evans AM, Dana R. Dry eye disease ranking among common reasons for seeking eye care in a large US claims database. *Clin Ophthalmol.* (2019) 13:225–32. doi: 10.2147/OPTH.S188314
3. Uchino M, Schaumberg DA, Dogru M, Uchino Y, Fukagawa K, Shimmura S, et al. Prevalence of dry eye disease among Japanese visual display terminal users. *Ophthalmology.* (2008) 115:1982–8. doi: 10.1016/j.ophtha.2008.06.022
4. Song P, Xia W, Wang M, Chang X, Wang J, Jin S, et al. Variations of dry eye disease prevalence by age, sex and geographic characteristics in China: a systematic review and meta-analysis. *J Glob Health.* (2018) 8:020503. doi: 10.7189/jogh.08.020503
5. Dana R, Bradley JL, Guerin A, Pivneva I, Stillman I, Evans AM, et al. Estimated prevalence and incidence of dry eye disease based on coding analysis of a large, all-age united states health care system. *Am J Ophthalmol.* (2019) 202:47–54. doi: 10.1016/j.ajo.2019.01.026
6. Stapleton F, Alves M, Bunya VY, Jalbert I, Lekhanont K, Malet F, et al. TFOS DEWS II epidemiology report. *Ocul Surf.* (2017) 15:334–65. doi: 10.1016/j.jtos.2017.05.003
7. Craig JP, Wang MTM, Ambler A, Cheyne K, Wilson GA. Characterising the ocular surface and tear film in a population-based birth cohort of 45-year old New Zealand men and women. *Ocul Surf.* (2020) 18:808–13. doi: 10.1016/j.jtos.2020.08.005
8. Malet F, Le Goff M, Colin J, Schweitzer C, Delyfer MN, Korobelnik JF, et al. Dry eye disease in French elderly subjects: the alienor study. *Acta Ophthalmol.* (2014) 92:e429–36. doi: 10.1111/aos.12174
9. Berg EJ, Ying GS, Maguire MG, Sheffield PE, Szczotka-Flynn LB, Asbell PA, et al. Climatic and environmental correlates of dry eye disease severity: a report from the dry eye assessment and management (DREAM) study. *Transl Vis Sci Technol.* (2020) 9:25. doi: 10.1167/tvst.9.5.25
10. Sayin N, Kara N, Pekel G, Altinkaynak H. Effects of chronic smoking on central corneal thickness, endothelial cell, and dry eye parameters. *Cutan Ocul Toxicol.* (2014) 33:201–5. doi: 10.3109/15569527.2013.832688
11. Porcar E, Pons AM, Lorente A. Visual and ocular effects from the use of flat-panel displays. *Int J Ophthalmol.* (2016) 9:881–5. doi: 10.18240/ijo.2016.06.16
12. Wang MTM, Muntz A, Mamidi B, Wolffsohn JS, Craig JP. Modifiable lifestyle risk factors for dry eye disease. *Cont Lens Anterior Eye.* (2021) 101409. doi: 10.1016/j.clae.2021.01.004 [Epub ahead of print].
13. Kastelan S, Lukenda A, Salopek-Rabatić J, Pavan J, Gotovac M. Dry eye symptoms and signs in long-term contact lens wearers. *Coll Antropol.* (2013) 37 (Suppl. 1):199–203.
14. Azuma M, Yabuta C, Fraunfelder FW, Shearer TR. Dry eye in LASIK patients. *BMC Res Notes.* (2014) 7:420. doi: 10.1186/1756-0500-7-420
15. Roszkowska AM, Biondi S, Chisari G, Messina A, Ferreri FM, Meduri A. Visual outcome after excimer laser refractive surgery in adult patients with amblyopia. *Eur J Ophthalmol.* (2006) 16:214–8. doi: 10.1177/112067210601600204
16. Man REK, Veerappan AR, Tan SP, Fenwick EK, Sabanayagam C, Chua J, et al. Incidence and risk factors of symptomatic dry eye disease in Asian Malays from the Singapore Malay eye study. *Ocul Surf.* (2017) 15:742–8. doi: 10.1016/j.jtos.2017.04.004
17. Meduri A, Urso M, Signorino GA, Rechichi M, Mazzotta C, Kaufman S. Cataract surgery on post radial keratotomy patients. *Int J Ophthalmol.* (2017) 10:1168–70. doi: 10.18240/ijo.2017.07.23
18. Fraunfelder FT, Sciubba JJ, Mathers WD. The role of medications in causing dry eye. *J Ophthalmol.* (2012) 2012:285851. doi: 10.1155/2012/285851
19. Roberti G, Tanga L, Manni G, Riva I, Verticchio AC, Berardo F, et al. Tear film, conjunctival and corneal modifications induced by glaucoma treatment. *Curr Med Chem.* (2019) 26:4253–61. doi: 10.2174/0929867326666190517111823
20. Simşek C, Dogru M, Kojima T, Tsubota K. Current management and treatment of dry eye disease. *Turk J Ophthalmol.* (2018) 48:309–13. doi: 10.4274/tjo.69320
21. Yu J, Asche CV, Fairchild CJ. The economic burden of dry eye disease in the United States: a decision tree analysis. *Cornea.* (2011) 30:379–87. doi: 10.1097/ICO.0b013e3181f7f363
22. Siffel C, Hennies N, Joseph C, Lascano V, Horvat P, Scheider M, et al. Burden of dry eye disease in Germany: a retrospective observational study using German claims data. *Acta Ophthalmol.* (2020) 98:e504–12. doi: 10.1111/aos.14300
23. McDonald M, Patel DA, Keith MS, Snedecor SJ. Economic and humanistic burden of dry eye disease in europe, north america, and asia: a systematic literature review. *Ocul Surf.* (2016) 14:144–67. doi: 10.1016/j.jtos.2015.11.002
24. Clegg JP, Guest JF, Lehman A, Smith AF. The annual cost of dry eye syndrome in France, Germany, Italy, Spain, Sweden and the United Kingdom among patients managed by ophthalmologists. *Ophthalmic Epidemiol.* (2006) 13:263–74. doi: 10.1080/09286580600801044
25. Galor A, Zheng DD, Arheart KL, Lam BL, Perez VL, McCollister KE, et al. Dry eye medication use and expenditures: data from the medical expenditure panel survey 2001 to 2006. *Cornea.* (2012) 31:1403–7. doi: 10.1097/ICO.0b013e31823cc0b7
26. Tachkov K, Vassilev A, Kostova S. Modeling the pharmacotherapy cost and outcomes of primary open-angle glaucoma with dry eye. *Front Public Health.* (2019) 7:363. doi: 10.3389/fpubh.2019.00363
27. Darbà J, Ascanio M. Economic impact of dry eye disease in Spain: a multicentre retrospective insurance claims database analysis. *Eur J Ophthalmol.* (2020) 31:328–33. doi: 10.1177/1120672120907315
28. Mizuno Y, Yamada M, Shigeyasu C. Annual direct cost of dry eye in Japan. *Clin Ophthalmol.* (2012) 6:755–60. doi: 10.2147/OPTH.S30625
29. Nagata T, Mori K, Ohtani M, Nagata M, Kajiki S, Fujino Y, et al. Total health-related costs due to absenteeism, presenteeism, and medical and pharmaceutical expenses in japanese employers. *J Occup Environ Med.* (2018) 60:e273–80. doi: 10.1097/JOM.0000000000001291

30. Waduthantri S, Yong SS, Tan CH, Shen L, Lee MX, Nagarajan S, et al. Cost of dry eye treatment in an Asian clinic setting. *PLoS ONE.* (2012) 7:e37711. doi: 10.1371/journal.pone.0037711
31. Yao W, Le Q. Social-economic analysis of patients with sjogren's syndrome dry eye in East China: a cross-sectional study. *BMC Ophthalmol.* (2018) 18:23. doi: 10.1186/s12886-018-0694-5
32. Luo Y, Yang W, Qi M, Wang Y, Li S, Wang M, et al. Annual direct economic burden and influencing factors of dry eye disease in Central China. *Ophthalmic Epidemiol.* (2021) 1–8. doi: 10.1080/09286586.2021.1959618
33. Nassiri N, Zhou XY, Torres YR, Meyer Z, Beyer MA, Mehregan CA, et al. Current and emerging therapy of dry eye disease. Part B: non-pharmacological modalities. *Expert Rev Ophthalmo.* (2017) 12:299–312. doi: 10.1080/17469899.2017.1344552
34. Gupta PK, Vora GK, Matossian C, Kim M, Stinnett S. Outcomes of intense pulsed light therapy for treatment of evaporative dry eye disease. *Can J Ophthalmol.* (2016) 51:249–53. doi: 10.1016/j.jcjo.2016.01.005
35. Uchino M, Yokoi N, Kawashima M, Ryutaro Y, Uchino Y, Tsubota K. Treatment trends in dry eye disease and factors associated with ophthalmic follow-up discontinuation in Japan. *J Clin Med.* (2019) 8:1120. doi: 10.3390/jcm8081120

21

Artificial Intelligence to Detect Meibomian Gland Dysfunction From *in-vivo* Laser Confocal Microscopy

Ye-Ye Zhang [1,2†]***, Hui Zhao*** [3†]***, Jin-Yan Lin*** [4]***, Shi-Nan Wu*** [5]***, Xi-Wang Liu*** [4,6]***, Hong-Dan Zhang*** [4,6]***, Yi Shao*** [5*] ***and Wei-Feng Yang*** [2,4,6*]

[1] Department of Electronic Engineering, School of Science, Hainan University, Haikou, China, [2] Department of Electronic Engineering, College of Engineering, Shantou University, Shantou, China, [3] Department of Ophthalmology, Shanghai First People's Hospital, Shanghai Jiao Tong University, National Clinical Research Center for Eye Diseases, Shanghai, China, [4] Research Center for Advanced Optics and Photoelectronics, Department of Physics, College of Science, Shantou University, Shantou, China, [5] Jiangxi Centre of National Ophthalmology Clinical Research Center, Department of Ophthalmology, The First Affiliated Hospital of Nanchang University, Nanchang, China, [6] Department of Mathematics, College of Science, Shantou University, Shantou, China

***Correspondence:**
Wei-Feng Yang
weifeng_yang@yeah.net
Yi Shao
freebee99@163.com

† These authors have contributed equally to this work

Background: In recent years, deep learning has been widely used in a variety of ophthalmic diseases. As a common ophthalmic disease, meibomian gland dysfunction (MGD) has a unique phenotype in *in-vivo* laser confocal microscope imaging (VLCMI). The purpose of our study was to investigate a deep learning algorithm to differentiate and classify obstructive MGD (OMGD), atrophic MGD (AMGD) and normal groups.

Methods: In this study, a multi-layer deep convolution neural network (CNN) was trained using VLCMI from OMGD, AMGD and healthy subjects as verified by medical experts. The automatic differential diagnosis of OMGD, AMGD and healthy people was tested by comparing its image-based identification of each group with the medical expert diagnosis. The CNN was trained and validated with 4,985 and 1,663 VLCMI images, respectively. By using established enhancement techniques, 1,663 untrained VLCMI images were tested.

Results: In this study, we included 2,766 healthy control VLCMIs, 2,744 from OMGD and 2,801 from AMGD. Of the three models, differential diagnostic accuracy of the DenseNet169 CNN was highest at over 97%. The sensitivity and specificity of the DenseNet169 model for OMGD were 88.8 and 95.4%, respectively; and for AMGD 89.4 and 98.4%, respectively.

Conclusion: This study described a deep learning algorithm to automatically check and classify VLCMI images of MGD. By optimizing the algorithm, the classifier model displayed excellent accuracy. With further development, this model may become an effective tool for the differential diagnosis of MGD.

Keywords: deep learning, meibomian gland dysfunction, convolution neural network, *in-vivo* confocal microscopy, DenseNet CNN

INTRODUCTION

The meibomian gland (MG) is a modified secretory sebaceous gland arranged vertically in the upper and lower eyelids and with openings at the eyelid edge (1). The MG can maintain the dynamic balance of the ocular surface by secreting lipids (meibum) into the tear film, thus helping to prevent tear evaporation, to lubricate the eye surface, and form barriers for protection from microbes and other environmental organisms (2–4). Meibomian gland dysfunction (MGD) is a chronic and diffuse meibomian gland disease, the main feature of which is the obstruction of the gland's terminal ducts and/or abnormal meibum secretion (5). The prevalence of MGD ranges from 46.2 to 68.0% in Asians (6). The earliest evaluation of meibomian gland function used the slit lamp and direct observation, but these evaluation methods are approximate. The later infrared imaging technology was effective in diagnosing MGD. It used infrared penetrating camera technology and enhanced contrast function to facilitate meibomian gland imaging (7). It allowed quantitative assessment of the meibomian glands (such as their presence or absence) but not morphological characteristics at the cellular level. In recent years, scholars have found that *in-vivo* laser confocal microscopy imaging (VLCMI) allows observation of the microscopic morphology of the meibomian glands *in-vivo* (8, 9) and investigation of the pathophysiological process of MGD, with particular significance for the diagnosis of MGD.

Artificial intelligence (AI) is a branch of computer science which uses logical operation methods to establish related databases and application models (10). Machine learning is an implementation method of artificial intelligence which extracts generalized rules from data through algorithms characterized by "learning" (11). These rules are represented by mathematical models, including a descriptive analysis of given data. At the same time, other automated methods required experts in the field to define the descriptive rules of the data after which they were implemented by computer programmers in the automated system. The clinical application of AI in ophthalmology diagnosis and treatment includes automatic detection and quantification of ocular lesions or features, automatic screening of ocular diseases, AI-based diagnostic grading, and clinical decision support in retinal treatment and prognostic disease models (12–14). A previous study showed that the application of AI technology in retinal disease was based on the detection of disease-related features on color fundus photography images. The primary retinal markers used in this procedure were large retinal blood vessels and optic discs, sometimes including foveal features, because these markers exist in every fundus image (15). So far, deep learning and other artificial intelligence methods have developed rapidly in ophthalmic research. Glushan's development and validation of deep learning detection algorithms for diabetic retinopathy has been fully recognized (16). Therefore, the development of a deep learning algorithm to automatically identify MGD may reduce the uncertainty of MGD screening and decrease the challenges for human assessors, reducing the need for medical resources and long-term finance.

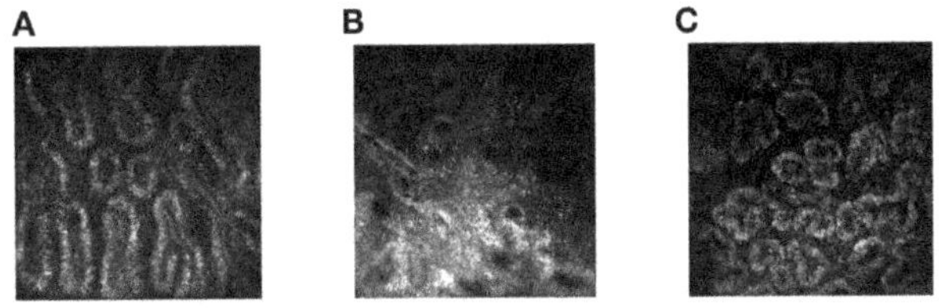

FIGURE 1 | *In-vivo* laser confocal microscope images of obstructive **(A)** and atrophic MGD **(B)** and healthy eyes **(C)**. MGD, meibomian gland dysfunction.

As far as we know, no diagnostic approach using AI technology for MGD morphological characteristics has been reported previously. Therefore, the purpose of this study was to assess the ability of AI models to detect different types of MGD using VICMIs.

METHODS

Study Subjects

The institutional review board of the First Affiliated Hospital of Nanchang University approved this study, which was conducted in accordance with the tenets of the Declaration of Helsinki. This was a single-center, clinical study. Eight thousand three hundred eleventh VLCMIs were included, among which 2,766 were from healthy controls, 2,744 for diagnosis of OMGD, and 2,801 for diagnosis of AMGD (**Figure 1**). All the subjects were recruited at the Ophthalmology Department of the First Affiliated Hospital of Nanchang University. Diagnoses were conducted by the ophthalmology expert team and the artificial intelligence screening system. Inclusion criteria for the healthy group were as follows: 1. 18–50 years of age; 2. No significant ocular discomfort and no apparent abnormalities on eyelid margin examination; 3. No eye diseases, no history of eye surgery or trauma and no contact lens wear; 4. No serious systemic disease and able to cooperate to undergo all examinations; 5. Voluntary participation in the study. Inclusion criteria for the MGD group were as follows: 1. Absence of meibomian glands; 2. Abnormal meibomian gland secretion and meibomian gland opening; 3. Changes in quantity and quality of meibomian gland secretions, and any of the above signs combined with symptoms can diagnose MGD. Exclusion criteria: 1. Age younger than 18 or older than 50 years; 2. Patients who are not newly diagnosed in our hospital or have undergone MGD related treatment; 3. Have a history of eye surgery; 4. Have a history of eye trauma; 5. Combined ocular inflammation (such as blepharitis, seborrheic dermatitis, etc.) or eyelid conjunctival scarring disease; 6. Contact lens wearer; 7. Unable to complete all inspections due to other factors; 8. Involuntary take part in this research.

In-vivo Laser Confocal Microscopy

All subjects were examined using the *in-vivo* confocal microscopy (IVCM; Heidelberg Retina Tomograph II-Rostock Cornea Module, Dossenheim, Germany) as previously described (17). Briefly, the subjects were under topical anesthesia, and the eyelid was everted. The center of the Tomo-Cap with comfort gel was placed onto the palpebral conjunctiva and gradually moved from the focal plane into the subconjunctival tissue until the glands were visualized. The images of the underlying meibomian glands were observed and captured by the software (Python 3.7.6; tensorflow GPU 2.0). We scanned the glands while moving the lens from the eyelid margins toward the fornix (vertical movements) and along the palpebral width (horizontal movements). During the examination, no subjects complained of discomfort. The images were two-dimensional with a 400 × 400μm field of view. For each subject, three high-quality digital images of nasal, middle, and temporal glands (total nine images of each eyelid) were selected.

Definition of Meibomian Gland Abnormalities

Normal meibomian glands were sebaceous glands situated vertically and parallel to each other. Each gland contained grape-like acini, connected by the duct. The acini had convoluted borders with large cells lining and a lumen consisting of fine cellular material (18). Previous study shows that the normal meibomian gland acinar unit density is 113 ± 36.6 glands/mm^2 (19). In MGD patients, any change in morphology and the number of acinar units may be observed. The diameter of obstructive meibomian acinus was larger than that of normal meibomian acinus, and the acinus contained eyelid fat blockage. Atrophic meibomian acinus was characterized by destruction of acinar epithelial cells with fibrosis (19–21). Based on such changes, we categorized the MGD group images as atrophic or obstructive. The atrophic meibomian glands were fibrosed with abnormal architecture and a reduced acinar unit density. The obstructive glands showed considerable acinar unit enlargement, with the acinar unit density again decreased.

All the subjects underwent evaluation by an ophthalmologist, including tear film breakup time and corneal fluorescein staining, in order to confirm the clinical diagnosis. The VLCMIs were classified by the ophthalmologist into three groups: normal, atrophic, and obstructive.

Model Construction

A total of 4,985 VLCMIs were used for training, and 1,663 VLCMIs were used to test the our deep learning system. **Figure 2** shows details of the training data set, the external test data set and the model construction process. We trained three types of network structures (DenseNet 121, DenseNet 169, and DenseNet 201) to classify the meibomian glands into one of the three classes: normal, atrophic, and obstructive. Sparse categorical cross-entropy was performed on the primary data set to differentiate between normal, atrophic, and obstructive. The training started with multiple iterations on a batch size of 16 images, with a learning rate of 0.001, and stopped at 200 epochs. Using the same thresholds, the diagnostic performance of the three classification models was assessed on the five independent external-testing data sets.

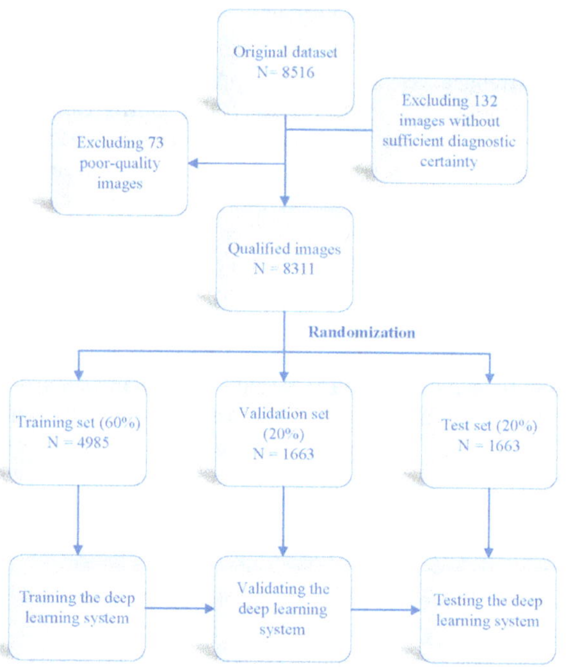

FIGURE 2 | Flow chart illustrating development of the deep learning system.

Statistical Analysis

We derived the receiver operating characteristic (ROC) curve by changing the thresholds of ratios of the images classified as different groups and the values output by the neural network. We calculated the area under the ROC curve (AUC). For the sensitivity and specificity, we considered the neural network answer as abnormal if the value output of the ratio of images classified as the two MGD groups was 0.5 or more and standard if the value was <0.5. Finally, we used confusion matrix analysis to evaluate the performance of the automated diagnosis based on the final test results of the three models.

RESULTS

Performance of Different Deep Learning Algorithms in the Test Datasets

The ROC curve was used to evaluate the accuracy of the machine model for autonomous recognition of VLCMIs for differential diagnosis between different types of MGD and differentiation between MGD and normal images. Accuracy of the DenseNet 169 model in differential diagnosis of OMGD, AMGD and healthy subjects was 97, 99 and 98%, respectively. The DenseNet 121 model showed accuracy of 94, 96, and 93%, respectively while the DenseNet 201 model showed 94, 97, and 94%, respectively (**Figure 3**). The DenseNet169 therefore showed highest accuracy. Compared with the correct recognition accuracy of medical experts, the correct recognition accuracy was 91%. The identification accuracy

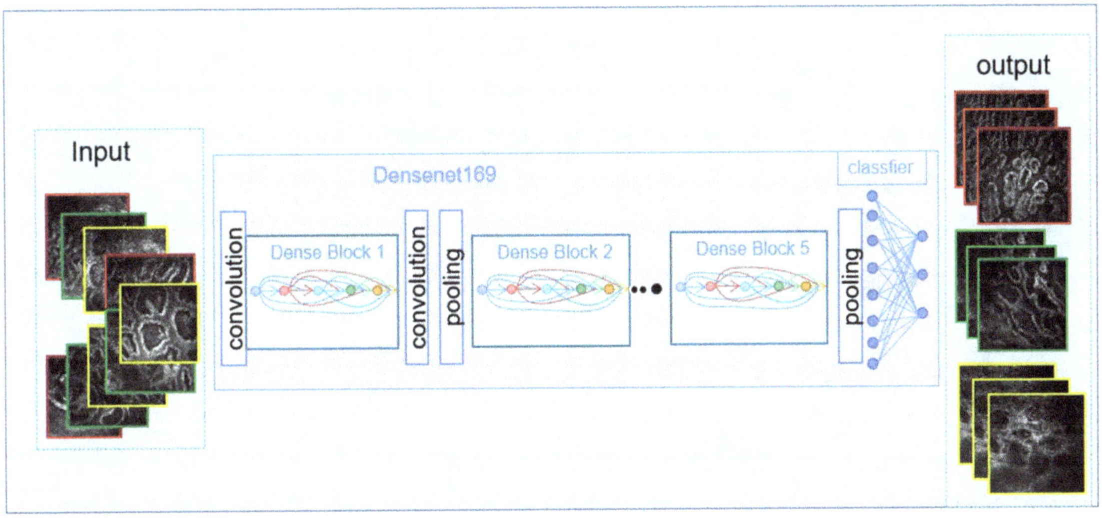

FIGURE 3 | The imaging images go through the deep learning algorithm and the output of the final results.

TABLE 1 | Performance of three deep learning algorithms in the test dataset.

Different deep learning models	Test dataset		
	Sensitivity (95% CI)	**Specificity (95% CI)**	**Accuracy (95% CI)**
DenseNet 169			
Obstructive MGD	88.8% (86.1–91.4%)	95.4% (94.2–96.6%)	97.3% (96.4–98.2%)
Atrophic MGD	89.4% (86.8–91.9%)	98.4% (97.6–99.1%)	98.6% (97.9–99.3%)
Healthy controls	94.5% (92.6–96.4%)	92.6% (91.0–94.1%)	98.0% (97.4–98.6%)
DenseNet 121			
Obstructive MGD	85.8% (82.9–88.8%)	87.1% (85.1–89.1%)	93.8% (92.7–95.0%)
Atrophic MGD	69.0% (65.2–72.8%)	99.5% (99.0–99.9%)	95.6% (94.3–96.9%)
Healthy controls	88.8% (86.1–91.4%)	85.2% (83.1–87.3%)	92.7% (91.2–94.1%)
DenseNet 201			
Obstructive MGD	89.3% (86.7–91.9%)	85.4% (83.3–87.5%)	94.2% (93.0–95.4%)
Atrophic MGD	70.6% (66.9–74.4%)	99.1% (98.5–99.7%)	96.7% (95.6–97.8%)
Healthy controls	86.4% (83.6–89.3%)	88.6% (86.8–90.5%)	94.1% (92.9–95.3%)

DenseNet 169 demonstrated the highest accuracy.
MGD, meibomian gland dysfunction; CI, confidence interval.

of the DenseNet 169 model was higher than that of the medical experts.

The DenseNet169 model showed sensitivity and specificity of 88.8 and 95.4%, respectively, and AUC of 97.3% for OMGD, 89.4 and 98.4%, respectively and AUC of 98.6% for AMGD, 94.5 and 92.6%, respectively with AUC of 98.0% in normal subjects. Further details and the sensitivities and specificities of the other two DenseNet models are shown in **Table 1**.

DISCUSSION

The aim of the present study was to evaluate performance of the deep learning system to detect different types of MGD in images obtained using an *in-vivo* laser confocal microscope. Our main finding was that the system based on a deep learning neural network can distinguish between OMGD, AMGD and normal subjects (**Figures 4**, **5**), the best performing algorithm being the DenseNet169, with differential diagnostic accuracy of 97 to 99%, sensitivity of over 88% and specificity over 95% (**Figure 6**).

MGD is a chronic, nonspecific inflammation of the meibomian gland, characterized by duct obstruction or abnormal secretion, and is an important cause of hyperevaporative dry eye (22). In addition, the symptoms of MGD have a significant impact on the quality of life of patients, not only causing eye irritation, but also leading to the sequelae of ocular surface inflammation and visual dysfunction (5). Age is a risk factor for MGD. With increasing age, atrophy of the meibomian gland acinar epithelial cells leads to the large-scale irreversible atrophy

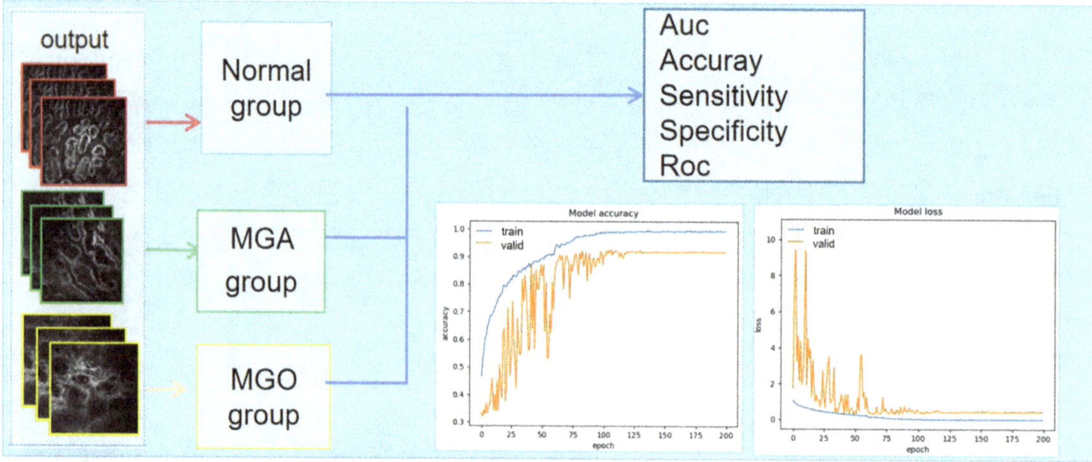

FIGURE 4 | The output of the discriminant result and the final classification accuracy vary with the number of iterations. MGA, atrophic meibomian gland; MGO, obstructive meibomian gland; AUC, area under the curve; ROC, receiver operating characteristic curve.

of the gland, with a decrease in lipid secretion (23). In recent years, the incidence of MGD in the population has increased, making it the most common disease in ophthalmology clinics. The estimated pooled prevalence of MGD worldwide was 35.8% (24). Consistent with this, a global survey of dry eye patients found that 35% of the population had dry eye, of which 53% were caused by MGD (25). Difficulties in the clinical diagnosis and treatment of MGD included extensive effort required for comprehensive ocular surface analysis and examination, low precision of examination results of MGD-related dry eye, low relevance of the severity of the disease to its management, and poor subjective perception of patient prognosis. At present ophthalmology clinic, the infrared meibography was performed with the Oculus Keratograph 5M® (Wetzlar, Germany) to evaluate the meibomian gland morphology. Images of meibomian glands in the entire lower eyelids were obtained. The meibomian gland function scores were graded according to the extent of the meibomian gland dropout. It was graded from 0 to 3 (0 = no gland loss; 1 = loss < 33%, 2 = loss between 33 and 66%, 3 = loss > 66%). This method can also evaluate MGD, but it can only evaluate the morphology of meibomian gland, not meibomian gland acinus (26). Meibomian gland acinus is a cell secreting palpebral fat, which can better represent the function of meibomian gland. However, conventional detection techniques could not directly observe the morphological and quantitative changes of meibomian acinus. These problems restrict the improvement of the diagnosis, treatment level and long-term management of MGD. In addition, due to the low medical and economic resources in underdeveloped and remote areas, the ophthalmologist to patient ratio is low, leading to delayed diagnosis and deterioration of MGD in some patients. For example, in Nigeria, reported physician to patient ratio is as low as 1:2,660 (27). An efficient and socially effective method for evaluating meibomian gland function is therefore needed urgently. The AI-assisted diagnosis of ophthalmic diseases such as cataract, early glaucoma, diabetic retinopathy, and age-related macular degeneration is undergoing rapid development (28–31), but there are few studies on artificial intelligence-assisted diagnosis or screening of dry eye or MGD. We aimed to make a preliminary attempt by studying deep-learning models and conducting a series of in-depth processing of meibomian gland images such as automatic segmentation of meibomian conjunctiva and meibomian glands, morphological feature extraction, and missing rate calculation. The evaluation duration was about 0.5 s, demonstrating sub-second analysis of the meibomian gland images.

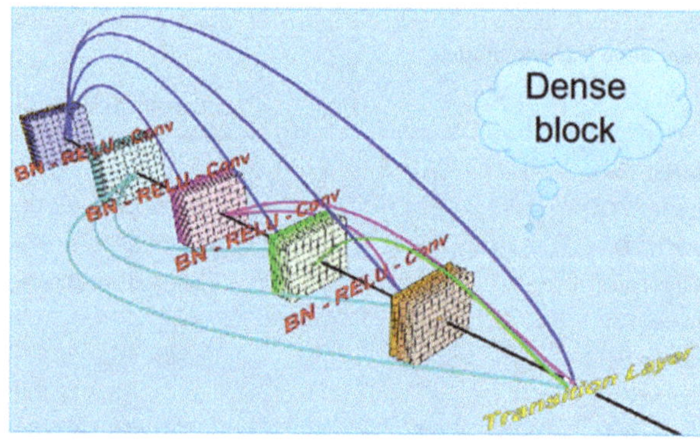

FIGURE 5 | Pooling process of deep learning algorithms.

To date, the IVCM has been used to qualitatively and quantitatively evaluate the posterior pole, including the optic disc (32). Recently, IVCM has played an increasingly important role in the evaluation of meibomian gland function (17, 33). The advantage of IVCM lies in its imaging of ocular surface tissue *in-vivo* at the cellular level, and its option to observe and measure the microstructure of meibomian glands (34), providing a new perspective from which to understand the pathophysiological mechanism of meibomian gland disease (33).

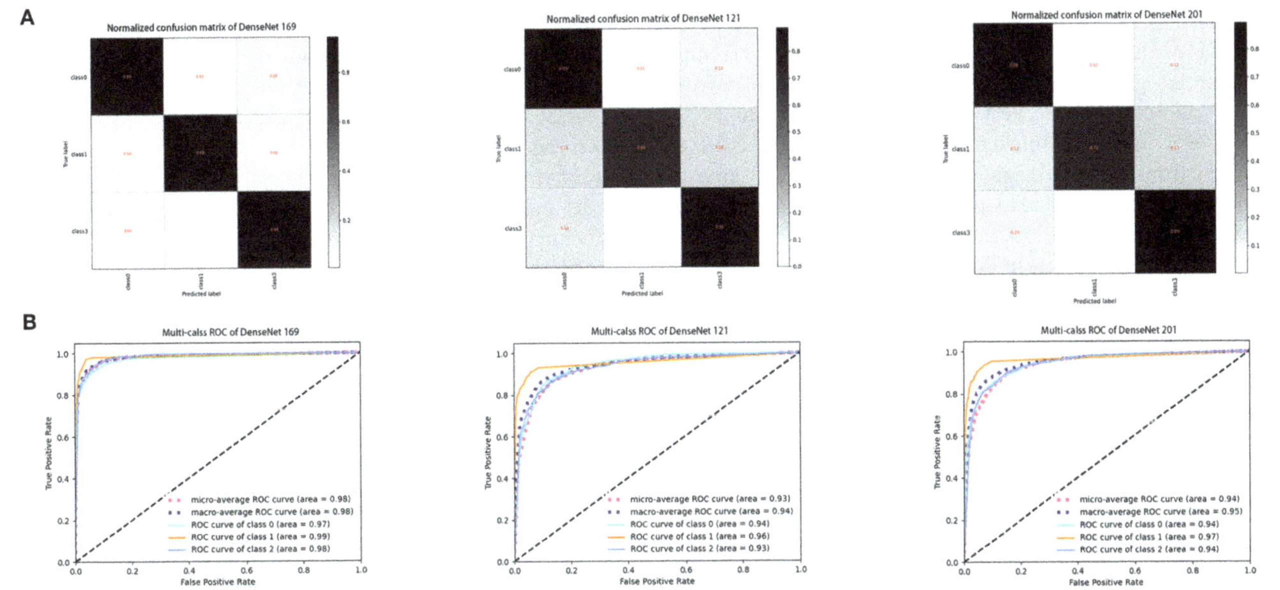

FIGURE 6 | Performance of three DenseNet deep learning algorithms in the test dataset. **(A)** Confusion matrices describing the accuracies of deep learning algorithms. **(B)** Receiver operating characteristic curves indicating the performance of each algorithm in diagnosis of obstructive MGD, atrophic MGD and healthy controls. DenseNet 169 model demonstrated the highest differential diagnostic accuracy. Class 0: obstructive MGD; class 1: atrophic MGD; class 2: healthy controls. MGD, meibomian gland dysfunction.

In addition, related studies have further confirmed that IVCM can be used for preclinical diagnosis before the significant loss of glands (18). The arrangement and specific number of acinar units can be observed using the IVCM, and nine confocal images at different angles can be obtained from one side of the eyelid (19). By carefully evaluating the confocal images, we can look for atrophy of acinar units, presence of inflammatory cells, and reduced acinar unit density in MGD patients. The IVCM allows the phenotypic changes in MGD to be described using new diagnostic parameters, such as acinar unit density and acinar unit diameter, reflecting histopathological changes such as glandular atrophy or ductal dilatation, respectively. Healthy control VLCMIs allow the morphological changes of meibomian gland acini to be identified at a preclinical stage, before the appearance of ocular symptoms and morphological changes of the meibomian gland opening. In MGD, there was more neutrophil infiltration into the conjunctiva and some Langerhans cells infiltration into the palpebral conjunctiva, suggesting that the occurrence of MGD was related to conjunctival inflammation. We believed that the micromorphological changes of meibomian glands were earlier than the loss of glands, and the absence of glands appeared ocular symptoms (i.e., MGD) to a certain extent. Therefore, the IVCM may play an important role in the accurate diagnosis of MGD. Combination of the deep learning module developed by our team provides a novel technique for diagnosis of MGD.

The term "DenseNets" reflects its dense connection method, which improves the backpropagation of the gradient, facilitating network training (35). Since each layer can directly reach the final error signal, implicit "deep supervision" is realized. The error signal can rapidly propagate to the earlier layers to obtain direct supervision from the final classification layer. The vanishing gradient is alleviated, and the problem of over-gradient disappearance is more likely to occur at greater network depth (36). This is because the input and gradient information are transferred between many layers, and now this kind of dense connection is equivalent to each layer directly connect the input and loss so that it can reduce the disappearance of the gradient so that the deeper network is not a problem. The number of parameters is reduced, and low-dimensional features are preserved. In a standard convolutional network, the final output will only be used to extract the highest-level features. DenseNet uses high and low feature levels and tends to give a smoother decision boundary, with good performance even with insufficient training data (37). The disadvantage of DenseNet is that due to the need to perform multiple concatenate operations, the data need to be copied multiple times, video memory is rapidly used and dedicated video memory optimization technology is required. In addition, DenseNet is a specialized network, while others such as ResNet are more generic with a broader range of applications. Related deep learning studies in dry eye diseases adopted a VCG19 model, which used machine algorithms to recognize the anterior segment optical coherence tomography images of subjects to independently distinguish dry eye patients from normal subjects, and its recognition sensitivity and specificity reached 86.36 and 82.35%, respectively (38). The advantages of deep learning algorithms in the differential diagnosis of ophthalmic diseases were independent, objective, rapid and non-invasive. With the further development and clinical testing of the model, our model can be used as an important auxiliary means for the diagnosis and screening of meibomian gland dysfunction. From our discussion above, confocal microscopy was very effective in evaluating MGD and dry eye. Artificial intelligence technology can assist in reading pictures, quickly diagnosed and classify them, improve doctors' work efficiency, and help Internet diagnosis and medical treatment in timeliness.

However, there are some limitations in our study. The present model tests the conditions of "meibomian gland atrophy" and "meibomian gland obstruction" only. The meibomian glands may also have structural abnormalities and missing structures, and the model's image recognition accuracy of the meibomian glands still needs to be further improved to detect these in clinical practice. We anticipate collaboration with other hospitals to establish a multi-center database to make data sources more universal and extensive, further improve the accuracy of model interpretation, and promote the further development of artificial intelligence in assisting the diagnosis of ocular surface diseases. In the future, while increasing the sample size, we will also combine other dry eye-related indicators such as the height of the tear meniscus, tear film break up time, and tear secretion to improve the model algorithm further.

In summary, we have found good accuracy of an image depth processing model to evaluate meibomian glands in MGD, and this method can assist clinicians in analyzing the examination results better and faster and provide a more reliable basis for diagnosis. It is of great value as a means to support individualized treatment of dry eye and chronic disease management. This model is most appropriate for general ophthalmology clinics with a low doctor to patient ratio. It can also be used for dry eye screening in the wider population and follow-up and efficacy observation in management of dry eye. Finally, the DenseNet169 model may assist ophthalmologists in the diagnosis of MGD, reducing their workload and pressure related to diagnosis.

ETHICS STATEMENT

The studies involving human participants were reviewed and approved by the Medical Ethics Committee of the Shanghai First People's Hospital and First Affiliated Hospital of Nanchang University. The patients/participants provided their written informed consent to participate in this study.

AUTHOR CONTRIBUTIONS

Y-YZ, S-NW, and HZ analyze and process data. HZ and J-YL wrote the manuscript. X-WL and H-DZ involved in the data curation. YS and W-FY involved in the study conceptualization, data curation, funding acquisition, and project administration. All authors have read and approved the final manuscript.

REFERENCES

1. Jester JV, Nicolaides N, Smith RE. Meibomian gland studies: histologic and ultrastructural investigations. *Invest Ophthalmol Vis Sci.* (1981) 20:537–47.
2. Willcox MDP, Argüeso P, Georgiev GA, Holopainen JM, Laurie GW, Millar TJ, et al. TFOS DEWS II tear film report. *Ocul Surf.* (2017) 15:366–403. doi: 10.1016/j.jtos.2017.03.006
3. Butovich IA. Meibomian glands, meibum, and meibogenesis. *Exp Eye Res.* (2017) 163:2–16. doi: 10.1016/j.exer.2017.06.020
4. Wang YC, Li S, Chen X, Ma B, He H, Liu T, et al. Meibomian gland absence related dry eye in ectodysplasin a mutant mice. *Am J Pathol.* (2016) 186:32–42. doi: 10.1016/j.ajpath.2015.09.019
5. Sabeti S, Kheirkhah A, Yin J, Dana R. Management of meibomian gland dysfunction: a review. *Surv Ophthalmol.* (2020) 65:205–17. doi: 10.1016/j.survophthal.2019.08.007
6. Amano S. Meibomian gland dysfunction: recent progress worldwide and in Japan. *Invest Ophthalmol Vis Sci.* (2018) 59: DES87–93. doi: 10.1167/iovs.17-23553
7. Adil MY, Xiao J, Olafsson J, Chen X, Lagali NS, Ræder S, et al. Meibomian gland morphology is a sensitive early indicator of meibomian gland dysfunction. *Am J Ophthalmol.* (2019) 200:16–25. doi: 10.1016/j.ajo.2018.12.006
8. Matsumoto Y, Ibrahim OMA. Application of *in vivo* confocal microscopy in dry eye disease. *Invest Ophthalmol Vis Sci.* (2018) 59: Des41–7. doi: 10.1167/iovs.17-23602
9. Vagge A, Bernabei F, Del Noce C, Pellegrini M, Giannaccare G, Senni C, et al. *In vivo* confocal microscopy morphometric analysis of meibomian glands in patients with graves ophthalmopathy. *Cornea.* (2021) 40:425–29. doi: 10.1097/ICO.0000000000002404
10. Kapoor R, Walters SP, Al-Aswad LA. The current state of artificial intelligence in ophthalmology. *Surv Ophthalmol.* (2019) 64:233–40. doi: 10.1016/j.survophthal.2018.09.002
11. Shouval R, Fein JA, Savani B, Mohty M, Nagler A. Machine learning and artificial intelligence in haematology. *Br J Haematol.* (2021) 192:239–50. doi: 10.1111/bjh.16915
12. Cheung CY, Tang F, Ting DSW, Tan GSW, Wong TY. Artificial intelligence in diabetic eye disease screening. *Asia Pac J Ophthalmol.* (2019). doi: 10.22608/APO.201976
13. Raman R, Srinivasan S, Virmani S, Sivaprasad S, Rao C, Rajalakshmi R. Fundus photograph-based deep learning algorithms in detecting diabetic retinopathy. *Eye.* (2019) 33:97–109. doi: 10.1038/s41433-018-0269-y
14. Ting DSW, Pasquale LR, Peng L, Campbell JP, Lee AY, Raman R, et al. Artificial intelligence and deep learning in ophthalmology. *Br J Ophthalmol.* (2019) 103:167–75. doi: 10.1136/bjophthalmol-2018-313173
15. Schmidt-Erfurth U, Sadeghipour A, Gerendas BS, Waldstein SM, Bogunović H. Artificial intelligence in retina. *Prog Retin Eye Res.* (2018) 67:1–29. doi: 10.1016/j.preteyeres.2018.07.004
16. Gulshan V, Peng L, Coram M, Stumpe MC, Wu D, Narayanaswamy A, et al. Development and validation of a deep learning algorithm for detection of diabetic retinopathy in retinal fundus photographs. *Jama.* (2016) 316:2402–10. doi: 10.1001/jama.2016.17216
17. Matsumoto Y, Sato EA, Ibrahim OM, Dogru M, Tsubota K. The application of in vivo laser confocal microscopy to the diagnosis and evaluation of meibomian gland dysfunction. *Mol Vis.* (2008) 14:1263–71.
18. Fasanella V, Agnifili L, Mastropasqua R, Brescia L, Di Staso F, Ciancaglini M, et al. *In vivo* laser scanning confocal microscopy of human meibomian glands in aging and ocular surface diseases. *Biomed Res Int.* (2016) 2016:7432131. doi: 10.1155/2016/7432131
19. Ibrahim OM, Matsumoto Y, Dogru M, Adan ES, Wakamatsu TH, Goto T, et al. The efficacy, sensitivity, and specificity of *in vivo* laser confocal microscopy in the diagnosis of meibomian gland dysfunction. *Ophthalmology.* (2010) 117:665–72. doi: 10.1016/j.ophtha.2009.12.029

20. Maruoka S, Tabuchi H, Nagasato D, Masumoto H, Chikama T, Kawai A, et al. Deep neural network-based method for detecting obstructive meibomian gland dysfunction with *in vivo* laser confocal microscopy. *Cornea.* (2020) 39:720–25. doi: 10.1097/ICO.0000000000002279
21. Randon M, Aragno V, Abbas R, Liang H, Labbé A, Baudouin C. *In vivo* confocal microscopy classification in the diagnosis of meibomian gland dysfunction. *Eye.* (2019) 33:754–60. doi: 10.1038/s41433-018-0307-9
22. Nichols KK, Foulks GN, Bron AJ, Glasgow BJ, Dogru M, Tsubota K, et al. The international workshop on meibomian gland dysfunction: executive summary. *Invest Ophthalmol Vis Sci.* (2011) 52:1922–9. doi: 10.1167/iovs.10-6997a
23. Knop E, Knop N, Millar T, Obata H, Sullivan DA. The international workshop on meibomian gland dysfunction: report of the subcommittee on anatomy, physiology, and pathophysiology of the meibomian gland. *Invest Ophthalmol Vis Sci.* (2011) 52:1938–78. doi: 10.1167/iovs.10-6997c
24. Hassanzadeh S, Varmaghani M, Zarei-Ghanavati S, Heravian Shandiz J, Azimi Khorasani A. Global prevalence of meibomian gland dysfunction: a systematic review and meta-analysis. *Ocul Immunol Inflamm.* (2021) 29:66–75. doi: 10.1080/09273948.2020.1755441
25. Murakami DK, Blackie CA, Korb DR. All warm compresses are not equally efficacious. *Optom Vis Sci.* (2015) 92:e327–33. doi: 10.1097/OPX.0000000000000675
26. Daniel E, Maguire MG, Pistilli M, Bunya VY, Massaro-Giordano GM, Smith E, et al. Grading and baseline characteristics of meibomian glands in meibography images and their clinical associations in the dry eye assessment and management (DREAM) study. *Ocul Surf.* (2019) 17:491–501. doi: 10.1016/j.jtos.2019.04.003
27. Zhang K, Liu X, Xu J, Yuan J, Cai W, Chen T, et al. Deep-learning models for the detection and incidence prediction of chronic kidney disease and type 2 diabetes from retinal fundus images. *Nat Biomed Eng.* (2021) 5:533–45. doi: 10.1038/s41551-021-00745-6
28. Russakoff DB, Lamin A, Oakley JD, Dubis AM, Sivaprasad S. Deep learning for prediction of AMD progression: a pilot study. *Invest Ophthalmol Vis Sci.* (2019) 60:712–22. doi: 10.1167/iovs.18-25325
29. Grzybowski A, Brona P, Lim G, Ruamviboonsuk P, Tan GSW, Abramoff M, et al. Artificial intelligence for diabetic retinopathy screening: a review. *Eye.* (2020) 34:451–60. doi: 10.1038/s41433-019-0566-0
30. Mursch-Edlmayr AS, Ng WS, Diniz-Filho A, Sousa DC, Arnold L, Schlenker MB, et al. Artificial intelligence algorithms to diagnose glaucoma and detect glaucoma progression: translation to clinical practice. *Transl Vis Sci Technol.* (2020) 9:55. doi: 10.1167/tvst.9.2.55
31. Goh JHL, Lim ZW, Fang X, Anees A, Nusinovici S, Rim TH, et al. Artificial intelligence for cataract detection and management. *Asia-Pacific journal of ophthalmology.* (2020) 9:88–95. doi: 10.1097/01.APO.0000656988.16221.04
32. Nguyen C, Midgett D, Kimball E, Jefferys J, Nguyen TD, Schaub J, et al. Age-related changes in quantitative strain of mouse astrocytic lamina cribrosa and peripapillary sclera using confocal microscopy in an explant model. *Invest Ophthalmol Vis Sci.* (2018) 59:5157–66. doi: 10.1167/iovs.18-25111
33. Wang Y, Le Q, Zhao F, Hong J, Xu J, Zheng T, et al. Application of *in vivo* laser scanning confocal microscopy for evaluation of ocular surface diseases: lessons learned from pterygium, meibomian gland disease, and chemical burns. *Cornea.* (2011) 30 Suppl 1:S25–8. doi: 10.1097/ICO.0b013e318227fcd9
34. Cheng S, Zhang M, Chen H, Fan W, Huang Y. The correlation between the microstructure of meibomian glands and ocular demodex infestation: a retrospective case-control study in a Chinese population. *Medicine.* (2019) 98:e15595. doi: 10.1097/MD.0000000000015595
35. Wang A, Wang M, Wu H, Jiang K, Iwahori Y. A novel LiDAR data classification algorithm combined capsnet with ResNet. (2020) 20:1151. doi: 10.3390/s20041151
36. Le WT, Maleki F, Romero FP, Forghani R, Kadoury S. Overview of machine learning: part 2: deep learning for medical image analysis. *Neuroimaging Clin N Am.* (2020) 30:417–31. doi: 10.1016/j.nic.2020.06.003
37. Chun J, Zhang H, Gach HM, Olberg S, Mazur T, Green O, et al. MRI super-resolution reconstruction for MRI-guided adaptive radiotherapy using cascaded deep learning: in the presence of limited training data and unknown translation model. *Med Phys.* (2019) 46:4148–64. doi: 10.1002/mp.13717
38. Chase C, Elsawy A, Eleiwa T, Ozcan E, Tolba M, Abou Shousha M. Comparison of autonomous AS-OCT Deep learning algorithm and clinical dry eye tests in diagnosis of dry eye disease. *Clin Ophthalmol.* (2021) 15:4281–89. doi: 10.2147/OPTH.S321764

22

Correlations Between Single-Photon Emission Computed Tomography Parameters of Salivary Glands and Dry Eye Tests in Patients With Sjögren's Syndrome

Xiaoyu Huang [1], Lingjuan Xu [1], Wei Wang [1], Weikun Hu [1], Xinyu Li [1], Hong Zhang [1], Jing Chen [2] and Guigang Li [1]*

[1] *Department of Ophthalmology, Tongji Medical College, Tongji Hospital, Huazhong University of Science and Technology, Wuhan, China,* [2] *Department of Nuclear Medicine, Tongji Medical College, Tongji Hospital, Huazhong University of Science and Technology, Wuhan, China*

***Correspondence:**
Guigang Li
guigli@163.com

Objective: To evaluate the correlations between Single-Photon Emission Computed Tomography (SPECT) parameters of salivary glands and dry eye parameters in patients with Sjögren's syndrome (SS).

Methods: A total of 28 patients with SS participated in this prospective study. Dry eye assessments include tear film break-up time (TBUT), corneal fluorescein staining scoring (CFS), Schirmer's I test (SIT) examination and SPECT of salivary gland. The following quantitative parameters were derived from SPECT imaging for salivary glands: Uptake index (UI), the time needed to achieve the minimum counts after Vit C stimulation (T_S), and excretion fraction (EF). The relation between the aforementioned parameters and TBUT, CFS and SIT were analyzed with SPSS 22.0 software.

Results: All the 28 eyes of the 28 subjects were examined. The mean SIT was 6.04 ± 4.64 mm/5 min (0–18 mm/5 min); the mean CFS was 3.07 ± 2.65 (0–10) and the mean BUT was 2.11 ± 1.97 s (0–9 s). The mean EF value was 0.52 ± 0.12 (0.26–0.75) in parotid glands and 0.45 ± 0.10 (0.30–0.67) in submandibular glands, respectively. The mean UI value was 9.33 ± 1.68 (6.03–13.20) in parotid glands and 9.92 ± 1.48 (7.08–12.60) in submandibular glands, respectively. The mean T_S (min) was 5.32 ± 3.01 (2.00–12.00) in parotid glands and 11.09 ± 7.40 (2.00- 29.00 min) in submandibular glands, respectively. It was found that EF positively correlates with SIT in patients with SS ($r = 0.499$ and 0.426 in parotid glands and submandibular glands, with $P < 0.05$), while no significant correlation was found between the UI, T_S and CFS, TBUT ($P > 0.05$).

Conclusions: The EF was positively correlated with SIT in patients with SS, it could reflex the dysfunction of salivary glands in SS patients. So, EF may be a valuable parameter for the diagnosis of SS patients with lacrimal gland secretion dysfunction.

Keywords: dry eye, Sjögren's syndrome, salivary glands, single photon emission computed tomography (SPECT), Schirmer's I test

INTRODUCTION

Sjögren's syndrome (SS) is a chronic autoimmune disorder that typically affects the exocrine glands (mainly salivary and lacrimal glands). Patients who suffer from this condition experience dry mouth and also very dry eyes. The estimated prevalence of this medical condition varies between 0.5 and 1% of the general population (1). Dry eye disease (DED) and dry mouth are typical symptoms of SS. It's reported that 11.6% of patients with clinically significant aqueous-deficient dry eye (ADDE) had SS in an prospective, industry-sponsored, multicentre clinical trial (2).

According to the SS diagnostic criteria of 2016 American College of Rheumatology/European League Against Rheumatism (ACR-EULAR) (3), ocular and oral problems are the main symptoms of SS patients. Ocular examination mainly includes the symptom of ocular dryness, ocular staining score and Schirmer's test (3). Gland biopsy is a method that can provide directly evidence of glandular inflammation, but it is invasive and cause discomfort to the patient, which make it challenging to get early diagnosis.

Single-Photon Emission Computed Tomography (SPECT) can detect nuclide radioactivity and generate images of the human body at both planar and three-dimensional levels. This type of scan has been suggested as a sensitive, dynamic, and objective alternative approach to functional and morphological evaluation of salivary glands of SS patients (4–7). However, the role of SPECT in the diagnosis of SS has been weakened (3, 8), mainly because of the lack of specific criteria for quantitative evaluation of salivary gland SPECT in patients under these conditions (9). The aim of this study is to evaluate the correlations between SPECT parameters of salivary glands and dry eye tests in patients with Sjögren's syndrome.

METHODS

The procedures conducted for study are consistent with the Helsinki Declaration and approved by the Ethics Committee of Tongji Hospital. All subjects have been informed of the aim of study, the principles of related examination methods and possible adverse consequences. Each individual signed an informed consent under totally comprehension.

Research Objects

Twenty eight patients with SS were enrolled in the study, consulting in the department of Ophthalmology, Rheumatology and Immunology at Tongji Hospital of Tongji Medical College, Huazhong University of Science & Technology (HUST).

Inclusion criteria:

1. 18 to 65 years old.
2. According to the 2016 ACR-EULAR (3), the criteria are based on five objective tests/items: labial salivary gland with focal lymphocytic sialadenitis and focus score of $\geq$1 foci/4 mm^2 (3 points), anti-SSA/Ro-positive (3 points), ocular staining score $\geq$5 (or van Bijsterveld score $\geq$4) in at least one eye (1 point), Schirmer's test $\leq$5 mm/5 min in at least one eye (1 point), unstimulated whole saliva flow rate $\leq$0.1 mL/min (1 point). Individuals are classified as having primary SS if they have a total score of $\geq$4.

Exclusion criteria:

1. 3 months before the screening visit with ocular trauma, inflammation of the eyelid infection.
2. Contact lens wearer.
3. Severe heart, lung, liver, kidney dysfunction.
4. Pregnant and lactating women. Psychopaths.

Research Methods

SPECT Examination of Salivary Glands

SPECT was performed with a dual-head Discovery NM/CT 670 SPECT/CT instrument (General Electric Medical Systems, Waukesha, WI, USA) fitted with a low energy, general-purpose, parallel-hole collimator with standard peak energy settings (20% at 140 keV). The subject remained in supine position, and the probe was positioned for an anterior head-and-neck projection. Dynamic images were immediately acquired in a 128 × 128-pixel matrix, at 1 min per frame. The process lasted for 30 min after a bolus intravenous injection of 370 MBq of 99 mTc-sodium pertechnetate. Fifteen minutes after the injection, each subject was administered 300 mg VitC (sublingual application) without moving, while imaging was continued.

Regions of interests (ROI) were drawn on the compressed dynamic images of the parotid and submandibular glands for both right and left sides. Time activity curves were generated for each gland (**Figure 1**). The following quantitative parameters were derived by nuclear medicine physicians from the department of Nuclear Medicine, Tongji Hospital, Tongji Medical College, HUST. Then, the mean values of each pair of glandular parameters were analyzed.

C_p = maximum counts before VitC stimulation.
C_0 = counts at 1st min.
C_v = minimum counts after VitC stimulation.
C_b = background count, obtained from the average count of bilateral frontal regions.
Uptake index (UI) = $(C_p\text{-}C_0)/C_0$.
The time after stimulation (T_s) = time needed to achieve the minimum counts after VitC stimulation.
Excretion fraction (EF) = $(C_p\text{-}C_v)/(C_p\text{-}C_b)$.

Dry Eye Assessments

The right eyes of all patients were included in the study. All enrolled patients were diagnosed with DED according to the Tear Film and Ocular Surface Society (TFOS) Dry Eye Workshop (DEWS) II (10). The dry eye assessments were performed in the order of tear film break-up time (TBUT), corneal fluorescein staining scoring (CFS), Schirmer's I test (SIT).

TBUT

The examiners pulled down the eyelid of the subject using the thumb or the index finger, infiltrated and touched the conjunctiva of lower eyelid with the sodium fluorescein test paper. The patient was required to look straight and blink 3–4 times. This allowed the examiner to observe the first dry spot (random

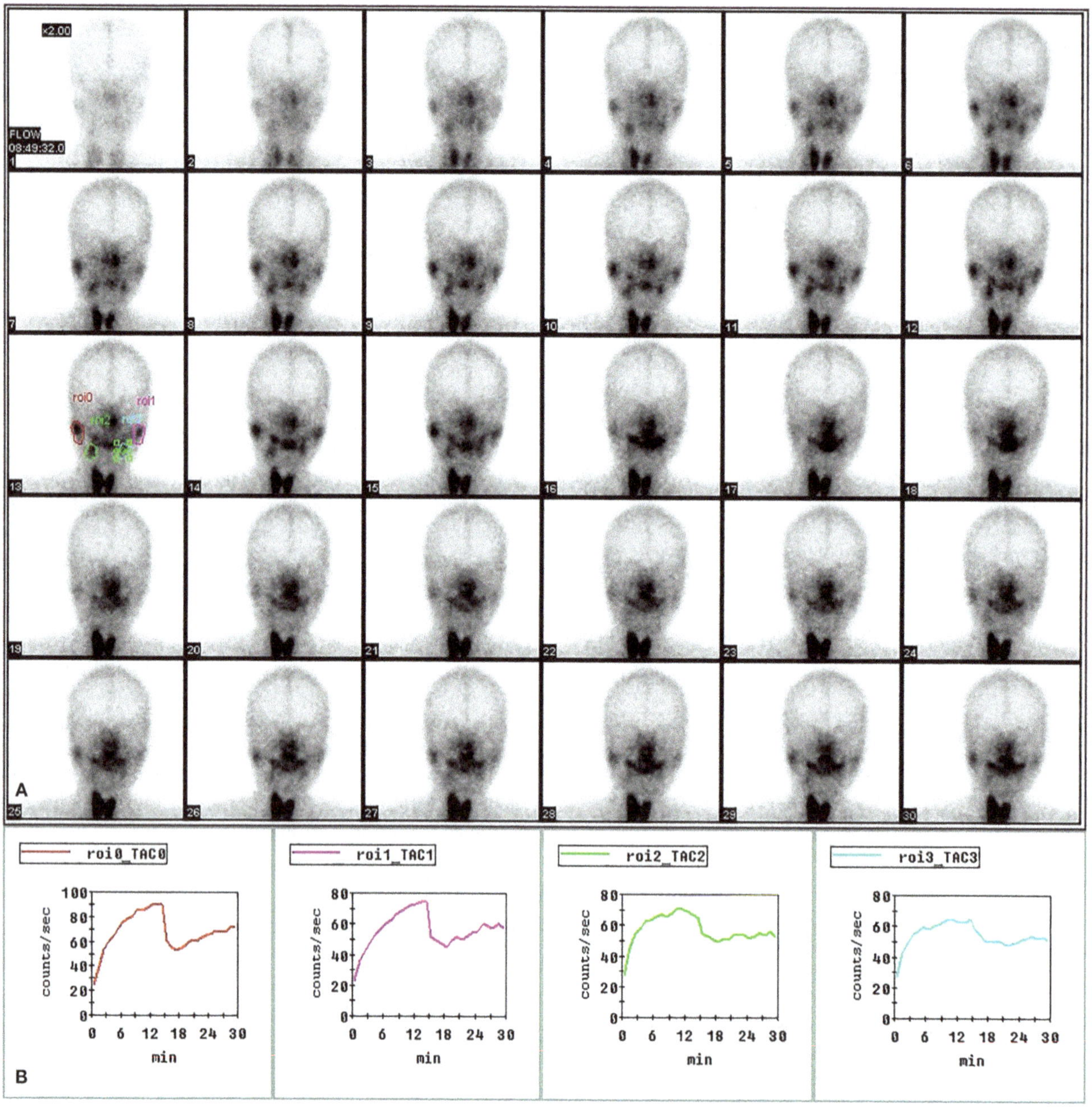

FIGURE 1 | Regions of interest (ROIs) in SPECT imaging of salivary gland. The images of bilateral parotid and submandibular glands at 1–30 min post injection of 370 MBq of 99 mTc-sodium pertechnetate in the upper panel **(A)**. The time-activity curves for right parotid gland (red), left parotid gland (purple), right submandibular gland (green) and left submandibular gland (blue) in the lower panel **(B)**.

position) in fluorescein on the tear film after the last blink by using the slit-lamp microscope.

CFS

One end of the sodium fluorescein test paper was infiltrated with aseptic saline. The examiners pulled the participants' eyelid down using the thumb or the index finger, and touched the lower eyelid conjunctiva of the subjects with the humid end. Then, the subjects were advised to lightly close the eyes to observe the staining of the corneal epithelium with the cobalt blue light of slit lamp. The examiner then divided the cornea into four quadrants when scoring (11). Each quadrant was divided into 0–3 points:

0: 0 dots
1: 1–5 dots
2: 6–30 dots
3: >30 dots

TABLE 1 | Demographic information of the patients with Sjögren's syndrome (SS).

The number of cases	Male (Cases)	Female (Cases)	Maximum age (years old)	Minimum age (years old)	Average age (years old)
28	3	25	65	18	46.30 ± 11.1

TABLE 2 | Summary of dry eye parameters in patients with Sjögren's syndrome (SS).

	Mean	SD	Maximum	Minimum
SIT (mm/5 min)	6.04	4.64	18.00	0.00
CFS	3.07	2.65	10.00	0.00
BUT (second)	2.11	1.97	9.00	0.00

Tear film break-up time (TBUT), corneal fluorescein staining scoring (CFS), Schirmer's I test (SIT).

The four quadrant areas were added and recorded based on a standard of 0–12 points. Corneal epithelial staining was performed by the same examiner.

SIT

The subjects were oriented to maintain a calm and natural state. The examiner took a 35 mm long/5 mm wide standard test paper, folded the upper end of the test paper backward, and placed it gently in the middle and outside (1/3) of the conjunctive sac of the subject's lower eyelid. The rest of the palpebral fissure naturally hanged out of the eyelid. The whole process was completed following the principles of asepsis. The inspected patient was required to lightly close the eyes and look up, and could blink freely, and then lightly pulled down the eyelids and took out the test paper after 5 min, reading after another 2 min, and posted it for preservation.

Statistical Methods

The result data were analyzed with SPSS 22.0 software. In this study, spearmen rank correlation was analyzed and correlation coefficients were calculated. $P < 0.05$ represents that the difference was statistically significant.

RESULTS

Twenty eight eyes of 28 subjects (25 females, 3 males; age range from 18 to 65 years old; averaged 46.3 ± 11.1 years old, **Table 1**) were examined. The mean SIT was 6.04 ± 4.64 mm/5 min (0–18 mm/5 min); the mean CFS was 3.07 ± 2.65 (0–10) and the mean BUT was 2.11 ± 1.97 s (0–9 s) (**Table 2**). The mean EF value was 0.52 ± 0.12 (0.26–0.75) in parotid glands and 0.45 ± 0.10 (0.30–0.67) in submandibular glands, respectively; the mean UI value was 9.33 ± 1.68 (6.03–13.20) in parotid glands and 9.92 ± 1.48 (7.08–12.60) in submandibular glands, respectively; the mean Ts (min) was 5.32 ± 3.01 (2.00–12.00) in parotid glands and 11.09 ± 7.40 (2.00–29.00 min) in submandibular glands, respectively (**Table 3**).

TABLE 3 | Summary of quantitative parameters of SPECT examination in salivary glands.

	Mean	SD	Maximum	Minimum
Parotid glands				
EF	0.52	0.12	0.75	0.26
UI	9.33	1.68	13.20	6.03
T_S (min)	5.32	3.01	12.00	2.00
Submandibular glands				
EF	0.45	0.10	0.67	0.30
UI	9.92	1.48	12.60	7.08
T_S (min)	11.09	7.40	29.00	2.00

Excretion fraction (EF). Uptake index (UI). The time needed to achieve the minimum counts after Vit C stimulation (T_S).

TABLE 4 | Correlation analysis of quantitative parameters of SPECT examination in salivary glands and dry eye tests.

SPECT parameters	SIT		CFS		BUT	
	r	*P*-value	r	*P*-value	r	*P*-value
Parotid glands						
EF	0.499	0.007*	−0.145	0.462	0.272	0.162
UI	−0.028	0.887	0.164	0.403	0.258	0.186
T_S (min)	0.034	0.865	0.313	0.105	−0.087	0.660
Submandibular glands						
EF	0.426	0.024*	−0.298	0.124	0.164	0.405
UI	−0.091	0.644	0.173	0.378	0.123	0.533
T_S (min)	0.078	0.724	0.275	0.204	−0.114	0.606

*r, Pearson correlation coefficient; *$P < 0.05$, the correlation was statistically significant. Excretion fraction (EF). Uptake index (UI). The time needed to achieve the minimum counts after Vit C stimulation (T_S).*

The SPECT parameters were compared with TBUT, CFS, and SIT, accordingly. The excretion fraction was correlated with SIT in patients with SS ($r = 0.499$ and 0.426 in parotid glands and submandibular glands and $P < 0.05$). It was verified that UI and Ts do not have a significant correlation with CFS and TBUT ($P > 0.05$) (**Table 4**; **Figures 2**, **3**).

DISCUSSION

The major characteristic of SS is the chronic autoimmune disorder of the exocrine glands with associated lymphocytic infiltrates of the affected glands (12). Sets of diagnostic criteria for SS have been proposed, the 2002 American-European Consensus Group (AECG) criteria (13) and 2012 American College of Rheumatology (ACR) criteria (14) were the most widely used in the medical community (15, 16) until 2016 ACR-EULAR criteria (3) was published. However, both the 2002 AECG criteria and 2012 ACR criteria have a high specificity (94.3% vs. 91.3%, respectively) but low sensitivity (61.6% vs. 62.3%, respectively) (17). We are constantly exploring new tests and methods for sensitive diagnose of SS.

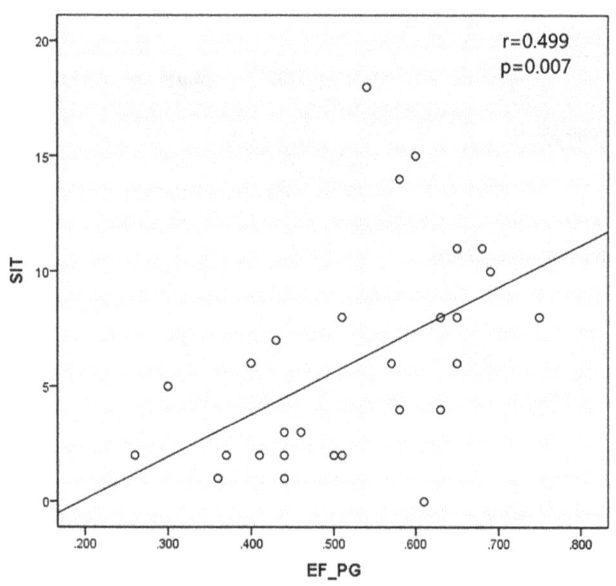

FIGURE 2 | Excretion fraction in parotid glands (EF_PG) was positively correlated with SIT.

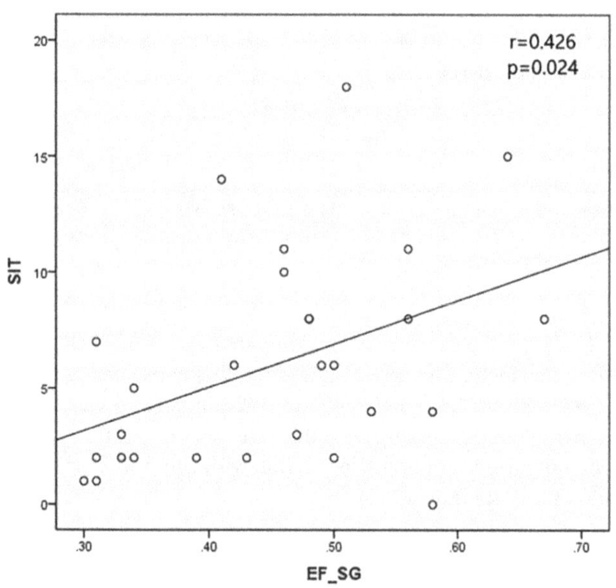

FIGURE 3 | Excretion fraction in submandibular glands (EF_SG) was positively correlated with SIT.

The functional tests for the salivary glands were not included in the 2012 ACR criteria. The assessment of salivary glands was limited to the results of a minor salivary gland biopsy. The pathological features of minor salivary glands in SS patients were not exactly the same as those of major salivary glands (18). Furthermore, since the labial glands biopsy procedure is invasive, some patients may refuse it thus resulting in failure of the SS diagnosis. SPECT is currently considered a well-recognized test for the investigation of multiple diseases affecting salivary glands (19). In fact, radionuclide imaging of salivary gland yields only relatively low effective radiation doses compared with computed tomography (CT) for sialography (20). This dynamic, non-invasive, and quantitative detection assesses the functional state and degree of injury to the salivary glands.

Recently, SPECT has been refined to provide quantitative information on changes in salivary function (4). The use of computer-assisted time-activity curves allows quantification of salivary gland radioactivity turnover in a defined time period. However, which quantification parameter of salivary gland is best for assessing salivary gland dysfunction in SS patients remains inconclusive.

Delayed tracer uptake and secretion in SS patients is a progressive decrease in the exocrine function of the major salivary glands. This happens due to morphological changes caused by chronic immune-mediated inflammation. In order to improve the specificities of SPECT, we chose UI, T_S, and EF as assessment parameters. The UI is defined as the tissue concentration of the tracer, measured by a scanner. It mainly assess the uptake function of the major salivary glands. T_S indicates how long the salivary glands secrete after acid stimulation. The EF value represents the secretory function of the salivary glands. In this study, decreased EF, UI and increased T_S are considered as a result of a progressive reduction in the exocrine function of the major salivary glands.

Schirmer's I test was developed nearly 100 years ago and the method has been widely used for evaluation of tear production. It is a well-standardized test that can be used to estimate stimulated reflex aqueous secretion (10) by observing the degree on the folded strip. The secretion disorder caused by the exocrine gland damage is the main pathological process of SS patients (12). The reduction of lacrimal gland secretion in SS patients leads to the decrease of SIT. The correlation between SIT and EF in this study may be due to the consistent degree of damage to the exocrine glands in SS. There is no significant correlation between SIT and T_S maybe because of the insensitivity of T_S as an indicator of salivary gland secretion. UI, as an indicator of uptake function, was not correlated with other indicators in this trial, possibly because the uptake function of the glands in SS patients was not much damaged. It's reported there's no difference in UI value between SS patients and non-SS patients (5). Studies involving more subjects are needed to confirm this conclusion.

Some other widely used diagnostic methods for dry eye are BUT and CFS. The BUT is defined as the time interval between a blink and the first occurrence of gaps or breaks in the tear film and it mainly assesses the tear film stability. The tear film lipid layer is derived from the meibum secreted from the lid margins and is spread onto the tear film after each blink. It plays an important role in stabilizing the tear film (21). Thus, the BUT has no significant correlation with the UI, T_S, and EF in our results.

Corneal and conjunctival staining are considered informative markers of severity degree in severe DED cases, whereas mild/moderate ocular surface staining is less associated with disease severity (22). Fluorescein sodium staining can be observed when the corneal epithelium is damaged. The classical theory is that the dye, which is dissolved in saline and is thus hydrophilic, is transported across altered tight junctions in diseased patients (23). A punctate cornea stain is actually a small lump of dye where cells are missing. Thus, CFS mainly reflects the integrity of the corneal epithelium rather than the secretion of tears. Hence, it is not significantly correlated with UI, Ts, and EF in our results.

SPECT has unique diagnostic advantages for patients with SS since it provides a non-invasive, dynamic, and quantitative measure of exocrine glands function. The lacrimal gland is a small part of the orbital structures, which makes it difficult to obtain biopsy materials. With the successful clinical application of positron emission tomography (PET)/CT in recent years, the next step is to produce a higher resolution SPECT/CT hybrid scanner (24). Then, the dynamic detection of lacrimal gland function will be possible.

CONCLUSION

SPECT can help examiners and doctors to better understand the decreased secretion velocity in the submandibular and parotid glands. The EF was positively correlated with SIT in patients with SS, and could reflex the dysfunction of salivary glands in SS patients. EF may be a valuable parameter for the diagnosis of SS patients with lacrimal gland secretion dysfunction.

ETHICS STATEMENT

The studies involving human participants were reviewed and approved by the Ethics Committee of Tongji Hospital, Tongji Medical College, Huazhong University of Science and Technology. The patients/participants provided their written informed consent to participate in this study. Written informed consent was obtained from the individual(s) for the publication of any potentially identifiable images or data included in this article.

AUTHOR CONTRIBUTIONS

XH: acquisition of data, conception and design of study, analysis and/or interpretation of data, and drafting the manuscript. GL and JC: revising the manuscript critically for important intellectual content. All authors contributed to manuscript revision, read, and approved the submitted version.

REFERENCES

1. Mavragani CP, Moutsopoulos HM. Sjogren's syndrome. *Annu Rev Pathol.* (2014) 9:273–85. doi: 10.1146/annurev-pathol-012513-104728
2. Liew MS, Zhang M, Kim E, Akpek EK. Prevalence and predictors of Sjogren's syndrome in a prospective cohort of patients with aqueous-deficient dry eye. *Br J Ophthalmol.* (2012) 96:1498–503. doi: 10.1136/bjophthalmol-2012-301767
3. Shiboski CH, Shiboski SC, Seror R, Criswell LA, Labetoulle M, Lietman TM, et al. 2016 American College of Rheumatology/European League Against rheumatism classification criteria for primary Sjogren's syndrome: a consensus and data-driven methodology involving three international patient cohorts. *Arthritis Rheumatol.* (2017) 69:35–45. doi: 10.1002/art.39859
4. Kim J, Lee H, Lee H, Bang JI, Kang YK, Bae S, et al. Quantitative single-photon emission computed tomography/computed tomography for evaluation of salivary gland dysfunction in Sjogren's syndrome patients. *Nucl Med Mol Imaging.* (2018) 52:368–76. doi: 10.1007/s13139-018-0547-4
5. Chen J, Zhao X, Liu H, Zhou S, Yang Y, Li S, et al. A point-scoring system for the clinical diagnosis of Sjogren's syndrome based on quantified SPECT imaging of salivary gland. *PLoS ONE.* (2016) 11:e155666. doi: 10.1371/journal.pone.0155666
6. Minami Y, Ogura I. A clinical pilot study of salivary gland secretion for xerostomia patients with Sjogren's syndrome using SPECT/CT. *Gerodontology.* (2021). doi: 10.1111/ger.12584. [Epub ahead of print].
7. Ninomiya K, Toya S, Ogura I. Single-photon emission computed tomography/computed tomography for evaluation of salivary gland dysfunction: preliminary study on diagnostic ability of maximum standardized uptake value. *Oral Radiol.* (2020) 36:163–67. doi: 10.1007/s11282-019-00393-2
8. Fox RI, Robinson CA, Curd JG, Kozin F, Howell FV. Sjogren's syndrome. Proposed criteria for classification. *Arthritis Rheum.* (1986) 29:577–85. doi: 10.1002/art.1780290501
9. Vivino FB, Hermann GA. Role of nuclear scintigraphy in the characterization and management of the salivary component of Sjogren's syndrome. *Rheum Dis Clin North Am.* (2008) 34:973–86. doi: 10.1016/j.rdc.2008.08.011
10. Wolffsohn JS, Arita R, Chalmers R, Djalilian A, Dogru M, Dumbleton K, et al. TFOS DEWS II diagnostic methodology report. *Ocul Surf.* (2017) 15:539–74. doi: 10.1016/j.jtos.2017.05.001
11. Keratology Group of Ophthalmology Branch of Chinese Medical Association. Expert consensus on clinical diagnosis and treatment of dry eye 2013. *Chin J Ophthalmol.* (2013) 49:73–5. doi: 10.3760/cma.j.issn.0412-4081.2013.01.020
12. Fox RI. Sjogren's syndrome. *Lancet.* (2005) 366:321–31. doi: 10.1016/S0140-6736(05)66990-5
13. Vitali C, Bombardieri S, Jonsson R, Moutsopoulos HM, Alexander EL, Carsons SE, et al. Classification criteria for Sjogren's syndrome: a revised version of the European criteria proposed by the American-European Consensus Group. *Ann Rheum Dis.* (2002) 61:554–8. doi: 10.1136/ard.61.6.554
14. Shiboski SC, Shiboski CH, Criswell L, Baer A, Challacombe S, Lanfranchi H, et al. American College of Rheumatology classification criteria for Sjogren's syndrome: a data-driven, expert consensus approach in the Sjogren's International Collaborative Clinical Alliance cohort. *Arthritis Care Res.* (2012) 64:475–87. doi: 10.1002/acr.21591
15. Bootsma H, Spijkervet FK, Kroese FG, Vissink A. Toward new classification criteria for Sjogren's syndrome? *Arthritis Rheum.* (2013) 65:21–3. doi: 10.1002/art.37701
16. Tincani A, Andreoli L, Cavazzana I, Doria A, Favero M, Fenini MG, et al. Novel aspects of Sjogren's syndrome in 2012. *BMC Med.* (2013) 11:93. doi: 10.1186/1741-7015-11-93
17. Hernandez-Molina G, Avila-Casado C, Nunez-Alvarez C, Cardenas-Velazquez F, Hernandez-Hernandez C, Luisa CM, et al. Utility of the American-European Consensus Group and American College of Rheumatology classification criteria for Sjogren's syndrome in patients with systemic autoimmune diseases in the clinical setting. *Rheumatology.* (2015) 54:441–8. doi: 10.1093/rheumatology/keu352
18. Guellec D, Cornec D, Jousse-Joulin S, Marhadour T, Marcorelles P, Pers JO, et al. Diagnostic value of labial minor salivary gland biopsy for Sjogren's syndrome: a systematic review. *Autoimmun Rev.* (2013) 12:416–20. doi: 10.1016/j.autrev.2012.08.001
19. Wu CB, Xi H, Zhou Q, Zhang LM. The diagnostic value of technetium 99m pertechnetate salivary gland scintigraphy in patients with certain salivary gland diseases. *J Oral Maxillofac Surg.* (2015) 73:443–50. doi: 10.1016/j.joms.2014.09.013

20. Brix G, Nekolla EA, Borowski M, Nosske D. Radiation risk and protection of patients in clinical SPECT/CT. *Eur J Nucl Med Mol Imaging.* (2014) 41(Suppl. 1):S125–36. doi: 10.1007/s00259-013-2543-3
21. Craig JP, Tomlinson A. Importance of the lipid layer in human tear film stability and evaporation. *Optom Vis Sci.* (1997) 74:8–13. doi: 10.1097/00006324-199701000-00014
22. Tomlinson A, Khanal S, Ramaesh K, Diaper C, McFadyen A. Tear film osmolarity: determination of a referent for dry eye diagnosis. *Invest Ophthalmol Vis Sci.* (2006) 47:4309–15. doi: 10.1167/iovs.05-1504
23. Norn MS. Micropunctate fluorescein vital staining of the cornea. *Acta Ophthalmol.* (1970) 48:108–18. doi: 10.1111/j.1755-3768.1970.tb06578.x
24. Suh MS, Lee WW, Kim YK, Yun PY, Kim SE. Maximum standardized uptake value of (99m)Tc hydroxymethylene diphosphonate SPECT/CT for the evaluation of temporomandibular joint disorder. *Radiology.* (2016) 280:890–6. doi: 10.1148/radiol.2016152294

23

TLR4-Dependent DUOX2 Activation Triggered Oxidative Stress and Promoted HMGB1 Release in Dry Eye

*Bowen Wang†, Hao Zeng†, Xin Zuo, Xue Yang, Xiaoran Wang, Dalian He and Jin Yuan**

State Key Laboratory of Ophthalmology, Zhongshan Ophthalmic Center, Guangdong Provincial Key Laboratory of Ophthalmology and Visual Science, Sun Yat-sen University, Guangzhou, China

***Correspondence:**
Jin Yuan
yuanjincornea@126.com

†These authors have contributed equally to this work and share first authorship

Dry eye disease (DED) is one of the most common ocular surface diseases worldwide. DED has been characterized by excessive accumulation of reactive oxygen species (ROS), following significant corneal epithelial cell death and ocular surface inflammation. However, the key regulatory factor remains unclear. In this study, we tended to explore whether DUOX2 contributed to DED development and the underlying mechanism. Human corneal epithelial (HCE) cells were treated with hyperosmolarity, C57BL/6 mice were injected of subcutaneous scopolamine to imitate DED. Expression of mRNA was investigated by RNA sequencing (RNA-seq) and quantitative real-time PCR (qPCR). Protein changes and distribution of DUOX2, high mobility group box 1 (HMGB1), Toll-like receptor 4 (TLR4), and 4-hydroxynonenal (4-HNE) were evaluated by western blot assays and immunofluorescence. Cell death was assessed by Cell Counting Kit-8 (CCK8), lactate dehydrogenase (LDH) release, and propidium iodide (PI) staining. Cellular ROS levels and mitochondrial membrane potential (MMP) were analyzed by flow cytometry. RNA-seq and western blot assay indicated a significant increase of DUOX2 dependent of TLR4 activation in DED both *in vitro* and *in vivo*. Immunofluorescence revealed significant translocation of HMGB1 within corneal epithelial cells under hyperosmolar stress. Interestingly, after ablated DUOX2 expression by siRNA, we found a remarkable decrease of ROS level and recovered MMP in HCE cells. Moreover, knockdown of DUOX2 greatly inhibited HMGB1 release, protected cell viability and abolished inflammatory activation. Taken together, our data here suggest that upregulation of DUOX2 plays a crucial role in ROS production, thereafter, induce HMGB1 release and cell death, which triggers ocular surface inflammation in DED.

Keywords: dry eye, DUOX2, oxidative stress, ROS, HMGB1, inflammation

INTRODUCTION

Dry eye disease (DED) is a global ocular surface disorder. The prevalence of DED worldwide ranged from 5 to 50% respectively (1). Generally, patients with DED frequently suffer from eye discomfort, dryness, and pain, which could influence work efficiency and finally vision-related quality of life (2). Until now, although the specific pathophysiological mechanism of DED is not fully established, one of the recognized core mechanisms is chronic ocular surface inflammatory responses (3). Therefore, targeting early inflammation activation may provide new therapeutic possibilities for DED treatment. Recently, several research have elucidated that consecutive damage of human corneal epithelium cells could give rise to ocular surface inflammation (4, 5).

Corneal epithelium is the outermost layer of the eye so that it sustains massive oxidative stress from the external environment (6). One of the outstanding characteristics of ocular surface oxidative stress is the overproduction of reactive oxygen species (ROS), particularly within human corneal epithelial (HCE) cells (7, 8). In our previous study, we have clarified that ROS accumulation in HCE cells could induce impaired autophagy, which further lead to cell death and the activation of inflammation (9). Whereas how risk factors of DED trigger oxidative stress accumulation and influence downstream cell viability remain uncertain.

Dual oxidase 2 (DUOX2) is a member of the nicotinamide adenine dinucleotide phosphate (NADPH) oxidase family that regulates the production of intracellular ROS, and plays diverse biological functional roles (10). DUOX2 is remarkably expressed in multiple epithelial cell types and has been implicated to perform host defense functions in various diseases (11, 12). DUOX2-mediated host defense is mainly derived from generating hydrogen peroxide and other oxides as well as inducing redox-dependent regulation of cellular responses (13, 14). Nevertheless, moderate activation of response pathway is beneficial to restore homeostasis, but excessive activation could conversely lead to the development of disease (15). It is remarkable, however, that the pathological effect of DUOX2 in ROS-cell death axis is still indistinct in DED.

High mobility group box 1 (HMGB1) is a highly conservative nucleoprotein (16). Nuclear HMGB1 serves in the regulation of DNA damage repair as a DNA chaperone. Interestingly, after post-translational modifications, HMGB1 could translocate from the nucleus to the cytoplasm, and thereby involved in cellular immune reaction (17, 18). Several research indicated that the elevation of HMGB1 within cytoplasm plays a key role in cell necrosis and production of pro-inflammation cytokine accelerating enormous inflammatory responses (19, 20). Though HMGB1 expression was found to be enhanced by dry eye conditions, the crosstalk between DUOX2-mediated excessive ROS release and HMGB1 during DED inflammation progression has not been previously investigated.

In the current study, we tended to explore the role of DUOX2 in DED and provide a novel therapeutic target for DED. As far as we are aware, our present research for the first time reveals that Toll-like receptor 4 (TLR4)-dependent increase of DUOX2 promotes oxidative stress in HCE cells, which triggers the cell death by means of enhancing translocation of HMGB1 and accelerates ocular surface inflammation in DED.

METHODS

Reagents

Dulbecco's modified Eagle's medium (DMEM)/F12 medium, fetal bovine serum (FBS), penicillin/streptomycin, 0.25% trypsin-EDTA, recombinant human epidermal growth factor (hEGF), and an insulin-transferrin-selenium supplement were obtained from Invitrogen/Gibco (Carlsbad, CA, USA). Additionally, 6-, 12-, 24-, and 96-well culture plates and cell culture dish were purchased from Corning (Corning, NY, USA). Cell Counting Kit-8 (CCK8) was gained from Dojindo Laboratories (Japan). A Pierce LDH Cytotoxicity Assay Kit was purchased from Thermo Fishier Scientific (Rockford, IL, USA). DCFDA/H2DCFDA-Cellular ROS Assay Kit (#ab113851) and the anti-HMGB1 (#ab18256) antibody were purchased from Abcam (Cambridge, UK). The anti-4-HNE (#MA5-27570) was purchased from Invitrogen. The anti-DUOX2 (#sc-398681) antibody was obtained from Santa Cruz Biotechnology (TX, USA). The antibody targeting TLR4 (#A11226) was purchased from ABclonal Biotech (Wuhan, China). The following antibodies were purchased from Cell Signaling Technology (Danvers, MA, USA): anti-β-actin (#3700), anti-GAPDH (#5174), horseradish peroxidase (HRP)-conjugated anti-rabbit IgG (#7076), HRP-conjugated anti-mouse IgG (#7072), Alexa Fluor 488-labeled donkey anti-rabbit IgG (#4412), Alexa Fluor 488-labeled donkey anti-mouse IgG (#4409), and DAPI (#4083). Scopolamine hydrobromide (#427039), Lipopolysaccharides (LPS, #8643), and other reagent-grade chemicals were purchased from Sigma-Aldrich (St. Louis, MO, USA) unless otherwise indicated.

Cell Culture and Development of Hyperosmolar Stress Model

Human SV40 immortalized corneal epithelial cell line [CRL-11135, human corneal epithelium (HCE2)] was purchased from ATCC (Manassas, VA, USA). HCE cells were cultured on culture dish in a humidified atmosphere of 5% carbon dioxide (CO_2) at 37°C. Then, 5 μg/ml insulin, 10 ng/ml human epidermal growth factor, 10% fetal bovine serum, 1% penicillin/streptomycin, and DMEM/F12 composed the culture medium. After adherence, HCE-2 cells were treated for iso- or hyperosmolar (312 or 500 mOsM, respectively) culture medium. The hyperosmolarity was implemented by adding 94 mM sodium chloride.

Cell Viability Assay

According to the protocol of manufacturer, CCK8 assay was used to detect cell viability. In brief, HCE cells were seeded in 96-well plates and exposed to a conditioned medium. After treatment, each well of the plates was added in 100 μl of a mixture of culture medium and CCK8 solution. The plate was incubated for 1–2 h in incubator (at 37°C and 5% CO_2) afterward. A microplate reader (BioTek Instruments, Winooski, VT, USA) was used to measure the absorbance at 450 nm.

Lactate Dehydrogenase Assay

Pierce^{TM} LDH Cytotoxicity Assay Kit (Thermo Scientific, #C20300) was applied to the measurement of lactate dehydrogenase (LDH) release. Briefly, HCE cells were cultured under a conditioned medium and equivoluminal of cell-free supernatant was added into a 96-well plate in triplicate. Then, LDH substrate mixture was added to each well and still standing at room temperature for 30 min. A microplate reader was used to evaluate the absorbance at 490 and 680 nm.

LDH release = $\frac{A_{490nm}\ of\ treated\ group - A_{680nm}\ of\ treated\ group}{A_{490nm}\ of\ control\ group - A_{680nm}\ of\ control\ group}$, where A is the absorbance.

ROS Measurement

The level of ROS was measured using a 2',7'-dichlorofluorescein diacetate (H2DCFDA) assay kit as described in our previous study (21). In brief, HCE cells were seeded in 6-well plates. After adherence, the culture medium was replaced by a conditioned medium. When confluent, the cells were rinsed and incubated with 10 μM of H2DCFDA at 37°C for 30–45 min. Subsequently, the reaction mixture was replaced by PBS. The fluorescence intensity was evaluated by flow cytometry (BD LSRFortessa™ cell analyzer, NJ, USA).

Mitochondrial Membrane Potential Assay

A TMRE-Mitochondrial Membrane Potential (MMP) Assay Kit (ab113852; Abcam) was used for MMP assay as described before (22). Briefly, after culture, cells were rinsed with PBS for 3 times and incubated with TMRE at 37°C for 15–30 min. Subsequently, the cells were resuspended with PBS and detected by flow cytometry.

RNA Interference

The HCECs were transfected using Lipofectamine™ RNAiMAX Transfection Reagent (Invitrogen, #13778150) with following siRNAs: siDUOX2, #1: sense, GGACAACAUAGUGGUUGA ATT, antisense, UUCAACCACUAUGUUGUCCTT; #2: sense, CAGUCAAUGUCUACAUCUUTT, antisense, AAGAUGUA GACAUUGACUGTT; #3: sense, CAAAUGCUGUGUAAGA AGATT; antisense, UCUUCUUACACAGCAUUUGTT; si-TLR4, #1: sense: GCAAUUUGACCAUUGAAGATT, antisense, UCUUCAAUG GUCAAAUUGCTT; #2: sense, CAUUGGAU ACGUUUCCUUATT, antisense, UAAGGAAACGUAUC CAAUGTT. #3: sense, GAAGUUGAACGAAUGGAAUTT, antisense, AUUCCAUUCGUUCAACUUCTT. Non-targeting scramble siRNA (si-NC) was applied as a negative control treatment. In brief, siRNA was dissolved in nuclease-free water to achieve a final concentration of 10 μM. Subsequently, siRNA and Lipofectamine RNAiMAX was added to Opti-MEM, respectively. Then, the solution of siRNA and Lipofectamine RNAiMAX was mixed. The mixture was maintained at room temperature for 5 min to form total complexed. After that, the mixture was added to the culture dish equally. The medium was replaced after 24 h.

Western Blot Analysis

The cells total protein was extracted by the Minute Total Protein Extraction Kit (Invent Biotechnologies, MN, USA, #SD001). The Bicinchoninic Acid (BCA) Protein Assay Kit (Millipore, Billerica, MA, USA) was used to measure the total protein concentration. Then, equal amounts of protein samples were loaded onto sodium dodecyl sulfate-polyacrylamide gels and electrophoresed. The separated proteins in the gels were transferred to polyvinylidene fluoride membranes (Millipore, Bedford, MA, USA). After blocking the membranes with 5% non-fat milk in Tris-buffered saline with Tween-20 for 1–2 h at room temperature, the membranes were incubated with the appropriate primary antibodies overnight. After the membranes were rinsed thoroughly, they were further incubated with secondary antibodies for 1 h at room temperature. The blots were visualized using an enhanced chemiluminescence (ECL) kit according to the instructions of manufacturer. Western-blot gray scale results were used to semiquantitative analysis by using Image J software (NIH, MD, USA).

Establishment of RNA Sequence Library and Data Processing

RNA extraction was performed according to the protocol of manufacturer by an RNeasy Plus Mini Kit (Qiagen, Valencia, CA, USA). The RNA sequence (RNA-seq) libraries were constructed with a TruSeq Stranded mRNA Library Prep kit (Illumina, CA, USA, #20020594) and sequenced on Illumina PE150 sequencers. Sequencing reads were mapped to hg19 using Star. Transcripts Per Million (TPM) values were called using RNA-Seq by Expectation-Maximization (RSEM). Differential gene expression was determined using DESeq2 and defined at $\log_2$-fold change >1 as well as $p < 0.01$.

Quantitative Real-Time PCR (QPCR)

Total RNA from HCECs or intact corneas were extracted by an RNeasy Plus Mini Kit (Qiagen, Valencia, CA, USA) according to the instructions of manufacturer. Total RNA was quantified with a spectrophotometer (NanoDrop ND-1000; Thermo Fisher Scientific, Waltham, MA, USA). After synthesized with the PrimeScript RT Master Mix (TaKaRa, Japan), the cDNA was amplified with SYBR Green Supermix (Bio-Rad Laboratories, Inc., CA, USA) using the Light Cycler 480 Real-Time PCR System and designed primers. Glyceraldehyde-3-phosphate dehydrogenase (GAPDH) served as an internal reference gene. The following sequences of the primers were used: DUOX2: Forward, 5′-CTGGGTCCATCGGGCAATC-3′, Reverse, 5′- GT CGGCGTAATTGGCTGGTA 3′; TLR4: Forward, 5′-AGACCT GTCCCTGAACCCTAT-3′, Reverse, 5′-CGATGGACTTCTAA ACCAGCCA-3′; HMGB1: Forward, 5′-TATGGCAAAAGCGG ACAAGG-3′, Reverse, 5′-CTTCGCAACATCACCAATGGA-3′; IL-1β: Forward, 5′-CCTGGAGAGAGCTCGGACT-3′, Reverse, 5′-TGTGTGCCAACCTGATGCAG-3′; IL18: Forward, 5′-TC TTCATTGACCAAGGAAATCGG-3′, Reverse, 5′-TCCGGGGT GCATTATCTCTAC-3′; NLRP3: Forward, 5′-GATCTTCGCT GCGATCAACAG-3′, Reverse, 5′-CGTGCATTATCTGAACCC CAC-3′; CASPASE1: Forward, 5′-TTTCCGCAAGGTTCGATT TTCA-3′, Reverse, 5′-GGCATCTGCGCTCTACCATC-3′; ASC: Forward, 5′-TGGATGCTCTGTACGGGAAG-3′, Reverse, 5′-CCAGGCTGGTGTGAAACTGAA-3′; TNF-α: Forward, 5′-CC TGGAGAGAGCTCGGACT-3′, Reverse: 5′-TGTGTGCCAACC TGATGCAG-3′; NF-κB: Forward, 5′-AACAGAGAGGATTTCG TTTCCG-3′, Reverse, 5′-TTTGACCTGAGGGTAAGACTTCT-3′; GAPDH: Forward, 5′-CTCATGACCACAGTCCATGC-3′, Reverse, 5′-TTCAGCTCTGGGATGACCTT-3′.

Immunofluorescence Staining

For cells immunofluorescence staining, HCECs were grown in 24-well-plates containing a glass sheet in each well. After different treatments, the cells were washed with PBS, fixed with 4% paraformaldehyde for 10 min, blocked with 3% BSA which contain 0.3% Triton X-100 for 1 h, and then, incubated overnight at 4°C with the primary antibodies. After washing, the cells were incubated for 1.5 h with secondary antibody. Images were observed with a confocal fluorescence microscope (LEICA DMi8, Germany).

For corneal immunofluorescence staining, mice were killed, and the eyeballs were excised. After fixed and embedded in paraffin, the eyeballs were sectioned. Slices were dewaxed by dimethylbenzene and then suffered high pressure for antigen retrieval. The remaining steps were performed as previously described in cells immunofluorescence staining.

Animal Model and Treatment

A total of 20 female C57BL/6j mice aged 6–8 weeks were purchased from Beijing Vital River Laboratory Animal Technology Co. Ltd (Beijing, China). The mice of dry eye model were maintained in an environmentally controlled room that was maintained at ≤30% humidity and were exposed to a continuous air draft created by fans. The mice were given subcutaneous scopolamine hydrobromide (1.5 mg/0.3 ml; Sigma-Aldrich) injections three times per day for 5 consecutive days, as previously described (9). Control mice matched for age and sex were maintained at environment of 50–75% relative humidity. All animal experiments complied with the Association for Research in Vision and Ophthalmology Statement for the Use of Animals in Ophthalmic and Vision Research and were approved by the Ethics Committee of Zhongshan Ophthalmic Center, Sun Yat-Sen University (Guangzhou, China; approval ID: 2020-138).

Sodium Fluorescein Staining of the Corneal Epithelium

Sodium fluorescein was administered to the inferior lateral conjunctival sac to evaluate the degree of corneal epithelial defects in the mice. The corneal epithelial images were acquired using a cobalt blue filter under a slit-lamp microscope image system (SL-D7/DC-3/MAGENet; Topcon, Tokyo, Japan) by two independent technicians. The quantification of corneal defects was carried out by Image J software. The covering area of corneal defects (%) = (fluorescein sodium positive area/the whole cornea) × 100%.

Statistical Analysis

All data are expressed as the mean ± SD. Statistical analyses were performed using GraphPad Prism. Student's *t*-test was used to compare differences between groups. One- or two-way ANOVA followed by Bonferroni's *post-hoc* test was used for comparisons among three or more groups. The $p < 0.05$ was considered to indicate statistical significance.

RESULT

DUOX2 Expression Is Increased in DED

Previous studies reported that excessive oxidative stress could lead to damage in HCE cell and contribute to DED development (23). Therefore, to further explore the key regulator of oxidative pathways in DED, we first carried out RNA-seq analysis in corneal epithelial cells exposed to hyperosmolarity. Our Gene Ontology (GO) analysis suggested that hyperosmolarity activated the regulation of body fluid levels, metal ion transporter activity, regulation of cellular component movement, and cellular response to hypoxia in HCE cells. Interestingly, we consistently found that there was a significant activated regulation of ROS metabolic process (**Figure 1A**). Moreover, in the detailed gene list, we discovered several oxidative-related regulators, such as DUOX2, YPEL2, and HSPA2, were greatly upregulated under hyperosmolarity comparing with the control group. Among them, the increase of DUOX2 was the most remarkably and stable during repeated experiment and then we chose DUOX2 for further investigation (**Figure 1B**). Moreover, we assessed the relative protein expression levels of DUOX2 using western blot, our results thereby confirmed an elevation of DUOX2 in HCE cells since 12 h after treatment of hyperosmolar stress (**Figure 1C**). In addition, immunofluorescence suggested a significant accumulation of DUOX2 after hyperosmolar treatment (**Figure 1D**). Then, to evaluate the change of DUOX2 *in vivo*, we used our established DED mouse model, which showed reduced tear aqueous secretion and significant decrease in the number of PAS-stained goblet cells in the conjunctiva (9). Consistently, we revealed DUOX2 was greatly increased within corneal epithelium in DED (**Figure 1E**). Taken together, our data here showed induction of DUOX2 in DED both *in vitro* and *in vivo*.

TLR4 Is Essential for DUOX2 Activation Under Hyperosmolarity

As several published papers have reported that induction of DUOX2 could be triggered *via* TLR4, which is a main modulator in cellular homeostasis (13). In our current study, RT-PCR and western blot showed that the expression of TLR4 was increased in HCE cells under hyperosmolarity (**Figures 2A,B**). Furthermore, immunofluorescence suggested that TLR4 was significantly activated in DED cell and mouse model (**Figures 2C,D**). Therefore, to test the crosstalk of TLR4 upon DUOX2, we tried to ablate TLR4 expression in HCE cells. After application of RNA interference system, in which control siRNA or three distinct human-specific siRNAs targeting different domains of TLR4 were transiently transfected into HCE cells. After 24 h following transfection, RT-PCR displayed that TLR4 siRNA knockdown TLR4 expression with high efficiency (**Supplementary Figure 1**). Interestingly, our data discovered that ablation of TLR4 was sufficient to suppress the increase of DUOX2 in HCE cells exposed to normal culture medium as well as hyperosmolarity, whereas control siRNAs had no inhibitory effects (**Figures 2E,F**). In contrary, we applied inducer of TLR4, LPS (1 μg/ml) to treated HCE cell. RT-PCR showed LPS could promote ~3-fold over the levels of DUOX2 in HCE cells comparing with the control group (**Supplementary Figure 2**). Together, our results indicated that TLR4 is necessary for synergistic increase of DUOX2 in DED.

Induction of DUOX2 Increases Oxidative Stress in HCE Cells

Considering the potential consequences of DUOX2 upon oxidative stress, we examined the time course of cellular ROS accumulation in DED. In response to hyperosmolar

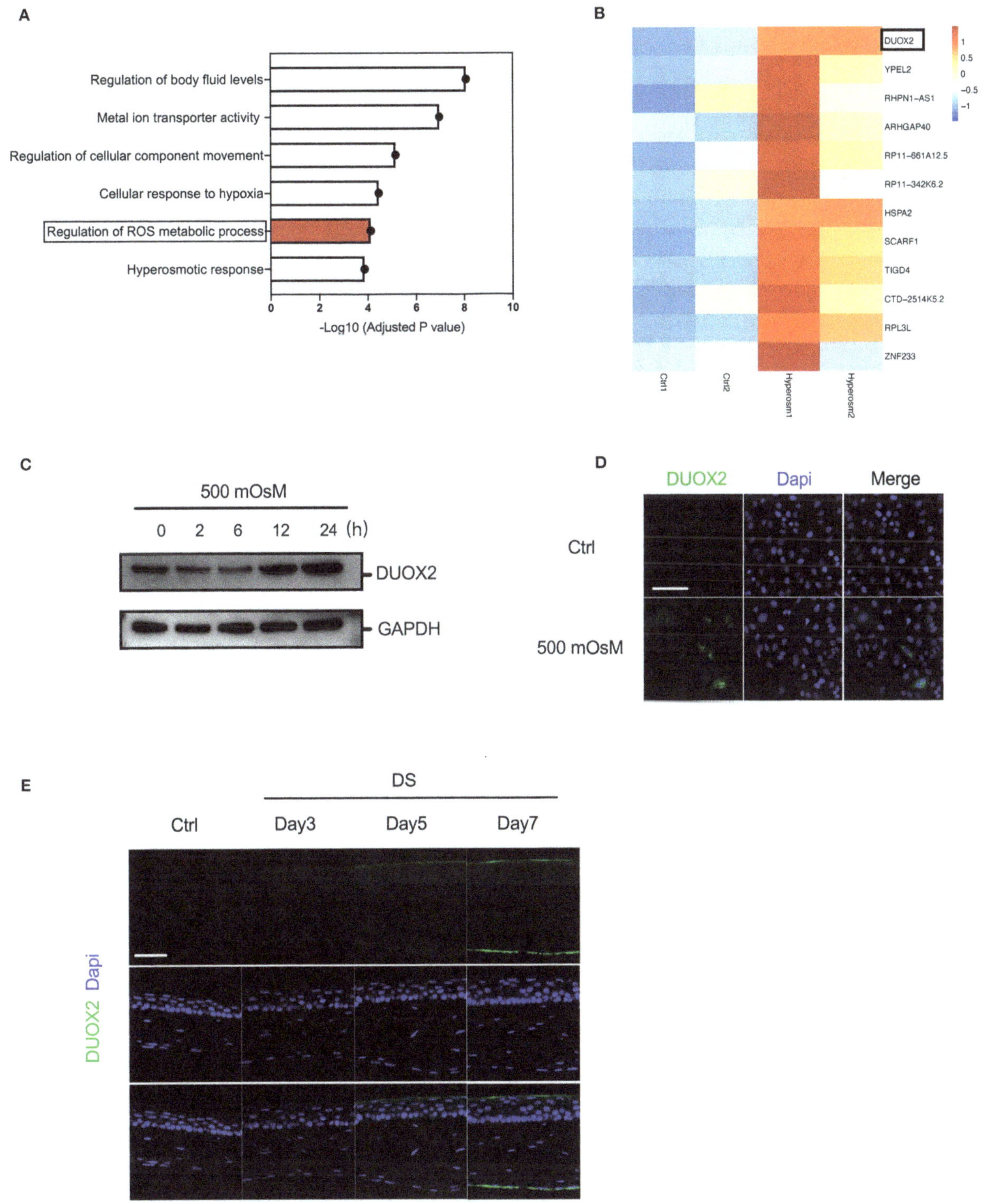

FIGURE 1 | Activation of dual oxidase 2 (DUOX2) in dry eye disease (DED). **(A,B)** RNA sequencing (RNA-seq) from human corneal epithelial cells (HCECs) treated with/without hyperosmolar stress (500 mOsM) for 24 h showed differentially expressed genes related to oxidative stress. Biological process terms overexpressed for the oxidative-related genes identified in hyperosmolar stress. Top overexpressed Gene Ontology (GO) terms according to their fold-enrichment are depicted **(A)**. Heatmap showed the fold change of oxidative-related genes in control (Ctrl) and hyperosmolarity (Hyperosm) groups **(B)**. (Two samples from each group) **(C,D)** Western blot and immunofluorescence showing the changes of DUOX2 expression in human corneal epithelial (HCE) cells exposed to hyperosmotic medium (500 mOsM) relative to that in normal medium over time. **(E)** Immunofluorescence results showing the changes in DUOX2 expression in the corneal epithelium of desiccation stress (DS) mice relative to those in untreated (UT) mice after 3, 5, and 7 days and 5 mice were included in each group. Scale bar = 100 μm. The data shown are representative of two or more independent experiments.

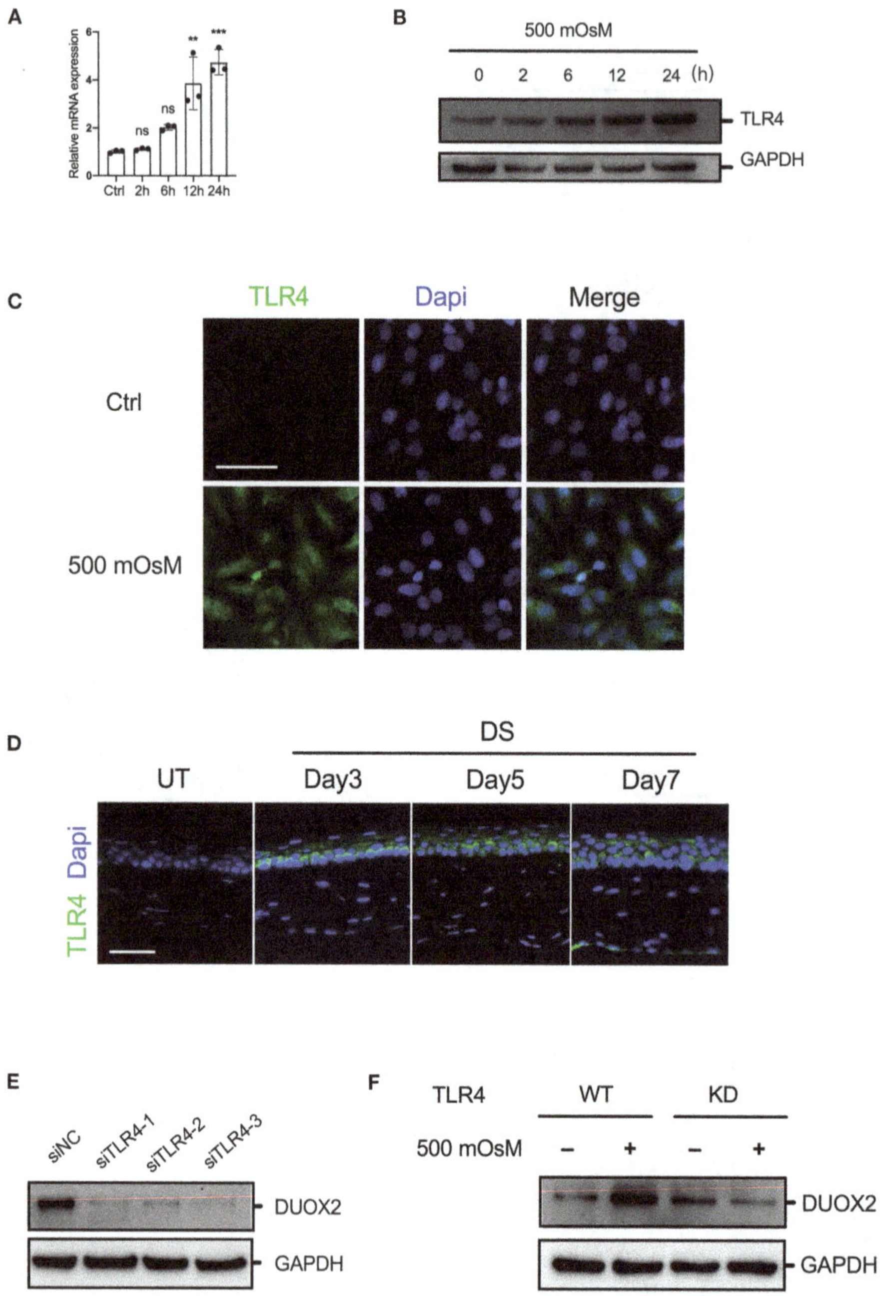

FIGURE 2 | TLR4 is essential for DUOX2 activation under hyperosmolarity. **(A,B)** Human corneal epithelial cells were treated by hyperosmolarity (500 mOsM) for indicated time. The expression of TLR4 was determined by RT-PCR and western blotting. **(C)** Representative fluorescence images showing the increased expression of TLR4 in HCE cells exposed to 500 mOsM or normal medium (Ctrl) after 6 h. **(D)** Immunofluorescence results showing the changes of TLR4 in the corneal epithelium of DS mice relative to those in UT mice after 3, 5, and 7 days and 5 mice were included in each group. **(E)** HCE cells were transfected with different siRNAs targeted to TLR4 or negative control (siNC) for 24 h. The expression of DUOX2 was determined by western blot. **(F)** Wild-type (WT) and TLR4-knockdown (KD) HCECs were exposed to hyperosmotic medium (500 mOsM) or normal medium (Ctrl) for 24 h. Expression levels of DUOX2 were measured by western blot assay. Scale bar = 100 μm. The data shown are representative of two or more independent experiments (mean ± SD). $^{**}p < 0.01$ and $^{***}p < 0.001$ vs. untreated controls.

culture medium, the ROS production of HCE cells steadily increased over time (**Figure 3A**). We next measured that when DUOX2 was knockdown in HCE cells, the ROS level was changed to a much lesser degree under hyperosmolar challenge (**Figures 3B,C**). In addition, we observed remarkable mitochondrial dysfunction under hyperosmolar condition, which was detected *via* decreased MMP level. Surprisingly, these decreases were profoundly reversed by DUOX2 ablation

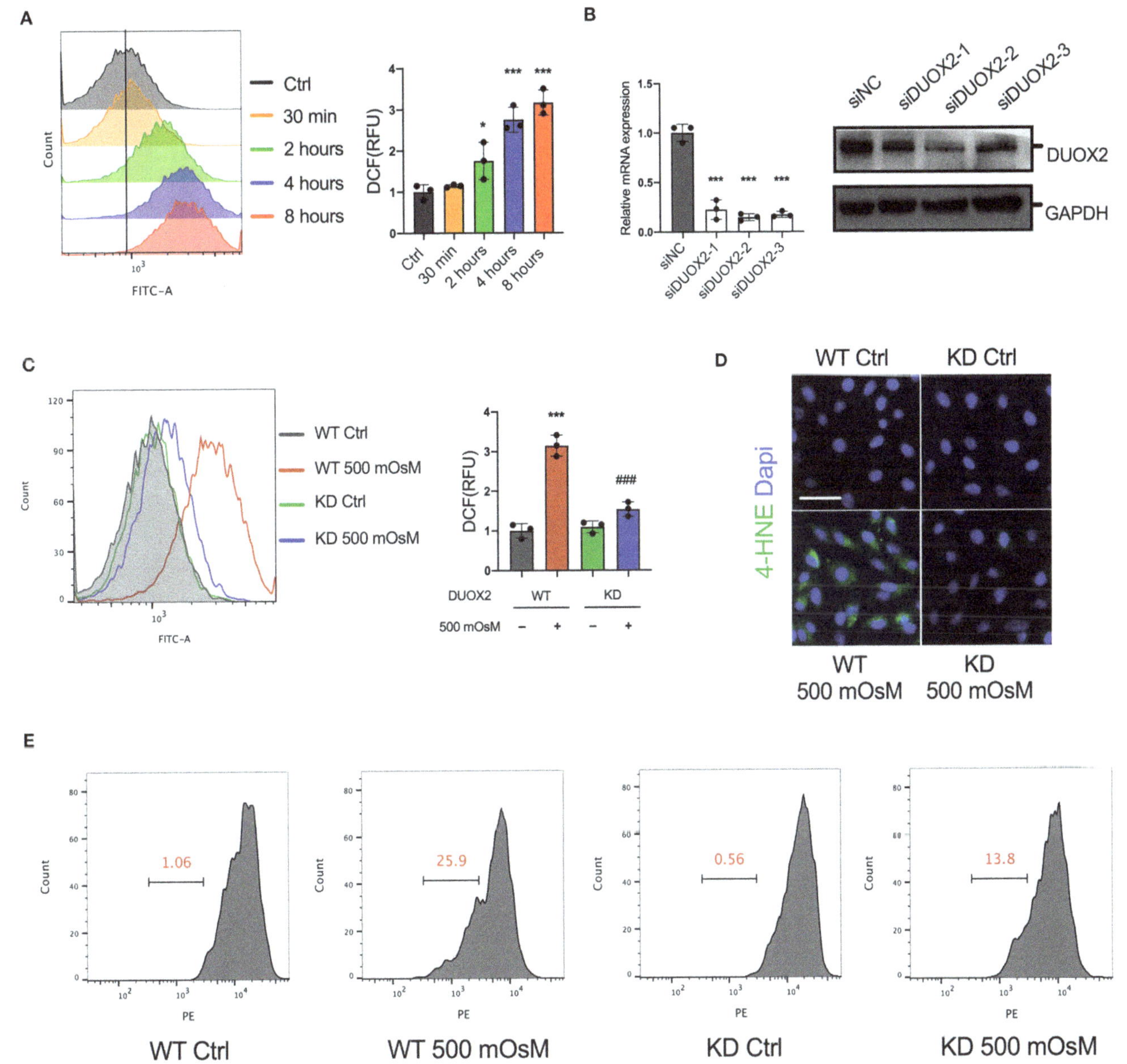

FIGURE 3 | Elevation of DUOX2 triggers oxidative stress in HCE cells. **(A)** Reactive oxygen species (ROS) levels were measured in HCE cells exposed to normal medium (Ctrl) or hyperosmotic medium (500 mOsM) for the indicated times by 2′,7′-dichlorofluorescein diacetate (H2DCFDA) using flow cytometry. Right: relative fluorescence units (RFUs) were monitored. **(B)** HCE cells were transfected with different siRNAs targeted to DUOX2 or negative control (siNC) for 24 h. The expression of DUOX2 was examined by RT-PCR and western blot. Wild-type (WT) and DUOX2-knockdown (KD) HCE cells were exposed to hyperosmotic medium (500 mOsM) or normal medium (Ctrl) for 6 h. **(C)** ROS levels were measured by flow cytometry. Right: RFUs were monitored. **(D)** Representative fluorescence images showing the change of 4-hydroxynonenal (4-HNE). **(E)** Mitochondrial membrane potential (MMP) was evaluated by TMRE staining using flow cytometry. Scale bar = 100 μm. The data shown are representative of three or more independent experiments (mean ± SD). $^{*}p < 0.05$ and $^{***}p < 0.001$ vs. untreated controls; $^{\#\#\#}p < 0.001$ vs. 500 mOsM(+) DDIT4 KD(−).

(**Figure 3E**). Additionally, 4-hydroxynonenal (4-HNE) was considered as a potential mechanism by which ROS can inflict cellular damage within peroxidation cycle. We next observed a great reduction of 4-HNE expression in DUOX2-KD HCE cells exposed to hyperosmolarity comparing with wild type group (**Figure 3D**). To further investigate whether the increase of DUOX2 participated in cell fate decision in DED, we used CCK8 and LDH assay (**Figures 4A,B**). Our results turned out to find that inhibition of DUOX2 could significantly protect cell viability (**Figures 4C,D**). Moreover, this protective effect was consistently confirmed by declining PI positive cells in DUOX2-KD as well as an established ROS inhibitor N-acetylcysteine (NAC) treated HCE cells, respectively (**Figure 4E**). Therefore, our experiments implied here that induction of DUOX2 in

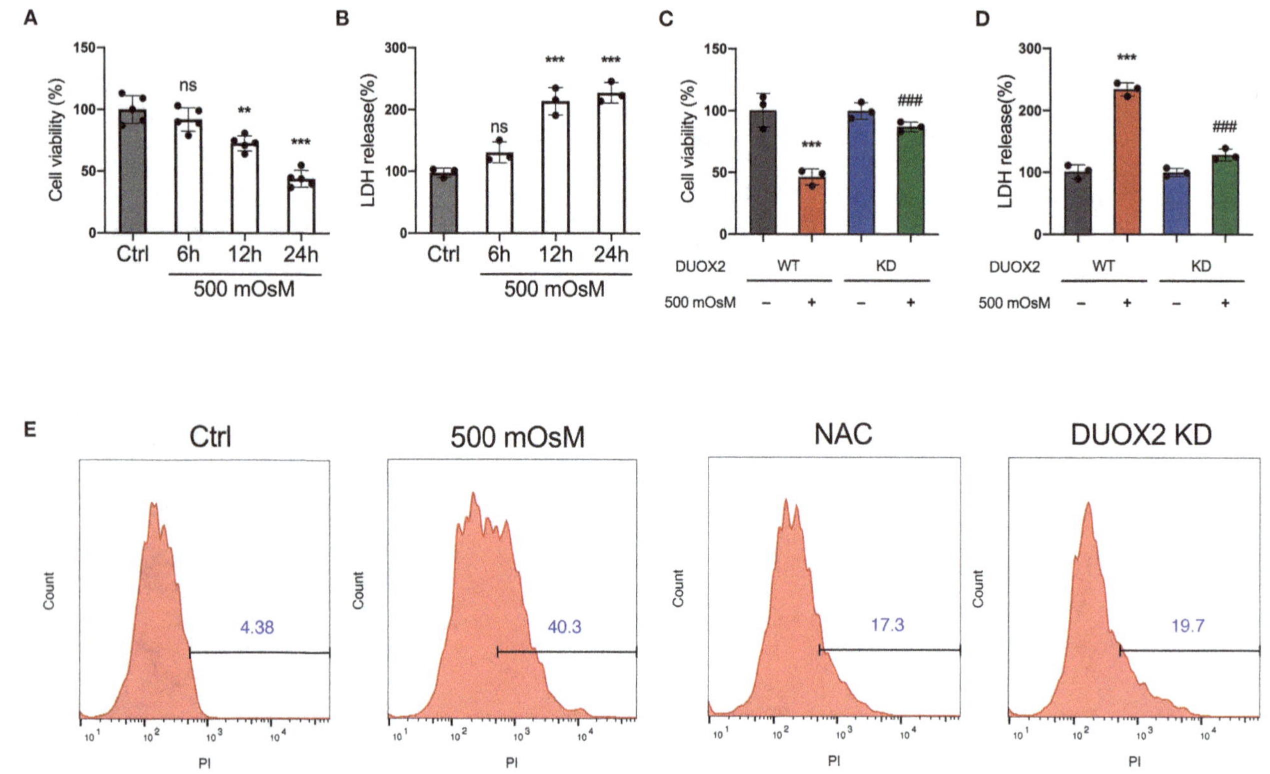

FIGURE 4 | Ablation of DUOX2 inhibits hyperosmolarity-induced cell death. HCE cells were treated with 500 mOsM or normal culture medium (Ctrl) for 6, 12, and 24 h. **(A)** Changes in cell viability were determined by Cell Counting Kit-8 (CCK8) assay. **(B)** Changes in LDH levels were monitored by LDH assay. HCE cells were transfected with control siRNA (WT) or DUOX2 siRNA (KD) for 24 h and then treated with 500 mOsM or normal culture medium (ctrl) for 24 h. **(C)** Changes in cell viability were determined by CCK8 assay. **(D)** Changes in lactate dehydrogenase (LDH) levels were monitored by LDH assay. **(E)** HCE cells were transfected with DUOX2 siRNA (DUOX2 KD) for 24 h and cultured in hyperosmotic medium (500 mOsM) for 18 h. Control siRNA transfected HCE cells were exposed to 500 mOsM and co-treated with N-acetylcysteine (NAC) or left untreated (Ctrl). Positive percentage of propidium iodide (PI) staining was monitored by flow cytometry. The data shown are representative of three or more independent experiments (mean ± SD). $^{**}p < 0.01$ and $^{***}p < 0.001$ vs. untreated controls; $^{\#\#\#}p < 0.001$ vs. 500 mOsM(+) DUOX2 KD(−).

DED had potential damage toward HCE cells through excessive oxidative stress.

DUOX2 Promotes Translocation of HMGB1 and Aggregates Inflammation

Multiple cellular mechanisms known to regulate cell death through releasing and translocation of HMGB1 (24). To assess whether DUOX2 actively contributes to the change of HMGB1 in HCE cells, we first evaluate HMGB1 expression in DED. Surprisingly, RT-PCR found there was no obvious increase of HMGB1 in DED (**Supplementary Figure 3**). However, our immunostaining results showed that hyperosmolar treatment could cause obvious leakage of HMGB1 from the nucleus to the cytoplasm in HCE cells. By contrast, after knockdown of DUOX2, this translocation was effectively prevented. Considering that the elevation of oxidative stress could be responsible for HMGB1 translocation. We revealed ROS scavenger NAC was able to prohibit HMGB1 moving into cytoplasm (**Figure 5A**). Furthermore, HMGB1 is a chromatin-binding protein that could function as pro-inflammatory cytokines when released into extracellular space, we then explored the impacts of DUOX2-HMGB1 axis on inflammation pathways. Notably, we discovered that the mRNA expression levels of NOD-, LRR- and pyrin domain-containing 3 (NLRP3), interleukin-1β (IL-1β interleukin-18 (IL-18) in HCE cells were significantly attenuated after DUOX2 inhibition (**Figure 5B**). Collectively, we indicated that DUOX2 has potent regulatory effects upon cell death *via* enhancing translocation of HMGB1 and promotes ocular surface inflammation in DED.

DISCUSSION

Although DED is still one of the most common chronic ocular surface diseases, the specific underlying mechanism of pathogenesis remains to be clearly elucidated. Recently, a variety of studies have suggested that ocular surface oxidative stress is involved in the DED development (25, 26). In the present study, we discover that TLR4-mediated DUOX2 increase as a key regulator among oxidant pathways in DED. Furthermore, DUOX2 promotes cell death and inflammation activation through the enhancing of HMGB1 translocation.

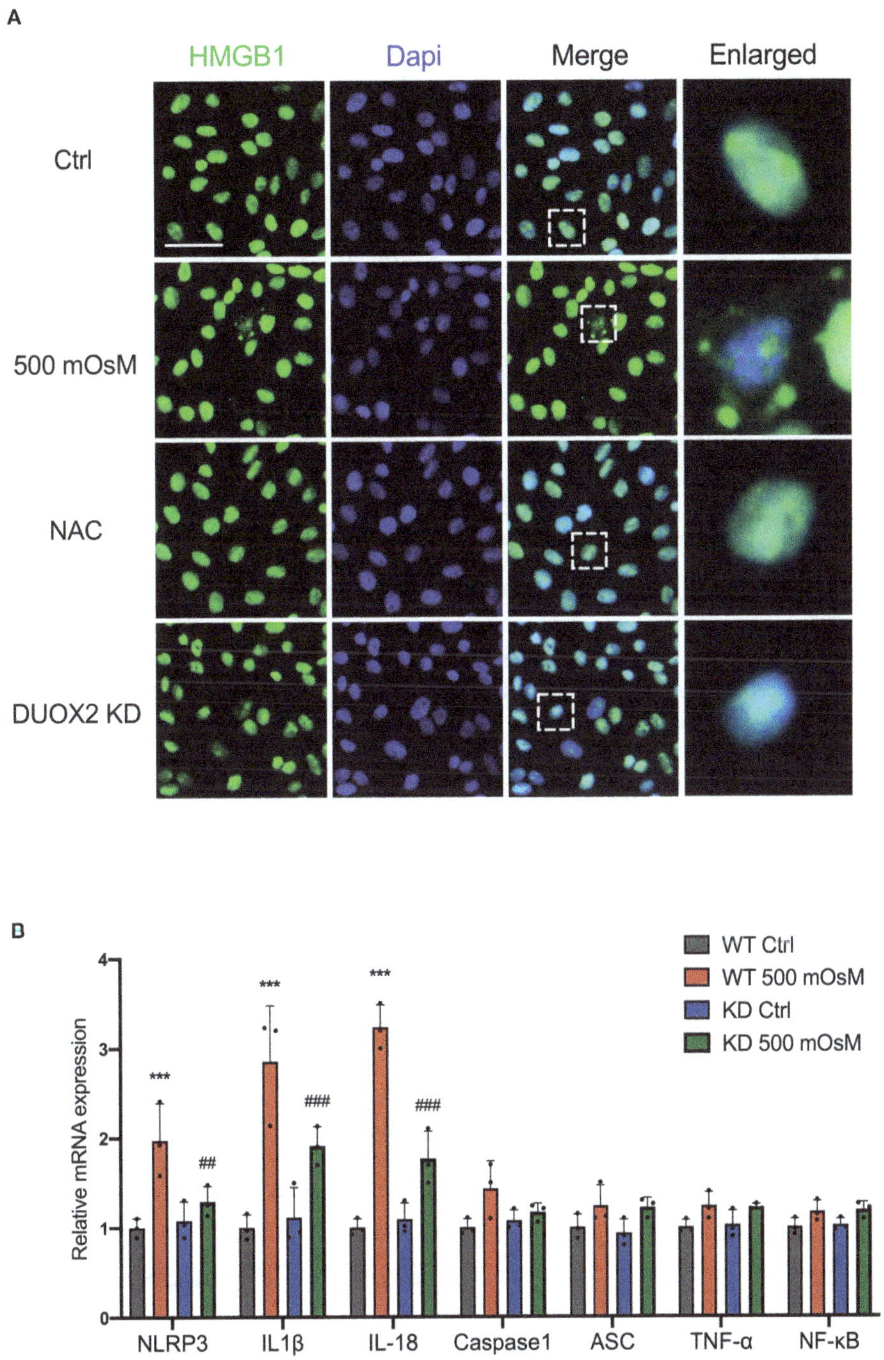

FIGURE 5 | DUOX2-related oxidative pathway promotes translocation of high mobility group box 1 (HMGB1) and aggregates inflammation. **(A)** HCE cells were transfected with DUOX2 siRNA (DUOX2 KD) for 24 hours and cultured in hyperosmotic medium (500 mOsM) for 18 hours. Control siRNA transfected HCE cells were exposed to 500 mOsM and co-treated with NAC or left untreated (Ctrl). Representative fluorescence images showing the translocation of HMGB1. **(B)** HCE cells were transfected with control siRNA (WT) or DUOX2 siRNA (KD) for 24 hours and then treated with 500 mOsM or normal culture medium (Ctrl) for 24 hours. The mRNA changes of representative inflammation pathway were detected by RT-PCR. Scale bar = 100 μm. The data shown are representative of three or more independent experiments (mean ± SD). $^{***}p < 0.001$ vs. untreated controls; $^{\#\#}p < 0.01$, $^{\#\#\#}p < 0.001$ vs. 500 mOsM(+) DUOX2 KD(−).

In previous study, we demonstrated that inhibition of ROS could alleviate cell death in HCE cells (9). Using RNA-seq, we further screened and found that DUOX2 was highly expressed among oxidant pathways in HCE cells under hyperosmolarity. Moreover, this was further supported by immunofluorescence in our DED mouse model. However, the specific trigger DUOX2 in DED has not been investigated. It has been observed that corneal epithelial cells expressing TLRs are capable of signal transduction through TLR-related pathways, which previously recognized to be an exclusive characteristic of immune cells (27, 28). Interestingly, researchers recently revealed that ablated TLR4 signaling in HCE cells significantly decreased the development of ROS production and cell death (29, 30). Therefore, these results encourage our evaluation of TLR4 activation on the formation of DUOX2 in DED. As expected, the requirement for upregulation of TLR4-related signaling in the control of DUOX2 expression by hyperosmolarity was substantiated by the RNA interference studies. We noticed that siRNAs targeting different sites on TLR4 not only decreased TLR4 expression but also greatly inhibited DUOX2 expression at the RNA level, as well as the expression of DUOX2 protein. On the other hand, a well-established TLR4 inducer, LPS was able to prompt DUOX2 expression. We then confirm that induction of DUOX2 requires TLR4-mediated signaling, which provides new clues for DUOX2 regulatory network in ocular surface diseases. It is worth noting that GO analysis indicated fluid regulation and metal transportation were upregulated in HCE cells under hyperosmolarity. We assumed that future studies are needed to clarify the pathological connection between DUOX2 oxidative signaling and these biological procedures in dry eye development.

Interestingly, DUOX2 has been reported to play a critical role in host defense system, especially during chronic inflammatory conditions (10). In addition, it is reported that increase of DUOX2 could directly mediate the production of ROS, therefore accelerate development of gastrointestinal and respiratory diseases and cancer (31, 32). Our latest study discovered that a proper level of ROS was necessary for cell homeostasis maintenance, which could become important therapeutic strategy in DED treatment (33). In this research, we consistently discovered DUOX2 overexpression accompanied by excessive ROS production. Moreover, after inhibition of DUOX2, ROS release could be greatly abolished. DUOX2 knockdown could rescue the decrease of MMP, which is necessary to maintain normal mitochondrial function. These findings strongly suggest that a DUOX2-ROS axis exists in DED. Considering that the uncontrolled ROS release has been frequently combined with impaired cell function and cell death (34). We then found that DUOX2 ablation was able to protect cell viability and inhibit PI-positive cells under hyperosmolarity. Admittedly, more animal studies of DUOX2 knockout are necessary to further clarify the specific effect of DUOX2 in DED. Nevertheless, this present study provides new insight into potential DUOX2-based agents for future DED precision treatment. Moreover, based on our current database of RNA-seq, our results suggested that other oxidative-related genes, such as YPEL2 and HSPA2 could become promising treatment targets in dry eye after systematic *in vitro* and *in vivo* studies.

Notably, previous *in vitro* DED studies have suggested the co-existence of apoptosis and necrosis in oxidant-induced HCE injury (35, 36). In this study, we performed LDH analysis and revealed LDH release was strongly increased after hyperosmolar treatment, which could be decreased sharply in DUOX2 knockdown group. Hence, we indicated that DUOX2 might participate in the necrosis process of HCE cells in DED. Several observations demonstrate that abnormal release HMGB1 is highly pathogenic in the context of necrosis (37, 38). Indeed, our results suggested that although there was no obvious increase of HMGB1 in mRNA level, hyperosmolar stimulus could lead to the translocation of HMGB1 from the nucleus to the cytoplasm in HCE cells. Importantly, ablation of DUOX2 could function to stop this trend. Furthermore, it has been shown that HMGB1 can exhibit proinflammatory role during ocular surface damage and dry eye-related inflammation *via* interacting with soluble PAMPs and binding to TLRs (39). Our data further evaluated that DUOX2 inhibition attenuated upregulation of NLRP3, IL-1β, and IL-18. By contrast, a latest study suggested that the release of HMGB1 did not mediate DED-related inflammation in the corneal epithelium by directly inducing inflammatory cytokine production (40). Based on our data, we suppose that the proinflammatory role of HMGB1 within the corneal epithelium could be dependent on other alarmins or inflammatory molecules derived from cell disruption. Chen et al. indicated that GSDMD-dependent pyroptosis, as one of the programmed cell necrosis, is pivotal for subsequent amplification of inflammatory cascades in DED (41). Further studies are needed to precisely determine the role of HMGB1 within interactions between specific mode of cell death and ocular surface inflammation.

Taken together, our work showed that corneal epithelial expression of DUOX2 was remarkably elevated in DED both *in vitro* and *in vivo*. Moreover, we implicated that TLR4 activation was necessary to enhance DUOX2 transcription. When DUOX2 was blocked in HCE cells, excessive ROS production and damaged mitochondrial function were greatly reversed. Lastly, our results suggested that the cytoprotective function of DUOX2 inhibition might rely on abolished HMGB1 translocation, which further prevented ocular surface inflammation. Consequently, this research for the first time provided the evidence that DUOX2 could be a key regulatory factor in DED and further elaborate the pathogenetic mechanisms. Admittedly, further work is required to identify safe and effective ways to target this novel pathway, which is a critical step in developing future DED therapies.

ETHICS STATEMENT

The animal study was reviewed and approved by Ethics Committee of Zhongshan Ophthalmic Center, Sun Yat-sen University.

AUTHOR CONTRIBUTIONS

BW and HZ performed the experiments, analyzed the data, and wrote the manuscript. XZ, XY, XW, and DH performed the experiments and interpreted the results. JY designed the study and reviewed and revised the paper. All authors contributed to the article and approved the submitted version.

REFERENCES

1. Stapleton F, Alves M, Bunya VY, Jalbert I, Lekhanont K, Malet F, et al. TFOS DEWS II epidemiology report. *Ocul Surf.* (2017) 15:334–65. doi: 10.1016/j.jtos.2017.05.003
2. Clayton JA. Dry Eye. *N Engl J Med.* (2018) 378:2212–23. doi: 10.1056/NEJMra1407936
3. Bron AJ, de Paiva CS, Chauhan SK, Bonini S, Gabison EE, Jain S, et al. TFOS DEWS II pathophysiology report. *Ocul Surf.* (2017) 15:438–510. doi: 10.1016/j.jtos.2017.05.011
4. Elbasiony E, Mittal SK, Foulsham W, Cho W, Chauhan SK. Epithelium-derived IL-33 activates mast cells to initiate neutrophil recruitment following corneal injury. *Ocul Surf.* (2020) 18:633–40. doi: 10.1016/j.jtos.2020.06.006
5. Lee HS, Han S, Seo JW, Jeon KJ. Exposure to traffic-related particulate matter 2.5 triggers th2-dominant ocular immune response in a murine model. *Int J Environ Res Public Health.* (2020) 17:2965. doi: 10.3390/ijerph17082965
6. Dogru M, Kojima T, Simsek C, Tsubota K. Potential role of oxidative stress in ocular surface inflammation and dry eye disease. *Inv Ophthalmol Visual Sci.* (2018) 59:DES163–8. doi: 10.1167/iovs.17-23402
7. Seen S, Tong L. Dry eye disease and oxidative stress. *Acta Ophthalmol.* (2018) 96:e412–20. doi: 10.1111/aos.13526
8. Huo Y, Chen W, Zheng X, Zhao J, Zhang Q, Hou Y, et al. The protective effect of EGF-activated ROS in human corneal epithelial cells by inducing mitochondrial autophagy via activation TRPM2. *J Cell Physiol.* (2020) 235:7018–29. doi: 10.1002/jcp.29597
9. Wang B, Peng L, Ouyang H, Wang L, He D, Zhong J, et al. Induction of DDIT4 impairs autophagy through oxidative stress in dry eye. *Inv Ophthalmol Visual Sci.* (2019) 60:2836–47. doi: 10.1167/iovs.19-27072
10. Bedard K, Krause KH. The NOX family of ROS-generating NADPH oxidases: physiology and pathophysiology. *Physiol Rev.* (2007) 87:245–313. doi: 10.1152/physrev.00044.2005
11. Grasberger H, Magis AT, Sheng E, Conomos MP, Zhang M, Garzotto LS, et al. DUOX2 variants associate with preclinical disturbances in microbiota immune homeostasis and increased inflammatory bowel disease risk. *J Clin Invest.* (2021) 13:e141676. doi: 10.1172/JCI141676
12. Geiszt M, Witta J, Baffi J, Lekstrom K, Leto TL. Dual oxidases represent novel hydrogen peroxide sources supporting mucosal surface host defense. *FASEB J.* (2003) 17:1502–4. doi: 10.1096/fj.02-1104fje
13. Burgueno JF, Fritsch J, Gonzalez EE, Landau KS, Santander AM, Fernandez I, et al. Epithelial TLR4 signaling activates DUOX2 to induce microbiota-driven tumorigenesis. *Gastroenterology.* (2021) 160:797–808 e6. doi: 10.1053/j.gastro.2020.10.031
14. Kim HJ, Seo YH, An S, Jo A, Kwon IC, Kim S. Chemiluminescence imaging of Duox2-derived hydrogen peroxide for longitudinal visualization of biological response to viral infection in nasal mucosa. *Theranostics.* (2018) 8:1798–807. doi: 10.7150/thno.22481
15. van der Vliet A, Danyal K, Heppner DE. Dual oxidase: a novel therapeutic target in allergic disease. *Br J Pharmacol.* (2018) 175:1401–18. doi: 10.1111/bph.14158
16. Lotze MT, Tracey KJ. High-mobility group box 1 protein (HMGB1): nuclear weapon in the immune arsenal. *Nat Rev Immunol.* (2005) 5:331–42. doi: 10.1038/nri1594
17. Wang S, Zhang Y. HMGB1 in inflammation and cancer. *J Hematol Oncol.* (2020) 13:116. doi: 10.1186/s13045-020-00950-x
18. Bianchi ME, Crippa MP, Manfredi AA, Mezzapelle R, Rovere Querini P, Venereau E. High-mobility group box 1 protein orchestrates responses t tissue damage via inflammation, innate and adaptive immunity, and tissue repair. *Immunol Rev.* (2017) 280:74–82. doi: 10.1111/imr.12601
19. Deng M, Tang Y, Li W, Wang X, Zhang R, Zhang X, et al. The endotox delivery protein HMGB1 mediates caspase-11-dependent lethality in sepsis. *Immunity.* (2018) 49:740–53 e7. doi: 10.1016/j.immuni.2018.08.016
20. Zhang S, Hu L, Jiang J, Li H, Wu Q, Ooi K, et al. HMGB1/RAGE axis mediates stress-induced RVLM neuroinflammation in mice via impairing mitophagy flux in microglia. *J Neuro.* (2020) 17:15. doi: 10.1186/s12974-019-1673-3
21. Wang B, Wang L, Gu S, Yu Y, Huang H, Mo K, et al. D609 protects retinal pigmented epithelium as a potential therapy for age-related macular degeneration. *Signal Transduct Target Ther.* (2020) 5:20. doi: 10.1038/s41392-020-0122-1 in
22. Troiano L, Ferraresi R, Lugli E, Nemes E, Roat E, Nasi M, et al. Multiparametric analysis of cells with different mitochondrial membrane potential during apoptosis by polychromatic flow cytometry. *Nat Protoc.* (2007) 2:2719–27. doi: 10.1038/nprot.2007.405
23. Jung SJ, Mehta JS, Tong L. Effects of environment pollution on the ocular surface. *Ocul Surf.* (2018) 16:198–205. doi: 10.1016/j.jtos.2018.03.001
24. Tang D, Loze MT, Zeh HJ, Kang R. The redox protein HMGB1 regulates cell death and survival in cancer treatment. *Autophagy.* (2010) 6:1181–3. doi: 10.4161/auto.6.8.13367
25. Kojima T, Dogru M, Kawashima M, Nakamura S, Tsubota K. Advances the diagnosis and treatment of dry eye. *Prog Retin Eye Res.* (2020) 78:100842. doi: 10.1016/j.preteyeres.2020.100842
26. Dai Y, Zhang J, Xiang J, Li Y, Wu D, Xu J. Calcitriol inhibits ROS NLRP3-IL-1beta signaling axis via activation of Nrf2-antioxidant signaling in hyperosmotic stress stimulated human corneal epithelial cells. *Redox Biol.* (2019) 21:101093. doi: 10.1016/j.redox.2018.101093
27. Roy S, Marla S, Praneetha DC. Recognition of corynebacterium pseudodiphtheriticum by Toll-like receptors and up-regulation of antimicrobial peptides in human corneal epithelial cells. *Virulence.* (2015) 6:716–21. doi: 10.1080/21505594.2015.1066063
28. Fitzgerald KA, Kagan JC. Toll-like receptors and the control of immunity. *Cell.* (2020) 180:1044–66. doi: 10.1016/j.cell.2020.02.041
29. Fu JY, Yu XF, Wang HQ, Lan JW, Shao WQ, Huo YN. MiR-205-3p protects human corneal epithelial cells from ultraviolet damage by inhibiting autophagy via targeting TLR4/NF-κB signaling. *Eur Rev Med Pharmacol Sci.* (2020) 24:6494–504. doi: 10.26355/eurrev_202006_21632
30. Gao X, Zhao G, Li C, Lin J, Jiang N, Wang Q, et al. LOX-1 and TLR4 affect each other and regulate the generation of ROS in A. fumigatu keratitis. *Int Immunopharmacol.* (2016) 40:392–9. doi: 10.1016/j.intimp.2016.09.027
31. Grasberger H, Gao J, Nagao-Kitamoto H, Kitamoto S, Zhang M, Kamada N, et al. Increased expression of DUOX2 is an epithelial response to mucosal dysbiosis required for immune homeostasis in mouse intestine. *Gastroenterology.* (2015) 149:1849–59. doi: 10.1053/j.gastro.2015.07.062
32. Gibson AR, O'Leary BR, Du J, Sarsour EH, Kalen AL, Wagner BA, et al. Dual oxidase-induced sustained generation of hydrogen peroxide contributes to pharmacologic ascorbate-induced cytotoxicity. *Cancer Res.* (2020) 80:1401–13. doi: 10.1158/0008-5472.CAN-19-3094
33. Wang B, Zuo X, Peng L, Wang X, Zeng H, Zhong J, et al. Melatonin ameliorates oxidative stress-mediated injuries through induction of HO-1 and restores autophagic flux in dry eye. *Exp Eye Res.* (2021) 205:108491. doi: 10.1016/j.exer.2021.108491
34. Dixon SJ, Stockwell BR. The role of iron and reactive oxygen species in cell death. *Nat Chem Biol.* (2014) 10:9–17. doi: 10.1038/nchembio.1416
35. Yang L, Zhang S, Duan H, Dong M, Hu X, Zhang Z, et al. Different effects of pro-inflammatory factors and hyperosmotic stress on corneal epithelial stem/progenitor cells and wound healing in mice. *Stem Cells Transl Med.* (2019) 8:46–57. doi: 10.1002/sctm.18-0005
36. Pflugfelder SC, de Paiva CS. The pathophysiology of dry eye disease: what we know and future directions for research. *Ophthalmology.* (2017) 124(Suppl. 11):S4–13. doi: 10.1016/j.ophtha.2017.07.010
37. Scaffidi P, Misteli T, Bianchi ME. Release of chromatin protein HMGB1 by necrotic cells triggers inflammation. *Nature.* (2002) 418:191–5. doi: 10.1038/nature00858
38. Hoste E, Maueroder C, van Hove L, Catrysse L, Vikkula HK, Sze M, et al. Epithelial HMGB1 delays skin wound healing and drives tumor initiation by priming neutrophils for NET formation. *Cell Rep.* (2019) 29:2689–701 e4. doi: 10.1016/j.celrep.2019.10.104
39. Han SJ, Min HJ, Yoon SC, Ko EA, Park SJ, Yoon JH, et al. HMGB1 in the pathogenesis of ultraviolet-induced ocular surface inflammation. *Cell Death Dis.* (2015) 6:e1863. doi: 10.1038/cddis.2015.199
40. Lema C, Reins RY, Redfern RL. High-mobility group box 1 in dry eye inflammation. *Inv Ophthalmol Visual Sci.* (2018) 59:1741–50. doi: 10.1167/iovs.17-23363
41. Chen H, Gan X, Li Y, Gu J, Liu Y, Deng Y, et al. NLRP12- and NLRC4-mediated corneal epithelial pyroptosis is driven by GSDMD cleavage accompanied by IL-33 processing in dry eye. *Ocul Surf.* (2020) 18:783–94. doi: 10.1016/j.jtos.2020.07.001

24

Mean Tear-Film Lipid Layer Thickness and Video Display Terminal Time as Risk Factors for Abnormal Blinking in Children

Hui Zhao [1†], Shi-Nan Wu [2,3†], Zhe Cheng [1], Dong Xiao [1], Hui-Ye Shu [2,3], Qian-Min Ge [2,3], Tian Tian [1] and Yi Shao [2,3*]*

[1] *Xinhua Hospital Affiliated to Shanghai Jiao Tong University School of Medicine, Shanghai, China,* [2] *Department of Ophthalmology, The First Affiliated Hospital of Nanchang University, Jiangxi Province Ocular Disease Clinical Research Center, Nanchang, China,* [3] *Department of Radiology, The First Affiliated Hospital of Nanchang University, Jiangxi Province Medical Imaging Research Institute, Nanchang, China*

Correspondence:
Hui Zhao
20887787@qq.com
Yi Shao
freebee99@163.com

These authors have contributed equally to this work and share first authorship

†

Objective: To explore the risk factors for abnormal blinking in children and the role of the tear-film lipid layer thickness (LLT) as a function of duration of video display terminal (VDT) use in children.

Methods: Children attending the Optometry Clinic of Xinhua Hospital affiliated with Shanghai Jiao Tong University were recruited for the study between June 2019 and June 2020. Time spent viewing a VDT (VDTt) over the previous 6 months was recorded. Incomplete blinking (IB) and blinking rate were measured over a 10 s period using the Lipiview® interferometer (Tear Science, Morrisville, NC, USA), and participants were allocated into groups with normal blinking (NBG, blink rate $<$ 20 blinks/min) and abnormal blinking (ABG, blink rate $\geq$ 20 blinks/min). *T*-test, chi-square test and Mann-Whitney *U*-test were used to compare the differences in tear film (TF) stability indexes and meibomian gland function indexes between the two groups. Binary logistic analysis was used to analyze the risk factors for abnormal blinking and protective factors related to children's use of VDT, and receiver operating characteristic (ROC) curve analysis was also conducted.

Results: A total of 167 children were included, with no statistically significant differences in age or sex between the two groups. According to the *t*-test, VDTt was significantly higher in ABG than NBG, while TF stability indices including tear break up time, LLT and the height of the tear meniscus, were significantly higher in NBG than ABG ($P < 0.001$). The results also showed better meibomian gland function in NBG than ABG ($P < 0.05$). Binary logistic analysis showed that VDTt is an important risk factor for abnormal blinking, and the average of LLT (AVG) was found to be an important protective factor for children using a VDT for long periods, with a cut-off value of 1.5 h and 57.5 nm, respectively. ROC curve analysis showed that the area under the curve value of VDTt and AVG was 0.833 and 0.969, respectively ($P < 0.001$).

Conclusion: In children, VDTt is an important risk factor for abnormal blinking, and the AVG is an important protective factor for children using VDT for long periods.

Keywords: children, abnormal blinking, video display terminal time, dry eye, tear film alteration

INTRODUCTION

A blink is a coordinated movement of eyelids closing and opening in a natural state. The normal blink rate is 10–15 blinks/min, each of 0.3–0.4 s duration, with inter-blink interval of 3–4 s. When the blink rate or amplitude exceeds an upper limit, it is considered abnormal. Abnormal blink as a chief complaint in children presenting at the ophthalmology clinic is most commonly secondary to other ocular abnormalities. In addition, some scholars have pointed out that abnormal blinks are closely related to the development of meibomian gland dysfunction (MGD) (1). Therefore, clinical optimization of blinking can effectively improve the symptoms of MGD patients. To date, some studies have shown that video display terminal (VDT) use is an important factor in dry eye (2). China has one of the highest portable VDT utilization rates in the world, with 847 million smart phone users in 2019, an average usage time of 27.9 h per week, 4% of users being children under the age of 10 and 16.9% being 10–19 years old, indicating that about 177 million children making extensive use of smart phones and VDTs (3). Long periods of VDT use are associated with discomfort symptoms such as dry eyes, ocular foreign body sensation, burning sensation and visual fatigue (4, 5). The various eye diseases related to VDT use are summarized in **Table 1** (6–12). Relevant studies have shown that dry eye patients often have ocular surface epithelial damage, abnormal blinking and other clinical symptoms. Therefore, children may be at risk of abnormal blinking and possibly MGD (13) after prolonged use of VDT. Fenga et al. reported that long-term VDT users accompanied by MGD were more likely to have symptoms of eye discomfort and go to ophthalmology (11), which was consistent with the results of other scholars' studies (14).

There are many other external factors that can cause abnormal blinking. It has been reported that the main factors determining blink frequency are stimuli external to the eye, such as the state of the tear film (TF) on the surface of the cornea and conjunctiva, the excitation state of relevant receptors and environmental factors (15). As the outermost layer between the eye and the external environment, the ocular lipid layer of the TF plays an important role in reducing tear evaporation, increasing the stability of the TF and promoting the formation of TF on the ocular surface. A series of studies have shown a significant correlation between dry eye symptoms and tear-film lipid layer thickness (LLT) (16). Previous studies have focused on dry eyes following VDT use in adults, but few reports on meibomian glands (MGs) have involved long-term use of VDT in children. In addition, the scale of children's use of VDTs in China is expanding, and the age at which children begin to use VDTs is increasingly early. Children are unable to accurately describe their subjective symptoms, so conditions such as MGD may be neglected in children with long-term use of VDT. Abnormal blinking is a sign which can be observed by the clinician and does not need to be reported by the child. However, there are no published reports of the correlation between abnormal blinking and the time spent using VDT (VDTt), and there is a lack of research on the relationship between LLT, dry eye and abnormal blinking. Through the analysis of the correlation among VDT, dry eye and abnormal blinking, to provide guidance for the prevention and control of abnormal blink and dry eye in advance. Therefore, the purpose of this study was to explore the correlation between blink abnormalities in children and VDTt, the functional state of the MGs and the TF stability represented by LLT.

METHODS

Patients and Examination

A total of 167 children aged 15 years or less attending ophthalmology outpatient clinics at Xinhua Hospital Affiliated to Medical College of Shanghai Jiao Tong University between June 2019 and June 2020 were enrolled. The blink rate was measured using the Lipiview® interferometer, and subjects with a blink rate of $\geq$20 blinks/min were allocated to an abnormal blinks group (ABG), while those with a blink rate of <20 blinks/min were allocated to a normal blinks group (NBG) (17). Some data results were shown as mean + standard deviation.

Participants were eligible if they met the following criteria: (1) no active inflammation of the eye and no eye drops used within the preceding three months; (2) no history of wearing corneal contact lenses, no history of laser or other ocular surgical operations, no history of ocular trauma, ocular chemical injury or burns; (3) no upper respiratory tract infection within the preceding two weeks; (4) no use of drugs affecting tears such as atropine, neostigmine or artificial tears within the last six months.

Children older than 15 years or with any of the following were excluded: (1) other ocular diseases that may cause ocular surface abnormalities such as abnormal eyelid position, proptosis, or

TABLE 1 | A variety of eye diseases caused by VDT.

References	Year	Corresponding population	Eye diseases
Moon et al. (6)	2016	Children	Dry eye
Ranasinghe et al. (7)	2016	Computer office workers	Computer Vision Syndrome
Basso et al. (8)	2006	VDT workers	Myopia
Ozawa et al. (9)	2015	Office workers aged 20–40 years	Eye fatigue
Lee et al. (10)	2016	Myopic patients with open-angle glaucoma	Visual field progression of open-angle glaucoma
Fenga et al. (11)	2008	VDT workers	Meibomian gland dysfunction
Chen et al. (12)	2017	Long term VDT user	Paracentral acute middle maculopathy

VDT, video display terminal.

TABLE 2 | General information.

Parameters	NBG	ABG	P value[c]
Age (years)[a]	7.82 ± 2.66	8.14 ± 3.01	0.462
Gender (F:M)[b]			0.941
Female	40 (48%)	40 (48%)	
Male	43 (52%)	44 (52%)	
Blinking rate[a]	14.60 ± 4.00	30.00 ± 7.62	<0.001
Incomplete blinking rate[a]	13.95 ± 7.20	23.71 ± 11.44	<0.001
VDTt (hours)[a]	1.03 ± 0.95	2.48 ± 1.08	<0.001

P < 0.05 indicates statistical significance.
[a]Independent sample T test.
[b]Chi-squared test.
[c]Comparison between the NBG and ABG.
Data showed as mean ± standard deviation or n.
NBG, normal blinking group; ABG, abnormal blinking group; VDTt, video display terminal time.

pterygium; (2) other systemic diseases such as hyperthyroidism that affect tear production; or (3) developmental abnormalities. The study was compliant with the tenets of the Declaration of Helsinki, was approved by the Xinhua Hospital ethics committee and was registered with the Chinese Clinical Trial Registry (trial registration number: ChiCTR2000038908 and the approved number: XHEC-D-2018-103). Prior to each subject's participation, a guardian signed a declaration of paper informed consent.

Eye examination and other procedures were conducted in the following order: (1) The child and/or guardian was asked about the child's duration of VDT use over the preceding six months; (2) Lipiview® measurements (including LLT and blink rate) were recorded; (3) tear meniscus height (TH) was measured and MG morphology was assessed using the Oculus Keratography 5M; (4) an ocular surface slit lamp examination was carried out to assess conjunctival congestion and fluorescein BUT, the Marx line (ML) score, MG expression and Meibum score, and corneal fluorescein staining score. All the examinations were finished in one day by the same ophthalmologist in the same dark room.

Measurement of Tear-Film Lipid Layer Thickness (LLT), Incomplete Blinks (IB) and Blink Rate

The LLT of the TF (minimum, maximum and average), number of incomplete blinks (IB) and the blink rate over a 10 s period were measured using a Lipiview® interferometer and during this procedure the child was encouraged to blink naturally (18). The equipment can automatically calculate the number of blinks per min and the number of abnormal blinks per min.

TH and MG Morphology by Oculus Keratography 5M

The TH was measured using the Oculus Keratograph 5M camera and related software (19). TH $\geq$ 0.2 mm indicates normal tear secretion, while TH < 0.2 mm indicates insufficient tear secretion. The upper and lower eyelids were inverted, the conjunctiva was fully exposed, and the images were recorded, analyzed and height calculated. MG dropout was scored using the same equipment according to the following scale: I (normal, with no MG deficiency); II (MG deficiency < 1/3); III (MG deficiency 1/3–2/3); IV (MG deficiency > 2/3) (20).

Slit Lamp Examination

To measure TF breakup time (BUT), 2 μL 1% sodium fluorescein preservative free solution was dropped into the lower conjunctival sac and the participant was instructed to blink several times for a few seconds. TBUT was measured three times, and the mean calculated.

Corneal fluorescence staining score (FL) was measured by considering the corneal surface as four quadrants: supra-nasal, infra-nasal, superior temporal, and inferior temporal, with each quadrant being scored I-IV for a total out of 12 points. Scoring criteria were: I (no staining; 0 point); II (mild scattered spot staining, 1–30 spots stained; 1 point); III (moderate staining, >30 spots stained but staining not fused; 2 points); IV (heavy staining or sheet staining of the entire cornea, spot staining fused, with filaments, or ulcers; 3 points) (21).

The Marx line (ML) score was calculated for the outer, middle, and inner thirds of the lower eyelid margin, and recorded as: I [entirely on the conjunctival side of the meibomian orifices (MOs)]; II (part of the ML touches the MOs); III (ML runs through all of the MOs); and IV (ML runs on the eyelid margin side of the MOs) (22–24).

To measure MG expression (MGE), the five glands at the center of the upper and lower eyelids were located and their orifices observed. Scores were based on the following scale: I (normal, meibum secretion from all glands with light pressure on the eyelid); II (secretion from 3 to 4 glands with light pressure on the eyelid; III (secretion from 1 to 2 glands with light pressure on the eyelid); IV: no secretion from any glands with light pressure on the eyelid) (25).

The quality of secreted meibum was scored (Meibum score) according to the following criteria: I (normal, clear, transparent lid ester); II (cloudy lid ester); III (cloudy lid ester with granules); IV (thick lid fat with a toothpaste-like consistency) (26).

Statistical Analyses

Statistical analysis was conducted using SPSS (version 25.0) and R (version 4.0.5; package pROC version 1.18.0; package ggplot2 version 3.3.5) to carry out *t*-tests, Chi-square test and Mann-Whitney U test between groups. Binary logistic analysis was performed on the related factors according to the grouping. Receiver operating characteristic (ROC) curves and the area under the curve (AUC) were used to analyze sensitivity and specificity of risk factors as diagnostic indicators. *P* values of <0.05 were considered statistically significant.

RESULTS

Patient Demographics

A total of 167 children aged 15 years or younger were included in this case-control study. And 167 right eyes were examined in the study. The NBG included 40 females and 43 males (mean age 7.82 ± 2.66 years; range 2–15 years) and the ABG included 40

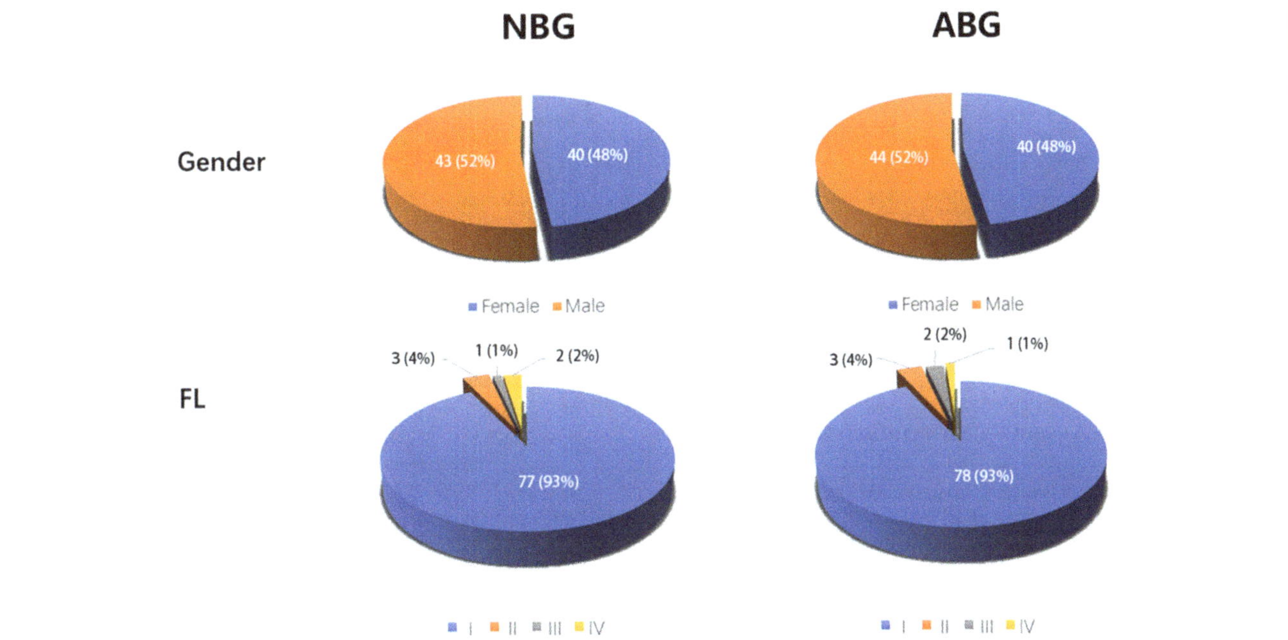

FIGURE 1 | Clinical characteristics of NBG and ABG. $N = 83$ in NBG, $n = 84$ in ABG. NBG, normal blinking group; ABG, abnormal blinking group; FL, corneal fluorescence staining score.

TABLE 3 | The index of tear film.

Parameters	NBG	ABG	Z[c]	P value[c]
FL[a]		−0.032	0.974	
I	77 (93%)	78 (93%)		
II	3 (4%)	3 (4%)		
III	1 (1%)	2 (2%)		
IV	2 (2%)	1 (1%)		
BUT(s)[b]	6.25 ± 2.63	4.79 ± 2.65	-	<0.001
TH (mm)[b]	0.21 ± 0.08	0.18 ± 0.07	-	<0.001
AVG[b]	70.70 ± 22.05	47.70 ± 16.88	-	<0.001
MIN[b]	63.81 ± 22.33	42.58 ± 16.40	-	<0.001
MAX[b]	81.25 ± 21.27	59.35 ± 20.18	-	<0.001

$P < 0.05$ indicates statistical significance.
[a]Mann-Whitney U test.
[b]Independent sample T test.
[c]Comparison between the NBG and ABG.
Data showed as mean ± standard deviation or n.
NBG, normal blinking group; ABG, abnormal blinking group; FL, corneal fluorescence staining score; BUT, tear film breakup time; TH, tear meniscus height; AVG, the average of tear film lipid layer thickness; MIN, the minimum of tear film lipid layer thickness; MAX, the maximum of tear film lipid layer thickness.

females and 44 males (mean age 8.14 ± 3.01 years; range 2–15 years). The two groups were statistically similar in age and gender ($P = 0.462$ and $P = 0.941$ respectively). The mean blink rate in the NBG was 14.60 ± 4.00, and this was significantly lower than the ABG blink rate of 30.00 ± 7.62 ($P < 0.001$). In addition, the frequency of incomplete blinking in ABG (23.71 ± 11.44) was significantly higher than that in NBG (13.95 ± 7.20; $P < 0.001$). The VDTt was also significantly different between the two groups, with longer times in ABG than in NBG ($P < 0.001$). Data are shown in **Table 2**; **Figure 1**.

Tear Film Stability

The TH measure provided an indication of the quantity of TF. The TH and BUT of ABG was significantly lower than NBG, (TH 0.18 ± 0.07 and 0.21 ± 0.08; BUT 4.79 ± 2.65 and 6.25 ± 2.63; $P < 0.001$) (**Table 3**). LLT was assessed using mean and range. All LLT indices were significantly lower in ABG than NBG (mean 47.70 ± 16.88 and 70.70 ± 22.05; minimum 42.58 ± 16.40 and 63.81 ± 22.33; and maximum 59.35 ± 20.18 and 81.25 ± 21.27, respectively; all $P < 0.001$). No significant between-groups difference was found in FL ($Z = -0.032$, $P = 0.974$, **Table 3**) (**Figure 2**).

Meibomian Gland Function

MG dropout, meibum score, MGE and ML were used to evaluate the morphology and function of MG. Although there was no significant difference in MG dropout between the two groups ($Z = -0.012$, $P = 0.990$). ML ($Z = -3.886$, $P < 0.001$), MGE ($Z = -3.798$, $P < 0.001$) and Meibum scores ($Z = -2.411$, $P = 0.016$) were lower in the NBG than in the ABG. More detailed information is shown in **Table 4**; **Figure 3**.

Binary Logistic and ROC Curve Analysis

Binary logistic multivariate analysis based on ABG and NBG grouping showed that VDTt was an important risk factor for abnormal blinking. Based on an odds ratio of 3.486, it can be inferred that the risk of abnormal blinking after long-term use

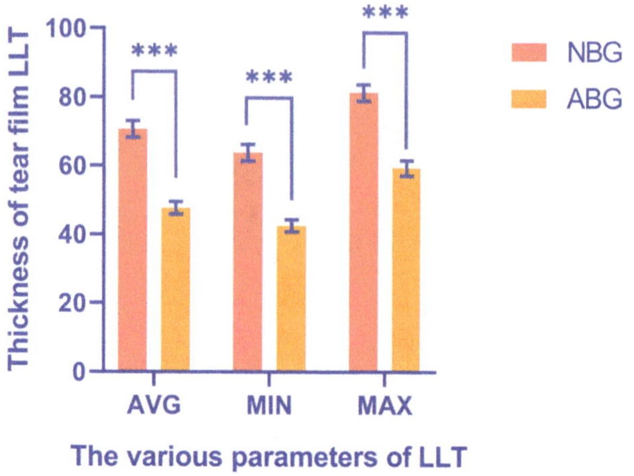

FIGURE 2 | The difference of tear film LLT between NBG and ABG. ***There was a significant difference between the two groups. LLT, lipid layer thickness; NBG, normal blinking group; ABG, abnormal blinking group; AVG, the average of tear film lipid layer thickness; MIN, the minimum of tear film lipid layer thickness; MAX, the maximum of tear film lipid layer thickness.

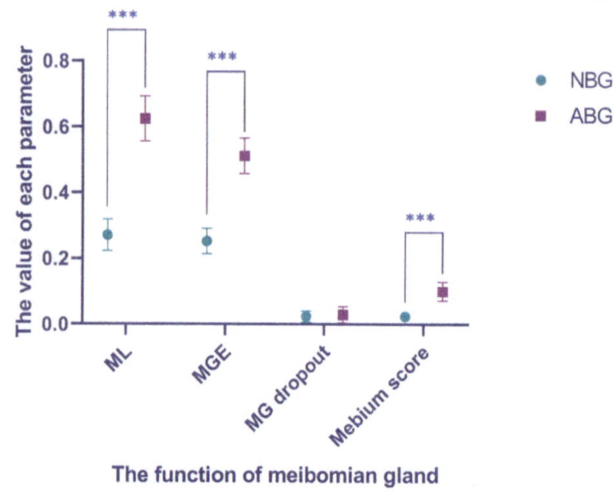

FIGURE 3 | Comparison of meibomian gland function between NBG and ABG. ***There was a significant difference between the two groups. NBG, normal blinking group; ABG, abnormal blinking group; ML, marx line; MGE, meibomian gland expression; MG dropout, meibomian gland dropout degree.

TABLE 4 | The function of meibomian gland.

Parameters	NBG	ABG	Z[b]	*P* value[b]
ML[a]			−3.886	<0.001
I	59 (71%)	36 (43%)		
II	3 (4%)	5 (6%)		
III	21 (25%)	36 (43%)		
IV	0 (0%)	7 (8%)		
MGE[a]			−3.798	<0.001
I	51 (61%)	28 (33%)		
II	22 (27%)	34 (40%)		
III	10 (12%)	18 (21%)		
IV	0 (0%)	4 (5%)		
MG dropout[a]			−0.012	0.990
I	81 (98%)	82 (98%)		
II	0 (0%)	1 (1%)		
III	2 (2%)	0 (0%)		
IV	0 (0%)	1 (1%)		
Mebium score[a]			−2.411	0.016
I	80 (97%)	72 (86%)		
II	2 (2%)	7 (8%)		
III	1 (1%)	5 (6%)		

$P < 0.05$ indicates statistical significance.
[a]Mann-Whitney U test.
[b]Comparison between the NBG and ABG.
NBG, normal blinking group; ABG, abnormal blinking group; ML, marx line; MGE, meibomian gland expression; MG dropout, meibomian gland dropout degree.

of VDT is 3.486 times higher than that of people who have not used VDT for a long time. ROC curve analysis was used to further explore this risk factor, and showed an AUC value for VDTt of 0.833. Based on the ROC curve, cut-off value of 1.5, sensitivity of 0.827, and specificity of 0.825 were determined ($P < 0.001$) (**Tables 5, 6; Figure 4A**).

Binary Logistic Analysis Results and ROC Curve With 1.5 h as Boundary-Value Grouping

In order to exclude the collinearity effect of VDTt on other covariates, data were grouped based on the 1.5 h cut off value, and binary logistic multivariate analysis was conducted. Mean LLT was found to be an important protective factor with an odds ratio of 0.762. To evaluate the clinical significance of mean LLT in differential diagnosis, further ROC curve analysis was performed. The AUC value corresponding to mean LLT was 0.969, with cut-off value of 57.5, sensitivity and specificity of 0.857 and 0.940 respectively ($P < 0.001$) (**Tables 5, 6; Figure 4B**).

DISCUSSION

The present study identified the amount of time spent using a VDT as an important risk factor for abnormal blinking in children, and that VDTt of <1.5 h per day may be more conducive to children's eye health than longer periods. Moreover, statistical analysis pointed to mean LLT as an important protective factor for long periods of VDT use, with a bound value of 57.5 nm. This indicates that mean LLT $\leq$ 57.5 nm found in clinical ophthalmological examination would require consideration of the child's use of VDT and its possible impact on TF stability (**Figure 5**). According to the above clinical indicators, ophthalmologists could play a further important role in guiding children's eye health.

Previous research has shown that prolonged use of VDT could cause musculoskeletal pain, poor mental performance and psychological distress, and most commonly eye irritation (27).

TABLE 5 | Binary logistic analysis results under different groups.

Factor	Cut-Off value	Sensitivity (%)	Specificity (%)	AUC	*P* value
VDTt[a]	1.5	82.7	82.5	0.833	<0.001
AVG[b]	57.5	85.7	94.0	0.969	<0.001

[a] *The results are grouped according to a bound of 20 blinks per min.*
[b] *The results are grouped according to a daily bound value of 1.5 h of VDT usage.*
$P < 0.05$ denoted statistical significance.
B, coefficient of regression; OR, odds ratio; CI, confidence interval; VDTt, video display terminal time; AVG, the average of tear film lipid layer thickness.

TABLE 6 | The Cut-off Value, sensitivity, specificity, and AUC of factors for the different grouping conditions.

Factors	B	OR	OR (95% CI)	*P* value
VDTt[a]	1.249	3.486	2.410–5.042	<0.001
AVG[b]	−0.272	0.762	0.687–0.845	<0.001

[a] *The results are grouped according to a bound of 20 blinks per min.*
[b] *The results are grouped according to a daily bound value of 1.5 h of VDT usage.*
$P < 0.05$ denoted statistical significance.
VDTt, video display terminal time; AVG, the average of tear film lipid layer thickness; AUC, area under the curve.

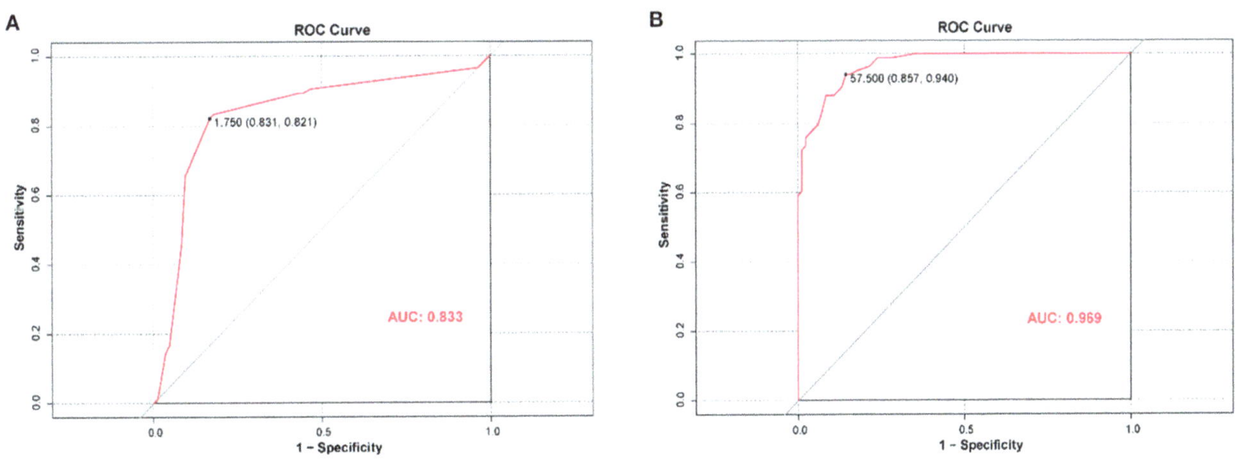

FIGURE 4 | (A) The receiver operating characteristics (ROC) curves of risk factors for detecting children with abnormal blinking. ROC curves of VDTt showed that the AUC value was 0.833 ($P < 0.001$). The sensitivity and specificity were 82.7 and 82.5%, respectively. **(B)** The receiver operating characteristics (ROC) curves for factors associated with prolonged use of VDT in children. ROC curves of AVG showed that the AUC value was 0.969 ($P < 0.001$). The sensitivity and specificity were 85.7 and 94.0%, respectively. VDTt, video display terminal time; AVG, the average of tear film lipid layer thickness; AUC, area under the curve.

In China, a high risk factor for myopia in children is the use of VDT in close proximity, especially long periods of smartphone use (28). However, to date, little research exists on the correlation between abnormal blinking and the use of VDT. Since it is difficult for children to clearly express their symptoms, and children with xerophthalmia may have allergic conjunctivitis to varying degrees, these diseases may be misdiagnosed clinically (29). In a prospective study of frequent blinking in children, the most common cause was abnormality of the anterior segment or eyelid (30), but diverse causative factors exist and most are related to benign or self-limiting conditions (see **Figure 6**) (31–33). Careful medical history and clinical examination are important to determine the corresponding etiology and to provide timely and targeted treatment.

In this study, a significant risk factor for excessive blinking in children was prolonged video device use. Some scholars have pointed out that the prolonged use of VDT is an important cause of dry eyes, and found that warming moist chamber goggles have an excellent curative effect (34). There is a time-dependent oxidative stress response in ocular surface tissue, but the VDT durations in the present study are not sufficient to discern any damage to the ocular surface. Longer periods of VDT use may cause damage to the ocular surface. Perhaps short periods of use cause the decline of MG secretion function and the thinning of

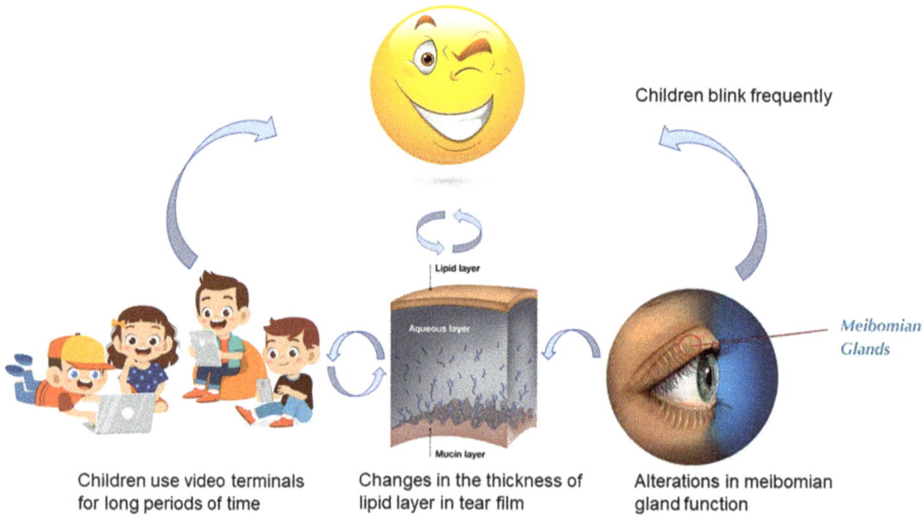

FIGURE 5 | Frequent blinking in children was associated with prolonged use of terminal devices, thickness of tear film lipid layer, and alterations in meibomian gland function.

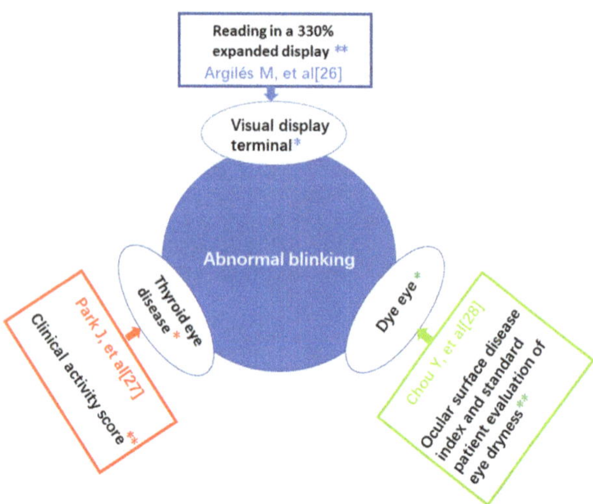

FIGURE 6 | Summary of risk factors leading to abnormal blinking and their important influencing factors. *Risk factors. **Important influencing factors.

TF lipid layer, which leads to the deterioration of TF stability, but not the loss of MGs.

Numerous studies have shown reduced blink rates in long-term VDT users, as low as 7–11 blinks/min, with a significant increase in the percentage of incomplete blinks (35, 36). In children, with highly appealing entertainment and materials available to view on VDTs, blink rate is lower still, with the orbicularis oculi and Riolan muscles in children contracting completely around the eyelid gland opening. MG acini constantly synthesize and secrete meibum, which leads to the abnormal discharge of meibum, a decrease in MG secretion capacity and obstruction of the meibum (37, 38). This may be alleviated by the patient squeezing the eyes hard and increasing blink frequency. Previous research has shown that 60% of people who use VDT for long periods have significantly decreased blink rates, which in turn can lead to MGD (39). We hypothesize that children are more sensitive than adults to MG and TF abnormalities, with associated increased blink rate and abnormal blinking habits, and these signs can be misdiagnosed by clinicians as Tourette's syndrome.

Interestingly, studies have shown that incomplete blinking is associated with a two-fold increased risk of dry eye disease in patients with poor LLT (40). The TF lipid layer is composed of lipids secreted by meibomian glands, is located in the outermost layer of the TF, and has thickness in the range of 20–180 nm. As the lipid contact surface between the eye and the external environment, TF lipid layer can assist other TF components to inhibit tear evaporation, stabilize the air-tear surface between eye opening and blinks, and play a role in the first line of defense against bacterial invasion (41). The thickness of TF lipid layer is affected by a decrease of eyelid lipid or a change of tear composition.

In a recent study using Lipiview®, LLT was positively correlated with the number of normally secreting MGs, with LLT $\leq$ 60 nm in adults with dry eye, indicating a clinical application of MG assessment (33). This evaluation method has important clinical application value. In our study, BUT, TH and LLT were significantly lower in ABG than NBG. These finding suggest poor TF stability and a possibility of evaporative dry eye in children with abnormal blinking. For those using VDT for long periods, maintaining appropriate LLT could be a significant protective factor for ocular health. According to our statistical analysis, when the average LLT is reduced to 57.5 nm or less, TF stability may be significantly reduced in children using VDTs.

There are some limitations to our study. Firstly, abnormal blinking was assessed using the blink rate and number of incomplete blinks, and excessive blinking was not studied. Secondly, ocular surface morphology was observed over a short period, and longer observation time would help to compare different research results and support the research conclusion. Thirdly, the sample size of each group in the study was small, and larger studies would provide more certainty about the effect of VDTt on TF stability in children. Finally, the children involved in this study were all from the eastern Chinese city of Shanghai, so it is difficult to exclude the effect of air pollution on the ocular surface (42).

ETHICS STATEMENT

The studies involving human participants were reviewed and approved by Xinhua Hospital Affiliated to Medical College of Shanghai Jiao Tong University. Written informed consent to participate in this study was provided by the participants' legal guardian/next of kin.

AUTHOR CONTRIBUTIONS

HZ and S-NW were involved in the data curation and writing of the original draft. ZC, S-NW, and DX performed the data curation and formal analysis and participated in the writing and editing of the manuscript. H-YS was involved in the study conceptualization and methodology design. Q-MG and TT were involved in data validation and visualization. YS and HZ were involved in the study conceptualization, data curation, funding acquisition, and project administration. All authors have read and approved the final manuscript.

REFERENCES

1. Wan T, Jin X, Lin L, Xu Y, Zhao Y. Incomplete blinking may attribute to the development of meibomian gland dysfunction. *Curr Eye Res.* (2016) 41:179–85. doi: 10.3109/02713683.2015.1007211
2. Tsubota K, Yokoi N, Shimazaki J, Watanabe H, Dogru M, Yamada M et al. New perspectives on dry eye definition and diagnosis: a consensus report by the Asia dry eye society. *Ocul Surf.* (2017) 15:65–76. doi: 10.1016/j.jtos.2016.09.003
3. *The 45th China Statistical Report on Internet Development.* China Internet Network Information Center.
4. Nakamura S. Approach to dry eye in video display terminal workers (basic science). *Invest Ophthalmol Vis Sci.* (2018) 59:DES130–7. doi: 10.1167/iovs.17-23762
5. Mehra D, Galor A. Digital screen use and dry eye: a review. *Asia Pac J Ophthalmol (Phila).* (2020) 9:491–7. doi: 10.1097/APO.0000000000000328
6. Moon JH, Kim KW, Moon NJ. Smartphone use is a risk factor for pediatric dry eye disease according to region and age: a case control study. *BMC Ophthalmol.* (2016) 16:188. doi: 10.1186/s12886-016-0364-4
7. Ranasinghe P, Wathurapatha WS, Perera YS, Lamabadusuriya DA, Kulatunga S, Jayawardana N, et al. Computer vision syndrome among computer office workers in a developing country: an evaluation of prevalence and risk factors. *BMC Res Notes.* (2016) 9:150. doi: 10.1186/s13104-016-1962-1
8. Basso A, Di Lorenzo L, Cramarossa AA, Corfiati M, Ria W, Bellino R, et al. Evaluation of myopia in a group of people working with video terminals: first results. *G Ital Med Lav Ergon.* (2006) 28:207–9.
9. Ozawa Y, Kawashima M, Inoue S, Inagaki E, Suzuki A, Ooe E, et al. Bilberry extract supplementation for preventing eye fatigue in video display terminal workers. *J Nutr Health Aging.* (2015) 19:548–54. doi: 10.1007/s12603-014-0573-6
10. Lee JR, Lee J, Lee JE, Lee JY, Kook MS. Optic disc tilt direction affects regional visual field progression rates in myopic eyes with open-angle glaucoma. *Graefes Arch Clin Exp Ophthalmol.* (2016) 254:2267–76. doi: 10.1007/s00417-016-3501-0
11. Fenga C, Aragona P, Cacciola A, Spinella R, Di Nola C, Ferreri F, et al. Meibomian gland dysfunction and ocular discomfort in video display terminal workers. *Eye (Lond).* (2008) 22:91–5. doi: 10.1038/sj.eye.6703025
12. Chen Y, Hu Y. The optical imaging of idiopathic paracentral acute middle maculopathy in a Chinese young man and review of the literature. *Photodiagn Photodyn Ther.* (2017) 19:383–7. doi: 10.1016/j.pdpdt.2017.07.004
13. Talens-Estarelles C, García-Marqués JV, Cervino A, García-Lázaro S. Use of digital displays and ocular surface alterations: a review. *Ocul Surf.* (2021) 19:252–65. doi: 10.1016/j.jtos.2020.10.001
14. Wu H, Wang Y, Dong N, Yang F, Lin Z, Shang X, et al. Meibomian gland dysfunction determines the severity of the dry eye conditions in visual display terminal workers. *PLoS ONE.* (2014) 9:e105575. doi: 10.1371/journal.pone.0105575
15. Collins MJ, Iskander DR, Saunders A, Hook S, Anthony E, Gillon R. Blinking patterns and corneal staining. *Eye Contact Lens.* (2006) 32:287–93. doi: 10.1097/01.icl.0000224551.58399.9a
16. Foulks GN. The correlation between the tear film lipid layer and dry eye disease. *Surv Ophthalmol.* (2007) 52:369–74. doi: 10.1016/j.survophthal.2007.04.009
17. Doughty MJ, Naase T. Further analysis of the human spontaneous eye blink rate by a cluster analysis-based approach to categorize individuals with 'normal' versus 'frequent' eye blink activity. *Eye Contact Lens.* (2006) 32:294–9. doi: 10.1097/01.icl.0000224359.32709.4d
18. Gulati S, Jain S. Ocular pharmacology of tear film, dry eye, and allergic conjunctivitis. *Handb Exp Pharmacol.* (2017) 242:97–118. doi: 10.1007/164_2016_73
19. Pérez Bartolomé F, Martínez de la Casa JM, Arriola Villalobos P, Fernández Pérez C, Polo V, Sánchez Jean R, et al. Ocular redness measured with the keratograph 5M in patients using anti-glaucoma eye drops. *Semin Ophthalmol.* (2018) 33:643–50. doi: 10.1080/08820538.2017.1395891
20. Wong S, Srinivasan S, Murphy PJ, Jones L. Comparison of meibomian gland dropout using two infrared imaging devices. *Cont Lens Anterior Eye.* (2019) 42:311–7. doi: 10.1016/j.clae.2018.10.014
21. Amparo F, Wang H, Yin J, Marmalidou A, Dana R. Evaluating corneal fluorescein staining using a novel automated method. *Invest Ophthalmol Vis Sci.* (2017) 58:BIO168–73. doi: 10.1167/iovs.17-21831
22. Schiffman RM, Christianson MD, Jacobsen G, Hirsch JD, Reis BL. Reliability and validity of the ocular surface disease index. *Arch Ophthalmol.* (2000) 118:615–21. doi: 10.1001/archopht.118.5.615
23. Yamaguchi M, Kutsuna M, Uno T, Zheng X, Kodama T, Ohashi Y. Marx line: fluorescein staining line on the inner lid as indicator of meibomian gland function. *Am J Ophthalmol.* (2006) 141:669–75. doi: 10.1016/j.ajo.2005.11.004
24. Rabensteiner DF, Aminfar H, Boldin I, Nitsche-Resch M, Berisha B, Schwantzer G, et al. Demodex mite infestation and its associations with tear film and ocular surface parameters in patients with ocular discomfort. *Am J Ophthalmol.* (2019) 204:7–12. doi: 10.1016/j.ajo.2019.03.007
25. Asbell PA, Stapleton FJ, Wickström K, Akpek EK, Aragona P, Dana R, et al. The international workshop on meibomian gland dysfunction: report of the clinical trials subcommittee. *Invest Ophthalmol Vis Sci.* (2011) 52:2065–85. doi: 10.1167/iovs.10-6997h
26. Cho BJ, Jee DH, Kim WJ, Shin MC, Kim EC, Kim MS, et al. Direct visualization of continuous meibum secretion from the orifices of meibomian glands to the tear film. *Cornea.* (2019) 38:1245–52. doi: 10.1097/ICO.0000000000002049
27. Utsunomiya T, Kawahara A, Hanada K, Yoshida A. Effects of diquafosol ophthalmic solution on quality of life in dry eye assessed using the dry

eye-related quality-of-life score questionnaire: effectiveness in patients while reading and using visual display terminals. *Cornea.* (2017) 36:908–14. doi: 10.1097/ICO.0000000000001241
28. Guo L, Yang J, Mai J, Du X, Guo Y, Li P, et al. Prevalence and associated factors of myopia among primary and middle school-aged students: a school-based study in Guangzhou. *Eye (Lond).* (2016) 30:796–804. doi: 10.1038/eye.2016.39
29. Kim TH, Moon NJ. Clinical correlations of dry eye syndrome and allergic conjunctivitis in Korean children. *J Pediatr Ophthalmol Strabismus.* (2013) 50:124–7. doi: 10.3928/01913913-20130108-01
30. Coats DK, Paysse EA, Kim DS. Excessive blinking in childhood: a prospective evaluation of 99 children. *Ophthalmology.* (2001) 108:1556–61. doi: 10.1016/S0161-6420(01)00644-3
31. Argilés M, Cardona G, Pérez-Cabré E, Rodríguez M. Blink rate and incomplete blinks in six different controlled hard-copy and electronic reading conditions. *Invest Ophthalmol Vis Sci.* (2015) 56:6679–85. doi: 10.1167/iovs.15-16967
32. Park J, Baek S. Dry eye syndrome in thyroid eye disease patients: The role of increased incomplete blinking and Meibomian gland loss. *Acta Ophthalmol.* (2019) 97:e800–6. doi: 10.1111/aos.14000
33. Chou YB, Fan NW, Lin PY. Value of lipid layer thickness and blinking pattern in approaching patients with dry eye symptoms. *Can J Ophthalmol.* (2019) 54:735–40. doi: 10.1016/j.jcjo.2019.03.005
34. Ren Y, Chen J, Zheng Q, Chen W. Short-term effect of a developed warming moist chamber goggle for video display terminal-associated dry eye. *BMC Ophthalmol.* (2018) 18:33. doi: 10.1186/s12886-018-0700-y
35. Kawashima M, Tsubota K. Tear lipid layer deficiency associated with incomplete blinking: a case report. *BMC Ophthalmol.* (2013) 13:34. doi: 10.1186/1471-2415-13-34
36. Portello JK, Rosenfield M, Chu CA. Blink rate, incomplete blinks and computer vision syndrome. *Optom Vis Sci.* (2013) 90:482–7. doi: 10.1097/OPX.0b013e31828f09a7
37. Nakamura S, Kinoshita S, Yokoi N, Ogawa Y, Shibuya M, Nakashima H, et al. Lacrimal hypofunction as a new mechanism of dry eye in visual display terminal users. *PLoS ONE.* (2010) 5:e11119. doi: 10.1371/journal.pone.0011119
38. Korb DR, Baron DF, Herman JP, Finnemore VM, Exford JM, Hermosa JL et al. Tear film lipid layer thickness as a function of blinking. *Cornea.* (1994) 13:354–9. doi: 10.1097/00003226-199407000-00012
39. Randolph SA. Computer vision syndrome. *Workplace Health Saf.* (2017) 65:328. doi: 10.1177/2165079917712727
40. Wang MTM, Tien L, Han A, Lee JM, Kim D, Markoulli M, et al. Impact of blinking on ocular surface and tear film parameters. *Ocul Surf.* (2018) 16:424–9. doi: 10.1016/j.jtos.2018.06.001
41. Georgiev GA, Eftimov P, Yokoi N. Structure-function relationship of tear film lipid layer: a contemporary perspective. *Exp Eye Res.* (2017) 163:17–28. doi: 10.1016/j.exer.2017.03.013
42. Jung SJ, Mehta JS, Tong L. Effects of environment pollution on the ocular surface. *Ocul Surf.* (2018) 16:198–205. doi: 10.1016/j.jtos.2018.03.001

25

Correlation Study Between Abnormal Morphology of Meibomian Glands and Meibum in Patients With Dry Eye Disease Under *in vivo* Confocal Microscopy

*Qian Zheng [1], Yuanyuan Xue [1], Xiaowei Zhong [1], Guangwei Li [1], Weiyun Shi [1,2,3] and Ting Wang [1,2,3]**

[1] Department of Ophthalmology, Eye Hospital of Shandong First Medical University, Shandong First Medical University and Shandong Academy of Medical Sciences, Jinan, China, [2] State Key Laboratory Cultivation Base, Shandong Provincial Key Laboratory of Ophthalmology, Shandong Eye Institute, Jinan, China, [3] School of Ophthalmology, Shandong First Medical University, Jinan, China

***Correspondence:**
Ting Wang
wt-ting@163.com

Objective: To observe differences in meibomian gland morphology among patients with meibomian gland dysfunction (MGD) with liquid meibum, with solid meibum, and a non-MGD group by laser scanning *in vivo* confocal microscopy (IVCM), and then analyze the correlation between meibomian gland abnormalities and dry eye disease.

Methods: Twenty-one patients with MGD (42 eyes) with liquid meibum, 21 patients with MGD (38 eyes) with solid meibum, and 24 non-MGD patients (39 eyes) were enrolled in the study. IVCM examination and Schirmer II test were performed, and non-invasive tear-film breakup time (NIBUT) was measured.

Results: Data obtained from all the patients were normally distributed; therefore, one-way analysis of variance was performed. The meibomian gland opening diameter and gland opening area of the patients with MGD were greater than those of the non-MGD patients, and values of the liquid meibum group were greater than those of the solid meibum group ($F = 17.96$, $p < 0.001$; $F = 8.84$, $p < 0.001$, respectively). Due to changes in meibomian gland opening diameter and dilation of meibomian gland acini, the acinar longest diameter and unit area of the patients with MGD were also greater than those of the non-MGD patients, and the values of the solid meibum group were greater than those of the liquid meibum group ($F = 36.52$, $p < 0.001$; $F = 27.81$, $p < 0.001$, respectively). In the aspect of acinar shortest diameter, there was no difference among the three groups ($F = 0.24$, $P > 0.05$). Highest inflammatory cell density was observed in the solid meibum group, followed by the liquid meibum group, and the non-MGD group ($F = 111.54$, $p < 0.001$). Similarly, the results of the Schirmer II test and NIBUT showed that the condition of the patients with MGD in the solid meibum group was worst, followed by that of the liquid meibum group and the non-MGD group ($F = 99.57$, $p < 0.001$; $F = 11.87$, $p < 0.001$, respectively).

Conclusions: The different meibum in the patients with MGD is accompanied by different meibomian gland morphologies. Compared with the patients with liquid meibum, those with solid meibum have more obvious dilatation of meibomian glands under confocal microscopy and in these patients, the density of inflammatory cells among glands is higher, and the quality of tears is worse.

Keywords: meibomian gland dysfunction, meibomian gland morphology, structure, function, abnormalities of meibum

INTRODUCTION

The prevalence of dry eyes is increasing day by day. In patients over age 40 years, the prevalence is as high as 75% (1), and the affected population is getting younger. Dry eye is a multifactorial disease of the ocular surface. It has been reported that the pathogenesis of dry eyes has a close relationship with meibomian gland dysfunction (MGD) (2, 3), which is the condition where the quantity and quality of lipid-rich secretion that is produced by meibomian glands (meibum) (4) are abnormal under influences of the eyes, whole body, medicine, external environment, and other factors (5). The meibum of patients with MGD may be clear and transparent liquid, cloudy liquid, cloudy and particulate fluid, or thick toothpaste-like solid (6). However, specific reasons for the different forms of meibum are still unclear. In this study, the patients with MGD are divided into two types: patients with liquid meibum and patients with solid meibum. In recent years, *in vivo* confocal microscopy (IVCM) has been performed to scan the structure of the ocular surface. The cell morphology of the cornea and meibomian gland can be determined. At cellular level, it has established a good connection between *in vitro* histology and *in vivo* ocular pathology (7, 8). In this study, IVCM was performed to detect the meibomian gland conditions of patients with different meibum qualities, and found that the gland morphology of patients with different meibum qualities was also different, which serves as an effective basis for in-depth research and treatment of MGD.

MATERIALS AND METHODS

General Information

A total of 66 patients who were treated in Eye Hospital of Shandong First Medical University from June 2020 to August 2021 were involved. First of all, the patients received a slit-lamp examination for observation of meibomian gland orifice obstruction, followed by Schirmer II test and NIBUT for diagnosis of MGD. Then, IVCM examination was carried out. Finally, after meibomian gland massage, the patients with MGD whose meibum was clear or cloudy were divided into the liquid meibum group (21 cases, 42 eyes; seven males, 14 females), and the patients whose meibum was opaque and toothpaste-like were divided into the solid meibum group (21 cases, 38 eyes; 12 males and nine females). Those without dry eye symptoms, and with normal BUT and tear secretion were included in the non-MGD group (24 cases, 39 eyes; four males and 20 females). Massage was not performed on the non-MGD patients. The average age of the liquid meibum group was 58.8 ± 11.66 years, that of the solid group was 52.71 ± 18.5 years, and that of the normal subjects was 61.29 ± 14.87 years.

The inclusion criteria of the groups with MGD were as follows: (a) patient complained of dry eyes, foreign body sensation, burning sensation, eye fatigue, soreness, red jelly, and conscious blurred vision; (b) Schiermer II test < 10 mm, NIBUT < 10 s; (c) after meibomian gland massage, the meibum expressed is liquid or solid; and (d) participation in the research is voluntary.

Exclusion criteria were : patients (a) wearing contact lenses, or (b) having a history of eye trauma (acid-base burns), or (c) having had an eye surgery recently (9), or (d) with congenital abnormality or dysplasia of meibomian glands, or (e) with eye tattoos, (f) with immune system diseases such as Sjogren's syndrome (10), or (g) who have had long-term meibomian gland massage or fumigation, or (h) who have taken hormone drugs for a long time were excluded from the study.

The inclusion criteria for the non-MGD group were as follows: there is no eye dryness, foreign body sensation, and other discomforts in daily life; and at the same time, Schiermer II test >10 mm, and NIBUT >10 s.

This study was approved by the Ethics Committee of the Eye Hospital of Shandong First Medical University. All the procedures adhered to the tenets of the Declaration of Helsinki. Written informed consent was obtained from each patient. The trial was registered in the Chinese Clinical Trial Registry (registration number: ChicTR2100050900).

Method

In vivo Confocal Microscopy (IVCM)

An Heidelberg hrt 3 (HRT 3) *in vivo* confocal microscope (Heidelberg Engineering, Heidelberg, Germany) was used to observe the morphological and structural characteristics of the meibomian glands at the center of the upper eyelid and eyelid margin after topical anesthesia (0.5% proparacaine hydrochloride) was instilled. The wavelength was 670 nm, field of view was 400 μm × 400 μm, resolution was 384 × 384 pixels, magnification was 800 times, and horizontal and vertical resolutions were both 1 μm. The center of the upper eyelid near the eyelid margin was scanned to observe meibomian gland opening, morphology of acini, and inflammatory cell infiltration.

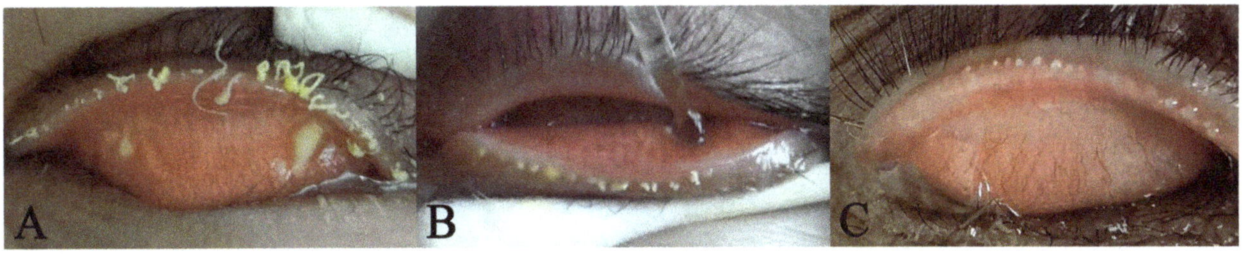

FIGURE 1 | (A) Solid meibum and yellow oil embolism. **(B)** Solid meibum. **(C)** Oily liquid meibum.

Image Evaluation

In view of the fact that imaging of the meibomian gland acini and openings can be in different shapes when scanning planes are different, we selected 3–5 images with the best quality for analysis, including clear meibomian gland openings (at least 1 per image), acini (at least 5 per image), palpebral conjunctival cell structure, and inflammatory cells as many as possible. The diameter of all the meibomian gland openings, area of the meibomian gland openings, acinar longest diameter, acinar shortest diameter, and acinar unit area in the confocal microscopy images were measured with the Image J software. The fused acinar was calculated as one acinar and the incomplete acinar in the image was excluded. After the measurement, the authors calculated the area using the following formula: actual area = area × 400 × 400/(384 × 384) μm^2. The number of inflammatory cells in the meibomian glands was measured using the Rostock Cornea Module. All the values were measured three times to get an average value.

Schirmer II Test

The lower eyelid of the patients was everted gently to instill topical anesthesia (0.5% proparacaine hydrochloride) and then, after a sterile filter paper strip was placed over the middle to lateral 1/3 of the lower eyelid, the patients were asked to close their eyes. The strip was removed after 5 min, and the length of tear wetting was measured.

Non-invasive Tear-Film Breakup Time (NIBUT)

Non-invasive tear-film breakup time (NIBUT) was evaluated with a Keratograph 5M ocular surface analyzer (10 times magnification). After two blinks, the patients were asked to focus on the target and keep the eyes open as long as possible to measure tear film breakup time.

Statistical Analysis

SPSS Version 23 was used for data analysis. The data obtained from patients in the three groups were normally distributed; therefore, one-way analysis of variance can be performed. $P < 0.05$ was regarded as statistically significant.

RESULTS

General Results

The average age of the liquid meibum group, solid meibum group, and non-MGD group had no significant difference (58.15 ± 11.66 vs. 52.71 ± 18.5 vs. 61.29 ± 14.87) ($F = 1.84$, $P > 0.05$). Therefore, the influence of age difference on the results was avoided.

According to the picture taken during meibomian glands massage, three of the 21 patients with solid meibum had light yellow oil embolism, which is the early state of a chalazion (**Figure 1**). The size of the toothpaste-like meibum in one patient was about 1 × 2 mm, and 0.5 × 1 mm in the other two patients.

IVCM Results

IVCM Meibomian Gland Opening Examination

In the patients with liquid meibum, the meibomian gland openings were round or oval, or nearly circular, surrounded by round and oval flat cells, and loosely arranged with irregular borders, similar to the surrounding conjunctival epithelial cells. The morphology of meibomian gland opening cells in the patients with solid meibum was different. The cells were irregularly long or diamond-shaped and more loosely arranged, and the number of goblet cells was increased. There was a small amount of scattered dendritic cells around, and more fibrotic tissues existed. The surrounding conjunctival epithelial cells had increased size and were arranged more irregularly, accumulating around the meibomian gland acini (**Figure 2**). A certain degree of blockage existed in the meibomian gland openings of patients with solid meibum. Compared with the two groups mentioned above, the meibomian gland of the non-MGD patients was round in shape, and had regular boundary and orderly cell arrangement. According to the results calculated with SPSS Version 23, the meibomian gland opening diameter and gland opening area of the patients with MGD were greater than those of the non-MGD patients, and the values of the liquid meibum group were greater than those of the solid meibum group. Statistical analysis of the opening diameter and opening area of the meibomian gland openings showed that there were statistically significant differences among the three groups. There were also statistical differences between any two groups (opening diameter: 39.47 ± 9.57 vs. 34.8 ± 9.98 vs. 26.21 ± 10.6; opening area: 1,861.47 ± 910.4 vs. 1,517.23 ± 713.12 vs. 1,188.96 ± 437.13) ($F = 17.96$, $p < 0.001$; $F = 8.84$, $p < 0.001$, respectively).

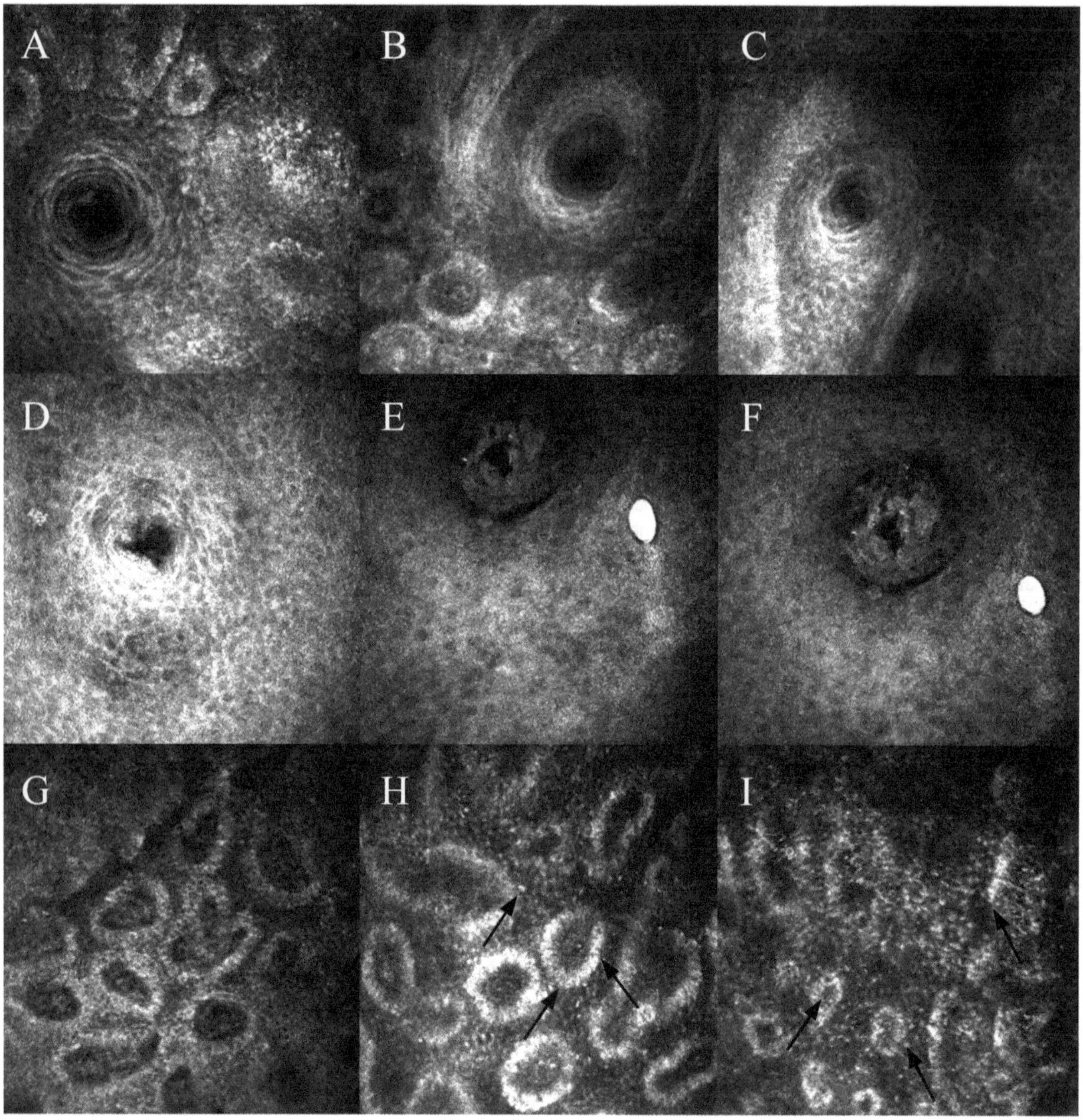

FIGURE 2 | (A–C) Meibomian gland openings of patients with liquid meibum. Cells surrounding the opening are arranged neatly, with regular borders. **(D–F)** Meibomian gland openings of patients with solid meibum. Morphology has changed, and the glands become blocked. The morphology of cells surrounding the opening has changed, and the arrangement is looser. **(G)** Image of a patient with liquid meibum. The glands have a certain degree of dilatation. **(H,I)** Images of patients with solid meibum. There is more dilatation and fusion between the acini. Black arrows indicate inflammatory cells.

Meibomian Gland Acini Examination Under IVCM

The acini of the meibomian gland were mostly round, oval, or irregular because of fusion, and each acinar unit was surrounded by cubic acinar cells. There was a connective tissue among the acini. Compared with the acini of patients with liquid meibum, the acini of patients with solid meibum had more obvious acinar dilatation and more fusion phenomena. Gland acinar shortest diameter in patients with liquid meibum, in patients with solid, and in the non-MGD group had no statistically significant difference (29.26 ± 8.23 vs. 28.04 ± 10.28 vs. 29.49 ± 10.6) ($F = 0.24$, $p > 0.05$). The acinar longest diameter and unit area of the patients with MGD were also greater than those of the non-MGD patients, and the values of the solid meibum group were greater than those of the liquid meibum group, with statistically significant differences. There were also statistical differences between any two groups (132.86 ±3 7.69 vs. 100.65 ± 25.54 vs. 77.07 ± 20.81; 4,804.49 ± 1,711.25 vs. 3,229.97 ± 1,108.35 vs. 2,639.89 ± 1,055.02) ($F = 36.52, p < 0.001; F = 27.81, p < 0.001$) (**Table 1**).

Inflammatory Cells Around the Meibomian Glands Under IVCM

The missing part of meibomian glands in the infrared imaging was manifested as atrophy and loss of meibomian acini under IVCM, or the acinar structure was replaced by a large number of cord- and grid-like structures and inflammatory cells. In the patients with MGD, there was often inflammatory cell infiltration among the acini. Highest inflammatory cell density was observed in the solid meibum group, followed by the liquid meibum group and the non-MGD group, with statistically significant differences. There were also statistical differences between any two groups (583.5 ± 103.42 vs. 395.11 ± 60.09 vs. 308.3 ± 80.78) ($F = 111.54, p < 0.001$) (**Table 1** and **Figure 1**).

Schirmer II Test

SPSS Version 23 was used to analyze the data obtained from the patients with solid meibum (21 cases, 42 eyes), patients with liquid meibum (21 cases, 38 eyes), and the non-MGD group (24 cases, 39 eyes). The parameter of the non-MGD group was the longest. The Schirmer II test results of the patients with liquid meibum were greater than those of the patients with solid meibum. The differences among the three groups were statistically significant. There were also statistical differences between any two groups (12.43 ± 2.76 vs. 6.6 ± 3.49 vs. 3.76 ± 1.56) ($F = 99.57, p < 0.001$) (**Table 2**).

Non-invasive Tear-Film Breakup Time (NIBUT)

The NIBUT in each group obtained with the Keratograph 5M was analyzed with SPSS Version 23. The NIBUT of the patients with liquid meibum was longer than that of the patients with solid meibum, and the time of the non-MGD group was longest, with statistically significant differences. There were also statistical differences between any two groups (9.3 ± 4.83 vs. 6.73 ± 3.69 vs. 12.43 ± 2.76) ($F = 11.87, p < 0.001$) (**Table 2**).

DISCUSSION

Meibomian glands, first described by Heinrich Meibom, a German anatomist, are the tarsal glands of the eyelids located between the massive connective tissue and elastic fibers (11), producing meibum to lubricate the surface of the lids. Meibum is the primary component of the surface lipid layer of the tear film, which lowers tear film surface tension to increase stability (12). MGD caused by abnormal secretion of meibum is the main cause of hyperevaporative dry eyes (13). Previous clinical studies have reported that there is a certain correlation between decline of meibomian gland function and morphological changes, but that exceptions also exist (14, 15). When several glands become blocked in an early stage, although the morphology and structure of the meibomian glands are normal, the meibum that is delivered to the ocular surface is reduced or completely inhibited. Under this circumstance, the function of the meibomian glands is weak. When meibomian gland atrophy appears, the morphology changes, and function decreases. At present, there are only few studies on the relationship between meibum status and morphology of the meibomian glands in patients with MGD. In this study, the relationship between meibum status and abnormal morphology of meibomian glands was analyzed by confocal microscopy for the first time.

The status of lipid secretion of the meibomian glands can roughly reflect the degree of meibomian gland dysfunction. According to the study conducted by Eom et al., the meibum expression was evaluated as follows: grade 1: cloudy meibum expressed with mild pressure; grade 2: cloudy meibum expressed with more than moderate pressure; and grade 3: toothpaste-like meibum (16). The higher the score, the more severe the dysfunction. That is, when the meibum score reaches grade 3, the meibomian gland acini have been extremely dilated, which is manifested by obvious increase in longest diameter and acinar area. Excessive dilation of ducts will reverse the pressure to the acini, which will result in acinar damage, meibomian gland atrophy, and destruction of acinar structures.

Conjunctival epithelial cells and subepithelial connective tissue layers can be observed by IVCM, among which are openings of the meibomian glands. In this study, meibomian gland opening diameter and area were studied in detail for the first time. Compared with the non-MGD group, the morphology of the meibomian glands in the MGD groups was changed. Consistent with the research findings by Yang et al., the results of this study showed that the meibomian gland openings in patients with liquid meibum were round or oval and surrounded by loosely-arranged flat cells (17), and high-reflective oil can occasionally be seen. While in the patients with solid meibum, the meibomian gland openings had obvious keratinization, damage, deformation, and unevenness, and were surrounded by increased inflammatory cells. The authors explored the reasons: heavily influenced by risk factors such as blockage, edema, inflammation, environmental stress, and stem cell aging (18), hyperkeratosis of the epithelium, and stagnant secretion of the meibum happened. The inability of the meibum to secrete normally promotes growth of bacteria, leading to the release of bacterial lipase secretion, which can break down the meibum. The increase of free fatty acids can change the viscosity of the meibum, which is originally clear liquid or oily, to granular or toothpaste-like solid secretions further, and consequently increases the difficulty of releasing meibum (19). In addition, after measuring the parameters of the patients included, the authors found that when suffering from MGD, the opening of the meibomian gland was dilated, but that the dilation in the patients with solid meibum was not as obvious as that in patients in the liquid meibum group, which was also unfavorable for releasing of solid meibum. The gradually increased pressure inside the blocked ducts led to the compensatory dilation of the acini and more fusions. The acinar longest diameter increased significantly, and so did the unit area (2). In turn, these processes promoted the inflammation and hyperkeratosis of the meibomian glands (20), which intensified the deformation

TABLE 1 | Parameters of the meibomian glands under a confocal microscope.

Group	Meibomian gland opening diameter /μm	Meibomian gland opening area /μm^2	Acinar longest diameter /μm	Acinar shortest diameter /μm	Acinar unit area/μm^2	Density of inflammatory cells/mm^2
Liquid meibum group	39.47 ± 9.57	1,861.47 ± 910.40	100.65 ± 25.54	29.26 ± 8.23	3,229.97 ± 1,108.35	395.11 ± 60.09
Solid meibum group	34.80 ± 9.98	1,517.23 ± 713.12	132.86 ± 37.69	28.04 ± 10.28	4,804.49 ± 1,711.25	583.50 ± 103.42
Non-MGD group	26.21 ± 10.60	1,188.96 ± 437.13	77.07 ± 20.81	29.49 ± 10.6	2,639.89 ± 1,055.02	308.30 ± 80.78
F	17.96	8.84	36.52	0.24	27.81	111.54
P	<0.001	<0.001	<0.001	0.78	<0.001	<0.001

TABLE 2 | Non-invasive tear breakup time and Schirmer II test results.

Group	Non-invasive tear break-up time (s)	Schirmer II test
Liquid meibum group	9.30 ± 4.83	6.60 ± 3.49
Solid meibum group	6.73 ± 3.69	3.76 ± 1.56
Non-MGD group	11.52 ± 4.27	12.43 ± 2.76
F	11.87	99.57
P	<0.001	<0.001

and atrophy of the meibomian gland openings in patients with solid meibum.

In healthy people, there is occasional infiltration of inflammatory cells in the acini and interstitium, about 300 cells/mm^2. In this study, the density of inflammatory cells in the patients with MGD was greater than that of the non-MGD patients, and the value of the solid meibum group was greater than that of the liquid meibum group (583.5 ± 103.42) cells/mm^2 vs. (395.11 ± 60.09) cells/mm^2, suggesting that when the condition got worse, the inflammation got more severe. In addition to the mentioned interactions among the abnormal meibum, etiology, and morphology of the meibomian glands, the density of inflammatory cells indicates the status of the meibum and development stage of the disease (21). Yang et al. established an animal model of MGD in mice and found that after Freund's adjuvant injection, ductal epithelial thickening, acinar cell atrophy, and increased inflammatory cell infiltration were observed. In the solid meibum group, although the meibomian acini had not fully developed to an atrophic state, there was a large number of scattered inflammatory cells among the acini and interstitium. The number of inflammatory cells in the patients with liquid meibum was less than that of the patients with solid meibum, but there was an increase in the number in the patients from both groups, which further proved that inflammation is a typical symptom of MGD. As the meibomian glands were continually in a microenvironment with inflammatory cell infiltration, stem cells that can undergo meiosis were senescent, and the morphology of the glands was also destroyed. In patients with severe symptoms, meibomian gland openings were more uneven, and cell arrangement was looser, with more fibrotic tissues. When meibomian gland dysfunction develops to a certain stage, inflammatory factors can cause corneal nerve damage and symptoms such as burning and tingling will become more obvious (22).

The results of the Schirmer II test showed the tear secretion condition. The amount of tear secretion in the solid meibum group, which was 3.76 ± 1.56 mm, was significantly lower than the 6.6 ± 3.49 mm in the liquid meibum group. Previous studies have confirmed that 10% of tears are discharged through evaporation, and that 90% are discharged through tear ducts (23). When the function of the meibomian glands is impaired, the tear film will also be affected, and the discharge of tears will mainly rely on evaporation. When lipid secretion is insufficient, the meibum cannot be distributed evenly on the surface of the tear film by blinking; therefore, the tear film is unstable, and tear evaporation is strong, leading to decrease in tear secretion. The tear secretion of patients with liquid meibum is close to that of healthy people, but the tear secretion of patients with solid meibum is obviously insufficient, which is also reflected in the following NIBUT research.

Non-invasive tear-film breakup time (NIBUT) is an objective test to evaluate the stability of the tear film. NIBUT > 10 s is generally considered as normal, while < 10 s is unstable. The physiological tear film is divided into an amucoaqueous-gel layer and a lipid layer, and the lipid layer is divided into polar and non-polar sublayers. The stability of the tear film depends on the function of mucoaqueous gel and lipid layers in the tear film. Meibum can reduce the surface tension of tears to facilitate the absorption of water into the tear film. As a result, the aqueous phase is thickened, and the tear film is more stable (24, 25). Lack of mucin in tear fluid indicates severe damage or loss of goblet cells. Changes in the lipid composition of the tear film can also contribute to increased instability of tears. An ocular surface analyzer can accurately record the specific location and time of tear film rupture in the form of corneal topography (26). First tear film rupture time is usually used as an indicator to evaluate the condition of MGD. In this study, the first tear film rupture time in the solid meibum group was shorter than that in the liquid meibum group ($F = 11.87$, $p < 0.001$), indicating that the tear film of the patients with solid meibum was more unstable. Therefore, the eyes were more likely to develop into dry eyes with excessive evaporation. When tear osmotic pressure continues to increase, it is more likely to result in ocular surface epithelial damage and lead to activation of inflammatory cells to release inflammatory factors (27), which, at the same time, indirectly explains why the patients with solid meibum have more inflammatory cells than the patients with liquid meibum.

From the perspective of the composition of meibum, lipid composition changes increase order degree and melting point. In patients with MGD, the viscosity of lipids increased because of composition changes in the meibomian glands. Meibum is divided into polar and -polar lipids, and polar lipids play an extremely important role in tear film stability (28). Sphingolipids, which are membrane lipids that exist in almost all cell types (29), account for 30% of polar lipids in meibomian glands and play a dominant role in cell signal transduction, inflammation, and apoptosis (30). Studies have shown that the clinical symptoms of patients with MGD are related to changes in the composition of sphingolipids, and that pro-apoptotic substances increase after the composition changes. We can boldly make a guess that under stimulation of pro-apoptotic substances, meibomian gland basal cells and the ductal epithelium of patients with solid meibum suffer from hyperkeratosis and apoptosis, which makes it difficult for the meibum to enter the central duct and accelerates changes in acinar morphology in patients with MGD. Therefore, with IVCM, we observed changes in the morphology of meibomian gland opening cells and increase in inflammatory cells. Different meibum status indicates different meibomian gland morphology, and different stages of inflammation, which are ultimately associated with clinical symptoms.

While conducting the study, it was expected that the number of patients with solid meibum would be higher. However, with the improvement of living standards in modern society, most patients seek medical attention in the early stage of MGD; therefore, fewer patients reach the clinical stage with solid meibum, so the solid meibum samples included in the study were limited. We will include more patients for further in-depth research in the future. In addition, most of the included patients were middle-aged and elderly people, especially in the non-MGD group, which may have an impact on the overall data (31).

With confocal microscopy, this study observed the meibomian gland morphology of patients with different meibum at the microscopic cellular level and gained a clearer understanding of the specific morphology and inflammation in patients with different meibum. The objective parameters obtained by observing different meibum status by confocal microscopy will help to divide the different stages of MGD in the future and guide the diagnosis and treatment of patients with MGD.

ETHICS STATEMENT

The studies involving human participants were reviewed and approved by the Ethics Committee of the Eye Hospital of Shandong First Medical University. The patients/participants provided their written informed consent to participate in this study.

AUTHOR CONTRIBUTIONS

TW, WS, and QZ contributed to the conception and design of the study and performed the statistical analysis. TW, QZ, YX, XZ, and GL organized the database. TW and QZ wrote the first draft of the manuscript. TW and WS reviewed and revised the manuscript. All the authors contributed to manuscript revision and read and approved the submitted version.

ACKNOWLEDGMENTS

The authors would like to thank Ms. Tong Liu for her linguistic and editorial assistance.

REFERENCES

1. Craig JP, Nichols KK, Akpek EK, Caffery B, Dua HS, Joo CK, et al. TFOS DEWS II definition and classification report. *Ocul Surf.* (2017) 15:276–83. doi: 10.1016/j.jtos.2017.05.008
2. Xiao J, Adil MY, Chen X, Utheim ØA, Ræder S, Tønseth KA, et al. Functional and morphological evaluation of meibomian glands in the assessment of meibomian gland dysfunction subtype and severity. *Am J Ophthalmol.* (2020) 209:160–7. doi: 10.1016/j.ajo.2019.09.005
3. Rouen PA, White ML. Dry eye disease: prevalence, assessment, and management. *Home HealthcNow.* (2018) 36:74–83. doi: 10.1097/NHH.0000000000000652
4. Butovich IA. Meibomian glands, meibum, and meibogenesis. *Exp Eye Res.* (2017) 163:2–16. doi: 10.1016/j.exer.2017.06.020
5. Cheriyan T, Schmid TM, Spector M. Presence and distribution of the lubricating protein, lubricin, in the meibomian gland in rabbits. *Mol Vis.* (2011) 17:3055–61.
6. Chinese Branch of the Asian Dry Eye Society, Ocular Surface and Tear Film Diseases Group of Ophthalmology Committee of Cross-Straits Medicine Exchange Association. Expert consensus on the diagnosis and treatment of meibomian gland dysfunction in China (2017). *Chin J Ophthalmol.* (2017) 53:657–61. doi: 10.3760/cma.j.issn.0412-4081.2017.09.005
7. Zhivov A, Stachs O, Kraak R, Stave J, Guthoff RF. *In vivo* confocal microscopy of the ocular surface. *Ocul Surf.* (2006) 4:81–93. doi: 10.1016/S1542-0124(12)70030-7
8. Wang Y, Le Q, Xu J. Application of *in vivo* laser scanning confocal microscopy for evaluation of ocular surface diseases: lessons learned from pterygium, meibomian gland disease, and chemical burns. *Cornea.* (2012) 31:968. doi: 10.1097/ICO.0b013e31824bd094
9. Donthineni PR, Das AV, Shanbhag SS, Basu S. Cataract surgery in dry eye disease: visual outcomes and complications. *Front Med.* (2020) 7:575834. doi: 10.3389/fmed.2020.575834
10. Wang Y, Qin Q, Liu B, Fu Y, Lin L, Huang X, et al. Clinical analysis: aqueous-deficient and meibomian gland dysfunction in patients with primary Sjogren's syndrome. *Front Med.* (2019) 6:291. doi: 10.3389/fmed.2019.00291
11. Ibrahim OM, Matsumoto Y, Dogru M, Adan ES, Wakamatsu TH, Shimazaki J, et al. *In vivo* confocal microscopy evaluation of meibomian gland dysfunction

in atopic-keratoconjunctivitis patients. *Ophthalmology.* (2012) 119:1961–8. doi: 10.1016/j.ophtha.2012.04.001
12. Borchman D, Ramakrishnan V, Henry C, Ramasubramanian A. Differences in meibum and tear lipid composition and conformation. *Cornea.* (2020) 39:122–8. doi: 10.1097/ICO.0000000000002095
13. Nelson JD, Shimazaki J, Benitez-del-Castillo JM, Craig JP, McCulley JP, Den S, et al. The international workshop on meibomian gland dysfunction: report of the definition and classification subcommittee. *Invest Ophthalmol Vis Sci.* (2011) 52:1930–7. doi: 10.1167/iovs.10-6997b
14. Chan TCY, Chow SSW, Wan KHN, Yuen HKL. Update on the association between dry eye disease and meibomian gland dysfunction. *Hong Kong Med J.* (2019) 25:38–47. doi: 10.12809/hkmj187331
15. Kim HM, Eom Y, Song JS. The relationship between morphology and function of the meibomian glands. *Eye Contact Lens.* (2018) 44:1–5. doi: 10.1097/ICL.0000000000000336
16. Eom Y, Choi KE, Kang SY, Lee HK, Kim HM, Song JS. Comparison of meibomian gland loss and expressed meibum grade between the upper and lower eyelids in patients with obstructive meibomian gland dysfunction. *Cornea.* (2014) 33:448–52. doi: 10.1097/ICO.0000000000000092
17. Yang L, Meng Z, Zhao J, Zhao S. Morphological evaluation of obstructive meibomian gland dysfunction by noninvasive Keratograph. *Chin J Exp Ophthalmol.* (2017) 35:458–62. doi: 10.3760/cma.j.issn.2095-0160.2017.05.01520
18. Hwang HS, Parfitt GJ, Brown DJ, Jester JV. Meibocyte differentiation and renewal: insights into novel mechanisms of meibomian gland dysfunction (MGD). *Exp Eye Res.* (2017) 163:37–45. doi: 10.1016/j.exer.2017.02.008
19. Obata H. Anatomy and histopathology of human meibomian gland. *Cornea.* (2002) 21(7Suppl.):S70–4. doi: 10.1097/01.ico.0000263122.45898.09
20. Baudouin C, Messmer EM, Aragona P, Geerling G, Akova YA, Benítez-del-Castillo J, et al. Revisiting the vicious circle of dry eye disease: a focus on the pathophysiology of meibomian gland dysfunction. *Br J Ophthalmol.* (2016) 100:300–6. doi: 10.1136/bjophthalmol-2015-307415
21. Lu Y, Yin Y, Gong L. Meibomian gland dysfunction model induced with complete Freund's adjuvant in C57BL/6 mice. *IntJ Ophthalmol.* (2020) 13:1705–12. doi: 10.18240/ijo.2020.11.04
22. Wei S, Ren X, Wang Y, Chou Y, Li X. Therapeutic effect of Intense Pulsed Light (IPL) combined with Meibomian Gland Expression (MGX) on Meibomian Gland Dysfunction (MGD). *J Ophthalmol.* (2020) 2020:3684963. doi: 10.1155/2020/3684963
23. Mishima S, Gasset A, Klyce SD Jr, Baum JL. Determination of tear volume and tear flow. *Invest Ophthalmol.* (1966) 5:264–76.
24. Mishima S, Maurice DM. The oily layer of the tear film and evaporation from the corneal surface. *Exp Eye Res.* (1961) 1:39–45. doi: 10.1016/S0014-4835(61)80006-7
25. Holly FJ. Physical chemistry of the normal and disordered tear film. *Trans Ophthalmol Soc.* (1985) 104:374–80.
26. Lemp MA, Holly FJ, Iwata S, Dohlman CH. The precorneal tear film. I. Factors in spreading and maintaining a continuous tear film over the corneal surface. *Arch Ophthalmol.* (1970) 83:89–94. doi: 10.1001/archopht.1970.00990030091017
27. Hong J, Liu Z, Hua J, Wei A, Xue F, Yang Y, et al. Evaluation of age-related changes in noninvasive tear breakup time. *Optom Vis Sci.* (2014) 91:150–5. doi: 10.1097/OPX.0000000000000126
28. Sawazaki R, Ishihara T, Usui S, Hayashi E, Tahara K, Hoshino T, et al. Diclofenac protects cultured human corneal epithelial cells against hyperosmolarity and ameliorates corneal surface damage in a rat model of dry eye. *Invest Ophthalmol Vis Sci.* (2014) 55:2547–56. doi: 10.1167/iovs.13-13850
29. Hetman ZA, Borchman D. Concentration dependent cholesteryl-ester and wax-ester structural relationships and meibomian gland dysfunction. *Biochem Biophys Rep.* (2020) 21:100732. doi: 10.1016/j.bbrep.2020.100732
30. Randon M, Aragno V, Abbas R, Liang H, Labbé A, Baudouin C. *In vivo* confocal microscopy classification in the diagnosis of meibomian gland dysfunction. *Eye.* (2019) 33:860. doi: 10.1038/s41433-019-0373-7
31. Nien CJ, Massei S, Lin G, Nabavi C, Tao J, Brown DJ, et al. Effects of age and dysfunction on human meibomian glands. *Arch Ophthalmol.* (2011) 129:462–9. doi: 10.1001/archophthalmol.2011.69

26

Effects of Sodium Hyaluronate Eye Drops With or Without Preservatives on Ocular Surface Bacterial Microbiota

Yanlin Zhong[1,2†], *Xie Fang*[1,2†], *Xuemei Wang*[1,2], *Yu-An Lin*[1,2], *Huping Wu*[1,2*] and *Cheng Li*[1,2*]

[1] *Eye Institute & Affiliated Xiamen Eye Center, School of Medicine, Xiamen University, Xiamen, China,* [2] *Fujian Provincial Key Laboratory of Ophthalmology and Visual Science & Ocular Surface and Corneal Diseases, Xiamen, China*

Correspondence:
Cheng Li
cheng-li@xmu.edu.cn
Huping Wu
wuhuping123@163.com

[†]*These authors have contributed equally to this work and share first authorship*

Purpose: This study aimed to determine the composition and diversity of bacterial communities on the ocular surface before and after the intervention with sodium hyaluronate eye drops (with or without preservatives) using 16S rRNA gene amplicon sequencing.

Methods: Sixteen healthy adults were randomly divided into two groups and treated with sodium hyaluronate eye drops with or without preservatives for 2 weeks. The individuals used the same artificial tears in both eyes. The microbial samples from the conjunctival sac of each participant were collected at baseline and 2 weeks after intervention. The diversity and taxonomic differences among different groups before and after intervention were compared by sequencing the V3–V4 region of the 16S rRNA gene.

Results: The similarity in the binocular microbial community was high in 1 of the 16 volunteers (Bray-Curtis dissimilarity score < 0.3). At the genus level, 11 bacteria were detected in all samples with an average relative abundance of more than 1%. The bacterial community changed significantly after the use of sodium hyaluronate eye drops (with or without preservatives), whether within individuals or between individuals in different groups ($P < 0.05$, PERMANOVA). Different dosage forms of sodium hyaluronate eye drops significantly decreased the relative abundance of *Flavobacterium caeni* and *Deinococcus antarcticus*, respectively ($P < 0.05$).

Conclusions: Healthy people had a rich diversity of the bacterial microbiota on the ocular surface, but the bacterial communities between the eyes were not completely similar. Irrespective of containing benzalkonium chloride (BAC), sodium hyaluronate eye drops can change the bacterial community on the ocular surface.

Keywords: microbiome, ocular surface bacterial microbiota, preservatives, 16S rRNA gene amplicon sequencing, sodium hyaluronate eye drops, benzalkonium chloride

INTRODUCTION

The ocular surface is a microecosystem in contact with the outside air and colonized by a specific microbial community (1). With the innovation of molecular biology techniques, such as polymerase chain reaction (PCR) and gene sequencing, it has been found that the total number of microorganisms is relatively small on the ocular surface compared with other parts of the body such as the intestinal tract, oral cavity, and skin, but they are quite abundant from the perspective of biodiversity (2–6). The ocular surface microbiota is mainly composed of bacteria, accounting for 98.15%, while fungi and viruses account for 0.94 and 0.91%, respectively (7). The ocular surface microbiota settles on the mucosal epithelium of the ocular surface and the tear film covering it. They form a dynamic balance microecosystem with the ocular surface tissue. The system is stable over time with low variability within an individual (8). However, differences exist among different individuals due to the influence of many factors. In healthy populations, age and region are the influencing factors for differences in microbial community (7, 9–12). Several studies have assessed the role of these microorganisms in ocular surface health and disease by characterizing ocular surface microbiota in patients under different disease conditions (13–19). Anthropogenic factors, such as the use of antibiotics (20) and the wearing of corneal contact lens (21, 22), also contribute to the changes in the microbiota on the ocular surface.

In recent decades, sodium hyaluronate eye drops have become an option for artificial tear therapy, thanks to sodium hyaluronate, a water-soluble polymer (23). Sodium hyaluronate not only has a strong water-retention function due to a large amount of negative charge, but also has high viscosity and affinity. It can stay on the ocular surface for a long time and lubricate the eye surface. It can also promote corneal epithelial extension and wound healing, reducing the adverse effects of preservatives in ophthalmic preparations (1). Sodium hyaluronate eye drops can be divided into single-dose and multi-dose types based on the presence of preservatives in them. Considering the risk of pollution, preservatives are added to many artificial tears to kill microbial vegetative forms and inhibit the growth of microorganisms for long-term preservation. Benzalkonium chloride (BAC) is the most common preservative. Several previous studies have found that BAC has a particular toxic effect on the ocular surface epithelium, and its toxicity is related to the frequency, concentration, tear secretion level, and severity of ocular surface diseases (24–27).

The ocular surface bacterial microbiota is the largest group in the ocular surface microbiota. Its colonization site is in the ocular surface epithelium and tear film, and therefore whether it is affected by the use of sodium hyaluronate eye drops is of great concern. Also, whether BAC affects the ocular surface bacterial community is not clear. To better understand the ocular surface bacteria and thus guide clinical medication, the present study aimed to (1) evaluate the diversity of ocular surface bacterial microbiota before and after the intervention with sodium hyaluronate eye drops using 16S rRNA gene amplicon sequencing and (2) compare the effects of different dose types with and without BAC on the diversity and composition of ocular surface bacterial microbiota.

MATERIALS AND METHODS

Study Population and Trial Groups

This study was designed as a randomized, parallel-group, open-label, controlled trial. It included 16 healthy volunteers (10 women and 6 men, aged 28.25 ± 3.51 years). The participants all lived in the same city and were the medical staff of the Xiamen Eye Center. They had no symptoms of ophthalmic surface disease and no more than 12 points on the Ophthalmic Surface Disease Index (OSDI) screening questionnaire. They underwent detailed eye examinations on the day before sampling, including intraocular pressure, tear meniscus height, non-invasive breakup time, and lipid layer analysis. **Table S1** shows the information of the included population and the measurements of ocular surface indicators. They did not have any systemic disease, ocular surface disease, uveitis, glaucoma, retinal disease, or a history of eye trauma/transplant; did not wear contact lenses; and did not use eye drops (artificial tears, antibiotics, steroids, and non-steroidal anti-inflammatory drugs) for 6 months. All the participants were randomly divided into two groups, each consisting of five women and three men. **Table 1** shows the statistical data of the included population; no statistically significant difference was found in the indicators between the two groups ($P > 0.05$, Mann–Whitney U test). The first group was given 0.3% sodium hyaluronate eye drops containing preservatives (Santen, Osaka, Japan), four times a day for 2 weeks in both eyes. The second group was given preservative-free 0.3% sodium hyaluronate eye drops (Santen, Osaka, Japan) with the same frequency and duration as the first group. The study plan was approved by the ethics committee of Xiamen Eye Center affiliated to the Xiamen University (Ethics Number: xmykzx-ky-2020-010). The study followed the principles of the Declaration of Helsinki. All participants provided a written informed consent document, and the participation was voluntary.

Sample Collection

The researchers took samples in a clean eye treatment room disinfected with ultraviolet light. The first sampling was done in the morning after the eye examination. The eyes were then treated with artificial tears and sampled again at the same time 2 weeks later. Based on the study by Shin et al. (22), topical anesthetics themselves could affect sequencing results. However, considering the previous reports of the differentiation between the superficial and deep microbiome (6), we used a single dose of anesthetic before sampling. Topical anesthetics allowed the subjects to cooperate fully by reducing blink reflexes and the discomfort of sampling. This ensured that sufficient and consistent pressure was taken during the sampling process to obtain high-quality samples. Meanwhile, it avoided the sample contamination caused by the accidental contact of the swab with the eyelid margin or the cornea, as well as the corneal epithelial injury caused by subjects' overreaction to the discomfort of sampling. After topical anesthesia with Proparacaine Hydrochloride Eye Drops (Alcon, TX, USA), a disposable sterile flocking cotton swab was used to wipe the upper and lower conjunctival sacs from the nasal side to the temporal side in a clockwise direction, and the intensity of the wiping was determined to avoid obvious discomfort. Care was taken not to touch the cornea, eyelid margin, or even eyelid skin throughout the process. Immediately after the collection, the swab was placed in a 1.5-mL sterile centrifuge tube (Axygen, CA, USA) and stored in an ultra-low temperature refrigerator at −80°C prior to DNA extraction, PCR amplification, and

TABLE 1 | Demographic and clinical characteristics of the cohort.

	All participants	Preservative-free group	Preservative-containing group	*P*-value*
No. of participants, *n*	16	8	8	–
Age, median (range)	29 (22-33)	29.5 (25-33)	27 (22-33)	ns
Female, % (*n*)	62.5 (10)	62.5 (5)	62.5 (5)	ns
Eyes, *n*	32	16	16	–
Ethnicity	Chinese (100%)	Chinese (100%)	Chinese (100%)	ns
IOP, mean ± SD	14.27 ± 2.73	13.89 ± 2.37	14.65 ± 3.08	ns
TMH, mean ± SD	0.23 ± 0.03	0.24 ± 0.03	0.23 ± 0.03	ns
NIBUT, mean ± SD	13.94 ± 2.55	14.04 ± 2.59	13.84 ± 2.59	ns
Avg ICU, mean ± SD	77.47 ± 11.37	75.75 ± 11.02	79.19 ± 11.80	ns
OSDI, mean ± SD	3.44 ± 2.00	3.25 ± 1.98	3.63 ± 2.13	ns

ICU, interferometric color units; IOP, intraocular pressure; NIBUT, non-invasive breakup time; ns, not significant; OSDI, ocular surface disease index; TMH, tear meniscus height.
Data presented as % (n) or mean (SD) or median (range).
**P-values based on Mann–Whitney U test comparing the preservative-free and preservative-containing groups.*

16S rRNA gene amplicon sequencing (Guangzhou Genedenovo Biotechnology Co., Guangzhou, China). To avoid contamination, topical anesthetics were injected into disposable sterile swabs and placed in sterile centrifuge tubes as blank controls.

DNA Extraction, PCR Amplification, and 16S rRNA Gene Amplicon Sequencing

The sample DNA was extracted using a HiPure soil DNA kit (Magen, Guangzhou, China) following the manufacturer's protocols. The blank samples were also fully extracted to exclude false-positive results from the process.

The V3–V4 region of 16S ribosomal RNA gene was amplified by PCR (94°C for 2 min, followed by 30 cycles at 98°C for 10 s, 62°C for 30 s, and 68°C for 30 s, and finally extended at 68°C for 5 min). Primers 341 F (5′- CCTAGGGNGGCWGCAG-3′) and 806 R (5′-GGACTACHVGGGTATCTAAT-3′) were used. PCR reactions were performed in triplicate in a 50-μL mixture containing 5 μL of 10× KOD buffer, 5 μL of 2 mM dNTPs, 3 μL of 25 mM $MgSO_4$, 1.5 μL of each primer (10 μM), 1 μL of KOD polymerase, and 100 ng of template DNA. The related PCR reagents were from Toyobo, Japan.

Amplicons were extracted from 2% agarose gels and purified using an AxyPrep DNA Gel Extraction Kit (Axygen Biosciences, CA, USA) following the manufacturer's protocols and quantified using an ABI StepOnePlus Real-Time PCR System (Life Technologies, CA, USA). Purified amplicons were pooled in equimolar amounts and paired-end sequenced (PE250) on an Illumina platform following the standard protocols. The raw sequence data were deposited into the Sequence Read Archive database (Accession Number: PRJNA720296).

Processing of 16S rDNA Dataset

Raw reads were further filtered using FASTP (28) (version 0.18.0) to obtain high-quality clean reads, according to the following rules: (1) removing reads containing more than 10% of unknown nucleotides (N) and (2) removing reads containing < 50% of bases with quality (Q-value) < 20. Paired-end clean reads were merged as raw tags using FLASH (version 1.2.11) with a minimum overlap of 10 bp and mismatch error rates of 2% (29). Noisy sequences of raw tags were filtered using the QIIME (30) (version 1.9.1) pipeline under specific filtering conditions (31) to obtain high-quality clean tags. The filtering conditions were as follows: (1) raw tags were broken from the first low-quality base site where the number of bases in the continuous low-quality value (default quality threshold, ≤3) reached the set length (default length, 3); (2) subsequently, tags whose continuous high-quality base length was <75% of the tag length were filtered. Clean tags were searched against the reference database (version r20110519, http://drive5.com/uchime/uchime_download.html) to perform reference-based chimera detection using the UCHIME algorithm (32). All chimeric tags were removed, and the finally obtained effective tags were used for further analysis. The UPARSE (33) (version 9.2.64) pipeline was used to cluster all effective tags, and the sequences with 97% similarity were grouped into operational taxonomic units (OTUs) (33). In each OTU, the absolute abundance of tags was calculated. The tag sequence with the highest abundance was selected as a representative sequence within each cluster. The representative sequences were classified into organisms by a naive Bayesian model using an RDP classifier (34) (version 2.2) based on the SILVA (35) database (version 132), with the confidence threshold value of 0.8.

Diversity and Statistical Analysis

The alpha diversity and beta diversity data of all populations before and after treatment were obtained through calculation and analysis. Observed-species index, Shannon index, and all other alpha diversity indices were calculated in QIIME (version 1.9.1) (**Table S2**). Rarefaction curves of alpha index and the stacked bar plot of the community composition were visualized in R project ggplot2 package (version 2.2.1). Unweighted UniFrac distance matrices were generated using the GUniFrac package (36) (version 1.0) in the R project. Bray-Curtis distance matrix was calculated in the R project Vegan package (version 2.5.3). Based on the distance index between samples, the Vegan package in the R project was used for the unweighted pair group method with arithmetic mean analysis (UPGMA), and the samples with smaller distance were merged into the same cluster. According to the study of Zilliox et al. (15), the similarity in ocular surface bacterial microbiota was high for Bray-Curtis dissimilarity scores < 0.30. The principal coordinate analysis (PCoA) of distance index and the statistical analysis of Adonis (also known as PERMANOVA) test were performed in the R project Vegan package (version 2.5.3) and plotted in the R project ggplot2 package (version 2.2.1). We used PCoA to evaluate the ocular surface microbiome at baseline and the differences in repeated samples after intervention. In GraphPad Prism (version 9.2.0), the box diagram was used to show the distribution of the relative abundance of bacteria in different samples. The top 10 at the phylum level and the top 20 at the genus level were shown. Kruskal-Wallis test and one-way analysis of variance were used to compare the differences in alpha diversity index and distance index before and after intervention in different groups. A scatter plot was drawn to visualize the average relative abundance of "core" bacteria at the genus level in each group after intervention. Based on the abundance and frequency of species in the sample, the indicator analysis was used to calculate the indicator value (IndVal) of each species in each group. The higher the value of IndVal, the more likely the species was to be the indicator species of the group. The labdsv package in the R project was used to calculate the indicator value of the species whose abundance value was >0 and the total proportion was >0.1% in each sample of the comparison group. We used cross-validation test to get the *P*-value. The biomarker of each group, shown in the bubble chart, could be found intuitively through the bubble size.

RESULTS

Sample Quality

The blank control samples used for monitoring DNA contamination did not produce 16S rRNA gene amplification products, indicating that the sampling process was controlled effectively. Then, 16S rDNA data were generated from 64 samples from 16 participants. A total of 6,870,617 reads were generated, with an average of 107,353.4 reads per sample. A total of 5,825,884 effective tags were generated after strict quality control of removing low-quality reads, tag mosaic, tag filtering, and tag de-chimerism. The total number of OTUs at 97% sequence similarity ranged from 674 to 2,127, with an average of 1,205.22 OTUs per sample and a total of 77,134 OTUs in all samples (**Table S3**). Rarefaction curves can directly reflect the rationality of sequencing data size by showing the variation trends in alpha diversity indices through a simulated resampling process and estimating the diversity of species in the environment. The curves reaching the saturation platform indicate that the sequencing data size is reasonable. The speed of the curve reaching the platform and the height of the curve reflect the difference in community alpha diversity among different groups. The value of Good's coverage equal to 1 indicates that all species in the sample have been detected. With the increase in the sequencing depth, the values of the Observed-species index, Shannon index, and Good's coverage increased, and later the curves gradually flattened (**Figure 1**). When the sequencing depth reached 50,000 tags/sample, these curves reached the saturated platform, and the average Good's coverage of all samples was 0.994 (**Table S2**), indicating that the sequencing had covered almost all species. The number of effective tags in this study was 91,029.44 tags/sample (**Table S3**), which showed that the depth of sequencing was sufficient for further analysis.

Composition Analysis of Ocular Surface Bacterial Microbiota

The results of each sample were first plotted to see whether a single individual had similar bacterial microbiota in both eyes before the artificial tears were used (**Figure 2A**). In the UPGMA analysis (**Figure 2B**), the samples with smaller distances between the eyes of volunteers 14 and 15 were merged into the same cluster. According to the study by Zilliox et al. (15), the Bray-Curtis dissimilarity score < 0.3 was considered to be high in similarity between the two samples. In our study, only 1 of the 16 volunteers had a high similarity in the microbiome between eyes (**Figure 2B**, Volunteer 14, Bray-Curtis dissimilarity score < 0.3). Using the single-sample *t*-test, the binocular Bray-Curtis

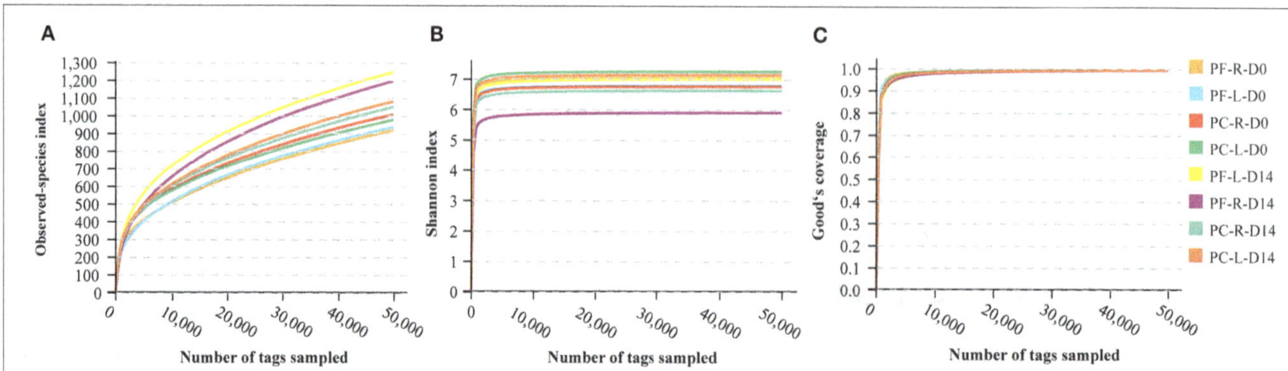

FIGURE 1 | Rarefaction curves computed for alpha diversity indices. **(A)** Observed-species index for reflection of the observed OTUs of individual sample. **(B)** Shannon indices for the species richness of samples. **(C)** Good's coverage reflected the sequencing saturation of samples. All rarefaction curves of samples from the volunteers reached the saturation platform, indicating that the sequencing data size was reasonable.

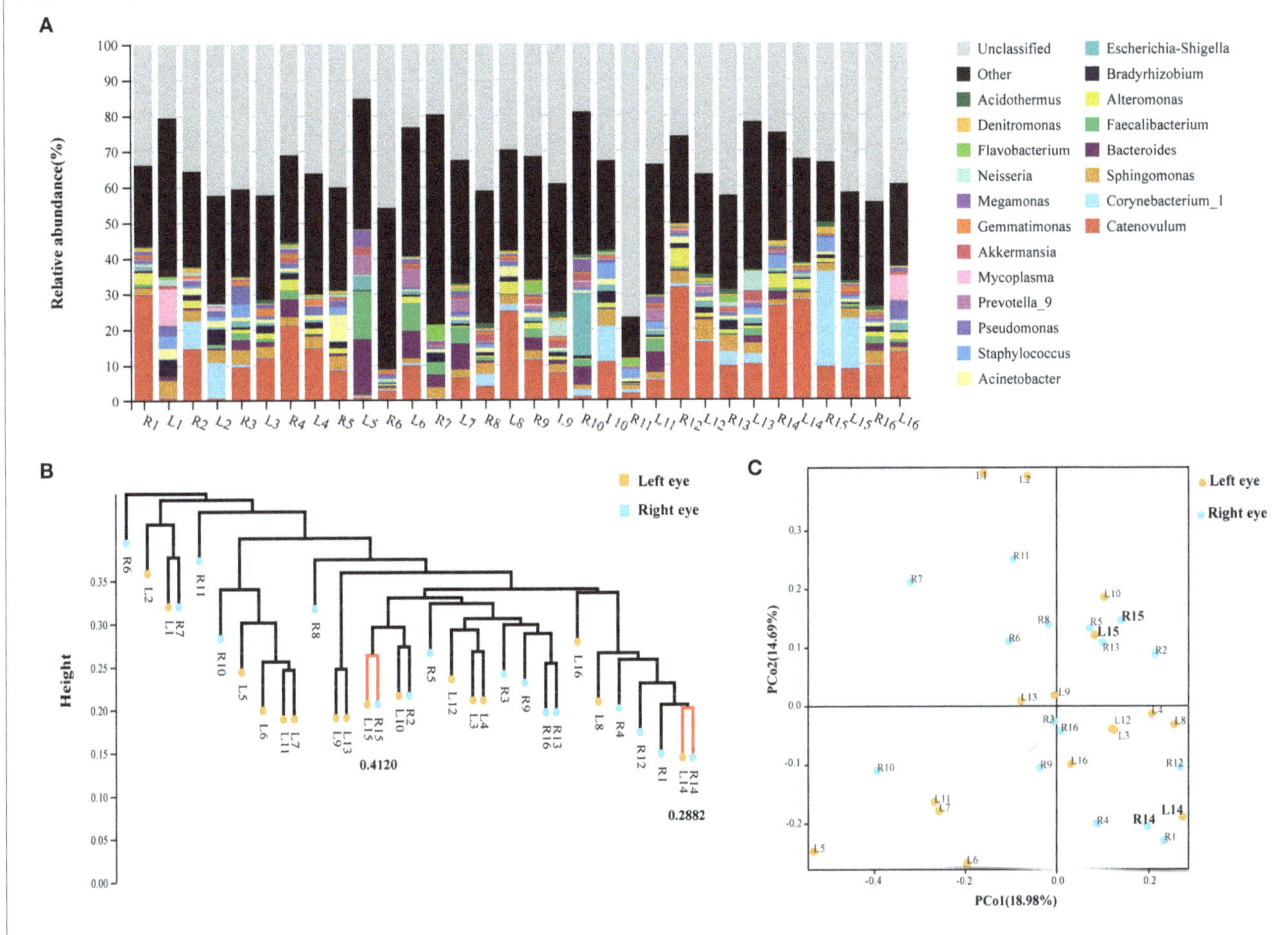

FIGURE 2 | Analysis of composition and dissimilarity of bacterial community between eyes within individual at baseline. **(A)** Stacking map of abundance of bacteria at baseline. 16S rRNA gene sequences were classified into genus levels. **(B)** Unweighted pair group method with arithmetic mean analysis (UPGMA) of all samples at baseline. **(C)** PCoA analysis between right (R) and left (L) eyes.

dissimilarity score was compared with the hypothetical value (the hypothetical value was set to 0.3). The average value of the sample was 0.6133, which was significantly different from the hypothetical value (**Figure S1**, $P < 0.0001$). The PCoA plot showed that none of the paired samples between eyes had an identical microbial composition (**Figure 2C**). Therefore, our study showed that the composition of ocular surface microbial community was not completely consistent between eyes and between different individuals. One volunteer had mainly *Catenovulum* in one eye and *Corynebacterium* in the second eye (**Figure 2A**, Volunteer 2). A second volunteer had *Catenovulum* in one eye and a variety of bacteria in the other eye, including *Sphingomonas*, *Comamonas*, *Bradyrhizobium*, *Acinetobacter*, *Staphylococcus*, *Pseudomonas*, and *Mycoplasma* (**Figure 2A**, Volunteer 1). In an individual, we treated one eye as an independent microhabitat. All further analyses were performed at the level of a single eye, rather than a combination for each participant.

At the phylum level, *Proteobacteria*, *Firmicutes*, *Actinobacteria*, and *Bacteroidetes* occupied the top four, which together accounted for 77.25% of all sequencing reads. They could be detected in all samples, and the relative abundance was more than 1% (**Figure 3A**; **Figure S2**). At the genus level, 11 bacterial genera had an average relative abundance of more than 1% in the population (**Figure 3B**). *Catenovulum* occupied the largest portion (0.2359–31.4431%), followed by *Corynebacterium* (0.1043–26.9518%), *Sphingomonas* (0.4794–5.5446%), *Bacteroides* (0.0879–15.6569%), *Faecalibacterium* (0.0268–13.3857%), *Alteromonas* (0.0179–5.2026%), *Escherichia-Shingella* (0.0812–17.4233%), *Bradyrhizobium* (0.1752–4.658%), *Acinetobacter* (0.1877–7.4161%), *Staphylococcus* (0.0398–4.523%), and *Pseudomonas* (0.1616–5.0249%). These bacteria were detected in the eyes of all participants, but the relative abundance values of different samples were significantly different. The proportion distribution of other bacteria was also different, but the range of relative abundance was smaller than that of the former two.

Sodium Hyaluronate Eye Drops Altered Ocular Surface Bacterial Microbiota

Multivariate statistical analysis was used to observe the changes in the ocular surface bacterial microbiota before and

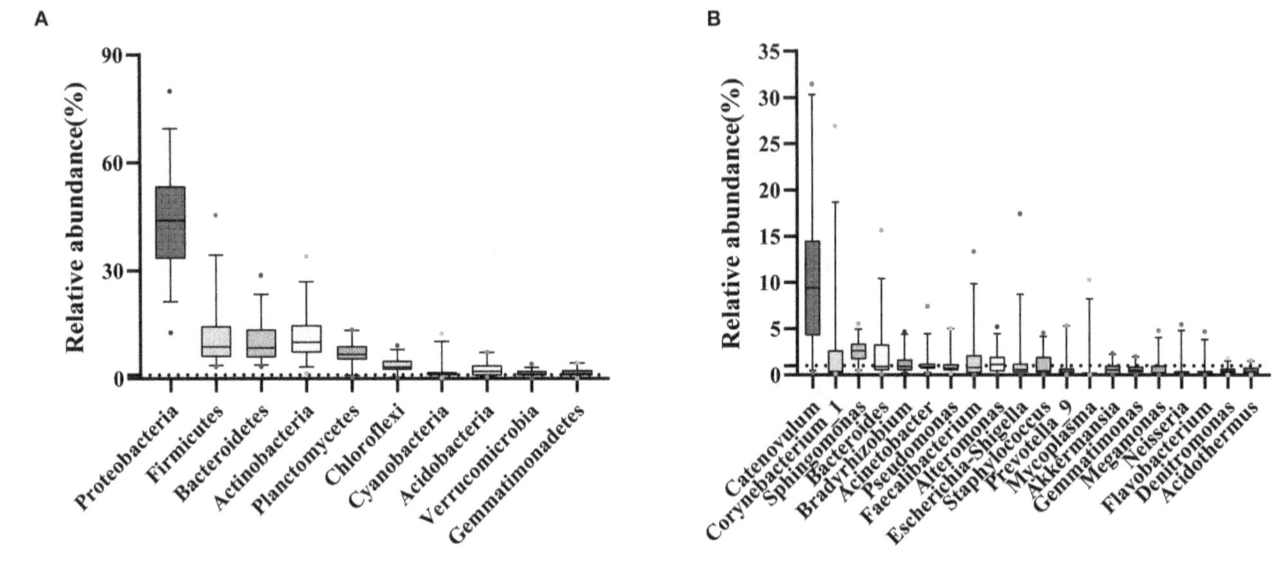

FIGURE 3 | Sample distribution of relative abundance of bacteria at different taxonomic levels. **(A)** Top 10 at phylum levels. **(B)** Top 20 at genus levels.

after intervention with different doses of sodium hyaluronate eye drops in different groups. The PCoA plot showed the relationships of bacterial microbiota among individual samples. The higher the similarity between the two samples, the closer the distance of the straight line projected in the graph. The PCoA plot based on the unweighted UniFrac distance index showed that the bacterial community on the ocular surface changed significantly after the use of sodium hyaluronate eye drops (with or without BAC), whether within individuals or between individuals in different groups (**Figure 4A**, $P < 0.05$, PERMANOVA). We analyzed the alpha and beta diversities of each group before and after intervention. We calculated the differences in the Shannon index before and after intervention in each group and compared them between groups. Whether within individuals or between individuals in different groups using different disposal methods, the use of sodium hyaluronate eye drops (whether containing BAC or not) did not cause a significant change in alpha diversity (**Figure 4B**, $P > 0.05$, Kruskal-Wallis test). We calculated the distance index between the repeated samples. Whether within individuals or between individuals in different groups, the distance index changed significantly after the use of sodium hyaluronate eye drops (whether containing BAC or not). The average distance index of repeated samples in each group was more than 0.6. However, no significant difference was found among the groups (**Figure 4C**, $P > 0.05$, one-way analysis of variance). Combined with the results of Shannon index analysis, no significant change was noted in species richness before and after intervention. The reason for the large distance index between repeated samples was probably that the composition and proportion of bacterial communities in each sample had changed.

To confirm our hypothesis, we first focused on 11 bacterial genera with an average relative abundance of more than 1% at baseline. These bacteria accounted for a relatively large proportion of the microbial community, and therefore the fluctuation in their relative abundance was bound to affect the composition of the whole bacterial community. We ranked the genera of bacteria in each group according to their relative abundance, as detailed in **Table S4**. These 11 genera of bacteria could be detected in all samples before and after intervention. The relative abundance of these bacteria was also ranked high among repetitive samples in different groups. Within and between individuals, the relative abundance of these bacteria fluctuated after the intervention of sodium hyaluronate eye drops (with or without BAC) (**Figure 5A**). Among these, four kinds of bacteria had an average relative abundance of more than 1% before and after the intervention; they were *Catenovulum*, *Bacteroides*, *Faecalibacterium*, and *Sphingomonas*. At the species level, we used the indicator analysis to find species with significant changes in relative abundance before and after intervention in different groups (**Figures 5B–E**; **Table S4**). The relative abundance of different species selected in each group was very low before and after intervention. The proportion of a few species was between 0.1 and 0.5%, and that of the rest was no more than 0.06%. A consistent and significant decrease in the relative abundance of *Flavobacterium caeni* in both eyes was found in the preservative-free group. In the preservative group, a consistent and significant decrease in intraocular relative abundance was observed with *Deinococcus antarcticus*.

DISCUSSION

Sodium hyaluronate eye drops are common artificial tears in China, accounting for about 60% of the dry eye market share, divided into single-dose and multi-dose packaging. Preservatives need to be added to conventional multi-dose artificial tears to prevent microbial growth. However, small bottles of artificial tears in single-dose packaging are discarded immediately after opening the bottle, and therefore preservatives are not required.

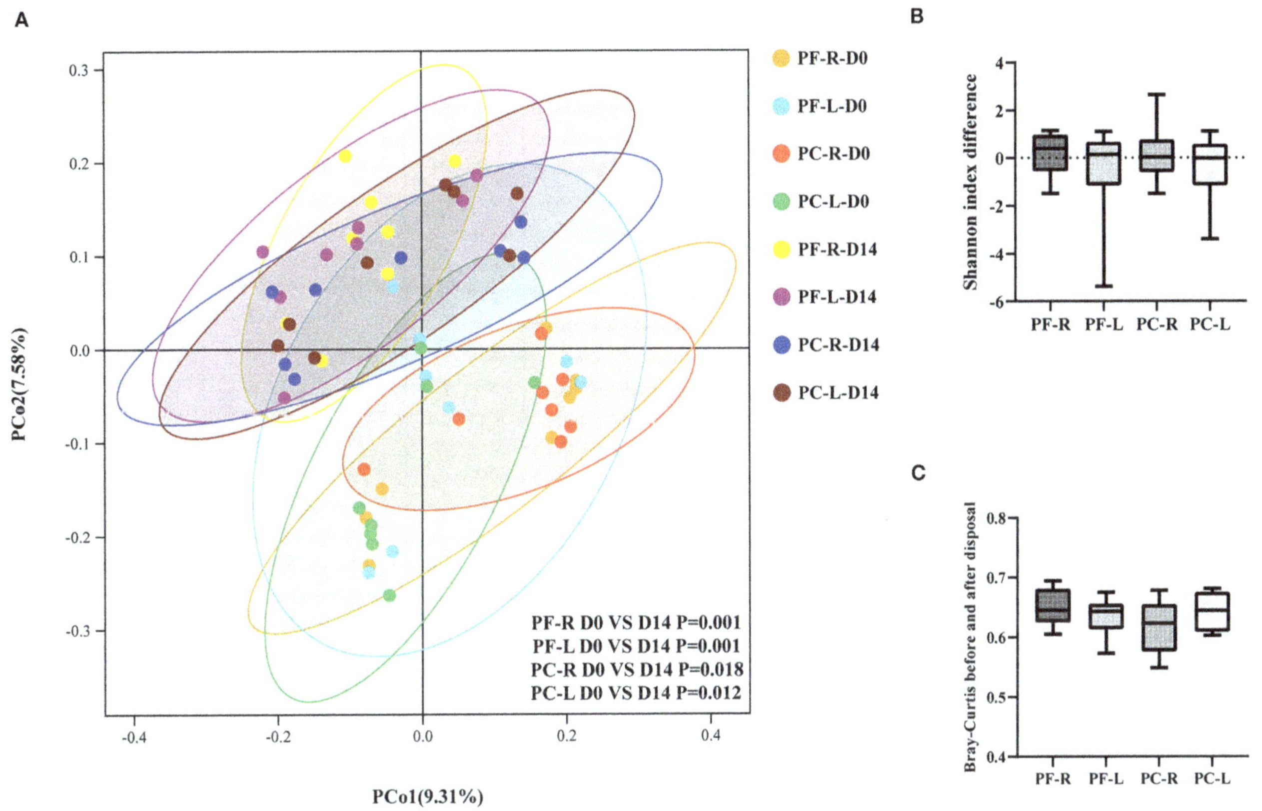

FIGURE 4 | Alpha and beta diversity analysis within the individuals and between the preservative-free (PF) and preservative-containing (PC) groups. **(A)** The PCoA plot based on the unweighted UniFrac distance index. **(B)** The differences in Shannon index between the repeated samples in each group. **(C)** Bray-Curtis indices between the repeated samples in different groups.

The tear film and the ocular surface epithelial cells are the physical barriers between the eye and the environment. As a part of the ocular surface microenvironment, ocular surface symbiotic bacteria also play an important role in ocular surface health, and the change in dynamic balance may be related to ocular pathology. The present study hoped to provide guidance for rational drug use by evaluating the effects of sodium hyaluronate eye drops and their different dosage types (with or without preservatives) on ocular surface bacteria. The traditional bacterial culture methods have obvious limitations in identifying conjunctival microflora. In this study, 16S rDNA sequencing was used to compare the conjunctival sac bacterial microbiota between single-dose and multi-dose sodium hyaluronate eye drops before and after the intervention. Our study found that healthy people had a rich diversity of ocular surface bacterial microbiota, but the bacterial communities between the eyes were not completely consistent. We also found that sodium hyaluronate eye drops, whether containing BAC or not, caused changes in the ocular surface bacterial community after treatment. The changes in the ocular surface microenvironment caused by sodium hyaluronate eye drops with different composition seemed to inhibit some bacteria.

Although previous studies compared ocular surface microbiota between eyes, the conclusion was controversial: previous studies found no significant difference in alpha diversity between left and right eyes (7, 10, 15); however, the present study found significant differences in genera and the relative abundance. The bacterial communities on the ocular surface between eyes were not entirely similar. The study by Zilliox et al. (15) supported the conclusion of this study. They found that half of the healthy people and patients with ocular surface diseases had different microbiota between their eyes. However, still, some differences were noted between the present study results and previous reports. Wen et al. (7) found no significant difference in the composition of microbial communities between the left and right eyes of the same volunteer. In addition, no significant difference was observed in the relative abundance of "core" species. This inconsistency was probably due to the differences in samples and methods used. The age range of the sample population in this study was 24–84 years. The conjunctival imprinting cytology technique was used to collect microorganisms on the conjunctival surface of the lower hemisphere, and the DNA shotgun sequencing was used for follow-up analysis. The beta diversity was analyzed by PCA analysis. PCA analysis was a direct projection of the species abundance data in the sample. The distance in different groups of samples reflected the community differences between the groups. This analysis was based on a linear model. The so-called linear

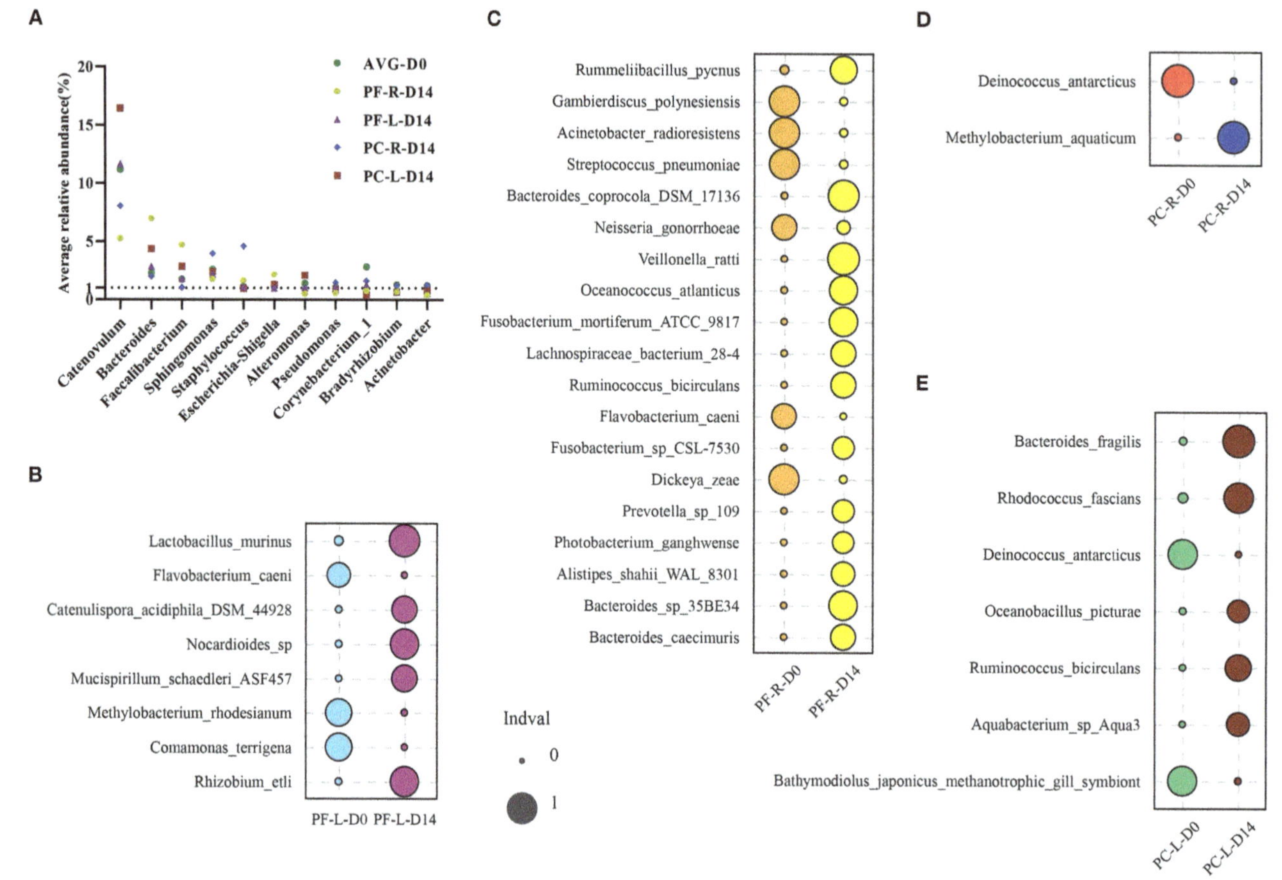

FIGURE 5 | Indicator analysis of repeated samples from the preservative-free (PF) and preservative-containing (PC) groups. **(A)** Changes in the average abundance of 11 "core" bacterial genera in each group before and after intervention. Indicator analysis of **(B)** PF-L group, **(C)** PF-R group, **(D)** PC-R group, and **(E)** PC-L group.

model assumed that species abundance changed linearly with the change in environmental variables. The scope of application of this model was limited. In real life, microbial abundance usually presents a unimodal model. Therefore, we thought that different raw data processing methods and statistical testing methods were also the reasons for the inconsistency between our conclusions and those of Wen et al. Differences existed in microbial communities among individuals, including many confounding factors. The limitation of our study and previous studies was in the lack of large-sample size data and data processing methods with gold standards. Larger-sample size research and recognized data research methods are needed to solve this controversial problem.

The core human microbiome is the set of genes present in a given habitat in all or the vast majority of humans (37). Dong et al. (3) identified the 10 most prevalent (defined as >1% of all detected genera) of the conjunctival microbiome, including *Pseudomonas*, *Bradyrhizobium*, *Propionibacterium*, *Corynebacterium*, and *Acinetobacter*. Zhou et al. (38) found 610 genera belonging to 22 phyla. Of the genera with a relative abundance > 1%, *Corynebacterium*, *Streptococcus*, *Propionibacterium*, *Staphylococcus*, *Bacillus*, and *Ralstonia* were present in 80% of the participants. Huang et al. (4) found that 10 bacterial genera that might represent the core genera accounted for more than 76% of the microbial community in the normal conjunctival sac. They were *Corynebacterium*, *Pseudomonas*, *Staphylococcus*, *Acinetobacter*, *Streptococcus Millisia*, *Anaerococcus*, *Finegoldia*, *Simonsiella*, and *Veillonella*. Ten genera were identified as common ocular bacteria in most participants (defined as >1% of all detected genera). Delbeke et al. (39) summarized the data on the ocular surface microbiome for a systematic review. In this study, the major phyla were found to be *Proteobacteria*, *Actinobacteria*, *Firmicutes*, and *Bacteroidetes*, with the first two being the most abundant. They defined the healthy adult core microbiome as genera present in minimum 5 out of the 11 published control cohorts with available raw data with a relative abundance of at least 1%. They found a core ocular surface microbiome comprising *Corynebacterium*, *Acinetobacter*, *Staphylococcus*, *Pseudomonas*, *Propionibacterium*, and *Streptococcus*. The present study also reported the core ocular surface bacterial microbiota in healthy adults. According to the definition in the previous literature, the core ocular surface microbiome, at the phylum level, includes *Proteobacteria*, *Firmicutes*, *Actinobacteria*, *Bacteroidetes*, *Planctomycetes*,

Chloroflexi, Cyanobacteria, Acidobacteria, Verrucomicrobia, and *Gemmatimonadetes*. The relative abundance of the first four items accounts for the largest proportion, which was consistent with previous findings (4, 39). However, at the genus level, the results were slightly different from the previous ones. The discrepancy in this series of results was due to the differences in swab pressure, amplification region, primer selection, detection platform, and database (8). Current microbiome analysis techniques have been developed for samples with high bacterial biomass (such as feces or soil), but not for samples with low bacterial content (such as ocular surface). The lack of standardization of the research workflow limited the repeatability and reliability of the study. It is worth noting that Ozkan et al. (5) assessed the time stability of ocular surface microbiota by sampling 43 participants at 3 time points. No single OTU was shown to be present in all participants at all times or at any given point in time. The possibility of individual-specific (or "minimal") core microbiomes was suggested. However, in our study, the 11 "core" genera were detected in all samples before and after intervention. Limited by the sample size, whether we have really defined the core ocular surface bacterial community of healthy people is debatable. Also, large differences in sample sizes existed in previous studies, and the conclusions thus obtained could not confirm the accurate definition of the core ocular surface microbiome. Future studies with larger sample sizes are needed to address this question.

Another finding of the present study was that the use of sodium hyaluronate eye drops, whether containing BAC or not, changed the ocular surface bacterial microbiota. Hyaluronic acid (HA) is a glycosaminoglycan polymerized by disaccharide units composed of glucuronic acid and N-acetyl glucosamine. It is the main component of the extracellular tissue and is abundant in synovial fluid, vitreous body, and aqueous humor of the joint cavity (40). Sodium hyaluronate is the second-generation product of HA. Using the first-generation common HA as the raw material, the low-molecular weight substances produced by mechanical, chemical, and biological enzyme-cutting methods are easier to absorb compared with the previous-generation products. The characteristic of sodium hyaluronate is that it can combine with ocular surface cells and form a regular, stable, and long-lasting water film on the ocular surface, which is not easy to wash off and promotes wound healing (41–44). The ocular surface microbiota settles on the mucosal epithelium of the ocular surface and the tear film covering it. The use of sodium hyaluronate eye drops resulted in a change in the microbial environment, which might be accompanied by an increase or decrease in nutrients. When two or more kinds of microorganisms have the same requirements for specific environmental factors, competition inevitably occurs. Certain bacteria that can adapt to the changes in the external environment stand out as the dominant species. Competition among species throughout the microecological environment creates this ebb and flow. It is also worth considering whether sodium hyaluronate itself is used as an energy source by some species to cause specific selection of microbial communities. Costagliola et al. (45) found that staphylococci and streptococci were obtained low-molecular weight sugars that could be used as nutrients by producing hyaluronidase in the presence of HA. Some bacteria such as *Pseudomonas aeruginosa* did not have the ability to produce hyaluronidase, thus limiting the benefit of sodium hyaluronate to them (46, 47). However, these results are not based on a complete microbiome, and therefore cannot explain whether this phenomenon occurs in the ocular surface microbiome.

Benzalkonium chloride (BAC) is used to avoid microbial contamination. It is also worth considering whether the environmental pressures imposed by BAC may cause some less tolerant species to fall behind in competition. However, how much it contributes to environmental change is unclear. The concentration of preservatives used in eye drops was very low, while the concentration of BAC in the present study was 0.003% (30 μg/mL). Tear dilution and blink scouring further weakened the effect of BAC. One study found that when 0.005% BAC (50 μg/mL) was injected into the eye for 1 min, the dilution multiple of BAC was 16 times, and the concentration of BAC after 5 min was negligible (48). BAC had neither the concentration nor the time (1 h) required to produce the antibacterial effect due to the rapid dilution of the tear film.

We analyzed differential species to explore whether single-dose and multi-dose sodium hyaluronate eye drops were selective for specific bacteria. According to the results of indicator analysis, no common and significant differences were found in 11 genera of "core" bacteria, either within individuals or between individuals in different groups. At the species level, most of the differential species selected in each group were those with an average relative abundance of <0.05%. In terms of relative abundance, we conjectured that even small fluctuations in bacteria with high values would have a significant impact on the values of the bacteria with low level in the bacterial community. However, sodium hyaluronate eye drops without BAC decreased the abundance of *F. caeni* between the eyes within the individual ($P < 0.05$). Meanwhile, the environmental pressure exerted by sodium hyaluronate eye drops containing BAC decreased the consistency of *D. antarcticus* between eyes. It seemed to suggest that these two specifications of sodium hyaluronate eye drops were selective for specific species ($P < 0.05$). However, it could not be ignored that the relative abundance of these two kinds of bacteria was not high; therefore, the reason for this phenomenon was likely to be consistent with our previous guess. Coupled with our sample size limit, we need more population samples for further research and analysis.

This study also had other limitations. First, gene sequencing could only detect the relative abundance of microorganisms and could not represent the true density of microorganisms in the environment. Hence, absolute quantitative indicators for the changes in the number of bacteria before and after the intervention were lacking, and the impact of differences in PCR amplification could not be ignored. Second, differences over the V3–V4 region were not enough to resolve everything to the species level. They were either identical or insufficiently different to identify a species within the genera. It limited the comprehensive analysis of the microbial community. Third, this study lacked the comparison of people of different ages. Hence, the impact of the same intervention on infants and even the elderly is worth in-depth exploration. Fourth, which environmental factors in the ocular surface microenvironment were changed by sodium hyaluronate eye drops was not clear. Fifth, what changes will occur once sodium hyaluronate eye drops are stopped or permanently used could not be predicted. We failed to indicate at what point in time the microbial community returned to the baseline level after stopping the use of sodium hyaluronate eye drops and whether the bacterial community really returned to it. Finally, the changes in ocular surface microbiota and the related mechanism in patients with different ocular surface diseases also needed to be further discussed.

In conclusion, 16S rDNA sequencing confirmed the rich diversity of the bacterial microbiota on the ocular surface of healthy people, but the bacterial communities between the eyes were not completely similar. Whether containing BAC or not, sodium hyaluronate eye drops could change the bacterial community on the ocular surface. These findings might help further understand the ocular surface bacteria and reasonably guide the use of drugs in the eye.

ETHICS STATEMENT

The studies involving human participants were reviewed and approved by the Ethics Committee of Xiamen Eye Center affiliated to Xiamen University. The participants provided their written informed consent to participate in this study.

AUTHOR CONTRIBUTIONS

CL and HW conceived and designed the experiments. YZ and XF collected samples and measured and analyzed data. XW and Y-AL analyzed the data. YZ wrote the manuscript. All authors read and approved the final manuscript.

ACKNOWLEDGMENTS

We are grateful to Guangzhou Genedenovo Biotechnology Co., Ltd. for assisting in sequencing and bioinformatics analysis.

REFERENCES

1. Zhang X, Qu Y, He X, Ou S, Bu J, Jia C, et al. Dry eye management: targeting the ocular surface microenvironment. *Int J Mol Sci.* (2017) 18:1398. doi: 10.3390/ijms18071398
2. Doan T, Akileswaran L, Andersen D, Johnson B, Ko N, Shrestha A, et al. Paucibacterial microbiome and resident DNA virome of the healthy conjunctiva. *Invest Ophthalmol Vis Sci.* (2016) 57:5116–26. doi: 10.1167/iovs.16-19803
3. Dong Q, Brulc JM, Iovieno A, Bates B, Garoutte A, Miller D, et al. Diversity of bacteria at healthy human conjunctiva. *Invest Ophthalmol Vis Sci.* (2011) 52:5408–13. doi: 10.1167/iovs.10-6939
4. Huang Y, Yang B, Li W. Defining the normal core microbiome of conjunctival microbial communities. *Clin Microbiol Infect.* (2016) 22:643.e7–e12. doi: 10.1016/j.cmi.2016.04.008
5. Ozkan J, Willcox MD. The ocular microbiome: molecular characterisation of a unique and low microbial environment. *Curr Eye Res.* (2019) 44:685–94. doi: 10.1080/02713683.2019.1570526
6. Zhou Y, Gao H, Mihindukulasuriya KA, La Rosa PS, Wylie KM, Vishnivetskaya T, et al. Biogeography of the ecosystems of the healthy human body. *Genome Biol.* (2013) 14:R1. doi: 10.1186/gb-2013-14-1-r1
7. Wen X, Miao L, Deng Y, Bible PW, Hu X, Zou Y, et al. The influence of age and sex on ocular surface microbiota in healthy adults. *Invest Ophthalmol Vis Sci.* (2017) 58:6030–7. doi: 10.1167/iovs.17-22957
8. Ozkan J, Nielsen S, Diez-Vives C, Coroneo M, Thomas T, Willcox M. Temporal stability and composition of the ocular surface microbiome. *Sci Rep.* (2017) 7:9880. doi: 10.1038/s41598-017-10494-9
9. Deng Y, Wen X, Hu X, Zou Y, Zhao C, Chen X, et al. Geographic difference shaped human ocular surface metagenome of young han Chinese From Beijing, Wenzhou, and Guangzhou Cities. *Invest Ophthalmol Vis Sci.* (2020) 61:47. doi: 10.1167/iovs.61.2.47
10. Cavuoto KM, Banerjee S, Miller D, Galor A. Composition and comparison of the ocular surface microbiome in infants and older children. *Transl Vis Sci Technol.* (2018) 7:16. doi: 10.1167/tvst.7.6.16
11. Cavuoto KM, Galor A, Banerjee S. Anatomic characterization of the ocular surface microbiome in children. *Microorganisms.* (2019) 7. doi: 10.3390/microorganisms7080259
12. Ozkan J, Willcox M, Wemheuer B, Wilcsek G, Coroneo M, Thomas T. Biogeography of the human ocular microbiota. *Ocul Surf.* (2019) 17:111–118. doi: 10.1016/j.jtos.2018.11.005
13. Dong X, Wang Y, Wang W, Lin P, Huang Y. Composition and diversity of bacterial community on the ocular surface of patients with meibomian gland dysfunction. *Invest Ophthalmol Vis Sci.* (2019) 6 0:4774–83. doi: 10.1167/iovs.19-27719
14. Ge C, Wei C, Yang BX, Cheng J, Huang YS. Conjunctival microbiome changes associated with fungal keratitis: metagenomic analysis. *Int J Ophthalmol.* (2019) 12:194–200. doi: 10.18240/ijo.2019.02.02
15. Zilliox MJ, Gange WS, Kuffel G, Mores CR, Joyce C, de Bustros P, et al. Assessing the ocular surface microbiome in severe ocular surface diseases. *Ocul Surf.* (2020) 18:706–12. doi: 10.1016/j.jtos.2020.07.007
16. Kang Y, Zhang H, Hu M, Ma Y, Chen P, Zhao Z, et al. Alterations in the ocular surface microbiome in traumatic corneal ulcer patients. *Invest Ophthalmol Vis Sci.* (2020) 61:35. doi: 10.1167/iovs.61.6.35
17. Yan Y, Yao Q, Lu Y, Shao C, Sun H, Li Y, et al. Association between demodex infestation and ocular surface microbiota in patients with demodex blepharitis. *Front Med.* (2020) 7:592759. doi: 10.3389/fmed.2020.592759
18. Li Z, Gong Y, Chen S, Li S, Zhang Y, Zhong H, et al. Comparative portrayal of ocular surface microbe with and without dry eye. *J Microbiol.* (2019) 57:1025–32. doi: 10.1007/s12275-019-9127-2
19. Shimizu E, Ogawa Y, Saijo Y, Yamane M, Uchino M, Kamoi M, et al. Commensal microflora in human conjunctiva; characteristics of microflora in the patients with chronic ocular graft-versus-host disease. *Ocul Surf.* (2019) 17:265–71. doi: 10.1016/j.jtos.2019.02.001
20. Fan C, Yang B, Huang Y. Efficacy of 0.5% levofloxacin and 5.0% povidone-iodine eyedrops in reducing conjunctival bacterial flora: metagenomic analysis. *J Ophthalmol.* (2020) 2020:1780498. doi: 10.1155/2020/1780498
21. Zhang H, Zhao F, Hutchinson DS, Sun W, Ajami NJ, Lai S, et al. Conjunctival microbiome changes associated with soft contact lens and orthokeratology lens wearing. *Invest Ophthalmol Vis Sci.* (2017) 58:128–36. doi: 10.1167/iovs.16-20231
22. Shin H, Price K, Albert L, Dodick J, Park L, Dominguez-Bello MG. Changes in the eye microbiota associated with contact lens wearing. *mBio.* (2016) 7:e00198. doi: 10.1128/mBio.00198-16
23. Craig JP, Nichols KK, Akpek EK, Caffery B, Dua HS, Joo C-K, et al. TFOS DEWS II definition and classification report. *Ocular Surface.* (2017) 15:276–83. doi: 10.1016/j.jtos.2017.05.008

24. Jaenen N, Baudouin C, Pouliquen P, Manni G, Figueiredo A, Zeyen T. Ocular symptoms and signs with preserved and preservative-free glaucoma medications. *Eur J Ophthalmol.* (2007) 17:341–9. doi: 10.1177/112067210701700311
25. Baudouin C, Labbé A, Liang H, Pauly A, Brignole-Baudouin F. Preservatives in eyedrops: the good, the bad and the ugly. *Prog Retin Eye Res.* (2010) 29:312–34. doi: 10.1016/j.preteyeres.2010.03.001
26. Chen W, Li Z, Hu J, Zhang Z, Chen L, Chen Y, et al. Corneal alternations induced by topical application of benzalkonium chloride in rabbit. *PLoS ONE.* (2011) 6:e26103. doi: 10.1371/journal.pone.0026103
27. Ye J, Wu H, Zhang H, Wu Y, Yang J, Jin X, et al. Role of benzalkonium chloride in DNA strand breaks in human corneal epithelial cells. *Graefes Arch Clin Exp Ophthalmol.* (2011) 249:1681–7. doi: 10.1007/s00417-011-1755-0
28. Chen S, Zhou Y, Chen Y, Gu J. fastp: an ultra-fast all-in-one FASTQ preprocessor. *Bioinformatics.* (2018) 34:i884–90. doi: 10.1093/bioinformatics/bty560
29. Magoc T, Salzberg SL. FLASH: fast length adjustment of short reads to improve genome assemblies. *Bioinformatics.* (2011) 27:2957–63. doi: 10.1093/bioinformatics/btr507
30. Caporaso JG, Kuczynski J, Stombaugh J, Bittinger K, Bushman FD, Costello EK, et al. QIIME allows analysis of high-throughput community sequencing data. *Nat Methods.* (2010) 7:335–6. doi: 10.1038/nmeth.f.303
31. Bokulich NA, Subramanian S, Faith JJ, Gevers D, Gordon JI, Knight R, et al. Quality-filtering vastly improves diversity estimates from Illumina amplicon sequencing. *Nat Methods.* (2013) 10:57–9. doi: 10.1038/nmeth.2276
32. Edgar RC, Haas BJ, Clemente JC, Quince C, Knight R. UCHIME improves sensitivity and speed of chimera detection. *Bioinformatics.* (2011) 27:2194–200. doi: 10.1093/bioinformatics/btr381
33. Edgar RC. UPARSE: highly accurate OTU sequences from microbial amplicon reads. *Nat Methods.* (2013) 10:996–8. doi: 10.1038/nmeth.2604
34. Wang Q, Garrity GM, Tiedje JM, Cole JR. Naive Bayesian classifier for rapid assignment of rRNA sequences into the new bacterial taxonomy. *Appl Environ Microbiol.* (2007) 73:5261–7. doi: 10.1128/AEM.00062-07
35. Pruesse E, Quast C, Knittel K, Fuchs BM, Ludwig W, Peplies J, et al. SILVA: a comprehensive online resource for quality checked and aligned ribosomal RNA sequence data compatible with ARB. *Nucleic Acids Res.* (2007) 35:7188–96. doi: 10.1093/nar/gkm864
36. Lozupone C, Knight R. UniFrac: a new phylogenetic method for comparing microbial communities. *Appl Environ Microbiol.* (2005) 71:8228–35. doi: 10.1128/AEM.71.12.8228-8235.2005
37. Turnbaugh PJ, Ley RE, Hamady M, Fraser-Liggett CM, Knight R, Gordon JI. The human microbiome project. *Nature.* (2007) 449:804–10. doi: 10.1038/nature06244
38. Zhou Y, Holland MJ, Makalo P, Joof H, Roberts CH, Mabey DC, et al. The conjunctival microbiome in health and trachomatous disease: a case control study. *Genome Med.* (2014) 6:99. doi: 10.1186/s13073-014-0099-x
39. Delbeke H, Younas S, Casteels I, Joossens M. Current knowledge on the human eye microbiome: a systematic review of available amplicon and metagenomic sequencing data. *Acta Ophthalmol.* (2021) 99:16–25. doi: 10.1111/aos.14508
40. Rah MJ. A review of hyaluronan and its ophthalmic applications. *Optometry.* (2011) 82:38–43. doi: 10.1016/j.optm.2010.08.003
41. Inoue M, Katakami C. The effect of hyaluronic acid on corneal epithelial cell proliferation. *Investig Ophthalmol Visual Sci.* (1993) 34:2313–15.
42. Stiebel-Kalish H, Gaton DD, Weinberger D, Loya N, Schwartz-Ventik M, Solomon A. A comparison of the effect of hyaluronic acid versus gentamicin on corneal epithelial healing. *Eye.* (1998) 12:829–33. doi: 10.1038/eye.1998.213
43. Gomes JAP, Amankwah R, Powell-Richards A, Dua HS. Sodium hyaluronate (hyaluronic acid) promotes migration of human corneal epithelial cells *in vitro*. *Br J Ophthalmol.* (2004) 88:821–5. doi: 10.1136/bjo.2003.027573
44. Camillieri G, Bucolo C, Rossi S, Drago F. Hyaluronan-induced stimulation of corneal wound healing is a pure pharmacological effect. *J Ocular Pharmacol Ther.* (2004) 20:548–53. doi: 10.1089/jop.2004.20.548
45. Costagliola C, Del Prete A, Winkler NR, Carpineto P, Ciancaglini M, Piccolomini R, et al. The ability of bacteria to use Na-hyaluronate as a nutrient. *Acta Ophthalmol Scand.* (1996) 74:566–8. doi: 10.1111/j.1600-0420.1996.tb00736.x
46. Ardizzoni A, Neglia RG, Baschieri MC, Cermelli C, Caratozzolo M, Righi E, et al. Influence of hyaluronic acid on bacterial and fungal species, including clinically relevant opportunistic pathogens. *J Mater Sci Mater Med.* (2011) 22:2329–38. doi: 10.1007/s10856-011-4408-2
47. Yadav MK, Chuck RS, Park CY. Composition of artificial tear solution affects in vitro Pseudomonas aeruginosa biofilm formation on silicone hydrogel lens. *J Ocul Pharmacol Ther.* (2013) 29:591–4. doi: 10.1089/jop.2012.0078
48. Friedlaender MH, Breshears D, Amoozgar B, Sheardown H, Senchyna M. The dilution of benzalkonium chloride (BAK) in the tear film. *Adv Ther.* (2006) 23:835–41.

Permissions

All chapters in this book were first published by Frontiers; hereby published with permission under the Creative Commons Attribution License or equivalent. Every chapter published in this book has been scrutinized by our experts. Their significance has been extensively debated. The topics covered herein carry significant findings which will fuel the growth of the discipline. They may even be implemented as practical applications or may be referred to as a beginning point for another development.

The contributors of this book come from diverse backgrounds, making this book a truly international effort. This book will bring forth new frontiers with its revolutionizing research information and detailed analysis of the nascent developments around the world.

We would like to thank all the contributing authors for lending their expertise to make the book truly unique. They have played a crucial role in the development of this book. Without their invaluable contributions this book wouldn't have been possible. They have made vital efforts to compile up to date information on the varied aspects of this subject to make this book a valuable addition to the collection of many professionals and students.

This book was conceptualized with the vision of imparting up-to-date information and advanced data in this field. To ensure the same, a matchless editorial board was set up. Every individual on the board went through rigorous rounds of assessment to prove their worth. After which they invested a large part of their time researching and compiling the most relevant data for our readers.

The editorial board has been involved in producing this book since its inception. They have spent rigorous hours researching and exploring the diverse topics which have resulted in the successful publishing of this book. They have passed on their knowledge of decades through this book. To expedite this challenging task, the publisher supported the team at every step. A small team of assistant editors was also appointed to further simplify the editing procedure and attain best results for the readers.

Apart from the editorial board, the designing team has also invested a significant amount of their time in understanding the subject and creating the most relevant covers. They scrutinized every image to scout for the most suitable representation of the subject and create an appropriate cover for the book.

The publishing team has been an ardent support to the editorial, designing and production team. Their endless efforts to recruit the best for this project, has resulted in the accomplishment of this book. They are a veteran in the field of academics and their pool of knowledge is as vast as their experience in printing. Their expertise and guidance has proved useful at every step. Their uncompromising quality standards have made this book an exceptional effort. Their encouragement from time to time has been an inspiration for everyone.

The publisher and the editorial board hope that this book will prove to be a valuable piece of knowledge for researchers, students, practitioners and scholars across the globe.

List of Contributors

Xiaoyu Zhang, Jiayu Bao and Ying Jie
Beijing Tongren Eye Center, Beijing Tongren Hospital, Beijing Institute of Ophthalmology, Capital Medical University, Beijing, China
Beijing Ophthalmology and Visual Sciences Key Laboratory, Beijing Tongren Hospital, Capital Medical University, Beijing, China

Lei Tian
Beijing Tongren Eye Center, Beijing Tongren Hospital, Beijing Institute of Ophthalmology, Capital Medical University, Beijing, China
Beijing Ophthalmology and Visual Sciences Key Laboratory, Beijing Tongren Hospital, Capital Medical University, Beijing, China
Beijing Advanced Innovation Center for Big Data-Based Precision Medicine, Beihang University & Capital Medical University, Beijing, China

Siyuan Li and Yiran Hao
Beijing Ophthalmology and Visual Sciences Key Laboratory, Beijing Tongren Eye Center, Beijing Institute of Ophthalmology, Beijing Tongren Hospital, Capital Medical University, Beijing, China

Wenxiu Song
Beijing Aier Intech Eye Hospital, Beijing, China

Shaohua Liu, Baihua Chen and Liwei Zhang
Department of Ophthalmology, The Second Xiangya Hospital of Central South University, Changsha, China
Hunan Clinical Research Centre of Ophthalmic Disease, Changsha, China

Shisheng Li, Mengmeng Li and Shiying Zeng
Department of Otorhinolaryngology, The Second Xiangya Hospital of Central South University, Changsha, China

Feng Wen and Hongfei Weng
The Affiliated Ningbo Eye Hospital of Wenzhou Medical University, Ningbo, China

Qinxiang Zheng and Wei Chen
The Affiliated Ningbo Eye Hospital of Wenzhou Medical University, Ningbo, China
Eye Hospital and School of Ophthalmology and Optometry, Wenzhou Medical University, Wenzhou, China

Saiqing Li Zhong Lin, Kemi Feng and Jie Bao
Eye Hospital and School of Ophthalmology and Optometry, Wenzhou Medical University, Wenzhou, China

Yexiang Sun, Peng Shen and Hongbo Lin
Department of Chronic Diseases and Health Promotion, Yinzhou District Center for Disease Control and Prevention, Ningbo, China

Qiankun Chen, Leying Wang, Xizhan Xu, Zhenyu Wei, Kai Cao, Zijun Zhang, Kexin Chen and Qingfeng Liang
Beijing Institute of Ophthalmology, Beijing Tongren Eye Center, Beijing Tongren Hospital, Capital Medical University, Beijing Key Laboratory of Ophthalmology and Visual Sciences, Beijing, China

Zhengjiang Wei
Beijing Miyun Mental Health Prevention and Treatment Hospital, Beijing, China

Panpan Zheng
National Center for Children's Health, Beijing Children's Hospital, Capital Medical University, Beijing, China

Yaying Wu and Wenbo Li
Eye Center, School of Medicine, The Second Affiliated Hospital of Zhejiang University, Hangzhou, China

Yu Zhang
Department of Ophthalmology, Peking University Third Hospital, Beijing, China
Eye Center, School of Medicine, The Second Affiliated Hospital of Zhejiang University, Hangzhou, China

Shuo Yang, ChunYang Wang and Xiuming Jin
Eye Center, Second Affiliated Hospital, School of Medicine, Zhejiang University, Hangzhou, China

Keiichi Fujimoto, Akie Midorikawa and Hurramhon Shokirova
Department of Ophthalmology, Juntendo University Graduate School of Medicine, Tokyo, Japan

Jun Zhu
Department of Ophthalmology, Juntendo University Graduate School of Medicine, Tokyo, Japan
Department of Ophthalmology, Northern Jiangsu People's Hospital, Yangzhou, China

Fang Chen
Department of Ophthalmology, Northern Jiangsu People's Hospital, Yangzhou, China

Ai Yanagawa
Department of Digital Medicine, Juntendo University Graduate School of Medicine, Tokyo, Japan

Yuichi Okumura, Kenta Fujio, Tianxiang Huang, Yasutsugu Akasaki, Maria Miura, Kunihiko Hirosawa, Mizu Kuwahara, Yuki Morooka and Akira Murakami
Department of Ophthalmology, Juntendo University Graduate School of Medicine, Tokyo, Japan
Department of Digital Medicine, Juntendo University Graduate School of Medicine, Tokyo, Japan

Ken Nagino
Department of Digital Medicine, Juntendo University Graduate School of Medicine, Tokyo, Japan
Department of Hospital Administration, Juntendo University Graduate School of Medicine, Tokyo, Japan

Akie Midorikawa-Inomata and Atsuko Eguchi
Department of Hospital Administration, Juntendo University Graduate School of Medicine, Tokyo, Japan

Kendrick Co Shih
Department of Ophthalmology, Li Ka Shing Faculty of Medicine, The University of Hong Kong, Pokfulam, Hong Kong SAR, China

Danyi Qin, Yingping Deng, Lixiang Wang and Hongbo Yin
Department of Ophthalmology, West China Hospital of Sichuan University, Chengdu, China

Wang, Xin Wang, Yujie Mou, Kelan Yuan and Xiaodan Huang
Eye Center, School of Medicine, 2nd Affiliated Hospital, Zhejiang University, Hangzhou, China

Haozhe Yu, Yifei Yuan, Wenyu Wu, Weizhen Zeng and Yun Feng
Department of Ophthalmology, Peking University Third Hospital, Beijing, China

Louis Tong
Singapore Eye Research Institute, Singapore, Singapore
Department of Cornea and External Diseases, Singapore National Eye Centre, Singapore, Singapore
Department of Ophthalmology, Duke-NUS Medical School, Singapore, Singapore

Yirui Zhu, Lin Lin and Mengshu Di
Eye Center, Affiliated Second Hospital, School of Medicine, Zhejiang University, Hangzhou, China

Ruida Chen
Eye Center, Affiliated Second Hospital, School of Medicine, Zhejiang University, Hangzhou, China
Eye Department, Affiliated Dongyang Hospital, Wenzhou Medical University, Dongyang, China

Fei Fang
Eye Center, Affiliated Second Hospital, School of Medicine, Zhejiang University, Hangzhou, China
Department of ENT, Wuning County People's Hospital, Jiujiang, China

Minjie Chen
Department of Ophthalmology, Eye and ENT Hospital, Fudan University, Shanghai, China

Yuhan Yang and Jiaxu Hong
Department of Ophthalmology, Eye and ENT Hospital, Fudan University, Shanghai, China
Department of Ophthalmology, The Affiliated Hospital of Guizhou Medical University, Guiyang, China

Hao Gu
Department of Ophthalmology, The Affiliated Hospital of Guizhou Medical University, Guiyang, China

Siyi Zhang, Yan Yan, Yixiong Zhou and Yao Fu
Department of Ophthalmology, Shanghai Ninth People's Hospital, Shanghai JiaoTong University School of Medicine, Shanghai, China
Shanghai Key Laboratory of Orbital Diseases and Ocular Oncology, Shanghai, China

Zhangling Chen
Department of Ophthalmology, Shanghai General Hospital of Nanjing Medical University, Shanghai, China
Department of Ophthalmology, Shanghai Songjiang District Central Hospital, Shanghai, China

Ying Xiao and Chenhao Yang
Department of Ophthalmology, Children's Hospital of Fudan University, Shanghai, China

Yu Qian, Qiurong Lin, Zhaoyu Xiang, Lipu Cui, Jiaqi Sun, Sicong Li and Xinran Qin
Department of Ophthalmology, Shanghai General Hospital, Shanghai Jiao Tong University School of Medicine, Shanghai, China

Songjiao Zhao
Department of Ophthalmology, Eye, Ear, Nose and Throat Hospital of Fudan University, Shanghai, China

Xiaoxia Niu
Department of Cornea and Ocular Surface Diseases, Harbin Aier Eye Hospital, Harbin, China

Haidong Zou
Department of Ophthalmology, Shanghai General Hospital of Nanjing Medical University, Shanghai, China
Department of Ophthalmology, Shanghai General Hospital, Shanghai Jiao Tong University School of Medicine, Shanghai, China
Shanghai Key Laboratory of Fundus Diseases, Shanghai, China
Shanghai Eye Diseases Prevention & Treatment Center, Shanghai Eye Hospital, Shanghai, China
National Clinical Research Center for Eye Diseases, Shanghai, China
Shanghai Engineering Center for Precise Diagnosis and Treatment of Eye Diseases, Shanghai, China

Nan Song
Department of Facial Plastic and Reconstructive Surgery, Eye, Ear, Nose and Throat Hospital of Fudan University, Shanghai, China

Pingjun Chang, Shuyi Qian, Feng Huang, Yinying Zhao, Zhangliang Li and Yun-e Zhao
Eye Hospital and School of Ophthalmology and Optometry, Wenzhou Medical University, Wenzhou, China
National Clinical Research Center for Ocular Diseases, Wenzhou, China
Eye Hospital of Wenzhou Medical University, Hangzhou Branch, Hangzhou, China

Zhizi Xu
Hangzhou Xiaoshan Liuliqiao Hospital, Hangzhou, China

Kangcheng Liu, Xia Peng, Ruolan Yuan, Min Liao, Jingwen Liang, Xiangbo Tang, Yi Xu, Yingjun Cai and Hua Wang
Eye Center of Xiangya Hospital, Hunan Key Laboratory of Ophthalmology, Central South University, Changsha, China,

Yau Kei Chan
Department of Ophthalmology, Li Ka Shing Faculty of Medicine, The University of Hong Kong, Hong Kong, China

Qiangxiang Li
Ningxia Geriatric Disease Clinical Research Center, People's Hospital of Ningxia Hui Autonomous Region, Yinchuan, China

Tong Lin, Wushuang Wang, Yang Lu and Lan Gong
Department of Ophthalmology, Eye, Ear, Nose, and Throat Hospital of Fudan University, Shanghai, China
NHC Key Laboratory of Myopia (Fudan University), Laboratory of Myopia, Chinese Academy of Medical Sciences, Shanghai, China
Shanghai Key Laboratory of Visual Impairment and Restoration, Fudan University, Shanghai, China

Wanju Yang, Shangcao Wu and Ying Zhang
Aier Eye Hospital of Wuhan University, Wuhan, China

Yanzhu Luo
Aier Eye Hospital of Wuhan University, Wuhan, China
Aier School of Ophthalmology, Central South University, Changsha, China
Department of Cornea and Ocular Surface Diseases, Wuhan Aier Hankou Eye Hospital, Wuhan, China

Chen Qiao, Wei Ming, Dan Chen, Mengying Qi, Lan Ke, Ying Wang , Liping Li and Haoyu Wang
Aier Eye Hospital of Wuhan University, Wuhan, China
Department of Cornea and Ocular Surface Diseases, Wuhan Aier Hankou Eye Hospital, Wuhan, China

Yanshuang Yan
Department of Cornea and Ocular Surface Diseases, Guangzhou Aier Eye Hospital, Guangzhou, China

Shaowei Li
Aier Cornea Institute, Beijing, China

Qingyan Zeng
Aier Eye Hospital of Wuhan University, Wuhan, China
Aier School of Ophthalmology, Central South University, Changsha, China
Department of Cornea and Ocular Surface Diseases, Wuhan Aier Hankou Eye Hospital, Wuhan, China
Aier Cornea Institute, Beijing, China
Aier School of Ophthalmology and Optometry, Hubei University of Science and Technology, Xianning, China

Ye-Ye Zhang
Department of Electronic Engineering, School of Science, Hainan University, Haikou, China
Department of Electronic Engineering, College of Engineering, Shantou University, Shantou, China

Hui Zhao
Department of Ophthalmology, Shanghai First People's Hospital, Shanghai Jiao Tong University, National Clinical Research Center for Eye Diseases, Shanghai, China

Jin-Yan Lin
Research Center for Advanced Optics and Photoelectronics, Department of Physics, College of Science, Shantou University, Shantou, China

Jing Chen
Department of Nuclear Medicine, Tongji Medical College, Tongji Hospital, Huazhong University of Science and Technology, Wuhan, China

Xi-Wang Liu, Hong-Dan Zhang and Wei-Feng Yang
Research Center for Advanced Optics and Photoelectronics, Department of Physics, College of Science, Shantou University, Shantou, China
Department of Mathematics, College of Science, Shantou University, Shantou, China

Xiaoyu Huang, Lingjuan Xu, Wei Wang, Weikun Hu, Xinyu Li, Hong Zhang and Guigang Li
Department of Ophthalmology, Tongji Medical College, Tongji Hospital, Huazhong University of Science and Technology, Wuhan, China

Bowen Wang, Hao Zeng, Xin Zuo, Xue Yang, Xiaoran Wang, Dalian He and Jin Yuan
State Key Laboratory of Ophthalmology, Zhongshan Ophthalmic Center, Guangdong Provincial Key Laboratory of Ophthalmology and Visual Science, Sun Yat-sen University, Guangzhou, China

Hui Zhao, Zhe Cheng, Dong Xiao and Tian Tian
Xinhua Hospital Affiliated to Shanghai Jiao Tong University School of Medicine, Shanghai, China

Shi-Nan Wu, Hui-Ye Shu, Qian-Min Ge and Yi Shao
Department of Ophthalmology, The First Affiliated Hospital of Nanchang University, Jiangxi Province Ocular Disease Clinical Research Center, Nanchang, China
Department of Radiology, The First Affiliated Hospital of Nanchang University, Jiangxi Province Medical Imaging Research Institute, Nanchang, China

Qian Zheng, Yuanyuan Xue, Xiaowei Zhong and Guangwei Li
Department of Ophthalmology, Eye Hospital of Shandong First Medical University, Shandong First Medical University and Shandong Academy of Medical Sciences, Jinan, China

Ting Wang and Weiyun Shi
Department of Ophthalmology, Eye Hospital of Shandong First Medical University, Shandong First Medical University and Shandong Academy of Medical Sciences, Jinan, China
State Key Laboratory Cultivation Base, Shandong Provincial Key Laboratory of Ophthalmology, Shandong Eye Institute, Jinan, China
School of Ophthalmology, Shandong First Medical University, Jinan, China

Yanlin Zhong, Xie Fang, Xuemei Wang, Yu-An Lin, Huping Wu and Cheng Li
Eye Institute & Affiliated Xiamen Eye Center, School of Medicine, Xiamen University, Xiamen, China
Fujian Provincial Key Laboratory of Ophthalmology and Visual Science & Ocular Surface and Corneal Diseases, Xiamen, China

Index

www.ingramcontent.com/pod-product-compliance
Lightning Source LLC
LaVergne TN
LVHW082135200926
848484LV00008B/2058
* 9 7 9 8 8 8 7 4 0 0 7 9 2 *